Home Parenteral Nutrition

2nd Edition

Home Parenteral Nutrition

2nd Edition

Edited by

Federico Bozzetti

Michael Staun

and

André Van Gossum

www.cabi.org

CABI is a trading name of CAB International

CABI
Nosworthy Way
Wallingford
Oxfordshire OX10 8DE
UK

Tel: +44 (0)1491 832111
Fax: +44 (0)1491 833508
E-mail: info@cabi.org
Website: www.cabi.org

CABI
38 Chauncy Street
Suite 1002
Boston, MA 02111
USA

T: +1 800 552 3083 (toll free)
E-mail: cabi-nao@cabi.org

A catalogue record for this book is available from the British Library, London, UK.

Library of Congress Cataloging-in-Publication Data

Home parenteral nutrition (Bozzetti)
Home parenteral nutrition/edited by Federico Bozzetti, Michael Staun and Andre Van Gossum. -- 2nd edition.
p. ; cm.
Includes bibliographical references and index.
ISBN 978-1-78064-311-3 (hbk : alk. paper)
I. Bozzetti, F. (Federico), editor. II. Staun, Michael, editor. III. Gossum, Andre van, editor. IV. Title.
[DNLM: 1. Parenteral Nutrition, Home. WB 410]

RM224
615.8'54--dc23

2014030464

ISBN-13: 978 1 78064 311 3

Commissioning editors: Rachel Cutts and David Hemming
Editorial assistant: Emma McCann
Production editor: Tracy Head

Typeset by AMA DataSet, Preston, UK.
Printed and bound by CPI Group (UK) Ltd, Croydon, CR0 4YY.

Contents

Contributors

Adjemian, Daniela, *University Health Network, Division of Gastroenterology, University of Toronto, Toronto, Ontario, Canada. E-mail: dadjemian@yahoo.com*

Agostini, Federica, *Center for Chronic Intestinal Failure, Department of Medical and Surgical Science, University of Bologna, Bologna, Italy. E-mail: federica.agostini@unibo.it*

Allard, Johanne P., *University Health Network, Division of Gastroenterology, University of Toronto, Toronto, Ontario, Canada. E-mail: Dr.Johane.Allard@uhn.ca*

Allison, Simon, *Clinical Nutrition Unit, University Hospital, Queen's Medical Centre, Nottingham, UK. E-mail: simonallison19@ntlworld.com*

Arvanitakis, Marianna, *Clinic of Intestinal Diseases and Clinical Nutrition, Hôpital Erasme, Free University of Brussels, Brussels, Belgium. E-mail: marianna.arvanitaki@erasme.ulb.ac.be*

Ball, Patrick, *Charles Darwin University, Darwin, Australia. E-mail: Patrick.Ball@cdu.edu.au*

Ballarin, Asuncion, *Hôpital Erasme, Brussels, Belgium. E-mail: asuncion.ballarin@erasme.ulb.ac.be*

Baxter, Janet P., *Ninewells Hospital and Medical School, Dundee, UK. E-mail: janetbaxter@nhs.net*

Beyer-Berjot, Laura, *Department of Colorectal Surgery, Beaujon Hospital, Assistance Publique – Hôpitaux de Paris, Université Paris VII, Clichy, France. E-mail: laura.beyer@ap-hm.fr*

Boeykens, Kurt, *AZ Nikolaas, Sint-Niklaas, Belgium. E-mail: kurt.boeykens@aznikolaas.be*

Bon Djemah, Vanessa, *Department of Gastroenterology and Nutrition Support, Beaujon Hospital, Assistance Publique – Hôpitaux de Paris, Université Paris VII, Clichy, France. E-mail: vanessabondjemah@gmail.com*

Bouhnik, Yoram, *Department of Gastroenterology and Nutrition Support, Beaujon Hospital, Assistance Publique – Hôpitaux de Paris, Université Paris VII, Clichy, France. E-mail: yoram.bouhnik@bjn.aphp.fr*

Bozzetti, Federico, *Faculty of Medicine, University of Milan, Milan, Italy. E-mail: federicobozzetti@gmail.com*

Buchman, Alan L., *Glencoe, Illinois, USA. E-mail: a.buchman@hotmail.com*

Colomb, Virginie, *French Association against Cystic Fibrosis 'Vaincre la mucoviscidose', Paris, France. E-mail: vcolomb@vaincrelamuco.org*

Corcos, Olivier, *Department of Gastroenterology and Nutrition Support, Beaujon Hospital, Assistance Publique – Hôpitaux de Paris, Université Paris VII, Clichy, France. E-mail: olivier.corcos@ap-hm.fr*

Cotogni, Paolo, *Anesthesiology and Intensive Care, Department of Medicine, S. Giovanni Battista Hospital, University of Turin, Turin, Italy. E-mail: paolo.cotogni@unito.it*

Cuerda, Cristina, *Nutrition Unit, Hospital General Universitario Gregorio Marañón, Madrid, Spain. E-mail: mcuerda.hgugm@salud.madrid.org*

Dupont, Benoît, *Service d'Hepato-Gastro-Entérologie et Nutrition, Centre Hospitalier Universitaire de Caen, Caen, France. E-mail: benoitdupont500@hotmail.com*

Elia, Marinos, *National Institute of Health Research Biomedical Research Centre (Nutrition), Faculty of Medicine, University of Southampton and University Hospital Southampton NHS Foundation Trust, Southampton, UK. E-mail: elia@soton.ac.uk*

Forbes, Alastair, *Norwich Medical School, University of East Anglia, Norwich, UK. E-mail: alastair.forbes@uea.ac.uk*

Gillanders, Lyn, *Auckland City Hospital, Auckland, New Zealand. E-mail: lyng@adhb.govt.nz*

Gomis, Pilar, *The Pharmacy Service, Hospital 12 de Octubre, Madrid, Spain. E-mail: pgomis.hdoc@salud.madrid.org*

Goulet, Olivier, *Pediatric Gastroenterology and Nutrition, Hôpital Necker-Enfants Malades, Paris, France. E-mail: olivier.goulet@nck.aphp.fr*

Hébuterne, Xavier, *Gastroenterology and Clinical and Nutrition Department, Archet Hospital University Hospital of Nice, Nice, France. E-mail: xavier.hebuterne@unice.fr*

Higashiguchi, Takashi, *Chairman of Japanese Society for Parenteral and Enteral Nutrition and Department of Surgery & Palliative Medicine, School of Medicine, Fujita Health University, Toyoake, Japan. E-mail: t-gucci30219@herb.ocn.ne.jp*

Ito, Akihiro, *Department of Surgery & Palliative Medicine, School of Medicine, Fujita Health University, Toyoake, Japan. E-mail: itoh@mctv.ne.jp*

Jeejeebhoy, Khursheed N., *St Michael's Hospital, Division of Gastroenterology, University of Toronto, Toronto, Ontario, Canada. E-mail: kushjeejeebhoy@compuserve.com*

Jeppesen, Palle B., *Department of Medical Gastroenterology, Rigshospitalet, Denmark. E-mail: Bekker@dadlnet.dk*

Joly, Francisca, *Department of Gastroenterology and Nutrition Support, Beaujon Hospital, Assistance Publique – Hôpitaux de Paris, Université Paris VII, Clichy, France, and Gastrointestinal and Metabolic Dysfunctions in Nutritional Pathologies, Inserm UMR 1149, Centre de Recherche sur l'Inflammation Paris Montmartre – UFR de Médecine Paris Diderot, Paris, France. E-mail: francisca.joly@gmail.com*

Jonkers-Schuitema, Cora F., *Home TPN and Intestinal Failure Team, Academic Medical Center, Amsterdam, The Netherlands. E-mail: c.f.jonkers@amc.uva.nl*

Joubert, Corinne, *Service d'Hepato-Gastro-Entérologie et Nutrition, Centre Hospitalier Universitaire de Caen, Caen, France. E-mail: joubert-c@chu-caen.fr*

Kelly, Darlene G., *Oley Foundation for Home Parenteral and Enteral Nutrition, Albany, New York, USA, and Mayo Medical School, Rochester, Minnesota, USA. E-mail: dgk28@chartermi.net*

Lal, Simon, *Intestinal Failure Unit, Salford Royal NHS Foundation Trust, Salford, UK. E-mail: simon.lal@srft.nhs.uk*

Lambe, Cécile, *Pediatric Gastroenterology and Nutrition, Hôpital Necker-Enfants Malades, Paris, France. E-mail: cecile.lambe@nck.aphp.fr*

Lauro, Augusto, *Liver and Multiorgan Transplant Unit, University of Bologna, St Orsola-Malpighi Hospital, Bologna, Italy. E-mail: augustola@yahoo.com*

Layec, Sabrina, *Intestinal Rehabilitation, Clinique Saint-Yves, Rennes, France. E-mail: sislayec@gmail.com*

Lievin, Viviane, *Department of Hospital Pharmacy, Hôpital Erasme, Brussels, Belgium. E-mail: viviane.lievin@erasme.ulb.ac.be*

Maggiori, Léon, *Department of Colorectal Surgery, Beaujon Hospital, Assistance Publique – Hôpitaux de Paris, Université Paris VII, Clichy, France. E-mail: leon.maggiori@bjn.aphp.fr*

Messing, Bernard, *Department of Gastroenterology and Nutrition Support, Beaujon Hospital, Assistance Publique – Hôpitaux de Paris, Université Paris VII, France. E-mail: bernard.messing@gmail.com*

Musikas, Marietta, *Service d'Hepato-Gastro-Entérologie et Nutrition, Centre Hospitalier Universitaire de Caen, Caen, France. E-mail: musikas-m@chu-caen.fr*

Nightingale, Jeremy, *St Marks Hospital, Harrow, UK. E-mail: jeremy.nightingale@nwlh.nhs.uk*

Oyanagi, Harumasa, *Former Chairman of Japanese Society for Parenteral and Enteral Nutrition. E-mail: ohyanagi@med.kindai.ac.jp*

Panis, Yves, *Department of Colorectal Surgery, Beaujon Hospital, Assistance Publique – Hôpitaux de Paris, Université Paris VII, Clichy, France. E-mail: yves.panis@bjn.aphp.fr*

Pinna, Antonio, *Liver and Multiorgan Transplant Unit, University of Bologna, St Orsola-Malpighi Hospital, Bologna, Italy. E-mail: tonyirc@yahoo.com*

Piquet, Marie-Astrid, *Service d'Hepato-Gastro-Entérologie et Nutrition, Centre Hospitalier Universitaire de Caen, Caen, France. E-mail: piquet-ma@chu-caen.fr*

Pironi, Loris, *Center for Chronic Intestinal Failure, Department of Medical and Surgical Science, University of Bologna, Bologna, Italy. E-mail: loris.pironi@unibo.it*

Pittiruti, Mauro, *Department of Surgery, Catholic University Hospital, Rome, Italy. E-mail: mauro.pittiruti@rm.unicatt.it*

van de Poll, Marcel C.G., *The University of Maastricht, Maastricht, The Netherlands. E-mail: mcg.vandepoll@maastrichtuniversity.nl*

Reimund, Jean-Marie, *Service d'Hépato-Gastroentérologie et d'Assistance Nutritive, Hôpitaux Universitaires de Strasbourg, Hôpital de Hautepierre, Strasbourg, France, and INSERM U1113, Laboratoire 'Voies de signalisation du développement et du stress cellulaire dans les cancers digestifs et urologiques', Faculté de*

Médecine, Université de Strasbourg, Strasbourg, France. E-mail: jm.reimund.gcb@gmail.com

Rye, Beth, *St Mark's Hospital, Harrow, UK. E-mail: bethrye@nhs.net*

Schneider, Stéphane, *Gastroenterology and Clinical and Nutrition Department, Archet Hospital, University Hospital of Nice, Nice, France. E-mail: stephane.schneider@unice.fr*

Scoppettuolo, Giancarlo, *Department of Infectious Diseases, Catholic University Hospital, Rome, Italy. E-mail: g.scoppettuolo@gmail.com*

Shaffer, Jon, *Intestinal Failure Unit, Salford Royal NHS Foundation Trust, Salford, UK. E-mail: jon.shaffer@srht.nhs.uk*

Shenkin, Alan, *Faculty of Medicine, University of Liverpool, United Kingdom. E-mail: shenkin@liv.ac.uk*

Soeters, Peter, *The University of Maastricht, Maastricht, The Netherlands. E-mail: pb.soeters@maastrichtuniversity.nl*

Staun, Michael, *Department of Medical Gastroenterology, Rigshospitalet, Copenhagen, Denmark. E-mail: staun@rh.dk*

Steiger, Ezra, *Center for Human Nutrition, The Cleveland Clinic, Cleveland, Ohio, USA. E-mail: steigee@ccf.org*

Tappy, Luc, *Department of Physiology, University of Lausanne and Division of Endocrinology, Diabetes and Metabolism, Lausanne University Hospital, Lausanne, Switzerland. E-mail: luc.tappy@unil.ch*

Tzakis, Andreas G., *Division of General Surgery, Cleveland Clinic Florida, Weston, Florida, USA. E-mail: agtzakis@med.miami.edu*

Van Gossum, André, *Clinic of Intestinal Diseases and Clinical Nutrition, Hôpital Erasme, Free University of Brussels, Brussels, Belgium. E-mail: andre.vangossum@erasme.ulb.ac.be*

Villares, Jose Manuel Moreno, *Unidad de Nutrición Clínica, Hospital Universitario 12 de Octobre, Madrid, Spain. E-mail: jmorenohdoc@salud.madrid.org*

Wang, Xinying, *Department of Surgery, Jinling Hospital, Nanjing University Medical School, Nanjing, People's Republic of China. E-mail: wxinying@263.net*

Wanten, Geert, *Radboud University Nijmegen Medical Centre, Nijmegen, The Netherlands. E-mail: geert.wanten@radboudumc.nl*

Preface

The second edition of this publication has been redesigned and updated to cover all aspects of home parenteral nutrition (HPN) on the basis of the evidence-based medicine, but also on the experience of worldwide experts in this field. We are deeply grateful to all the contributors – physicians, surgeons, nurses, dieticians, pharmacists – who contributed to the realization of this book.

HPN was initiated by some pioneers in the early 1970s in North America and Europe and was initially conceived to provide nutrition to patients who were suffering life-threatening chronic intestinal failure. Progressively, HPN use was extended to patients with advanced cancer who were unable to eat. HPN being at the edge of medical, ethical and psychological issues, a multidisciplinary approach is mandatory for taking care of these patients.

For these reasons, we felt it relevant to collect all the knowledge in this field – covering all aspects of the treatment – in a publication. The main objective of this book is to share the knowledge and the expertise of clinical researchers in this field with all the teams following patients on HPN in order to improve the quality of care.

Part I provides an overview on the history of HPN and the epidemiology in different areas around the world, raising some differences in the use of HPN throughout various countries.

Part II deals with the most frequent clinical conditions in which HPN can be initiated, from the short bowel syndrome to the cancer patient.

Part III is devoted to HPN complications, but mainly conceived to provide recommendations for preventing these complications.

In Part IV, the authors detail practical issues – requirements, teaching, monitoring, etc. – of HPN including the contribution of pharmacists, dieticians, nurses and physicians.

A special section (Part V) is reserved for HPN in children. Indeed, the use of HPN in the paediatric population – infants or adolescents – has its specific concerns. Exchange of knowledge between paediatricians and physicians for adults is important for transitioning patients from paediatric to adult care.

Finally in Part VI, some miscellaneous issues (quality of life, legislation, ethical issues) of HPN are debated. A special interest has been given to intestinal transplantation that is considered in some patients who are on HPN; progress in this field could change our strategy in the future.

This publication is also dedicated to our HPN patients who – in some way – also participated to improve the practice of HPN by sharing their experience and feelings with the nutrition teams.

We also underline the role of the ESPEN-Home Artificial Nutrition and Chronic Intestinal Failure working group that supported the project of this book, but also provided the opportunity to create a network on HPN in Europe and a worldwide collaboration.

Finally, we wish to thank all contributing authors and also CABI for the joint effort to produce a modern and updated publication that – we hope – will be of interest for those involved in a HPN programme. We are thankful for the financial support provided by the European Society for Parenteral and Enteral Nutrition (ESPEN).

Federico Bozzetti
Michael Staun
André Van Gossum

I Parental Nutrition: An Overview

1 History of Parenteral Nutrition

MARINOS ELIA*

National Institute of Health Research Biomedical Research Centre (Nutrition), Faculty of Medicine, University of Southampton and University Hospital Southampton NHS Foundation Trust, Southampton, UK

Introduction

Although the modern era of home parenteral nutrition (HPN), using central venous catheters to treat patients with disease, began almost four decades ago, its origins are almost four centuries old. A number of authors, including several pioneers in the field, have reviewed various aspects of parenteral nutrition (PN): some focused on nutrients and nutritional requirements (Levenson *et al.*, 1984; Shils, 1984; Winters *et al.*, 1984), others on pharmaceutical developments (Hardy, 1995), fluid administration (Barsoum and Kleeman, 2002), access routes, paediatric PN (Winters *et al.*, 1984) or a combination of these (Meng, 1976; Dudrick, 1977; Macht, 1980; Rhoads *et al.*, 1981; Hartmann, 1985; Wretlind and Szczygiel, 1998; Vinnars and Wilmore, 2003). Here a very brief overview is provided, with a focus on HPN.

Terminology

PN involves the administration of nutrients using routes other than the gut. This could include infusion of nutrients into veins, arteriovenous shunts, subcutaneous tissue, muscle and bone. Although all of these access routes have been tried at one time or another, PN usually involves the intravenous route, and for patients on HPN it almost invariably involves central venous catheters. The term hyperalimentation, introduced by Jonathan Rhoads in the USA, implies that patients can be given nutrients in excess of their normal requirements, even if they are sick or unconscious. The term 'artificial gut' was used by Scribner *et al.* in 1970 (Scribner

*E-mail: elia@soton.ac.uk

et al., 1970) to describe the use of PN to treat patients with intestinal failure (analogous to renal failure or cardiac failure).

Early Historical Developments

Since venous access is of key importance to the practice of PN, its history can be justifiably said to begin with the discovery, in 1628, of the circulatory system (Harvey, 1628) by William Harvey. By 1658 Sir Christopher Wren and colleagues had reported the effects of infusing ale, wine, opium and oil into dogs, using hollowed-out goose quills, which acted as needles/catheters, and a pig's bladder to act as a reservoir. For example, Sir Christopher Wren wrote: 'I injected wine and ale into the mass of blood of a living dog by vein in good quantities, till I made it drunk'. Some key historical events leading to the successful introduction of PN, first in hospital, and then in the community, are summarized in Table 1.1. The developments are listed in Table 1.1 under different headings ('General developments', 'Venous access', 'Macronutrients' (fats, carbohydrates, proteins/amino acids and alcohol) and 'Other nutrients'), although the developments overlapped in time and were interdependent. Developments in PN, and ultimately HPN, were facilitated by a better understanding of the metabolic response to trauma, sepsis and other diseases, as well as a better understanding of the nutritional fluid and electrolyte needs of these conditions and their effects on acid–base regulation. Understanding the chemical structure, stability and biological effects of a variety of nutrients that were discovered in the latter part of the 19th century and first half of the 20th century was also very important. However, before PN could become widespread and used to treat patients at home, it was essential that the nutrients could be delivered in a safe and predictable way.

Table 1.1. Some key chronological developments leading to PN and HPN.

General	
1628	Discovery of the circulatory system reported by William Harvey
1658	Intravenous infusion of alcohol, lipid and opium into animals reported (experiments began in 1656)
1831	Successful intravenous administration of a solution (essentially saline solution) for treating excessive fluid losses due to cholera (Latta, 1831)
1923	Seibert's work on pyrogens (Seibert, 1923, 1963) led to the subsequent description of principles and methods for providing pyrogen-free intravenous fluids
1904	Subcutaneous PN (fat, glucose, electrolytes and peptones) in humans (Freidreich, 1904)
1955–1965	Peripheral and sometimes central PN was used by clinicians for limited periods (5% or 10% glucose, protein hydrolysates and intravenous fat) (Levenson *et al.*, 1984)
1967	Successful intravenous nutrition over prolonged periods, allowing normal growth in beagle puppies (Dudrick *et al.*, 1967)
1967	Successful prolonged central venous PN with 20–25% dextrose and 4–5% amino acid solution

Table 1.1. *Continued.*

1969	Home PN in USA (Shils *et al.*, 1970)
1970	Home PN in Canada (Langer *et al.*, 1973)
1970s	Home PN in several European and other countries (see text)
1972	Introduction of the 'all-in-one' bag for long-term use, which is now routinely used in HPN (Romieu *et al.*, 1972)
1970–present	Evolution of HPN in different ways in various countries (Elia, 1995; Elia and Baldwin, 1999; Moreno *et al.*, 2001) (see text)
2003	International Organization for Standardization (ISO) produced a document (ISO 14698-1) outlining a strategy for implementing ISO 14644 (limits to particles and bacteria in the environment). This development arose from an outbreak of bacterial contamination of PN bags
2008 (updated 2014)	Introduction of the Pharmaceutical Inspection Co-operation Scheme (PIC/S) Guide to Good Manufacturing Practice for Aseptic Preparation in European Hospitals (PE 010-1, current version PE 010-4) (Pharmaceutical Inspection Co-operation Scheme, 2014)
Venous access	
1658	Hollowed-out goose quills used as needles for intravenous infusions
1940s	Variable success at administrating 15–20% dextrose solutions to humans (Dennis, 1944; Dennis *et al.*, 1948); phlebitis was a problem
1949	Hypertonic dextrose and protein solutions given successfully through central venous catheters in dogs (Meng and Early, 1949; Rhode *et al.*, 1949)
1952	Description of central (subclavian) vein cannulation (Aubaniac, 1952), although catheters threaded centrally had been reported as early as 1944 (Levenson *et al.*, 1984)
1967	Use of a technique for placement of central venous catheters for hypertonic PN in humans (Dudrick *et al.*, 1968, 1969)
1969	Arteriovenous shunt used for venous access in the first patients on HPN in the USA (Shils *et al.*, 1970)
Macronutrients	
Carbohydrate	
1843	Claude Bernard showed that sugar solutions could be safely given parenterally to animals (Foster, 1899) (later, he injected glucose into one of his own veins)
1887	Landner proposed that glucose could be used as part of a regimen for 'artificial nutrition'
1896	Successful intravenous infusion of glucose in man (Biedl and Kraus, 1896)
1915	Woodyatt *et al.* reported that up to ~0.85 g glucose/kg body weight/h could be supplied intravenously to humans without glycosurea (Woodyatt *et al.*, 1915)
1967	Long-term hypertonic glucose infusions in humans (Dudrick *et al.*, 1968)
Protein/amino acids	
1870–1900	Infusions of milk into man, but severe systemic reactions could occur
1913	Successful infusion of non-allergenic protein hydrolysate to nourish a goat for 16 days (Henreiques and Anderson, 1913)
1937	Similar and more extensive successes with protein hydrolysates in animals (Elman, 1937)

Continued

Table 1.1. *Continued.*

1939	A solution of 2% casein hydrolysate and 8% dextrose was infused into a patient without reactions (Elman and Weiner, 1939)
1940	Synthetic crystalline amino acids infused into infants reported (Schohl and Blackfan, 1940)
1964	Crystalline amino acid solution introduced in Germany (Bansi *et al.*, 1964)
1970s	Crystalline amino acids replaced commercial protein hydrolysates
1980s	Dipeptides such as glycylglutamine and alanyltyrosine were developed to stabilize unstable amino acids (e.g. glutamine) and solubilize amino acids with poor solubility (e.g. tyrosine). These are used in some commercial preparations today
Fat	
1678	Intravenous administration of lipid in animals reported by Christopher Wren
1869	Subcutaneous injection of fat in dogs without adverse effects (Menzel and Perco, 1869)
1869	Subcutaneous injection of fat into man suffering from malnutrition and Pott's disease
1915	First fat emulsion given intravenously to animals (Murlin and Riche, 1915)
1920	First fat emulsions given intravenously to paediatric patients in the USA (Rhoads, 1975)
1961	Safe and effective intravenous lipid emulsion (Intralipid) developed by Wretlind in Sweden (Schuberth and Wretlind, 1961). This was approved in most European countries by 1963, but not in North America until 1977
1964	Food and Drug Administration in the USA banned fat emulsions derived from castor oil and cotton seed oil due to adverse reactions
1980–present	New types of lipid emulsions developed, including those containing medium-chain triacylglycerols, fish oils and structured lipids, but these have not been widely used
Alcohol	
1658	Alcohol infused in animals
1970s	Alcohol was included in some commercial PN preparations, and used widely in some centres
1980–present	Intravenous nutritional products containing alcohol were withdrawn at a time when HPN was growing in many countries
Other nutrients	
	See text

Patients and Indications

The first case of home PN took place in 1969, and was managed by Shils and colleagues in New York, USA (Shils *et al.*, 1970). It involved a 37-year-old woman with short bowel syndrome, who was given PN for a period of 7 months. She was readmitted for small bowel transplantation, but she died from post-operative complications (see Chapter 3 of this volume). This patient was infused through an arteriovenous shunt, which became infected and blocked. Most of the subsequent cases of HPN in the USA and other countries involved central venous catheters.

The first patient to receive HPN in Canada started treatment in 1970, following an almost complete bowel resection due to mesenteric vessel thrombosis (Langer *et al.*, 1973). The patient survived for 20 years. Another patient, who started HPN in Canada in 1972, probably holds the record for being on HPN the longest (over 32 years; see Chapter 4 of this volume).

Following these landmark events, HPN began to be practised in the 1970s more widely in North America, and for the first time in several European and other countries, such as Australia. With the exception of Solassol and co-workers in France, who by 1973 had already reported the use of long-term intravenous feeding in 75 patients (Solassol *et al.*, 1974), HPN in Europe was generally slow to develop. For example, in Britain, the reports of HPN appeared in the late 1970s.

The commonest indication for HPN in different countries, which mainly involved adults, was the short bowel syndrome due to surgical resection in patients with Crohn's disease and mesenteric vascular disease. Over time, the age distribution of patients increased to encompass more (often younger) children and older adults; trends that are continuing in several countries today. At the same time, the indications for HPN widened. HPN began to be used for an increasing number of paediatric conditions, such as autoimmune enteropathy, necrotizing enterocolitis and congenital malformations. In some countries, such as the USA, it was also used for a growing number of patients with HIV, and in both the USA and many other countries it began to be used increasingly to support patients with malignant conditions.

However, international differences in the indications for HPN became apparent and they have changed over time. For example, in the UK the proportion of patients with malignant disease at a given point in time (point prevalence) has increased steadily from <5% in the period 1996–2000 (Elia *et al.*, 2001) (and earlier) to 7.8% in 2010. During 2010, 14% of all patients who received HPN had malignancy (period prevalence) (Smith *et al.*, 2011). The Canadian HPN Registry indicated that 7.1% of patients between 2004 and 2006 used HPN because of cancer (Raman *et al.*, 2007). In several other countries the proportion of patients with cancer receiving HPN was much higher: 57% during 1984–1992 according to the Italian Registry (De Francesco *et al.*, 1995) and 49% during 1985–1992 according to the North American HPN Registry (Howard *et al.*, 1995); and a high 88% of the patients started on HPN during 2000–2003 in a regional centre in Italy (Violante *et al.*, 2006). This great variation in practice (5 to 60%) is supported by a survey of newly registered patients: France, 16%; UK, 5%; Belgium, 23%; Denmark, 8%; The Netherlands, 60%; and Spain, 39%.

It also became apparent that the prevalence of HPN (per million of the population) varied considerably between countries (Elia, 1995; Elia and Baldwin, 1999) and was related to economy in HPN programmes in different European countries in 1997 (van Gossum *et al.*, 1999), which ranged from factors: lowest in low-income countries, such as several African countries and India, intermediate in Western European countries and highest in the USA.

The success of PN in human patients led to its use in animal patients (veterinary medicine), such as dogs and horses, although this practice has not extended into the community.

Developments in Preparation, Setting Up and Infusing PN

In the 1970s the administration of PN, including HPN, often involved multiple bottles (dextrose, amino acids, saline, fat emulsion). This was tedious, time consuming and increased the risk of errors and complications, such as catheter-related infections. In addition, the composition of vials containing vitamins and micronutrients was not optimal for long-term intravenous use. For example, the first patient on HPN (Shils *et al.*, 1970) was reported to receive four different commercial vials of vitamins, which were believed to be necessary, as well as eight other types of solution (a fat emulsion was not included in the initial formulation). Infusion schedules were also frequently complex.

Commercial companies took up the challenge to produce new formulations that simplified the administration. Such developments, which took place since the 1970s, were also made possible by pharmaceutical developments and appreciation of specific patient needs:

1. Large plastic bags ('all-in-one' bags), which allowed nutrients to be mixed together and delivered simultaneously over a prescribed period of time. Although the use of all-in-one bags in the community was first reported in 1972 (Romieu *et al.*, 1972), their use did not become widespread until the 1980s. The compatibility of nutrients had to be carefully assessed, to avoid, for example, precipitation of calcium phosphate or destabilization of lipid emulsions by divalent cations. This field of investigation led to the development of pre-nutrients, such as organophosphates, which were stable and soluble and did not cause precipitation. Once within the body, the organophosphates, such as glucose phosphate or glycerol phosphate, are hydrolysed to yield free phosphate and either glucose or glycerol.

2. Multilayered bags, which were studied in the 1990s, were found to limit the diffusion of oxygen, which was responsible for degradation of: (i) some amino acids, such as cysteine; (ii) some vitamins, such as vitamin C, especially in the presence of the catalytic effect of copper; and (iii) some drugs, such as ranitidine. Such bags are now routinely used for HPN in many countries.

3. Backpacks and plastic 'vests', which allowed the infusate to be carried in a plastic vest or backpack while the patient remained mobile, e.g. able to work outside his/her home. The infusate is delivered into a central vein via a lightweight portable infusion pump, which is also carried in the backpack.

4. Infusion pumps. Many of the initial infusion pumps, which were designed for use on hospital wards, were bulky, noisy and not ideal for home use. Therefore, new ambulatory pumps were designed that were smaller, lighter and more user friendly for home use.

5. Administration stands. Some of the stands were found to be unsuitable for use over certain surfaces in the home. For example, they were bulky, had small wheels and could not easily be moved up or down different floors, or across surfaces covered with certain types of carpet. In the UK, a patient organization, 'PINNT' (Patients on Intravenous and Nasogastric Nutrition Therapy), identified these problems and designed its own stand and pump system. Now, many patients use this tailor-made portable, lightweight and practical system.

Delivery of feeds and accessories

The feed and administration sets were initially delivered to the patients' home from hospital, although in many countries this practice has been largely taken over by commercial companies, whose role varies from delivery of feeds and accessories to total care, including clinical/nursing care. To allow international travel, some companies have established a network of care, so that patients can travel abroad to work or have holidays. Feeds and accessories are delivered according to individual patient specifications.

Nutrients

Key developments in the use of macronutrients (amino acids, carbohydrate, fat and alcohol) in HPN are summarized in Table 1.1. The trends in the 1970s were to replace protein hydrolysates with mixtures of amino acids (D- and L-amino acids gave way to L-amino acids), and to replace alternative carbohydrates, such as fructose (and to a much more limited extent other carbohydrates, such as sorbitol), with glucose, which was always the most widely used carbohydrate. In the USA, the adverse effects of administering castor and cottonseed oils (fever, coagulation problems, back pain, jaundice) led to their ban in 1964. This also led to slower introduction and use of smaller quantities of lipid emulsions compared with many European countries, when a safe lipid preparation emerged from Sweden in 1961 (Schuberth and Wretlind, 1961). Later, alcohol was introduced but withdrawn from commercial intravenous preparations, mainly in the 1970s, because of concern about potential adverse effects on the liver and brain.

A historical review of other nutrients in HPN is beyond the scope of this brief article, but three points are summarized below:

1. The quantity of some nutrients delivered to patients on PN (including HPN) was sometimes less than the amount prescribed. This was due to degradation (e.g. due to oxidation of vitamin C) or adsorption of nutrients on to the bags. It was found that photo-degradation of certain vitamins, notably vitamin A, could be reduced by administering the infusion overnight, covering the bag with a light-impermeable material and by using all-in-one bags containing lipid emulsions, which limited the transmission of light.
2. The profile of trace elements and minerals for PN use was different from that for oral nutrition due to their variable absorption, which in healthy subjects ranges from less than 10% (e.g. chromium, manganese) to almost 100% (e.g. sodium, potassium fluoride). A range of nutrient deficiencies and some toxicities, due to inadequate or excess provision of the nutrients, were described within a few years of introduction of PN in hospital and at home.
3. The term 'total parenteral nutrition' (TPN) is still used today, but has now largely been replaced by the term 'parenteral nutrition' (PN) since it was recognized that several nutrients were not (and are still not) included in routine PN, e.g. carotenoids, choline, taurine, glutamine, fructose and certain fish oils.

Finally, in some patients the 'artificial gut' (PN) has been replaced by a transplanted gut (Shils, 1984; Winters *et al.*, 1984; Fishbein, 2009; Desai *et al.*, 2012; Mercer *et al.*, 2014). This practice has been largely restricted to a small group of patients with irreversible intestinal failure in whom long-term PN is likely to be impossible, for example due to lack of venous access, or associated with poor survival and poor quality of life. Intestinal Transplant Registry reports (www.intestinaltransplant.org) and recent reviews suggest that the rates of 1- and 5-year graft survival range from 65 to 80%, with adult recipients generally performing better. The outcome is to a large extent determined by the status of the patient at the time of transplantation and tissue rejection. New strategies to facilitate graft acceptance while reducing the need for immunosuppression are in need of development (Pirenne and Kawai, 2009). In subjects surviving more than a year, the simultaneous transplantation of the liver confers some survival advantage, but this does not match the outcomes of other organ transplants such as kidney transplants that are now routinely undertaken in many countries. Advances in various fields, especially immunology, may allow intestinal transplantation to become a much more common and realistic option for many patients on long-term HPN (see Chapter 24 of this volume).

References

Aubaniac, R. (1952) L'injection intraveineuse sous calviculaire. Avantage et technique. *La Presse Médicale* 60, 1456.

Bansi, H.W., Jürgens, P., Müller, G. and Rostin, H. (1964) Der Stoffwechsel bei intravenöser. Applikation von Nährlösungen, insbeson dere synthetisczusammengestellter. *Klinische Woschenschrift* 42, 332–352.

Barsoum, N. and Kleeman, C. (2002) Now and then; the history of parenteral fluid administration. *American Journal of Nephrology* 22, 284–289.

Biedl, A. and Kraus, R. (1896) Uber intravenose Traubenzuckerinfusionen an Menschen. *Wiener Klinische Wochenschrift* 9, 55–58.

De Francesco, A., Fadda, M., Malfi, G., De Magistris, A., Da Pont, M.C. and Balzola, F. (1995) Home parenteral nutrition in Italy: data from the Italian National Register. *Clinical Nutrition* 14(Suppl. 1), 6–9.

Dennis, C. (1944) Preoperative and postoperative care for the bad-risk patient. *Minnesota Medicine* 27, 538–543.

Dennis, C., Eddy, F.D., Frykman, H.M., McCarthy, A.M. and Westover, D. (1948) The response to vagotomy in idiopathic ulcerative colitis and regional enteritis. *Annals of Surgery* 128, 479–496.

Desai, C.S., Khan, K.M., Girlanda, R. and Fishbein, T.M. (2012) Intestinal transplantation: a review. *Indian Journal of Gastroenterology* 31, 217–232.

Dudrick, S.J. (1977) The genesis of intravenous hyperalimentation. *JPEN Journal of Parenteral and Enteral Nutrition* 1, 23–29.

Dudrick, S.J., Wilmore, D.W. and Vars, H.M. (1967) Long-term total parenteral nutritional growth in puppies and positive nitrogen balance in patients. *Surgical Forum* 18, 356–357.

Dudrick, S.J., Wilmore, D.W., Vars, H.M. and Rhoads, J.E. (1968) Long-term total parenteral nutrition with growth, development, and positive nitrogen balance. *Surgery* 64, 134–142.

Dudrick, S.J., Wilmore, D.W., Vars, H.M. and Rhoads, J.E. (1969) Can intravenous feeding as the sole means of nutrition support growth in the child and restore weight loss in an adult? An affirmative answer. *Annals of Surgery* 169, 974–984.

Elia, M. (1995) An international perspective on artificial nutritional support in the community. *The Lancet* 345, 1345–1349.

Elia, M. and Baldwin, C. (1999) Nutritional support in the home setting. In: Sadler, M.J., Strain, J. and Caballero, B. (eds) *Encyclopedia of Human Nutrition.* Academic Press, London, pp. 1405–1413.

Elia, M., Russell, C. and Stratton, R. (2001) *Trends in Artificial Nutrition Support in the UK during 1996–2000. A Report by the British Artificial Nutrition Survey (BANS).* BAPEN, Redditch, UK.

Elman, R. (1937) Amino acid content of the blood following intravenous injection of hydrolysed casein. *Proceedings of the Society for Experimental Biology and Medicine* 37, 437–440.

Elman, R. and Weiner, D.O. (1939) Intravenous alimentation with special reference to protein (amino acid) metabolism. *Journal of the American Medical Association* 112, 796–802.

Fishbein, T.M. (2009) Intestinal transplantation. *New England Journal of Medicine* 361, 998–1008.

Foster, M. (1899) *Claude Bernard.* Longmans, New York/London.

Freidreich, P.L. (1904) Die kunstliche subcutane ernahrung in der praktuschen chirurgie. *Archives fur Klinische Chirurgie* 73, 507–516.

Hardy, G. (1995) Pharmaceutical aspects of parenteral nutrition: a historical perspective. *Nutrition* 11, 767–768.

Hartmann, G. (1985) History of parenteral nutrition. *Bibliotheca Nutritio et Dieta* 35, 1–8.

Harvey, W. (1628) *Exercitatio Anatomica de Motu Cordis et Sanguinis in Animalibus.* Sumptibus F. Fitzeri, Francofurti, Italy.

Henreiques, V. and Anderson, A.C. (1913) Uber parenterale Ernahrung durch intra-venose Injektion. *Hoppe Seyler's Zeitschrift fur Physiologische Chemie* 88, 357–369.

Howard, L., Ament, M., Fleming, C.R., Shike, M. and Steiger, E. (1995) Current use and clinical outcome of home parenteral and enteral nutrition therapies in the United States. *Gastroenterology* 109, 355–365.

Langer, B., McHattie, J.D., Zohrab, W.J. and Jeejeebhoy, K.N. (1973) Prolonged survival after complete small bowel resection using intravenous alimentation at home. *Journal of Surgical Research* 15, 226–233.

Latta, T. (1831) Affording a view of the rationale and results of his practice in the treatment of cholera in aqueous and saline injection (letter to the Secretary of the Central Board of Health, London). *The Lancet* 2, 274–277.

Levenson, S.M., Hopkins, B.S., Waldron, M., Canham, J.E. and Seifter, E. (1984) Early history of parenteral nutrition. *Federation Proceedings* 43, 1391–1406.

Macht, S.D. (1980) Three hundred years of parenteral nutrition: the history of intra-venous nutritional therapy. *Connecticut Medicine* 44, 27–30.

Meng, H.C. (1976) History and basic concepts of parenteral nutrition. *Acta Chirurgica Scandinavica* 466, 2–5.

Meng, H.C. and Early, F. (1949) Study of complete parenteral alimentation in dogs. *Journal of Laboratory and Clinical Medicine* 34, 1121–1132.

Menzel, A. and Perco, H. (1869) Uber die Resortpion von Nahrungsmitteln vom Unterhautzellgewebe aus. *Wiener Klinische Wochenscrift* 19, 517.

Mercer, D.F., Iverson, A.K. and Culwell, K.A. (2014) Nutrition and small bowel transplantation. *Nutrition in Clinical Practice* published online 19 June, pii: 0884533614539354.

Moreno, J.M., Shaffer, J., Staun, J., Hebuterne, X., Bozzetti, F., Pertkiewicz, M., Thul, P. and Van Gossum, A.; Home Artificial Nutrition Working Group–ESPEN (2001) Survey on

legislation and funding of home artificial nutrition in different European countries. *Clinical Nutrition* 20, 117–123.
Murlin, F.R. and Riche, J.A. (1915) Blood fat in relation to heat production and depth of narcosis. *Proceedings of the Society for Experimental Biology and Medicine* 13, 7–8.
Pharmaceutical Inspection Co-operation Scheme (2014) PIC/S Guide to Good Practices for the Preparation of Medicinal Products in Healthcare Establishments, version PE 010-4. Available at: http://www.picscheme.org/publication.php?id=8 (accessed 5 July 2014).
Pirenne, J. and Kawai, M. (2009) Intestinal transplantation: evolution in immunosuppression protocols. *Current Opinion in Organ Transplantation* 14, 250–255.
Raman, M., Gramlich, L., Whittaker, S. and Allard, J.P. (2007) Canadian home total parenteral nutrition registry: preliminary data on the patient population. *Canadian Journal of Gastroenterology* 21, 643–648.
Rhoads, J.E. (1975) History of parenteral nutrition. In: Solassol, C., Joyeux, H. and Astrue, B. (eds) *Manual of Surgical Nutrition, American College of Surgeons.* W.B. Saunders, Philadelphia, Pennsylvania, pp. 1–12.
Rhoads, J.E., Vars, H.M. and Dudrick, S.J. (1981) The development of intravenous hyperalimentation. *Surgical Clinics of North America* 61, 429–435.
Rhode, C.M., Perkins, W.M. and Vars, H.M. (1949) Nitrogen balances in dogs continuously infused with 50% glucose and protein preparations. *American Journal of Physiology* 159, 415–425.
Romieu, C., Solassol, C., Pujol, H., Serrou, B. and Joyeux, H. (1972) Long-term parenteral hypernutrition. Use in cancerous cachexia. *Chirurgie* 98, 600–605.
Schohl, A.T. and Blackfan, K.D. (1940) Intravenous administration of crystalline amino acids in infants. *Journal of Nutrition* 20, 305–316.
Schuberth, O. and Wretlind, A. (1961) Infusion of fat emulsions, phosphatides and emulsifying agents. *Acta Chirurgica Scandinavica* 278, 1–21.
Scribner, B.H., Cole, J.J., Christopher, T.G., Vizzo, J.E., Atkins, R.C. and Blagg, C.R. (1970) Long-term total parenteral nutrition. The concept of an artificial gut. *Journal of the American Medical Association* 212, 457–463.
Seibert, F.B. (1923) Fever producing substance found in some distilled waters. *American Journal of Physiology* 64, 90–104.
Seibert, F.B. (1963) Pyrogens from an historical perspective. *Transfusion* 3, 245–249.
Shils, M.E. (1984) Historical aspects of minerals and vitamins in parenteral nutrition. *Federation Proceedings* 43, 1412–1416.
Shils, M.E., Wright, W.L., Turnbull, A. and Brescia, F. (1970) Long-term parenteral nutrition through an external arteriovenous shunt. *New England Journal of Medicine* 283, 341–344.
Smith, T., Micklewright, A., Hirst, A., Stratton, R. and Baxter, J. (2011) *Annual BANS Report, 2011. Artificial Nutrition Support in the UK, 2000–2010.* BAPEN, Redditch, UK.
Solassol, C., Joyeux, H., Etco, L., Pujol, H. and Romieu, C. (1974) New techniques for long-term intravenous feeding: an artificial gut in 75 patients. *Annals of Surgery* 179, 519–522.
Van Gossum, A., Bakker, H., Bozzetti, F., Staun, M., Leon-Sanz, M., Hebuterne, X., Beau, P., Guedon, C., Schmit, A., Tjellesen, L., Messing, B. and Forbes, A.; ESPEN-Home Artificial Nutrition Working Group (1999) Home parenteral nutrition in adults: a European multicentre survey in 1997. *Clinical Nutrition* 18, 135–140.
Vinnars, E. and Wilmore, D. (2003) Jonathan Roads Symposium Papers. History of parenteral nutrition. *JPEN Journal of Parenteral and Enteral Nutrition* 27, 225–231.
Violante, G., Alfonsi, L., Santarpia, L., Cillis, M.C., Negro, G., De Caprio, C., Russo, N., Contaldo, F. and Pasanisi. F. (2006) Adult home parenteral nutrition: a clinical evaluation after a 3-year experience in a Southern European centre. *European Journal of Clinical Nutrition* 60, 58–61.

Winters, R.W., Heird, W.C. and Dell, R.B. (1984) History of parenteral nutrition in paediatrics with emphasis on amino acids. *Federation Proceedings* 43, 1407–1411.

Woodyatt, T.T., Sansum, W.D. and Wilder, R.M. (1915) Prolonged and accurately timed intravenous injections of sugar. A preliminary report. *Journal of the American Medical Association* 65, 2067–2070.

Wretlind, A. and Szczygiel, B. (1998) Total parenteral nutrition. History. Present time. Future. *Polski Merkuriusz Lekarshi* 4, 181–185.

2 Home Artificial Nutrition in Europe

André Van Gossum* on behalf of the ESPEN Home Artificial Nutrition and Chronic Intestinal Failure (HAN & CIF) group

Clinic of Intestinal Diseases and Clinical Nutrition, Hôpital Erasme, Free University of Brussels, Brussels, Belgium

History and Epidemiology

The use of parenteral nutrition started in the early 1960s. It is commonly cited that Shils *et al.* were the first in North America to report their experience of maintaining a patient at home on parenteral nutrition (Shils *et al.*, 1970). However, we should remember that Solassol and Joyeux were at the same period the pioneers of home parenteral nutrition (HPN) in Europe (Montpelier, France) (Solassol and Joyeux, 1976).

Although Shils' first patient survived only a few months, several teams in North America and Europe initiated a programme of HPN during the 1970s. Subsequently, HPN programmes were progressively launched in several Western European countries. Interestingly, Shils reported the advent of home parenteral nutrition support, enlightening some key developments of this method (Shils, 2010).

After a few years of practice, several European teams reported their experience in HPN, describing a low incidence of complications and good survival rate (Jarnum and Ladefoged, 1981; Mughal and Irving, 1986; Messing *et al.*, 1988).

Since 1990, a few people originating from different European countries who were interested in the field of HPN merged together for creating the Home Artificial Nutrition (HAN) working group that was further officially recognized as a working group of the European Society for Parenteral and Enteral Nutrition (ESPEN) in 1997. This group has recently been re-named as the Home Artificial Nutrition and Chronic Intestinal Failure (HAN & CIF) ESPEN Special Interest Group. Since its launch, the ESPEN HAN & CIF group has published numerous studies in the field of HPN.

*E-mail: andre.vangossum@erasme.ulb.ac.be

The main goals of the ESPEN-HAN group were to perform epidemiological surveys throughout Europe, to harmonize the use of HPN and to generate recommendations for good practice.

The ESPEN-HAN working group performed multicentre surveys in 1993, 1997 and 2003, respectively (Van Gossum *et al.*, 1997, 1999; Staun *et al.*, 2004). Between 1 January 1997 and 31 December 1997, a total of 494 patients were registered as having started HPN in 73 centres from nine European countries (Van Gossum *et al.*, 1999). On 1 January 1998, there were 756 patients receiving HPN from these centres. Incidence and prevalence could be estimated in seven out of nine countries. At this time, the incidence was estimated to be $3/10^6$/year in France, $1.2/10^6$/year in the UK and $0.7/10^6$/year in Spain. The highest prevalence was described in Denmark ($13/10^6$/year) (Ugur *et al.*, 2006), while it reached about $4/10^6$ in the UK and in France. So, it was easily apparent that the prevalence of HPN patients was the highest in countries having the longest duration of HPN experience (Denmark, France and the UK).

Since 1997, data about HPN incidence have been available only in a few European countries. In the UK, a national register was started by the British Artificial Nutrition Survey (BANS) in 1996 (Glencorse *et al.*, 2003). The number of adults on HPN registered with BANS has grown progressively since 1996. In 2010, 228 new adult patients were registered with BANS, compared with 148 in 2009 and 157 in 2008. Expressed in terms of population size, the prevalence of new HPN cases was 3.66 per million of the UK population, with a period prevalence of ten cases per million. However, the BANS committee recognizes that there is a considerable under-reporting and therefore these data need to be interpreted very cautiously.

In Scotland, all patients receiving HPN have been identified with the development of the Managed Clinical Network (MCN) and data from 2001 found the point prevalence to be 12 patients per million of the population (Baxter and McKee, 2003). The figure exceeds the overall UK rate of about eight patients per million of the population. Within the UK, further regional variation has also been identified.

In Spain, data are collected annually through a designed questionnaire (Planas *et al.*, 2004) and reported by the NADYA-SENPE Group (an annual registry of Home Artificial Nutrition in Spain). During the period from December 2009 to December 2010, there were 148 patients registered from 23 hospitals. The average age of the adult patients ($n = 139$) was 53 ± 15 years. The average duration of HPN was 316 days/patient. The indication for HPN was short bowel syndrome in 47%. Twenty-nine patients (19.5%) were patients with advanced cancer who received HPN as palliative care (Wanden Berghe *et al.*, 2011).

In France, a national HPN registry was opened in 2001 (Joly *et al.*, 2004). Between June 2001 and June 2004, 413 adults were included in the registry; the estimated incidence was three newly enrolled patients per million inhabitants per year.

There are no strong data for Italy; in 2005 the regional coordinators of the Italian Society for Parenteral and Enteral Nutrition (SINPE) recorded all the cases of home artificial nutrition (HAN), including enteral and parenteral nutrition. HAN prevalence was 152, but with 16.1% of HPN. At this time a HAN regulation was present in 11 out of 20 regions; a positive association ($P = 0.012$) was found between the number of years since the regulation was issued and the HAN prevalence. Santarpia *et al.* (2013) recently published an update seven years after the regional regulation, showing that the specific regional regulation in Campana has contributed to increase the prescription of HPN (156 in April 2005 to 306 in April 2012) and to improve the quality of care.

In 2012, Baxter *et al.* performed a survey as an international benchmarking exercise that provides a global figure of HPN use in Europe (Baxter *et al.*, 2012). This survey showed there is a wide range in HPN prevalence figures and that the existence of organized care varies across the countries studied. It is recognized that several countries under-reported the HPN prevalence, as registries are not fully available or used. Period prevalence figures ranged from 3.25 to 66 per million of the population (Table 2.1).

Underlying Diseases and Indications

The European survey performed in 1997 showed that, overall, the distribution of underlying diseases requiring HPN was quite similar in Europe and the USA (Van Gossum *et al.*, 1999; Howard and Ashley, 2003). At this time, cancer had already become the largest single worldwide indication for HPN (40%). Crohn's disease, mesenteric vascular diseases, radiation enteritis and disorders of intestinal motility remain the most frequent benign conditions requiring long-term HPN. HPN is also used in AIDS patients with intractable diarrhoea. However, the number of AIDS patients receiving HPN has decreased recently since the introduction of more efficacious triple therapy. We have to underline that 25% of HPN patients suffer from 'miscellaneous' diseases, including chronic pancreatitis, intestinal mucosa atrophy, anorexia nervosa, cachexia, etc.

However, the distribution of underlying diseases in HPN patients varies among the different European countries (Van Gossum *et al.*, 1999) (Table 2.2). In 1997, Crohn's disease accounted for 44% of indications in the UK but only for 13% in The Netherlands; in contrast, cancer represented 60% of indications in The Netherlands and 5% in the UK. An earlier survey performed in 1993 showed that cancer was the main indication for HPN in Italy (67%) (Van Gossum *et al.*, 1997). A team based in Naples (Italy) reported 159 patients who were discharged on HPN for at least 4 weeks from January 2000 to December 2002. In all, 140 (88%) were cancer and 19 (12%) non-cancer patients. The main indications were carcinomatosis in 68 and hypophagia/dysphagia in 62 patients. If we consider the benign diseases, the most common indications are small bowel resection, digestive fistula and motility disorders. According to data published in the UK in 2010, the vast majority of new and established HPN patients are under 71 years of age; more than two-thirds of patients are between 41 and 70 years of age (BAPEN report). Short bowel syndrome remains the commonest indication for new HPN patients (54.4%). Fistula is cited as the main reason in 17.1%, malabsorption in 13.6%, gastrointestinal obstruction in 9.6%, to 'improve nutrition' in 2.2% and swallowing disorder in 0.4%. For cancer patients, the main indication is intestinal obstruction, which is common in the case of peritoneal carcinomatosis.

Table 2.1. The populations, period and point prevalence data, the number of HPN centres and whether referral pathways and organized care are in place. (From Baxter *et al.*, 2012.)

					Organized care		
Country	Population (millions)	2010 period prevalence (millions)	31 Dec. 2010 point prevalence (millions)	No. of HPN centres	Referral pathways	Education programme	National guideline used
Australia	22.2	6.7	5.1	9	No	Yes	AuSPEN
Belgium	10.5	11 (estimate)	8 (estimate)	7	No	No	ESPEN
Denmark	5.3	66	47	3	Yes	Yes	ESPEN
Republic of Ireland	4.2	10.1	7.5	0	No	No	ESPEN/NICE
England	51.8	10	8.3 (estimate)	21	No	Yes	ESPEN/NICE
France	63.1	6	unknown	>14	No	Emerging	ESPEN
Germany	82	Unknown	49 (estimate)	few	No	No	ESPEN
Israel	7.85	25.5	–	4	No	Yes	ESPEN
Italy	60	33.3 (estimate)	Unknown	90 (estimate)	No	Yes	ESPEN
Netherlands	17	14.7	Unknown	2	Yes	Yes	ESPEN
Northern Ireland	1.7	18.8	14.1	1	No	Yes	ESPEN
New Zealand	4.2	7.2	5.3	1	No	Yes	AuSPEN
Poland	38.2	25	22.3	26	Yes	Yes	None
Scotland	5.3	23	17.5	11	Yes	Yes	Standards
Spain	46.2	3.25	2.7	7	No	Yes	ESPEN
Wales	3.0	18	21	2	Yes	Yes	Standards

AuSPEN, Australasian Society for Parenteral and Enteral Nutrition; ESPEN, European Society for Parenteral and Enteral Nutrition; NICE, National Centre for Health and Clinical Excellence.

Table 2.2. Indications for HPN in seven different European countries (1997) where reporting was assumed to be more than 80% of patients. (From Van Gossum *et al.*, 1999.)

	Patients (*n*)	Crohn's disease (%)	Vascular (%)	Cancer (%)	Radiation (%)	AIDS (%)	Others (%)
France	173	16	23	27	15	0.5	18.5
UK	72	44	14	5	2	–	35
Belgium	26	12	15	23	15	35	–
Denmark	15	20	13	8	26	–	33
The Netherlands	45	13	11	60	–	–	16
Spain	31	16	13	39	–	6	25
Poland	14	14	50	–	14	–	22

In the UK, according to the last data available, Crohn's disease still is the most common underlying diagnosis, representing 18.4% of new registrations in 2010 (BAPEN report, unpublished data; www.bapen.org.uk). However, the point prevalence data for Crohn's disease decreased from 44% of HPN patient registrations in 1996 to 29% in 2010. In 2010, cancer represented 14% of new registrations compared with 5% in 1997.

In 2006, the ESPEN-HAN working group collected a cohort of patients with benign diseases who were on HPN in order to assess the percentage of patients who were likely to be candidates for intestinal transplantation (Pironi *et al.*, 2006). This cohort included 688 adults and 166 children. For adults, the main primary diseases were mesenteric ischaemia, Crohn's disease and radiation enteritis (Table 2.3). Short bowel syndrome was the indication in 75% of the adult patients. For children, underlying diseases were heterogeneous but short bowel was the indication in 52%.

Perfusion Regimen

In the 1997 survey, in the majority of the cases (69%), administration of nutritional solutions was performed through a subcutaneous tunnelled catheter positioned in the vena cava via the internal jugular vein or the subclavian vein, preferentially on the right side (Van Gossum *et al.*, 1999). Based on the reports of the North America Registry on HPN and the European surveys, the use of subcutaneous reservoirs (port-a-cath) is growing (Van Gossum *et al.*, 1999; Howard and Ashley, 2003). This trend is due, on one hand, to its wide use in cancer patients who receive chemotherapy and, on the other hand, to the preference of some patients for implantable catheters for functional and aesthetic reasons, for instance for practising aquatic sports or for taking a shower. In the more recent survey that was performed in 2003, 26% out of 1117 HPN patients had an implanted port (Staun *et al.*, 2004).

The number of perfusions that are administered per week may vary in time as a function of intestinal adaptation capacities. The European survey showed that the percentage of bags/week was as follows: 7 (67%), 6 (9%), 5 (12%), 4 (8%) and 3 or less (4%) (Van Gossum *et al.*, 1999).

Table 2.3. Characteristics of the patient populations on HPN in Europe. (From Pironi *et al.*, 2006.)

	Adult (*n*=688)	Paediatric (*n*=166)
Sex		
Males/Females (*n*)	293/395	87/79
Age (years)		
Mean ± standard deviation (range)	52.9 ± 15.2 (18.5–88.0)	6.1 ± 5.1 (0.2–18.0)
Duration of HPN (years)		
Mean ± standard deviation (range)	5.5 ± 5.4 (0.1–29.0)	3.9 ± 4.1 (0.1–18.0)
*Primary disease (*n *(%))*		
Mesenteric ischaemia	185 (26.9)	1 (0.6)
Crohn's disease	159 (23.1)	6 (3.6)
Radiation enteritis	73 (10.6)	0
Chronic intestinal pseudo-obstruction	72 (10.5)	29 (17.4)
Cancer	17 (2.5)	0
Surgical complications	55 (8.0)	1 (0.6)
Familial polyposis	21 (3.0)	2 (1.2)
Connective disease	13 (1.9)	0
Volvulus	12 (1.7)	13 (16.5)
Ulcerative colitis	9 (1.3)	1 (0.6)
Protein-losing enteropathy	9 (1.3)	5 (3.0)
Chronic pancreatitis	7 (1.0)	0
Immunoglobulin deficiency	5 (0.7)	3 (1.8)
Congenital mucosal disease	5 (0.7)	24 (14.5)
Congenital short bowel	3 (0.4)	42 (25.3)
Hirschsprung's disease	2 (0.3)	9 (5.4)
Necrotizing enterocolitis	2 (0.3)	13 (7.8)
Others	39 (5.7)	8 (4.8)
*Cause of intestinal failure (*n *(%))*		
Short bowel syndrome	514 (74.7)	87 (52.4)
Motility disorder	124 (18.0)	38 (22.9)
Fistula	15 (2.2)	0
Extensive parenchymal disease	35 (5.1)	41 (24.7)

Oral feeding is not only allowed but also encouraged in patients without bowel obstruction or need for bowel rest. It has been shown that patients with short bowel are in fact hyperphagic. In the 1997 European survey, 50% of patients had free oral intakes, 27% had limited oral intakes, while 23% ingested nothing (Van Gossum *et al.*, 1999).

In the ESPEN-HAN group's survey that included only long-term HPN patients, the median duration of HPN was 7 years (range 2–24 years) (Van Gossum *et al.*, 2001). At the time of evaluation, the mean weekly number of nutritional bags was 5.6 (range 1–7), with a mean of 1.6 lipid-based bags per week. The regimen of perfusion was cyclical nocturnal in 224 patients, cyclical diurnal in two and over 24 h in two. Intravenous (IV) catheter care was performed by patients (94%), community nurses (4%) or by relatives (2%). Oral food intake was unlimited in 81%, restricted in 17% and nil in 2% of patients.

In this population, the composition of the nutritional support was conventional, with a mean number of 5.6 bags supplied weekly and a predominance of cyclical nocturnal regimen and autonomous manipulation. The provision of bags containing lipid-emulsions was however quite low (1.6 bags/week); this could be explained by the fact that low caloric supplementation is needed in some patients with a short gut because of the capability of energy absorption of the colon, as well as the hyperphagic behaviour of these patients who nearly all – in this series – had unlimited oral intake. It is also probable that some teams limited the administration of lipid emulsion because they were concerned about hepatic changes.

Training

In the 73 centres that reported their training technique in 1997, 75% had a nutrition support team and 76% had an HPN training programme (Van Gossum *et al.*, 1999). Seventy per cent of the patients were trained in hospital, while 30% were trained outside hospital. After training, 48% of patients were self-caring. Otherwise, the care was provided by relatives (10%) and community nurses (35%).

In a more recent survey that was also performed by the ESPEN-HAN group in 51 centres in seven European countries, one or more of the following criteria were used by 62% of the centres to exclude patients from their HPN programme: intellect (33%), physical disability (24%), social situation (25%), underlying diseases (18%) and age (16%) (Wegner *et al.*, 2003). Generally, hospital nurses/clinical nurse specialists (84%) and/or doctors (39%) trained two or more people in an in-patient setting over 1–2 weeks. In the international benchmarking survey published by Baxter *et al.* (2012), most of the reporting centres had an education programme and used published guidelines (see Table 2.1).

Prognosis

The ESPEN HAN & CIF group performed a longitudinal survey on a large cohort of patients on HPN with benign diseases. The primary goal of this study was to assess the adequacy of the criteria that are proposed for intestinal transplantation. The first step of this work was to estimate the number of ongoing HPN patients who fit the criteria for intestinal transplantation. Afterwards, a follow-up was performed after 3 years and after 5 years, respectively (Pironi *et al.*, 2008, 2011).

Globally, this study showed that HPN is still the first-line treatment for patients and that the survival on HPN is good. Moreover, this study discriminated some criteria for elective intestinal transplantation; this will be detailed elsewhere in this volume (Chapter 38). The global survival rate at 5 years was 60% but reached 90% for young adults with Crohn's disease.

HPN-related Complications

The ESPEN-HAN group also focused on HPN-related complications in the survey that was performed in 2001 (Van Gossum *et al.*, 2001). Within the 12-month period prior to evaluation, the mean number of hospitalizations was 2.7 (range 0–12), corresponding to a mean period of 23 days (range 0–270 days). Reasons for hospitalization were related to the underlying diseases in 27% of days admitted to hospital, to HPN complications in 48% or to other medical reasons in 25%. Of the HPN complications, catheter-related sepsis accounted for 61%, metabolic disorders for 27% and venous access thrombosis for 12%.

One of the main goals of HPN is, by definition, to avoid prolonged or recurrent hospitalizations. When we consider the 12-month period before the evaluation, the mean time of hospitalization corresponded to 8% of the year. This seems acceptable for patients with life-threatening intestinal failure. However, we have to accept that a few patients stayed much longer in hospital (up to 270 days). The mean number of central venous catheters used during the total HPN period was 3 (range 1–17), with a mean survival time per catheter of 34 months (range 4–245 months). During the 12-month period before evaluation, an episode of catheter-related sepsis occurred in 31% of the patients. Central venous thrombosis was reported in 9% and vascular access problems in 13% of the patients. These percentages of complications and hospitalization have been confirmed by the prospective surveys (Pironi *et al.*, 2008, 2011).

Rehabilitation Status and Quality of Care

When comparing the rehabilitation score before HPN and at the time of evaluation, it appears that the percentage of HPN patients who are capable of coping with a job is about 65% (Van Gossum *et al.*, 2001). Nevertheless, there is a sharp decrease in this percentage in favour of part-time work when on HPN. This can be easily explained by limitations due to the time spent taking parenteral nutrition. On the other hand, it clearly appears that the percentage of grade IV (bedridden at home) patients decreased significantly, meaning that HPN may improve the status of patients who have a very low rehabilitation score before starting HPN. This study also confirmed a 30% prevalence of analgesics and opiates dependence that has previously been reported to predict a poor outcome for HPN patients. Interestingly, depression was noted in 17% of the patients. Eight per cent of HPN patients claimed willingness for intestinal transplantation, while it was considered by the medical team in 10% of the patients.

In 2013, Dreesen and co-workers showed that the most important outcome indicators for adult patients on HPN with a benign underlying disease were: (i) incidence of catheter-related infections; (ii) incidence of readmission and quality of life (shared second place); and (iii) incidence of dehydration (Dreesen *et al.*, 2013a). For cancer patients on HPN, the most important outcome indicators were: (i) quality of life; (ii) incidence of hospital readmission; and (iii) incidence of catheter-related infections (Dreesen *et al.*, 2013b).

Legislation and Funding

The ESPEN-HAN working group has also performed a survey on the different legislations and modes of funding for HAN throughout Europe (Moreno *et al.*, 2001). There is legal coverage for HPN in many Western European countries. Except in Italy, where it has a regional scope, the rules apply nationwide. There are different levels of regulation of HPN with restrictions either to certain hospitals or to use in patients with specific diagnoses.

In all of the countries with regulations, the funding for HPN is provided by a national health service. Hospital pharmacies, private pharmacists and home care companies are involved to a different degree among the various countries in providing and distributing solutions and disposables.

Conclusions and Perspectives

The use of HPN started about 45 years ago in a few European centres – as in North America – on the impulse of some enthusiast physicians, pharmacists and nurses who were dealing with patients suffering from life-threatening intestinal insufficiency. Since this time, the central IV line is considered to be an 'artificial gut'.

In most Western European countries, HPN was initiated in specialized centres that developed growing expertise down the years. In the meantime, the number of HPN centres has increased, with a high variable number of patients from one centre to another. A recent survey in Europe showed that 50% of 41 centres followed fewer than ten HPN patients (Pironi *et al.*, 2006). There is a potential risk of loss of expertise. Indeed, it has been observed that both the percentage of HPN complications and the need for intestinal transplantation (due to HPN complications) is inversely related to the experience of the HPN centres. The use of prefilled nutrition bags (three chambers) may certainly contribute to the wide spread of HPN. That may be beneficial in extending the use of HPN for some patients, but should not hide the need for specific prescription of parenteral support that should be adapted to each individual by specialized nutrition teams.

In the beginning, HPN was exclusively reserved for patients with intestinal insufficiency related to benign diseases such as Crohn's disease or mesenteric vascular disorder. Short bowel syndrome was the main indication. Since the 1990s, HPN has been more and more used for patients with intestinal insufficiency related to an advanced cancer, mainly carcinomatosis. Cancer has become the largest indication for HPN in many European countries as well as in North America. However, the use of HPN for cancer patients is highly variable from one to another country throughout Europe, with a north–south gradient. This is probably due to medical, cultural, religious and economic factors. The global approach to cancer patients who need to be parenterally fed for a short period requires specific considerations that are – in some ways – different from those for long-term HPN patients with benign disorders.

Legislation and funding for HPN have been progressively adopted in several Western European countries. However, the use of HPN is still problematic in many previous so-called Eastern countries. There is still a need for expanding expertise and supporting legislation and funding in some European countries.

References

Baxter, J.P. and McKee, R.F. (2003) The Scottish home parenteral nutrition managed clinical network: one year on. *Clinical Nutrition* 22, 501–504.

Baxter, J.P., Gillanders, L., Angstmann, K., Staun, M., O'Hanlon, C., Smith, T., Joly, F., Thul, P., Jonkers, C., Wanten, G., Gardiner, K., Klek, S., Cuerda, C., Magambo, W., Hawthorne, A.B., Lukes, A., Van Gossum, A., Theilla, M., Singer, P., Shamir, R. and Pironi, L. (2012) Home parenteral nutrition: an international benchmarking exercise. *e-SPEN Journal* 7, 211–214.

Dreesen, M., Foulon, V., Vanhaecht, K., Hiele, M., De Pourcq, L., Pironi, L., Van Gossum, A., Wanten, G., Baxter, J., Joly, F., Cuerda, C. and Willems, L. (2013a) Development of quality of care interventions for adult patients on home parenteral nutrition (HPN) with a benign underlying disease using a two-round Delphi approach. *Clinical Nutrition* 32, 59–64.

Dreesen, M., Foulon, V., Hiele, M., Vanhaecht, K., De Pourcq, L., Pironi, L., Van Gossum, A., Arends, J., Cuerda, C., Thul, P., Bozzetti, F. and Willems, L. (2013b) Quality of care for cancer patients on home parenteral nutrition: development of key interventions and outcome indicators using a two-round Delphi approach. *Supportive Care in Cancer* 21, 1373–1381.

Glencorse, C., Meadows, N. and Holden, C. (2003) Trends in Artificial Nutrition Support in the UK between 1996 and 2002. BANS report.

Howard, L. and Ashley, C. (2003) Management of complications in patients receiving home parenteral nutrition. *Gastroenterology* 124, 1651–1661.

Jarnum, S. and Ladefoged, K. (1981) European experience of home parenteral nutrition. *Acta Chirurgica Scandinavica* 507, 128–139.

Joly, F., Fouche, W. and Messing, B. (2004) A website for descriptive epidemiological studies in HPN patients. *Clinical Nutrition* 23, 1468 (abstract).

Messing, B., Landais, P., Goldfarb, B., Lemann, M., Joyeux, H., Gouttebel, M.C., Robert, D., Bouletreau, P., Matuchansky, C. and Beau, P. (1988) Home parenteral nutrition for adults. Results of a multicenter survey in France. *La Presse Médicale* 17, 845–849.

Moreno, J.M., Shaffer, J., Staun, M., Hebuterne, X., Bozzetti, F., Pertkiewicz, M., Thul, P. and Van Gossum, A.; Home Artificial Nutrition Working Group–ESPEN (2001) Survey on legislation and funding of home artificial nutrition in different European countries. *Clinical Nutrition* 20, 117–123.

Mughal, M. and Irving, M. (1986) Home parenteral nutrition in the United Kingdom and Ireland. *The Lancet* 16, 383–387.

Pironi, L., Hebuterne, X., Van Gossum, A., Messing, B., Lyszkowska, M., Forbes, A., Micklewright, A., Moreno Villares, J., Bozzetti, F., Goulet, O. and Staun, M. (2006) Candidates for intestinal transplantation: a multicentre survey in Europe. *American Journal of Gastroenterology* 101, 1633–1643.

Pironi, L., Forbes, A., Joly, F., Colomb, V., Lyszokowska, M., Van Gossum, A., Baxtyer, J., Thul, P., Hebuterne, X., Gambarara, M., Gottrand, F., Moreno Villares, J., Messing, B., Goulet, O. and Staun, M. (2008) Survival of patients identified as candidates for intestinal transplantation: a 3 year prospective follow-up. *Gastroenterology* 135, 61–71.

Pironi, L., Joly, F., Forbes, A., Colomb, V., Lyszkowska, M., Baxter, J., Gabe, S., Hebuterne, X., Gambarara, M., Gottrand, F., Cuerda, C., Thul, P., Messing, B., Goulet, O., Staun, M. and Van Gossum, A. (2011) Long-term follow-up of patients on home parenteral nutrition in Europe: implications for intestinal transplantation. *Gut* 60, 17–25.

Planas, M., Castella, M., Moreno, J.M., Pita, A.M., Pedron, C., Gomez Candela, C., Gomez Enterria, P., de la Cuerda, C., Perez de la Cruz, A., Forga, M.T., Marti, E., Garde, C., Carrera, J.A., Garcia Luna, P.P., Ordonez, J., Bonada, A., Pares, R.M. and Rodriguez, A. (2004) Parenteral nutrition at home: NADYA register for the year 2001. *Nutrición Hospitalaria* 19, 139–143.

Santarpia, L., Pagano, M.C., Pasanisi, F. and Contaldo, F. (2013) Home artificial nutrition: an update seven years after the regional regulation. *Clinical Nutrition* published online 16 Oct, doi: 10.1016/j.clnu.2013.10.005.

Shils, M.E. (2010) The advent of home parenteral nutrition support. *Annual Review of Nutrition* 30, 1–12.

Shils, M.E., Wright, W.L., Turnbull, A. and Brescia, F. (1970) Long-term parenteral nutrition through external arteriovenous shunt. *New England Journal of Medicine* 283, 341–344.

Solassol, C. and Joyeux, H. (1976) Ambulatory parenteral nutrition. In: Manni, C., Magolini, S. and Scrascia, E. (eds) *Parenteral Alimentation: The International Symposium on Intensive Therapy*. Elsevier, New York, pp. 138–152.

Staun, M., Moreno, J., Bozzetti, F., Pertkiewicz, A., Van Gossum, A., Micklewright, A. and Thul, P. (2004) Home parenteral nutrition in adults: a European survey in 2003. *Clinical Nutrition* 23, 916 (abstract 326).

Ugur, A., Marashdeh, B., Gottschalck, I., Brobech Mortensen, P., Staun, M. and Bekker Jeppessen, P. (2006) Home parenteral nutrition in Denmark in the period 1996 to 2001. *Scandinavian Journal of Gastroenterology* 41, 401–407.

Van Gossum, A., Bakker, H., De Francesco, A., Ladefoged, K., Leon-Sanz, M., Messing, B., Pironi, L., Pertkiewicz, M., Shaffer, J., Thul, P. and Wood, S. (1997) Home parenteral nutrition in adults: a multicentre survey in Europe in 1993. *Clinical Nutrition* 15, 53–58.

Van Gossum, A., Bakker, H., Bozzetti, F., Staun, M., Pertkiewicz, M., Shaffer, J., Hebuterne, X., Beau, P., Guedon, C., Schmit, A., Tjellesen, L., Messing, B. and Forbes, A. (1999) Home parenteral nutrition in adults: a European multicentre survey in 1997. *Clinical Nutrition* 18, 135–140.

Van Gossum, A., Vahedi, K., Abdel-Malik, Staun, M., Pertkiewicz, M., Shaffer, J., Hebuterne, X., Beau, P., Guedon, C., Schmit, A., Tjellesen, L., Messing, B. and Forbes, A.; ESPEN-HAN Working Group (2001) Clinical, social and rehabilitation status of long-term parenteral nutrition patients: results of a European multicentre survey. *Clinical Nutrition* 20, 205–210.

Wanden Berghe, C., Gomez Candela, C., Chicharro, L. and Grupo NADYA-SENPE (2011) Home parenteral nutrition registry in Spain for the year 2010: NADYA-SENPE Group. *Nutrición Hospitalaria* 26, 1277–1282.

Wegner, A., Micklewright, A., Hébuterne, X., Bozzetti, F., Moreno, J., Pertkiewicz, M., Van Gossum, A., Thul, P. and Staun, M. (2003) Monitoring patients on home parenteral nutrition in Europe. *Clinical Nutrition* 22(Suppl. 1), S87–S88.

3 Home Parenteral Nutrition in the USA

DARLENE G. KELLY*

Oley Foundation for Home Parenteral and Enteral Nutrition, Albany, New York, USA and Mayo Clinic and Foundation, Rochester, Minnesota, USA

Introduction

The aim of this chapter is to highlight differences in home parenteral nutrition history and practice between the USA and other areas of the world.

Brief History

Although the earliest central parenteral infusions compounded with 5–10% glucose, protein hydrolysates and lipids were used between 1955 and 1965 (Elia, 2006), long-term central venous nutrition in the USA was first tested in the laboratory of Rhoads in 1967. The study demonstrated that these nutrients supported normal growth in beagle puppies (Dudrick *et al.*, 1967). Subsequently, Shils described the use of home parenteral nutrition (HPN) in a female patient who started the therapy in 1967 (Shils *et al.*, 1970). Because of concern about the low likelihood of long-term survival with HPN, it was decided to send her for intestinal transplantation. Unfortunately, she died of post-operative complications (Howard, 2006). Rhoads' group reported successful use of HPN in a child for supporting growth and in adults for correcting weight loss (Dudrick *et al.*, 1969). Over the following years several large HPN programmes were developed in the USA by many pioneers in the field: Howard, Fleming, Ament, Steiger, Bistrian, Broviac and others. Devices for central venous access, infusion pumps, acceptable formulas and better clinical support have advanced over time in the USA, as they have in Europe.

*E-mail: dgk28@chartermi.net

Development of a Unique HPN Support Organization

In 1983, Dr Lyn Howard and one of her patients, Clarence (Oley) Oldenburg, established a non-profit organization for individuals on home parenteral and enteral nutrition (HPEN). It was named the Oley Foundation to recognize that patient's family, who provided the start-up finances. At its outset, the foundation was a unique organization for persons on HPEN. It was located at Albany Medical Center in New York and initially was primarily a social and educational gathering for HPEN patients in Dr Howard's practice. The Lifeline Foundation, which had been started by a patient and her husband, was subsequently absorbed by Oley, expanding the membership to a few hundred consumers. Rapidly, Oley became involved in a large variety of projects, including management of the HPEN registry, provision of support and access to information on these therapies to consumers and clinicians, venues for HPEN consumers to network among themselves either face-to-face or through telephone contact (and later social networking), printed educational materials (bimonthly *LifeLineLetter*) and eventually electronic education materials (HPN and home enteral nutrition (HEN) complications charts, HPN management modules, etc.) and annual meetings throughout North America with several travel scholarships to these meetings. The mission statement is as follows: 'the Oley Foundation enriches the lives of those requiring home intravenous and tube feeding through education, outreach, and networking' (www.oley.org). Perhaps the most unique aspect of this patient support organization is that while it has strong consumer direction and professional input, it has a small paid staff that ensures its continuum (L. Howard, New York, 2013, personal communication).

The membership of Oley includes consumers of HPEN, clinicians involved in HPEN practices and businesses who provide HPEN products and supplies. As of January 2013, the membership is 12,570 (C. Harrington, New York, 2013, personal communication). Membership is free to persons on parenteral and enteral nutrition. It continues to grow as awareness of the foundation increases. There is a Board of Directors consisting of five HPEN consumers, five clinicians and five members-at-large. The President and Vice President are always consumers. The Board provides oversight and direction for Oley programmes. Financial support is obtained from private donors and corporate grants. There are approximately 63 HPN and HEN consumers or parents distributed across the country who are designated as regional volunteers and are listed on the website. They are available by telephone or e-mail to provide support to individuals with questions or simply to listen to them as needed. At the annual meetings there are lectures by HPEN clinicians, legislative representatives, psychologists, sociologists and experienced consumers. HPEN consumers have opportunities to spend time with speakers not only in question-and-answer sessions but also in social settings, at meals and during walks. For many consumers the meeting offers the first opportunity to interact with other consumers of HPEN. This is a very strong benefit for building self-confidence and for avoiding complications and depression, as demonstrated by Smith and colleagues in studies supported by the National Institutes of Health (Smith *et al.*, 2002). Many HPEN consumers attend the annual meetings repeatedly and maintain friendships with others who have the same experiences.

Since the Oley Foundation was begun there have been similar groups started in other countries: in the UK, PINNT (Patients on Intravenous Nutrition and Nasogastric Therapy); in Sweden, Svenska HPN-Föreningen Barn & Ungdom; in France, LaVie Par Un Fil; in Norway, Norwegian Association for Home Parenteral Nutrition; in Germany, Kinder and Schweiriger Emaehrungssituation V; in Poland, Lifeline Foundation and Parenteral Nutrition in Poland; in New Zealand and Australia, Parenteral Nutrition Down Under; in Italy, Un Filo per la Vita; and in Spain, Aepannupa. On the website of the Oley Foundation (www.oley.org) there are links to many of these organizations. At a recent meeting of several of these organizations it was decided that these groups would work together to share resources and develop programmes to connect members with each other and ultimately enhance the lives of all members (J. Bishop, New York, 2013, personal communication).

HPN Consumer Registry

The first registry of HPEN for the USA and Canada was established in 1978 at the New York Academy of Medicine and was later transitioned to the Oley Foundation with support from the American Society for Parenteral and Enteral Nutrition (A.S.P.E.N.), where it continued from 1984 until 1992 (Shils, 2010). During the latter years data were submitted by 217 programmes throughout North America characterizing the number of persons on HPEN, underlying diagnoses, gender and age distributions, survival, degree of rehabilitation and rate of complications (Howard, 2006). It was clear that the numbers of consumers of HPEN increased over the period studied and that the diagnostic distribution changed (notably malignancy increased from 17% in 1978 to 42% in 1985–1992). This registry was discontinued in 1993 because the annual information gathered was unchanging, and there were limits to the extent to which it could be demonstrated to be a randomized sample. In hindsight, changes in medical delivery that restricted patient referrals to centres with HPN experience may have worsened outcome, especially for long-term patients, i.e. Crohn's disease with short bowel syndrome. This might have been demonstrated by an ongoing registry (L. Howard, New York, 2013, personal communication). Currently A.S.P.E.N. has launched an endeavour to start a new registry of US HPN consumers, which has been named Sustain™, LLC (http://www.nutritioncare.org/sustain/). This project is made difficult by the fact that although many consumers are managed by larger HPN programmes, there is no requirement in the USA to have patients entered into a registry. Another barrier involves the US Health Insurance Portability and Accountability Act of 1996 (HIPAA). It is increasingly difficult for patients to identify a physician who has experience with HPN or to receive care from an experienced centre. For all of these reasons collecting data from a randomized sample of HPN consumers is more difficult than ever (L. Howard, New York, 2013, personal communication).

Insurance Coverage for US HPN Consumers

Another issue that varies between the USA and other parts of the world is insurance reimbursement for these rather expensive therapies. Early in the history of HPN in the USA there was not standardized insurance coverage, and companies negotiated coverage on a case-by-case basis (Howard, 2006). When it became apparent that the cost of delivering HPN was about half of that for receiving parenteral nutrition in hospital, the agreement to provide insurance coverage became more common. In 1976 Medicare started covering HPN under the prosthetic device benefit. It was not altogether nonsensical, since HPN is an artificial gut prosthesis. Subsequently, Medicare developed a set of criteria that must be met if it is to reimburse for HPN. A high percentage of HPN consumers are Medicare recipients either because of age over 65 years or medical disability. Medicare coverage for HPN requires two basic criteria: (i) intestinal failure; and (ii) permanence – at least 3 months' duration is the expected requirement in best medical judgement (https://www.noridianmedicare.com/dme/coverage/docs/trees/tpn_policy_decision_tree.pdf). For cases of malnutrition related to various diagnoses, documentation of weight loss of at least 10% of body weight within the prior 3 months and serum albumin of less than 3.4 g/dl are required. Then there are additional criteria for short bowel syndrome (resection within the prior 3 months leaving <152 cm residual small intestine), small intestinal dysmotility (no contrast or radionuclide in right colon within 6 h of oral ingestion, but excluding gastroparesis), severe malnutrition resulting from malabsorption (72 h faecal fat ≥50% of ≥50 g ingested long-chain lipid and urine output <1 l daily) and need for bowel rest for at least 3 months (e.g. in severe pancreatitis, obstructive Crohn's disease or proximal enterocutaneous fistula). Furthermore, Medicare requires that the HPN formula provides 20–35 kcal/kg body weight, 0.8–1.5 g protein/kg body weight and ≥10% dextrose content. Formulas outside these levels must be documented and explained to Medicare in writing. It is of note that Medicare does not reimburse for hydration fluids.

Medicare also has specific required charges for HPN, which in many cases are in excess of the price charged to patients with private insurance. Medicare covers 80% of this amount and the consumer or a supplemental/secondary insurance policy covers the balance. The charges for HPN for non-Medicare insurance recipients vary markedly, and the consumer's responsibility for the cost likewise is greatly different. Many private insurers have negotiated special contracts for their recipients arranged through infusion companies.

Drug Shortages in the USA

Over the past several years, drug shortages have been problematic in the USA. A pharmacist, Joseph Nadeau, RPh (Mayo Clinic Rochester), found that 22 of the necessary parenteral products have been in limited supply for variable durations (J. Nadeau, Minnesota, 2013, personal communication). The website listing the current shortages is http://www.fda.gov/Drugs/DrugSafety/DrugShortages/default.htm. Three of the most concerning shortages in the USA, as of January 2013, are parenteral vitamins, selenium and parenteral lipid emulsions. This lipid shortage was just announced, and it is complicated by the fact that emulsions of soybean and safflower oil are the only lipid products currently approved in the USA. The soybean and safflower oil emulsion, Liposyn®, has been temporarily withdrawn from the market, leaving Intralipid® as the only available lipid product that is approved by the Food and Drug Administration (FDA). The FDA had previously banned fat emulsions from castor oil and cottonseed oil in 1964 because of adverse reactions. Prior to the approval of these lipid emulsions many patients on HPN received maize oil that was slathered on the skin (C.R. Fleming, Minnesota, 1983, personal communication) to prevent essential fatty acid deficiency (Miller *et al.*, 1987). The lack of available lipids will make prescription of HPN extremely difficult, as lipids allow clinicians to limit the amount of carbohydrates needed for calories, thus decreasing the complication of hyperglycaemia and avoiding the need for insulin in most HPN consumers.

In the case of selenium shortage, this mineral has been unavailable or available in only very limited quantities for at least 6 months. Individuals on HPN who have not received selenium have developed symptoms of selenium deficiency (personal clinical experience). The most severe sequela of this deficiency is dilated cardiomyopathy, which can be a fatal complication, particularly in areas of the world where the soil is nearly devoid of selenium (Lei *et al.*, 2011).

Multivitamins have also been in very limited supply for many months. This has resulted in using oral vitamins in persons who can take oral products, but in many of these cases absorption cannot be assured. The most rapidly depleted vitamin is thiamin (Centers for Disease Control and Prevention, 1989) and in those who have had long-term malabsorption because of disease or short bowel syndrome, the fat-soluble vitamins (A, D, E and K) are frequently at inadequate levels (Thompson, 1989).

In a prior drug shortage several years ago involving parenteral multiple vitamins, supplies were obtained from companies in Canada and France. Although this approach has been proposed, to date it has not occurred. In addition, the US Congress has passed a bill to address drug shortages, but this does not appear to have affected the products needed to compound adequate HPN formulas. In two recent A.S.P.E.N.-supported conference publications (American Society for Parenteral and Enteral Nutrition, 2009; Vanek *et al.*, 2012) the current status of micronutrients has been reviewed. Looking to the future, it would seem important to standardize these micronutrient products for the USA and Europe, providing a bigger market and potentially broadening their availability.

Conclusion

This chapter has attempted to address HPN as practised in the USA and to emphasize those practices and problems that are unique to this country.

Acknowledgements

The author is grateful to the following Oley Foundation staff members who have provided details of the history of the foundation: Dr Lyn Howard, Medical Director; Joan Bishop, Executive Director; Roslyn Dahl, Communications & Development Director; Lisa Crosby Metzger, Editor, *LifelineLetter*; and Cathy Harrington, Executive Assistant.

References

American Society for Parenteral and Enteral Nutrition (2009) Proceedings from the A.S.P.E.N. Research Workshop 'Micronutrients in Parenteral Nutrition: Too Little or Too Much?' *Gastroenterology* 137, 1–109.

Centers for Disease Control and Prevention (1989) Deaths associated with thiamine-deficient total parenteral nutrition. *MMWR Morbidity and Mortality Weekly Report* 38(3), 43–46.

Dudrick, S.J., Wilmore, D.W. and Vars, H.M. (1967) Long-term total parenteral nutritional growth in puppies and positive nitrogen balance in patients. *Surgical Forum* 18, 356–357.

Dudrick, S.J., Wilmore, D.W., Vars, H.M. and Rhoads, J.E. (1969) Can intravenous feeding as the sole means of nutrition support growth in the child and restore weight loss in an adult? An affirmative answer. *Annals of Surgery* 169, 974–984.

Elia, M. (2006) History of parenteral nutrition. In: Bozzetti, F., Staun, M. and Van Gossum, A. (eds) *Home Parenteral Nutrition*, 1st edn. CAB International, Wallingford, UK, pp. 3–11.

Howard, L. (2006) Home parenteral nutrition in the USA. In: Bozzetti, F., Staun, M. and Van Gossum, A. (eds.) *Home Parenteral Nutrition.* CAB International, Wallingford, UK, pp. 23–35.

Lei, C., Niu, X., Ma, X. and Wei, J. (2011) Is selenium deficiency really the cause of Keshan disease? *Environmental Geochemistry and Health* 33, 183–188.

Miller, D.G., Williams, S.K., Palombo, J.D., Griffin, R.E., Bistrian, B.R. and Blackburn, G.L. (1987) Cutaneous application of safflower oil in preventing essential fatty acid deficiency in patients on home parenteral nutrition. *American Journal of Clinical Nutrition* 46, 419–423.

Shils, M.E. (2010) The advent of home parenteral nutrition. *Annual Review of Nutrition* 30, 1–12.

Shils, M.E., Wright, L.M., Turnbull, A. and Brescia, F. (1970) Long-term parenteral nutrition through an external arteriovenous shunt. *New England Journal of Medicine* 283, 324–344.

Smith, C.E., Curtas, S.L., Werkonitch, M., Kleinbect, S. and Howard, L. (2002) Home parenteral nutrition: does affiliation with a nutritional support and education organization improve patient outcome? *JPEN Journal of Parenteral and Enteral Nutrition* 26, 159–163.

Thompson, G.R. (1989) Lipid related consequences of intestinal malabsorption. *Gut Festschrift* 30, 29–34.

Vanek, V.W., Borum, P., Buchman, A., Fessler, T.A., Howard, L., Jeejeebhoy, K., Kochevar, M., Shenkin, A., Valentine, C.J., Novel Nutrient Task Force, Parenteral Multi-Vitamin and Multi–Trace Element Working Group and American Society for Parenteral and Enteral Nutrition (A.S.P.E.N.) Board of Directors (2012) A.S.P.E.N. position paper: recommendations for changes in commercially available parenteral multivitamin and multi-trace element products. *Nutrition in Clinical Practice* 27, 440–491.

4 Home Parenteral Nutrition in Canada: An Update

Daniela Adjemian[1], Khursheed N. Jeejeebhoy[2] and Johanne P. Allard[1]*

[1]*University Health Network, Division of Gastroenterology, University of Toronto, Toronto, Ontario, Canada;* [2]*St Michael's Hospital, Division of Gastroenterology, University of Toronto, Toronto, Ontario, Canada*

Introduction

Based on data of current health service providers, it is estimated that approximately 520 patients receive home total parenteral nutrition (HTPN) in Canada. In order to assess this patient population, a Canadian HTPN Registry was created in 2006 and HTPN programmes across Canada were invited to participate. The HTPN registry was designed to assess HTPN patient demography, indications for HTPN, clinical outcomes and factors affecting survival, complications and parenteral nutrition (PN) dependency (Raman *et al.*, 2007; Fernandes *et al.*, 2012). Data on the first 150 patients entered in the registry were published in 2007 (Raman *et al.*, 2007). Afterwards, a validation study was conducted followed by a cohort study, based on a second set of data entries performed in 2008–2009, which was published in 2012 (Fernandes *et al.*, 2012). Since then, several other studies, most based on data from the HTPN registry, have been published. In addition, several HTPN programmes have conducted studies on their own. This chapter provides a summary of these studies.

Canadian HTPN Registry and Participating Centres

The HTPN website-based registry was created in 2006 with the purpose of assessing and monitoring the Canadian patient population receiving HTPN as well as to determine the factors affecting survival, complications and HTPN dependency. In addition, it was planned to document the practice of HTPN administration for quality assurance purposes (Raman *et al.*, 2007).

*E-mail: Dr.Johane.Allard@uhn.ca

This registry collects data on patient demography, gastrointestinal anatomy, indications for HTPN, nutritional assessment, vascular access and complications (Raman *et al.*, 2007). To see if the information entered in the registry was reliable, we performed a study to validate the data entry (Fernandes *et al.*, 2012). This was done by blinded individuals with no access to the original registry forms or online information. They performed chart review for a second time and re-entered the baseline data in the web-based registry. This validation process was performed in two of the participating centres: University Health Network and St Michael's Hospital (Fernandes *et al.*, 2012). Most of the data had significant correlations and agreements between the two entries, indicating that the data collection on the website registry was valid for most parameters. However, parameters such as amount of chromium in the PN solution, plasma levels of sodium and chloride and clinical data such as documentation of vascular access, line infections, diagnoses of liver disease and number of hospitalizations were less reliable. For the clinical data, the most likely explanation was poor documentation due to the fact that many patients live far away and are hospitalized in peripheral institutions, making it more difficult to access data.

After this validation study (Fernandes *et al.*, 2012), baseline and follow-up data from four of the six participating centres were assessed. The follow-up data had been entered in 2008–2009, 2–4 years after the baseline entry (Fernandes *et al.*, 2012).

With the purpose of describing better the population on HTPN, we will mention some of the findings of the first 150 patients entered in the registry, based on the cross-sectional study of Raman *et al.* (2007) and we will also describe the findings of the patients who had follow-up at 2.24 ± 0.11 years after baseline ($n = 96$) (Fernandes *et al.*, 2012).

HTPN Registry Cross-sectional Study

Demography and gastrointestinal anatomy

At the time that the registry was created in 2006, there were approximately 400 patients receiving HTPN in Canada. The first 150 patients entered in the registry constituted 37.5% of the total number of patients on HTPN in Canada (Raman *et al.*, 2007). The five participating programmes at the time were: from Ontario, University Health Network and St Michael's Hospital in Toronto as well as McMaster Health Sciences Centre in Hamilton; from British Columbia, the Parenteral Nutrition Program in Vancouver; and from Alberta, the Capital Health/University of Alberta in Edmonton. For some of the subsequent studies, Winnipeg St Boniface Hospital in Manitoba and Calgary Foothills Medical Centre in Alberta participated. McGill University Program in Montreal, Quebec is currently entering patients.

The majority of the 150 patients from the initial five programmes were female (62.1%), the mean age was 53.0 ± 14 years and the mean duration that patients were on HTPN was 70.1 ± 78.1 months. The mean body mass index (BMI) before the start of HTPN was $19.8 \pm 5.0\,kg/m^2$. The main indication for HTPN was short bowel syndrome (SBS) in over 60% of the cases. The most common aetiology of SBS was Crohn's disease (51.1%) followed by mesenteric ischaemia (23.9%). Other indications for HTPN included pseudo-obstruction, mucosal disease, fistulas, cancer, unexplained nausea and vomiting, and mechanical obstruction. By the time the follow-up was done, SBS kept being the first indication for HTPN.

HTPN was associated with complications such as: catheter sepsis (28.6%); catheter change (50%); abnormal liver enzymes (27%); metabolic bone disease (60%); and PN-related hospitalizations (44%) (Raman *et al.*, 2007).

HTPN Registry Cross-sectional, Cohort and Other Studies

Among the 150 patients entered at baseline (Raman *et al.*, 2007), 96 had follow-up data entry at 2.24±0.11 years. Among these 96 patients, 19.8% had discontinued HTPN, 44.8% were still on HTPN and 35.4% were deceased.

Over the 2-year follow-up period, body weight remained stable. For those remaining on HTPN, PN was cycled to an average of 12 h/day and over time some of the components of PN had decreased (amino acids, dextrose, fat emulsions, calories and PN days/week), suggesting weaning. Over that period of time, most of the bloodwork remained stable except for potassium and platelets which were significantly lower but still within normal range (Fernandes *et al.*, 2012).

Complications

Vascular access

Based on the cross-sectional study, most of the patients had a tunnelled catheter with a single lumen and results showed that 28.6% of the patients had at least one episode of catheter sepsis over the previous year; double-lumen catheters had significantly more episodes of catheter sepsis per patient than single-lumen catheters (Raman *et al.*, 2007). Results from the cohort study showed that the number of line sepsis events had decreased since 2006 from 0.55±0.12 to 0.30±0.08 per year and the most common cause for change in vascular access was line sepsis (56%), followed by line breakage (24%) and line occlusion (20%) (Fernandes *et al.*, 2012).

Liver enzymes

From the cross-sectional study, abnormal liver enzymes were found in 27.4% of the patients: most of the patients were female and the mean number of months on HTPN was 68.34±71.09. The main histological finding was cholestasis (92%), followed by steatosis (8%) (Raman *et al.*, 2007). When the HTPN composition was compared with that of patients with normal liver enzymes, the dextrose content was higher but the amount prescribed was within recommended ranges. In the 96 patients who had the 2-year follow-up data entry, no significant changes in liver enzymes were documented besides a non-significant trend towards an elevated bilirubin (Fernandes *et al.*, 2012).

Metabolic bone disease

Metabolic bone disease (MBD) is another common complication in patients requiring HTPN. Data regarding MBD were available in 69 patients in the study published by Raman *et al.* (2007). In this sample, 60% of patients had MBD (46% osteoporosis and 18% osteopenia) and the primary indication for HTPN in these patients was SBS. In the cohort study (Fernandes *et al.*, 2012) data were available both for baseline and follow-up for 34 of the 96 patients. There was a significant decline in spine T score between 2006 and 2009 and an overall trend towards a decline for hip and neck T score. Further analyses showed that those who were on pamidronate at baseline had a higher T and Z scores for spine, neck and hip at the follow-up than those who were not on pamidronate.

Another study (Aljarallah *et al.*, 2012), based on the HTPN registry, also indicates that vitamin K could play a role in bone mineral density (BMD). This study evaluated 189 HTPN patients; of them, 78 (41.3%) received vitamin K supplementation in the form of 10 mg intravenously once weekly and 111 patients (58.7%) did not receive supplementation but got some vitamin K from lipid emulsion prescribed as part of their HTPN. Both groups were comparable in terms of PN phosphate, magnesium, calcium, BMI and amounts of lipids in the total parenteral nutrition (TPN) bags. The mean BMI in the patients supplemented with vitamin K was in fact trending lower, at 20 kg/m^2 versus 21 kg/m^2 in the non-supplemented ones. Data analyses showed that patients supplemented with vitamin K had higher BMD on lumbar spine and hip T scores compared with those who were not supplemented and in a general linear model adjusted for BMI, age, PN magnesium, phosphate, calcium and bisphosphonate intake, there was a trend towards higher T scores for the hip, but not the spine, in supplemented patients ($P=0.063$). The authors suggested that more studies are needed to address the role of vitamin K supplementation as there is evidence that it plays a role in bone metabolism. Vitamin K supplementation has been shown to reduce bone loss and decrease fractures (Cockayne *et al.*, 2006) and the proposed mechanism is that vitamin K is a coenzyme for glutamate carboxylase that mediates the conversion of glutamate to g-carboxyglutamic acid (Gla). Some Gla proteins, such as osteocalcin, matrix Gla proteins and periostin are expressed in bones and play an important role in its metabolism (Vermeer *et al.*, 2004).

In terms of bone health, another important vitamin that deserves consideration in HTPN patients is vitamin D since these patients are at risk of vitamin D deficiency because of insufficient intake or malabsorption. Routinely, these patients receive 5 µg (200 IU) of vitamin D as part of an intravenous multivitamin supplementation but this may not be sufficient. Levels of vitamin D and responses to oral supplementation were evaluated by the HTPN programme in Calgary (Kumar *et al.*, 2012). This was a study evaluating retrospectively 14 patients receiving HTPN for longer than 6 months. Five of these patients had SBS and insufficient levels of 25-hydroxyvitamin D (27.5–75 nmol/l), while the other nine individuals with different indications for HTPN had mixed vitamin D status (some normal and some low). Patients were provided with various amounts of oral vitamin D supplementation in an attempt to correct the vitamin D levels. Two SBS patients responded well to the oral supplementation and increased their serum vitamin D into the normal range. Their daily average vitamin D supplementation was ~68.7 µg (2748 IU). However, the other SBS patients did not respond adequately to vitamin D supplementation despite high doses. One patient's vitamin D status improved with an intake of 550 µg/day (22,000 IU/day) but the others had declining, persistently borderline or deficient vitamin D levels or became deficient. The authors suggested to adequately monitor vitamin D and consider adding supplementation orally, in the form of capsules or drops, or ultraviolet light therapy, or intravenously. High doses may be needed (Kumar *et al.*, 2012). Another programme from Winnipeg (Thomson and Duerksen, 2011) stated that all patients receiving HTPN should receive supplementation first in a dose of 25 µg/day (1000 IU/day) up to 1250 µg/week (50,000 IU/week) to correct vitamin D levels. Further studies are required to assess clinical outcomes.

Survival

Based on the HTPN registry and the cohort of 96 patients who were followed for about 2 years, 53 were no longer on HTPN (Fernandes *et al.*, 2012). Of these, 19 discontinued PN and 34 died. Data showed that ten deaths were PN-related (one had line sepsis and nine secondary to PN-related liver disease). Other deaths were related to underlying medical conditions. The combined mean survival was 17.67 ± 1.89 years (95% confidence interval (CI) 13.96–21.38 years). The probability of survival at 5 and 10 years on HTPN was 82% and 60%, respectively. Oncology patients had a significantly lower survival at 2.22 ± 1.43 years (95% CI 0.00–5.03 years) when compared with the other patients at 18.7 ± 1.97 years (95% CI 14.85–22.57 years) ($P < 0.0001$).

Quality of life

The cohort study (Fernandes *et al.*, 2012) also showed that the quality of life, based on the Karnofsky score, decreased significantly. In 2006 it was 79.56 ± 1.64 and in 2009 it decreased to 61.83 ± 5.01 ($P < 0.001$). It was not stated if the reason for this was HTPN or the underlying disease.

Trace Elements in HPN

There is much debate regarding the optimal supplementation of trace elements (TEs) in PN. With the aim of reviewing the practice of TE supplementation in HTPN in Canada, Abdalian *et al.* from the University Health Network programme retrospectively studied 135 patients from five Canadian HTPN programmes who were entered in the HTPN registry during 2005–2006 (Abdalian *et al.*, 2013a). In clinical practice in Canada, a standardized multiple-TE admixture is typically added to PN formulations. Various commercially available preparations exist, but some do not adhere to TE supplementation guidelines.

The authors found an excessive supplementation of some TEs compared with the American Medical Association (AMA) guidelines and the A.S.P.E.N. guidelines.

Zinc exceeded both guidelines, manganese and copper exceeded the A.S.P.E.N. but not the AMA recommendations and selenium exceeded only the A.S.P.E.N. guidelines. When they studied if there was a difference by diagnosis with respect to SBS versus others, there was no difference between groups except that SBS patients received less selenium and iodine compared with non-SBS patients. In addition, there were no significant differences between patients who had received nil by mouth compared with those who were on oral diet or enteral nutrition. Patients' underlying anatomy or indication for HTPN did not significantly influence decisions regarding replacement standards. Therefore HTPN TE supplementation in Canadian HTPN programmes needs to be reviewed and adjusted according to most current guidelines. This may require a re-evaluation of the commercial TE preparations currently available in Canada and potential new products worldwide to avoid over-supplementation and potential toxicity.

Excessive supplementation from commercial TE preparations may lead to toxicity. Recently, hypermanganesaemia and potential neurological toxicity were reported in the literature. The University Health Network programme (Abdalian *et al.*, 2013b) assessed manganese status in a convenience sample of 16 HTPN patients, using bloodwork and magnetic resonance imaging (MRI). They found that the mean daily manganese supplementation from the commercial preparation used at the time was 7.28 μmol/day, which was within the AMA Nutrition Advisory Group guidelines of 2.73–14.56 μmol/day but exceeded the A.S.P.E.N. 2002 recommendations of 1.09–1.82 μmol/day. The mean whole blood level was 1.38 ± 0.29 times the upper limit of normal (ULN) and eight of 14 patients with blood measurements had levels above the ULN. On MRI 81% of patients had high signals on T1-weighted images suggesting manganese deposits in the basal ganglia. Two of these patients had a clinical diagnosis of Parkinson's disease and multiple neuropsychiatric complaints were reported. These results suggest that manganese supplementation should be used with caution and attention should be paid to manganese content in multi-TE supplements. Most of the TE formulations are standardized and there is not enough flexibility in TE commercial preparations.

HPN in Cancer

There is evidence that cancer patients are at high risk of malnutrition. A multicentre study reported that weight loss is present in over 50% of patients with gastrointestinal, breast and pulmonary malignancies (DeWys *et al.*, 1980). Of all the cancers, gastrointestinal malignancies and advanced disease are the most commonly associated with malnutrition (DeWys *et al.*, 1980; Segura *et al.*, 2005).

There is controversy in Canada regarding the use of HTPN in patients with advanced, incurable cancer. Some support the use of HTPN on the basis that patients should not die of malnutrition, even if they have a non-curable disease (Mackenzie and Gramlich, 2008; Soo and Gramlich, 2008). In Canada, there is a big variation in the prevalence of HTPN use in patients with advanced cancer and in fact, in some programmes, the diagnosis of advanced cancer may be a contraindication to HTPN therapy (Mackenzie and Gramlich, 2008).

Table 4.1. Northern Alberta HTPN Program eligibility criteria. (From Mackenzie and Gramlich, 2008.)

Eligibility criteria for oncology patients
1. Selection criteria: nutritional diagnosis (obstruction, fistula); life expectancy of at least 6–12 weeks; reasonable quality of life (Karnofsky performance status > 50)
2. Medical stability
3. Venous access
4. Psychological considerations
5. Ability to learn

The Northern Alberta Home Total Parenteral Nutrition Program, along with the Regional Palliative Care Program and the Cross Cancer Institute, has developed clinical guidelines for the use of HTPN in advanced cancer. The main objective of these guidelines is to provide selection criteria for referral of patients with advanced cancer for HTPN. Table 4.1 lists the programme eligibility criteria for oncology patients to be able to receive HTPN (Mackenzie and Gramlich, 2008).

In a retrospective cohort study of all advanced cancer patients enrolled in the Northern Alberta Home Parenteral Nutrition Program in Canada, the authors found that from 1999 to 2006, 38 advanced cancer patients received HTPN (Soo and Gramlich, 2008) and accounted for 24% of all HTPN patients in Northern Alberta in the years mentioned, and also there was a 3% average annual increase when compared with all other indications for HTPN (Soo and Gramlich, 2008).

In this study (Soo and Gramlich, 2008), the most common malignancy was ovarian cancer and the main indication for HTPN was bowel obstruction. The mean length of survival in this sample was approximately 5 months; this is more than expected if the patient did not receive nutritional therapy. Also, 13.3% of the patients experienced complications, but there was no relationship between complications and mortality. This study concluded that there might be a subgroup of patients with advanced cancer who may benefit from HTPN therapy. An important marker may be the Karnofsky performance status > 50 to anticipate benefit from this therapy (Soo and Gramlich, 2008).

HPN in Systemic Sclerosis

Among the HTPN population, there is a small group of patients with systemic sclerosis who require HTPN because of intestinal pseudo-obstruction. These patients are frequently referred to us with significant malnutrition. The University Health Network programme evaluated the effect of HTPN on the nutritional status and the quality of life of a subset of these patients, using the HTPN registry (Jawa *et al.*, 2012). Twelve subjects were assessed and were found to have a significant and progressive improvement in their BMI from $16.95 \pm 0.80\,kg/m^2$ at baseline to $20.43 \pm 0.75\,kg/m^2$ at 12 months with improvements in albumin levels from 31.17 ± 1.78 g/l to 36.07 ± 2.30 g/l. However, the quality of life remained poor and the 2-year survival was 58%.

Cost Analysis

PN is a life-saving, but expensive therapy. The total annual cost for HTPN therapy is not precisely known, but the nutrition solution and infusion equipment alone account for US$70,000 to US$120,000 per year. In Canada, the cost is between CAN$60,000 and CAN$100,000 per year (Raman *et al.*, 2007). Management of complications requires additional costs and hospitalizations for serious complications can cost between US$10,000 and US$50,000. In Canada it is estimated to be the same (Raman *et al.*, 2007). In comparison to in-patient PN, HTPN reduces costs significantly. In a study done by the Hamilton programme in 29 of their patients, the authors found that the net savings per patient with HTPN after the first month of discharge from hospital was estimated to be CAN$4860, and these savings increased in patients with underlying malignancies and among those aged 55 years or older (Marshal *et al.*, 2005).

Telehealth and HTPN

The University Health Network programme assessed the use of telehealth to monitor HTPN patients living in remote areas (Saqui *et al.*, 2007). Telehealth has been a cost-saving alternative modality of care since the programme started using it in 2002. It allows the follow-up of patients with HTPN who live in remote areas of the province of Ontario. Patients who reside a mean of 611 km from Toronto would cost a mean of CAN$724.00 for flights and accommodations to have an appointment at the clinic in Toronto, while using telehealth would require to drive a mean of 14 km to the nearest telehealth site in the community and would cost only a mean of CAN$7.00 for parking and fuel. Patient satisfaction was also assessed and all patients were extremely satisfied with this modality. Clinical outcome was not different from the rest of the HTPN population.

The Canadian HTPN Registry in 2013

We have now seven participating centres: (i) University Health Network (Toronto); (ii) British Columbia Parenteral Nutrition Program (Vancouver); (iii) Foothills Medical Centre (Calgary); (iv) St Michael's Hospital (Toronto); (v) Hamilton Health Sciences (Hamilton); (vi) Capital Health/University of Alberta (Edmonton); and (vii) St Boniface Hospital (Manitoba). All of the centres follow adult patients except for British Columbia, where paediatric patients are included. The HTPN staff includes a nurse, dietician, pharmacist (in some of the centres) and a physician who is usually a gastroenterologist. The Ministry of Health from each province gives the funding for HTPN. This funding is distributed to home care services and hospitals to cover solutions, supplies and salaries. Each centre follows a standard HTPN teaching protocol with its patients, which can be slightly different from centre to centre. Most include a teaching period of 1–3 weeks as in-patients and patients may be followed by home care services or may be completely autonomous with the administration of TPN.

As of 2013, we have data on 369 HTPN patients (61% female; mean age 52.7 ± 14.2 years; range 18–87 years) entered in the registry since 2006, which include those who were weaned from TPN or deceased: 97.8% (n = 361) of the patients have a baseline assessment, 40.6% (n = 150) have a 2-year follow-up, 14.1% (n = 52) have a 4-year follow-up and 0.5% (n = 2) have a 6-year follow-up.

Of the total number of patients who are presently on HTPN across Canada (approximately 520), 250 patients currently receive HTPN from the participating centres. The main diagnosis of the current patients with HTPN (n = 250) remains short bowel syndrome (55.2%). Other indications for HTPN are: motility disorder (19.6%); mucosal defect (8.8%); cancer (8.4%); Crohn's other than due to short bowel syndrome (3.2%); and others (4.8%).

Conclusion

The Canadian HTPN Registry is a valid tool to report and follow several clinical parameters as well as monitor long-term outcomes and impact of therapy in this patient population. It also allows to assess HTPN prescriptions and to evaluate if changes in practice are required to optimize the treatment of these patients. Finally, it brings together HTPN teams from across the country, facilitating networking between the programmes to improve practice and formulate research questions. In that regard, the HTPN programmes across Canada have been very productive.

References

Abdalian, R., Fernandes, G., Duerksen, D., Jeejeebhoy, K., Whittaker, S., Gramlich, L. and Allard, J. (2013a) Prescription of trace elements in adults on home parenteral nutrition: current practice based on the Canadian home parenteral nutrition registry. *JPEN Journal of Parenteral and Enteral Nutrition* 37, 410–415.

Abdalian, R., Saqui, O., Fernandes, G. and Allard, J.P. (2013b) Effects of manganese from a commercial multi trace element supplement in a population sample of Canadian patients on long-term parenteral nutrition. *JPEN Journal of Parenteral and Enteral Nutrition* 37, 538–543.

Aljarallah, B., Fernandes, G., Jeejeebhoy, K.N., Gramlich, L., Whittaker, J.S., Armstrong, D., Duerksen, D.R. and Allard, J.P. (2012) The Canadian home total parenteral nutrition (HPN) registry: vitamin K supplementation and bone mineral density. *JPEN Journal of Parenteral and Enteral Nutrition* 36, 415–420.

Cockayne, S., Adamson, J., Lanham-New, S., Shearer, M., Gilbody, S. and Torgerson, D. (2006) Vitamin K and the prevention of fractures. *Archives of Internal Medicine* 166, 1256–1261.

DeWys, W.D., Begg, C., Lavin, P.T., Band, P.R., Bennet, J.M., Bertino, J.R., Cohen. M.H., Douglass, H.O., Enstrom, P.F., Ezdinli, E.Z., Horton, J., Johnson, G.J., Moertel, C.G., Oken, M.M., Perlia, C., Rosenbaum, C., Siverstein, M.N., Skreel, R.T., Sponzo, R.W. and Tomey, D.C. (1980) Prognostic effect of weight loss prior to chemotherapy in cancer patients. *American Journal of Medicine* 69, 491–497.

Fernandes, G., Kaila, B., Jeejeebhoy, K.N., Gramlich, L., Armstrong, D. and Allard, J. (2012) Canadian home total parenteral nutrition (HPN) registry: validation and patient outcomes. *JPEN Journal of Parenteral and Enteral Nutrition* 36, 407–414.

Jawa, H., Fernandes, G., Saqui, O. and Allard, J.P. (2012) Patients with systemic sclerosis receiving home parenteral nutrition improve their nutritional status but not their quality of life. *The Journal of Rheumatology* 39, 1004–1007.

Kumar, P.R., Fenton, T.R., Abdel, S. and Raman, M. (2012) Prevalence of vitamin D deficiency and response to oral vitamin D supplementation in patients receiving home parenteral nutrition. *JPEN Journal of Parenteral and Enteral Nutrition* 36, 463–469.

Mackenzie, M. and Gramlich, L. (2008) Home parenteral nutrition in advanced cancer: where are we? *Applied Physiology, Nutrition and Metabolism* 33, 1–11.

Marshall, J.K., Gadowsky, S.L., Childs, A. and Armstrong, D. (2005) Economic analysis of home vs hospital-based parenteral nutrition in Ontario, Canada. *JPEN Journal of Parenteral and Enteral Nutrition* 29, 266–269.

Raman, M., Gramlich, L., Whittaker, S. and Allard, J. (2007) Canadian home total parenteral nutrition registry: preliminary data on the patient population. *Canadian Journal of Gastroenterology* 21, 643–648.

Saqui, O., Chang, A., McGonigle, S., Purdy, B., Fairholm, L., Baun, M., Yeung, M., Rossos, P. and Allard, J. (2007) Telehealth videoconferencing: improving home parenteral nutrition patient care to rural areas of Ontario, Canada. *JPEN Journal of Parenteral and Enteral Nutrition* 31, 234–239.

Segura, A., Pardo, J., Jara, C., Zugazabeitia, L., Carulla, J., de Las Penas, R., Garcia-Cabrera, E., Luz Azuara, M., Casadó, J. and Gomez-Candela, C. (2005) An epidemiological evaluation of the prevalence of malnutrition in Spanish patients with locally advanced or metastatic cancer. *Clinical Nutrition* 24, 801–814.

Soo, I. and Gramlich, L. (2008) Use of parenteral nutrition in patients with advanced cancer. *Applied Physiology, Nutrition, and Metabolism* 33, 102–106.

Thomson, P. and Duerksen, D. (2011) Vitamin D deficiency in patients receiving home parenteral nutrition. *JPEN Journal of Parenteral and Enteral Nutrition* 35, 499–504.

Vermeer, C., Shearer, M.J., Zittermann, A., Bolton-Smith, C., Szulc, P., Hodges, S., Walter, P., Rambeck, W., Stöcklin, E. and Weber, P. (2004) Beyond deficiency: potential benefits of increased intakes of vitamin K for bone and vascular health. *European Journal of Nutrition* 43, 325–335.

5 Home Parenteral Nutrition in Australia and New Zealand

LYN GILLANDERS[1]* AND PATRICK BALL[2]

[1]*Auckland City Hospital, Auckland, New Zealand;* [2]*Charles Darwin University, Darwin, Australia*

Introduction

Australia and New Zealand have both had home parenteral nutrition (HPN) provision to patients in the community since about 1980. Services initially were provided on an ad hoc basis but in recent years have become much more organized within states in Australia; and in New Zealand, a new New Zealand National Intestinal Failure Service (NZ NIFS) has been approved in 2012. The Australasian Society for Parenteral and Enteral Nutrition (AuSPEN) has played a significant role in this improved organization through publication of Australasian HPN Guidelines and the development of the Australasian HPN Register and encouraging networking across state and country boundaries.

National Profiles

Australia and New Zealand have their own identities and cultures but also share much in common. Travel and kinship between both countries are common. The majority of the Caucasian population has Anglo-European roots but Asian immigrants are an increasing feature together with Pacific Islanders in both countries, while in New Zealand the Maori population is increasing together with a smaller increase in the Aboriginal population in Australia. New Zealand is a single country but Australia is a Commonwealth of eight states and territories with both federal (national) and state-funded health services. Fundamentally, primary care is federal and hospital care is state-based, so the latter is the predominant funder. The health service in both countries is based on public health funding and HPN is funded from the public purse.

*E-mail: lyng@adhb.govt.nz

In Australia this funding is linked to institutions through state health funding and may not necessarily be portable between states (although this may change shortly). Before an application for funding can occur, the patient's admixtures and consumables must be costed and quoted on an annual basis by the company that is supplying the products, thus this is a case-by-case situation. New Zealand has a Pharmaceutical Management Agency (Pharmac) that secures pharmaceutical treatments for eligible New Zealanders (pursuant to the New Zealand Public Health and Disability Act, 2000). This enables New Zealanders to have a nationally funded service for consumables and solutions.

Both Australia and New Zealand have a low population density because much of the land area is desert or mountainous, respectively. Major centres of health care consequently tend to be clustered primarily in the large urban centres along the eastern seaboard of Australia and in the major cities in New Zealand, with smaller provincial hospitals providing a range of general services. This has resulted in some inequality of service, particularly with regard to HPN provision.

Climate

Both countries span considerable variations in climate from tropical to temperate and uniform service delivery protocols do not always apply. This has implications for patients, with a number of centres reporting patients from the northern (hotter) areas requiring additional infusions of fluids and electrolytes or their formula being modified during the summer months. It is also relevant to maintenance of the cold chain, with extended transit times and lack of access to refrigerated vehicles in remote areas. At least one hospital in northern Australia reported having experienced problems with maintaining the cold chain for delivery to rural HPN patients, while another in southern New Zealand reported having a patient's HPN bags arrive part frozen one winter morning.

HPN History

The history of HPN in both countries is similar and comparable to European and North American experience. Technical advances in medicine and surgery resulted in a number of patients with long-term chronic intestinal failure requiring long-term parenteral nutrition to survive and in some cases achieve intestinal rehabilitation. Some notable centres including Professor Graham Hill's Body Composition Unit at Auckland Hospital (New Zealand) became involved at a pioneering and research level early in the development of parenteral nutrition as a viable technique. Similarly, Professor David Russell at the Royal Melbourne Hospital was an early leader in Australia and these initiatives underpinned the consequent development of these as early centres of service provision.

In Australia, the Australian (now Australasian) Society for Parenteral and Enteral Nutrition (AuSPEN) was the first of the Parenteral and Enteral Nutrition societies to be formed in 1974 (www.auspen.org.au). Membership is now drawn from Australia, New Zealand and the Asia-Pacific region. AuSPEN hosts an annual scientific meeting that enables research conducted in the region to be presented, including an increasing body of data emanating from the HPN AuSPEN Group who maintain the HPN Register for both countries and conduct research on this patient population. For the last 5 years AuSPEN has been affiliated with the European Society for Parenteral and Enteral Nutrition (ESPEN) and this has resulted in enhanced opportunities for attendance at ESPEN scientific meetings and membership of the ESPEN Home Artificial Nutrition and Chronic Intestinal Failure (HAN & CIF) Group with ongoing collaboration in HPN-related research.

Early surveys of HPN practice and outcomes of HPN patients in Australia and New Zealand are sparse. A report from Auckland Hospital (New Zealand) in 1991 indicated that in the previous 2.5 years six patients had been sent home on HPN (Stokes and Hill, 1991). Four were continuing after periods of 1–30 months. There had been one death and one patient had developed catheter sepsis. The paper reported that quality of life (QoL) on HPN had, in general, been very good. This paper was ground-breaking for its time in that the Department of Surgery at Auckland was pioneering methods in measuring body composition. Studies on this small cohort had shown that normal body composition could be maintained while on HPN.

An Australian group (Jones *et al.*, 1995) reviewed the outcomes in 14 patients treated with HPN at the Royal Prince Alfred Hospital in Sydney between 1978 and 1994. The median time of HPN therapy was 468 days (range 7–5352 days) and seven patients continued on HPN at the time of review. They reported that the majority of patients had been able to resume a reasonable place in society for varying periods and four of the patients had returned to work. They concluded that their experience indicated that HPN was a cost-effective treatment in selected patients with chronic intestinal failure.

The AuSPEN HPN Register

The AuSPEN HPN Group was established in 2006. Terms of reference are:

- to maintain the AuSPEN HPN Register;
- to collate and publish regular reports of practice and outcomes for HPN patients (including diagnosis, access, infection rates, professional care);
- to benchmark across New Zealand and Australia with international HPN organizations that agree to collaboration; and
- to allow audit of practice and outcomes and hence provide a basis for improving HPN quality of care.

Five AuSPEN HPN Register annual reports (2007–2011) and the current Register data were examined for patient numbers, patient characteristics and professional care across Australia and New Zealand. Data collection for the Register is continuous through a network of health professional reporters in Australia and

New Zealand. The HPN Group has published annual reports midway through each calendar year (www.auspen.org.au) to enable internal and external benchmarking.

Child and adult data were amalgamated in 2007 and 2008, with some missing data; hence trends from those years need to be interpreted with caution. Children's data from 2009 to 2011 were collated and held on a separate register and these data are now reported separately.

Overall 5-year data are summarized in Table 5.1. Children's data for 2009–2011 are summarized in Table 5.2. Pseudo-obstruction/motility disorders are the major diagnostic category for adults across the 5-year period and cancer accounts for ≤10% of patients.

Consistent trends indicate increasing patient numbers with most patients enjoying independence and normal activities of daily living (ADLs). Period prevalence indicates some regions of higher activity but patient numbers remain significantly lower than in many other contemporary HPN Register reports (see later).

Obstructing cancer remains a minor diagnostic category as an indicator for adult HPN in Australia and New Zealand, in contrast to many European centres (except the UK) (Puiggros *et al.*, 2011; Smith *et al.*, 2011). This may account for some of the disparities in point and period prevalence.

Average age, HPN days per week and average duration of HPN remain fairly consistent over the 5-year period for adults but use of tunnelled lines and ability to perform normal activity (ADLs) have declined. Reduced ADLs may be due to

Table 5.1. AuSPEN HPN Register 2007–2011: overall results.

	2007[a]	2008	2009	2010	2011
Total patients, Australia (*n*)	53	86	88	125	122
Total patients, New Zealand (*n*)	34	19	27	31	141
Average age, adults (years)	50	52	48	52	53
HPN days per week, adults	5.8	5.4	5.1	6.1	6.0
Average duration of HPN, adults (years)	7.9	4.8	6.4	6.0	5.8
Tunnelled central venous access device (%)	96	73	78	69	67
Normal activities of daily living, adults (%)	88	66	77	70	64

[a]Some missing data from Victoria and Western Australia.

Table 5.2. AuSPEN HPN Register 2007–2011: children's results.

	2009	2010	2011
Total patients, Australia (*n*)	26	26	24
Total patients, New Zealand (*n*)	10	5	10
Average age, children (years)	6.9	6.2	6.8
HPN days per week, children	6.4	6.0	6.1
Average duration of HPN, children (years)	3.7	3.0	3.5
Tunnelled central venous access device (%)	80	71	82

provision of HPN therapy to people with greater disabilities or co-morbidities but this warrants further investigation. The children's data show consistency over the 3-year reporting period. The AuSPEN HPN Register remains the key marker in defining the population with long-term intestinal failure in Australia and New Zealand. Comparison with industry data shows that there is <5% missing data in the AuSPEN HPN Register.

Standards of Service Provision

Evidence-based guidelines for HPN were commissioned by AuSPEN and developed by a multidisciplinary group drawn from practitioners in both Australia and New Zealand associated with long-established multidisciplinary nutrition support teams (NSTs) including dedicated nurse specialists. Despite the geographical separation, Australian states and territories and New Zealand have enjoyed a collaborative relationship regarding development of nutrition policy and joint standards for parenteral and enteral nutrition through AuSPEN. This led to publication of a clinical practice guideline for HPN patients in Australia and New Zealand that informs practice for clinicians caring for these patients (Gillanders *et al.*, 2008a). This guideline uses focused clinical questions to make recommendations in four domains: (i) patient selection; (ii) patient training; (iii) formulation and monitoring regimens; and (iv) preventing and managing complications. One recommendation noted that access devices should be selected for lowest risk of complications including occlusion, sepsis and breakage and be managed by early diagnosis and treatment. Although there are existing guidelines (Gillanders *et al.*, 2008a; Staun *et al.*, 2009) for the prevention and management of some aspects of these complications, the scope of the problem remained difficult to quantify. Limitations such as retrospective methodology (Bozzetti *et al.*, 2002; Shirotani *et al.*, 2006), skewed patient groups (Crispin *et al.*, 2008) and older data (Reimund *et al.*, 2002) precluded a reflection of contemporary practice and an examination of Australasian practice and outcomes.

The AuSPEN HPN Group conducted a prospective observational study over a 1-year period in 2009 to provide evidence on management of central vascular access device (CVAD)-related complications in Australia and New Zealand. Approaches to CVAD infections are broadly similar in both countries with local therapy being used for exit-site infections without systemic consequences and systemic therapy, with or without line removal, being used for bacteraemia and other severe infections.

HPN patients in Australia and New Zealand are self-caring in their own home with rare exceptions. Patients are taught in hospital to manage their own CVAD; sometimes another family member may also be involved in the home care. Discharge to a home setting is achieved after demonstrated competency in self-management of the CVAD. Written guidelines including emergency plans and open admission letters form part of this standard of care. Home care companies are not involved in post-discharge care of HPN patients in Australia or New Zealand, with the exception of some nurses employed by the parenteral solution manufacturing pharmacy to provide advice about the home infusion pump. Aftercare including regular review and management of complications remains the responsibility of the hospital-based multidisciplinary team.

Four tertiary referral centres caring for HPN patients in Australia and New Zealand (Flinders Medical Centre in Adelaide, Royal North Shore Hospital in Sydney, Royal Children's Hospital in Melbourne and Auckland City Hospital in Auckland) participated in the data collection for the study of CVAD-related complications. The four centres care for almost half of the HPN patients in Australia and New Zealand and all have long-established multidisciplinary NSTs including dedicated nursing specialists.

Results from the CVAD-complications study (Gillanders *et al.*, 2012) showed that over 2009, of 53 patients (42 adults and 11 children), 27 suffered a total of 49 episodes of CVAD-associated complications (line infection 36, catheter blockage 5, line fracture 1, line migration 7), giving an incidence of 3.6 catheter complications overall per 1000 CVAD-days (11.6 per 1000 in patients with multi-use CVAD). Thirty-seven episodes resulted in hospital admission for a median duration of 8 days (range 1–29 days). Responsible microbes were mainly enteric with *Klebsiella* spp. being the most commonly isolated organism (ten episodes).

The average cost of care per episode of CVAD-associated complication requiring in-patient admission was AU$9710 (€6480 approximately).

It was concluded that CVAD complications, in particular line infection, were still a major source of potentially avoidable HPN morbidity and mortality with a high cost to the healthcare system. The predominance of enteric organisms in the series raised the possibility of bacterial translocation as a significant component of the pathogenesis of line sepsis in HPN patients.

Patient Selection for HPN

Overall the accepted indication for HPN in Australia and New Zealand is for benign disease leading to intestinal failure and the major diagnostic categories are for Crohn's disease, short bowel syndrome from vascular occlusive disease and dysmotility syndromes. Children's indications are a little different, reflecting congenital disorders or severe and permanent diseases of early onset. Obstructing cancers such as peritoneal carcinomatosis (in contrast to some other countries) are rarely considered indications. The AuSPEN HPN Guideline made some recommendations for clinician consideration prior to embarking on HPN for patients with obstructing cancer:

- likelihood of response to oncologic treatment;
- patient awareness of the diagnosis and likely prognosis;
- QoL; and
- end-of-life issues, withdrawal of treatment.

The 2012 AuSPEN HPN Report (www.auspen.org.au) showed that pseudo-obstruction and motility disorders remain the major diagnostic category closely followed by short bowel due to vascular occlusive disease and then Crohn's disease. In contrast, the UK 2011 BANS Report indicated that in 2010 short bowel was the major reason for HPN (Smith *et al.*, 2011).

Only three people across both countries appeared to have obstructing cancers, but this distinction may not have been realized by all reporters and should be interpreted with caution.

International Benchmarking

Australia and New Zealand are geographically isolated but have similar health services to many European countries and in particular England and Scotland. Benchmarking with similar countries delivering similar services has been recognized as an essential tool to maintain and improve service delivery. Early collaboration with the Scottish HPN Managed Clinical Network, and in particular Janet Baxter who managed the network, was valuable in building the service locally.

An early joint study examined patients receiving HPN in Scotland and New Zealand. Patients in both countries were tracked through HPN registers which enabled clinical audit for identifying important variations in practice. Scotland and New Zealand have similar demographics, healthcare systems and populations (Scotland 5.1 million, New Zealand 4.1 million in 2005). The HPN registers for Scotland and New Zealand for 2005 were examined for patients who received HPN during 2005, together with the diagnostic category identified (World Health Organization International Classification of Diseases version 10; ICD-10) that resulted in provision of HPN. The diagnostic categories for the 2005 HPN patients were similar in both countries but rates of provision were much higher in Scotland (71 patients versus 14 patients) (Gillanders *et al.*, 2008b). Despite similar demographics, healthcare systems and population size, HPN was utilized to a significantly lesser extent in New Zealand. The reasons for this were not clear; however it was concluded that it is possible there is a lack of recognition of the need for HPN and/or under-provision of HPN in New Zealand, which may lead to poorer treatment outcomes.

QoL assessment tools have recently been developed and validated specifically for this patient population; previous studies have used generic instruments or techniques not validated in HPN. The assessment of QoL should produce clinically relevant data reflecting patients' issues. This is particularly important in more isolated countries such as Australia and New Zealand where patient care may be spread over vast geographical distances and rates of provision are low. The HPN-QoL study was designed to assess the QoL of HPN patients and used patient sampling from the UK and New Zealand. The purpose of this study was to test the hypothesized scale structure of the questionnaire with regard to reliability and validity in a sample of HPN patients (Baxter *et al.*, 2010a). Participation in this validation study enabled local perspectives to be formed regarding patient-centred care by focusing on the patient's experience and expectations with regard to outcome of treatment.

A further benchmarking study in 2007 (Gillanders and Baxter, 2008) found that in New Zealand the rates of provision for HPN within District Health Board regions varied from 25 patients per million to none. Twelve of 21 District Health Board regions in New Zealand including the two largest had no HPN patients. In contrast, in Scotland only three (the smallest) of the 14 Health Boards had no HPN patients. Rates of provision of HPN in Scotland varied from 57 patients per million to none within Health Board regions.

Referral pathways for HPN patients in Denmark, Scotland and New Zealand were examined in 2009 and the register data reporting period prevalence, again in very similar countries, appeared to confirm inequality of access to HPN in New Zealand (Baxter *et al.*, 2010b). Period prevalence rates are largely the same in Australia, so by extension the same conclusions probably apply.

An extended benchmarking exercise involving many of the European centres as well as Australia and New Zealand was recently published (Baxter *et al.*, 2012) which confirmed there is a wide range in HPN prevalence figures and that the existence of organized care varies across the countries studied.

Most countries either had developed their own clinical guidelines or standards or had adopted an international society guideline to improve patient care. It is recognized that several countries have under-reported the HPN prevalence as registries are not fully available or used. These benchmarking studies have been invaluable for Australia and New Zealand: on the one hand, they have a robust and well-maintained HPN Register with a local contemporary HPN Guideline that provides a standard of care for the region. On the other hand, provision of HPN is lagging when compared with countries with similar healthcare systems and provision of HPN for benign disease.

Patient Support Group

The important role of patient support groups has been widely acknowledged and Australia and New Zealand are now served by Parenteral Nutrition Down Under (PNDU) who recently celebrated their fourth birthday. Their informative website can be found at http://parenteral-nutrition-down-under.webs.com/.

Conclusion

HPN in Australia and New Zealand has made steady progress in terms of published standards, service delivery and collaborative research including international benchmarking. The recent establishment of the NZ NIFS and an Intestinal Transplant Service for Australia and New Zealand at the Austin Hospital in Melbourne will lead to further advances for HPN patients in both countries, underpinned by engagement with the international HPN clinical community.

References

Baxter, J.P., Fayers, P.M. and McKinlay, A.W. (2010a) The clinical and psychometric validation of a questionnaire to assess the quality of life of adult patients treated with long-term parenteral nutrition. *JPEN Journal of Parenteral and Enteral Nutrition* 34, 131–142.

Baxter, J., Gillanders, L., Rasmussen, H., Wilson, B., Perry, B. and Staun, M. (2010b) Comparison of referral pathways for patients on home parenteral nutrition in Scotland, New Zealand and Denmark. *Clinical Nutrition* 5, 146.

Baxter, J., Gillanders, L., Angstmann, K., Staun, M., O'Hanlon, C., Smith, T., Joly, F., Thul, P., Jonkers-Schuitema, C.F., Wanten, G., Gardiner, K., Klek, S., Cuerda, C., Magambo, W., Hawthorne, A., Lukes, A., van Gossum, A., Theilla, M., Singer, P., Shamir, R. and Pironi, L. (2012) Home parenteral nutrition: an international benchmarking exercise. *e-SPEN Journal* 7, 211–214.

Bozzetti, F., Mariani, L., Bertinet, D.B., Chiavenna, G., Crose, N., De Cicco, M., Gigli, G., Micklewright, A., Moreno Villares, J.M., Orban, A., Pertkiewicz, M., Pironi, L., Vilas, M.P., Prins, F. and Thul, P. (2002) Central venous catheter complications in 447 patients on home parenteral nutrition: an analysis of over 100,000 catheter days. *Clinical Nutrition* 21, 475–485.

Crispin, A., Thul, P., Arnold, D., Schild, S. and Weimann, A. (2008) Central venous catheter complications during home parenteral nutrition: a prospective pilot study of 481 patients with more than 30,000 catheter days. *Onkologie* 31, 605–609.

Gillanders, L. and Baxter, J. (2008) Equity of care for home parenteral nutrition patients in New Zealand and Scotland. *Clinical Nutrition* 3, 159.

Gillanders, L., Angstmann, K., Ball, P., Chapman-Kiddell, C., Hardy, G., Hope, J., Smith, R., Strauss, B. and Russell, D. (2008a) AuSPEN clinical practice guideline for home parenteral nutrition patients in Australia and New Zealand. *Nutrition* 24, 998–1012.

Gillanders, L., Baxter, J., Ball, P., Merrie, A. and McKee, R.F. (2008b) Benchmarking home parenteral nutrition in Scotland and New Zealand: disparities revealed. *New Zealand Medical Journal* 121, 28–33.

Gillanders, L., Angstmann, K., Ball, P., O'Callaghan, M., Thomson, A., Wong, T. and Thomas, M. (2012) A prospective study of catheter-related complications in HPN patients. *Clinical Nutrition* 31, 30–34.

Jones, L., Ramsey-Stewart, G. and Storey, D. (1995) Home parenteral nutrition: the Royal Prince Alfred Hospital experience. *Australian Journal of Advanced Nursing* 12, 22–25.

Puiggros, C., Gomez-Candela, C., Chicharro, L., Cuerda, C., Virgili, N., Martinez, C., Moreno, J.M., Perez de la Cruz, A., Alvarez, J., Luengo, L.M., Ordonez, J., Wanden-Berghe, C., Cardona, D., Laborda, L., Garde, C., Pedron, C., Gomez, L., Penacho, M.A., Martinez-Olmos, M.A., Apezetxea, A., Sanchez-Vilar, O., Canovas, B., Garcia, Y., Forga, M.T., Gil, C. and Grupo, N.S. (2011) Home parenteral nutrition (HPN) registry in Spain for the years 2007, 2008 and 2009 (NADYA-SENPE group). *Nutrición Hospitalaria* 26, 220–227.

Reimund, J.M., Arondel, Y., Finck, G., Zimmermann, F., Duclos, B. and Baumann, R. (2002) Catheter-related infection in patients on home parenteral nutrition: results of a prospective survey. *Clinical Nutrition* 21, 33–38.

Shirotani, N., Iino, T., Numata, K. and Kameoka, S. (2006) Complications of central venous catheters in patients on home parenteral nutrition: an analysis of 68 patients over 16 years. *Surgery Today* 36, 420–424.

Smith, T., Micklewright, A., Hirst, A., Stratton, R. and Baxter, J. (2011) Annual BANS Report, 2011 Artificial Nutrition Support in the UK 2000–2010. Available at: http://www.bapen.org.uk/pdfs/bans_reports/bans_report_11.pdf (accessed 17 December 2012).

Staun, M., Pironi, L., Bozzetti, F., Baxter, J., Forbes, A., Joly, F., Jeppesen, P., Moreno, J., Hébuterne, X., Pertkiewicz, M., Mühlebach, S., Shenkin, A. and Van Gossum, A. (2009) ESPEN guidelines on parenteral nutrition: home parenteral nutrition (HPN) in adult patients. *Clinical Nutrition* 28, 467–479.

Stokes, M.A. and Hill, G.L. (1991) Home parenteral nutrition at Auckland hospital. *New Zealand Medical Journal* 104, 208–210.

6 Home Parenteral Nutrition in China

Xinying Wang*

Department of Surgery, Jinling Hospital, Nanjing University Medical School, Nanjing, People's Republic of China

By the intravenous route, parenteral nutrition (PN) support can supply carbohydrate, fat, protein, multiple vitamins, electrolytes, trace elements and fluid to those patients who cannot meet their nutritional requirements by oral or enteral intake. Home parenteral nutrition (HPN) support can offer PN therapy to patients with stable clinical status outside of the acute care setting, which provides a life-saving therapy for patients with irreversible intestinal failure.

As a novel treatment modality, HPN was introduced primarily for the treatment of chronic intestinal failure in patients with benign disease in the early 1970s. In China, HPN was first utilized as a practical therapy in Shanghai for a female patient with short bowel syndrome (SBS) in 1986. The patient's total small intestine and right half of the colon were resected because of intestinal volvulus and necrosis. After 5 years of HPN, she had a pregnancy and gave birth to a healthy baby. This is the first case of successful HPN reported in China (Wu *et al.*, 2002). Soon after, another case of HPN for a male patient with SBS was successfully applied in Nanjing in 1987. He also suffered from intestinal volvulus and necrosis and has survived by means of HPN for 27 years now. Afterwards, HPN was gradually accepted in China.

Intestinal failure is defined as intestinal structural and/or functional damage that leads to obstacles in digestion and absorption of nutrition and/or the mucosal barrier function (Li, 2004). It is often caused by dysmotility, obstruction, disease-associated malabsorption, surgical resection or a congenital defect. It is characterized by the inability to maintain a protein–energy balance, fluid balance, electrolyte balance or micronutrient balance when on a conventionally accepted normal diet or enteral nutrition. Total parenteral nutrition (TPN) can solve the nutritional deficiencies due to indigestion and malabsorption well, although it is not yet perfect. HPN greatly improves nutritional supplementation

*E-mail: wxinying@263.net

especially in those who have permanent impairment of their intestinal digestion and absorption functions. In China, we have reported that rehabilitation therapy for SBS with enteral nutrition can effectively improve nutritional status and promote intestinal adaptation in patients with a segment of small bowel longer than 70 cm and a partial colon, or with a segment of small bowel longer than 30 cm and an intact colon (Zhu *et al.*, 2002). Most of these patients could finally cast off TPN after rehabilitation therapy. So the SBS patients at risk of needing HPN are those with a segment of small bowel less than 70 cm and a partial colon or those with less than 30 cm of small bowel and an intact colon in continuity, or those who fail the rehabilitation therapy.

Therefore, the most common underlying diseases needing HPN in China are inflammatory bowel disease, complications following surgery, mesenteric vascular disease and chronic small bowel disease with severe malabsorption and dysmotility syndromes. Those with a stoma or fistula output greater than 1.5 l/day are also indications for HPN. HPN for cancer patients has generally been accepted recently for the high incidence of malnutrition in patients receiving oncologic therapy, or if the patient suffers severe complications following chemotherapy, radiation therapy or surgery, such as radiation enteritis. Data from Jinling Hospital in Nanjing on HPN patients showed that 28% had SBS, 12% inflammatory bowel disease, 2% intestinal fistula and 52% had radiation enteritis (Zhou *et al.*, 2005; Huang *et al.*, 2012). The Shanghai Zhongshan Hospital reported that HPN patients included 50% with SBS and 50% with intestinal obstruction because of cancer (Huang *et al.*, 1993). Incurable cancer is not considered a contraindication for HPN even if oncologic treatment has been stopped. Patients having undernutrition or starvation not directly progressing from the underlying malignant disease, in whom death is not imminent, should be enrolled in an HPN programme. Certainly their other organ functions and life expectancy should be estimated in the meantime.

The relatively low morbidity and mortality associated with HPN has encouraged its widespread use in Western countries. However, HPN is at the early stage in China although it has been utilized. National differences in the organization of care and inclusion of different patient categories in studies of HPN make it difficult to estimate how commonly it is used. Uniform enrolment criteria and a national survey are still absent. It is estimated that about one to ten patients per million patients need HPN every year. But there are only several reports about the application of HPN; for example, eight HPN cases reported in Shanghai, 16 HPN patients in Nanjing and the other 47 cases in other centres. The current cumulative clinical reports of 71 HPN cases include 40 males and 31 females. Except one case report without detail, the remaining 70 cases had the accumulated HPN time of 7875 days and the average HPN time of 112 days per person. The HPN complications include 11% catheter infection, 3% catheter occlusion, 3% zinc deficiency and 3% cholestasis. Most of the HPN (72%) patients died due to the primary diseases (Huang *et al.*, 1993; Tu *et al.*, 2004; Zhou *et al.*, 2005; Huang *et al.*, 2012).

In 2003, the first HPN team was reported to be set up in Jinling Hospital, Nanjing. This team was made up of a physician, a dietician, a pharmacist and nurses. They need to evaluate the patients' nutritional status, prescribe the TPN formula, establish the intravenous catheters, monitor and prevent the complications (Huang *et al.*, 2012). In most of the hospitals in China, there are physicians and nurses in charge of HPN management but no special HPN team. Intervals between monitoring visits vary according to the patients' clinical status, but will typically be 3 months. The patient who is clinically unstable or is at the initial stage of HPN will need more attention. Monitoring usually takes place at the supervising hospital or a home care agency by the HPN team. The team will measure anthropometry (body weight, body composition, hand-grip strength, upper-arm muscle circumference and resting energy expenditure) and biochemistry (electrolytes, kidney function, liver function, glucose, haemoglobin, iron, albumin and C-reactive protein) at all visits. Measurement of trace elements, vitamins and nitrogen balance is recommended at intervals of 6 months. Bone mineral density assessment by dual-energy X-ray absorptiometry scanning is recommended annually. By 2014, there were nearly 2000 home enteral nutrition patients and about 50 HPN patients in Jinling Hospital.

Because of the limitation of medical insurance and home care condition, HPN is still at the initial stage in China. There is a considerable number of patients needing HPN. The national survey and the uniform enrolment criteria need to be established in the future.

References

Huang, D., Wu, Z. and Wu, Z. (1993) The home parenteral nutrition in 8 cases. *Chinese Journal of Practical Surgery* 13(2), 93–95.

Huang, Y., Wang, X. and Peng, N. (2012) The nine cases of home parenteral nutrition through PICC in one center. *Journal of Qilu Nursing* 18(5), 99.

Li, J. (2004) The concept of intestinal failure, nutrition support and protection of intestinal barrier. *JPEN Journal of Parenteral and Enteral Nutrition* 11, 65–67.

Tu, J., Fang, P. and Hou, J. (2004) The home parenteral nutrition in cancer patients. *Chinese Journal of Clinical Practice Medicine* 3, 342.

Wu, G., Wu, Z. and Wu, Z. (2002) The long-term home parenteral nutrition in the patients after the resection of total small intestine (six cases). *JPEN Journal of Parenteral and Enteral Nutrition* 9, 70–72.

Zhou, Z., Po, P., Ni, Y., Peng, N., Li, N. and Li, J. (2005) The home nutrition support and nursing of cancer ileus. *Journal of Clinical Medicine in Practice* 9, 17–18.

Zhu, W., Li, N., Ren, J., Gu, J., Jiang, J. and Li, J. (2002) Rehabilitation therapy for short bowel syndrome. *Chinese Medical Journal* 115(5), 776–778.

7 Home Parenteral Nutrition in Japan

Akihiro Ito[1*], Takashi Higashiguchi[2] and Harumasa Oyanagi[3]

[1]*Department of Surgery & Palliative Medicine, School of Medicine, Fujita Health University, Toyoake, Japan;* [2]*Chairman of Japanese Society for Parenteral and Enteral Nutrition, Department of Surgery & Palliative Medicine, School of Medicine, Fujita Health University, Toyoake, Japan;* [3]*Former Chairman of Japanese Society for Parenteral and Enteral Nutrition*

Introduction

To reform the medical system and improve quality of life (QoL) in Japan, home healthcare has recently been established as a third form of medical care, alongside in-patient care and out-patient care. Home parenteral nutrition (HPN) is a method of providing nutrition parenterally at home, to free patients from the hospital setting and allow them to return to their homes, lead a more normal daily life and resume their roles in society. When HPN is used in home healthcare, HPN is highly dependent on medical technology. In other words, HPN utilizes equipment and instruments ordinarily used in a hospital.

Parenteral nutrition is the only treatment by which patients with severe small bowel dysfunction such as short bowel syndrome (SBS) can receive adequate nutrition. HPN has been covered by medical insurance in Japan since 1985 and is now in wide use. HPN can safely be implemented if properly managed by patients and their families based on guidance from medical staff. This chapter presents an overview of HPN in Japan, including its indications, medical insurance coverage and increasing use.

Indications for HPN

HPN is generally indicated for diseases, regardless of medical insurance coverage, in which nutrition support is difficult to maintain other than by total parenteral nutrition (TPN) and for which a medical doctor judges that HPN is necessary. HPN is generally contraindicated in patients with chronically impaired oral intake

*E-mail: itoh@mctv.ne.jp

due to cerebrovascular disease, however, in whom digestion and absorption is not otherwise impaired. The indicated diseases can be broadly divided into two categories:

1. Benign diseases requiring long-term TPN. When the patient's condition is stable and life at home is not medically inconvenient.
2. Incurable end-stage malignancies when life at home would improve QoL. End-stage patients in Japan can spend time at home when their condition is stable, but a deterioration in general condition may require transfer to a medical facility such as a palliative care unit or provision of further caregiving at home.

Criteria for HPN

Guidelines (Shirotani, 2006) for parenteral and enteral nutrition by the Japanese Society for Parenteral and Enteral Nutrition (JSPEN) specify criteria for using HPN in adults and children. HPN is implemented based on these guidelines in Japan.

Criteria in adults

HPN is implemented based on these guidelines in adults as follows:

1. Home nutritional therapy should be implemented with the informed consent of not only the patients themselves, but also their caregivers (including family).
2. It is important that patients themselves or their caregivers are able to reliably implement the procedures for HPN.
3. If home nutritional therapy is necessary, enteral nutrition is preferable. In patients with digestive dysfunction in whom enteral nutrition cannot be adequately managed, parenteral nutrition is indicated.
4. Nutritional therapy should be monitored regularly.

Criteria in children

HPN is implemented based on these guidelines in children as follows:

1. If continued nutritional therapy is required in children whose disease is stable, HPN is indicated even for children.
2. HPN in children should be implemented in a suitable environment by caregivers or specialty medical staff who can provide nutritional management at home nearly equivalent to that in a hospital.
3. For HPN in children, caregiver education should begin before hospital discharge, and education and guidance should be continued even after the child is sent home.
4. For HPN in children, monitoring and nutritional assessment should be performed regularly, with particular attention on growth and development.

5. For HPN in children, a tunnelled silicone rubber catheter (Broviac catheter) is associated with fewer complications than a totally implantable port.

Prerequisites for implementation

The guidelines for HPN (Onodera, 2001) in Japan also recommend the following as prerequisites for implementation:

1. A decision should be made that in-patient treatment for the underlying disease is not necessary, that the condition is stable and that HPN will improve QoL.
2. The ability of medical staff to provide guidance on HPN must be sufficient and a system for managing HPN both within and outside the hospital must be established.
3. Both the patient and family should thoroughly understand the principles of TPN and the need for HPN, and both should then request HPN. A decision should be made that: (i) HPN can be implemented at home without problems adjusting intravenous fluids; (ii) infusions can safely be managed; and (iii) the risk of complications is low.

Contraindications for HPN

HPN is not indicated in patients with chronically impaired oral intake due to cerebrovascular disease, but in whom gastrointestinal function is otherwise normal, including:

- patients with senile dementia;
- patients with sequelae of stroke, intracerebral haemorrhage or post-traumatic head injury;
- patients in a vegetative state; and
- patients with amyotrophic lateral sclerosis, muscular dystrophy or Parkinson's disease.

TPN is generally contraindicated in patients with these diseases and conditions. Instead, enteral nutrition is indicated. HPN is also contraindicated:

- when a disease is unstable.

With fever due to intraperitoneal abscesses, gastrointestinal fistulas, urinary tract infections, respiratory tract infections or unknown cause, it is safer not to transfer patients to HPN. In addition, HPN should not be implemented when insulin control is unstable, such as in severe diabetes.

Treatment Reimbursement in Japan

As of 2008, reimbursement from the Social Insurance/Elderly Health Insurance systems is calculated as follows.

For HPN

Among patients with extensive intestinal resection or bowel dysfunction due to various causes, HPN is a method of nutrition implemented by patients themselves at home after discharge from a hospital in stable condition. These patients, regardless of the causative disease, have difficulty maintaining nutrition other than by HPN and a medical doctor has judged HPN as necessary. Specifically, 30,000 yen (US$340.40)/month is provided as a guidance and management fee, 20,000 yen (US$226.90)/month when a fluid administration set is used and 12,500 yen (US$141.80) when an infusion pump is used.

For HEN

Among patients who are unable to tolerate oral intake or have difficulty with oral intake due to various causes, home enteral nutrition (HEN; elemental diet by tube feeding) is a method of nutrition implemented by patients themselves at home. Items providing clearly nutritional components (amino acids, dipeptides, tripeptides mainly as proteins; not including indigestible proteins) are eligible for reimbursement. These patients, regardless of the causative disease, have difficulty maintaining nutrition other than by HEN and a medical doctor has judged HEN as necessary. Specifically, 25,000 yen (US$283.60)/month is a guidance and management fee, 20,000 yen (US$226.90)/month for when a fluid administration set is used and 12,500 yen (US$141.80) for when an infusion pump is used.

Status of HPN Use in Japan

Trends in use of HPN and HEN

According to excerpts from medical reimbursement fee statistics by the Ministry of Health, Labour and Welfare (a 1-month period during June each year) (http://www.e-stat.go.jp/SG1/estat/GL02020101.do), in 2002, 5344 patients/month were using HPN in Japan. With an increase in enteral nutrition in response to the rapid spread of nutrition support teams (NSTs) in Japan, these figures decreased to 2240 patients/month in 2006 and 1680 patients/month in 2008. However, this trend reversed with an increase to 3962 patients/months in 2009 and widespread use in 7412 patients/month in 2011. HEN was used by 4856 patients/month in 2002, steadily increased to 6847 patients/month in 2006 and 7715 patients/month in 2008, and reached 10,125 patients/month in 2011. These figures suggest a steady promotion of home medical care by NST members, because the number of NSTs has been increasing; in 2013, there were more than 1700 (>20% of total number of hospitals) in Japan (Higashiguchi, 2011).

Use of HPN by age group

Among the 7412 patients using HPN during a 1-month period in June 2011, the breakdown by age groups was: 0–19 years, 164 (22.1%); 20–39 years, 232 (31.3%); 40–59 years, 3222 (43.5%); 60–79 years, 2462 (33.2%); and ≥80 years, 1332 (18.0%). The highest use of HPN was in middle-aged adults (40–59 years old), but a high 18.0% of the total represented elderly patients at least 80 years of age. This is a distinct feature in Japan.

Diseases in which HPN is used, HPN duration and return to society

Surveys on diseases in which HPN is used and patient return to society have not been conducted since 2000 in Japan. In a survey of 355 patients in 2000, HPN was most often used for malignant diseases, in 202 patients (56.9%). Only 12% of patients with malignant diseases returned to society, and mean duration of HPN use was short (139 days). Some 153 patients with benign diseases such as inflammatory bowel disease, ischaemic bowel disease and bowel motility disorders received HPN. A relatively high rate of about 60% of these patients returned to society. The mean duration of HPN was long (1969 days). Sixty-nine patients (19.4%) had SBS and 65% returned to society (Table. 7.1) (Takagi, 2003).

Major disease indications for HPN in Japan

SBS

SBS is also defined in Japan as a condition in which intestinal absorption is decreased due to intestinal resection or dysfunction of the residual intestine; and in which the required intake of fluids, electrolytes, major nutrients, trace elements and vitamins cannot be achieved using standard oral intake or enteral nutrition.

CAUSATIVE DISEASES There are various causative diseases, but large-scale detailed surveys on their incidence have not been conducted in Japan. Vascular disorders

Table 7.1. HPN implementation and return of patients to society. (From Takagi, 2003.)

Disease	Number of patients	Number returning to society (%)	Mean number of days of HPN
Overall	355	115 (32)	855
Malignancies	202	25 (12)	139
Benign diseases	153	88 (59)	1969
Inflammatory bowel disease	36	24 (67)	1888
Ischaemic bowel disease	38	28 (74)	2616
Bowel motility disorder	34	23 (68)	2170
Others	45	15 (33)	1337
Short bowel syndrome	69	45 (65)	–

of the intestine include: SMA (superior mesenteric artery) occlusion, SMV (superior mesenteric vein) occlusion, small bowel torsion, strangulation ileus, incarcerated hernia and intussusception. Inflammatory diseases of the intestine include: Crohn's disease, intestinal Behçet's disease, intestinal tuberculosis and intestinal ulcers. Other causes include tumours, trauma, adhesion ileus and proximal intestinal fistulas. However, SMA occlusion is the most common cause of SBS, accounting for about 40% of cases in Japan (Hatakeyama, 1993).

CRITERIA Massive resection of the small bowel in Japan is defined as up to 75 cm of residual intestine in children, up to 150 cm of residual intestine in adults or generally up to one-third the residual intestine (Takagi and Okada, 1996).

CLINICAL COURSE AND NUTRITIONAL MANAGEMENT The clinical course after small bowel massive resection is divided into three periods (Koyama *et al.*, 1984). Nutritional management corresponding to each period (Table 7.2) is required.

Period I (immediate post-operative period). This period is further divided into paralytic ileus (2–7 days post-operatively (PO)) and increased intestinal peristalsis (3–4 weeks PO). During paralytic ileus, attention must be paid to fluid and electrolyte management. During increased intestinal peristalsis, watery diarrhoea frequently occurs. Because this can easily lead to loss of all nutrition, particularly electrolytes, TPN is required for at least a month in many patients. In patients with normal nutritional status, energy (calories) can gradually be increased starting on day 2–3 PO, aiming at about 40 kcal/kg body weight/day. Amino acids (1–1.5 g/kg body weight/day), fats at about 20–30% of total calories, multivitamins and trace element preparations should also be given. Watery diarrhoea requires long-term control. If an anti-diarrhoea drug such as loperamide (4–16 mg/day) proves ineffective, a prescription narcotic anti-diarrhoea drug should be given. In addition, an H2 blocker or proton pump inhibitor will reduce gastric secretions and is useful to reduce diarrhoea.

Period II (recovery and adaptation period; a few months to 12 months PO). During the recovery and adaptation period, because absorption from the residual intestine improves and the frequency of watery diarrhoea gradually decreases, enteral

Table 7.2. Nutritional management after extensive small bowel resection. (From Koyama *et al.*, 1884.)

Period	Calories (kcal/kg body weight/day)	Residual intestine (cm) 0	~30	30–70	≥70
I	40–50	TPN	TPN	TPN	TPN
II	30–40	TPN Home TPN	TPN ED Home TPN Home ED	TPN LRD Home TPN Home LRD	ED LRD Normal diet
II	30–50	Home TPN	Normal diet Home ED Home LRD	Normal diet Home ED Home LRD	Normal diet

ED, elemental diet; LRD, low-residue diet.

nutrition is started. From the perspective of reducing diarrhoea associated with decreased pancreatic enzyme activity and fat malabsorption, an elemental diet is often started in Japan. However, elemental diets have high osmotic pressure, which can lead to abdominal symptoms that include diarrhoea. Dilution of an elemental diet and a slower rate of administration when starting may be necessary. In addition, an elemental diet can lead to a deficiency in essential fatty acids, so periodic intravenous administration of lipid emulsions is necessary. While the clinical course is monitored, an elemental diet can be switched to a low-residue diet if possible, with the goal of transition to oral intake.

Period III (stabilized period; for a few years after period II). The compensatory level of the residual intestine has reached near maximum, so symptoms like diarrhoea are controlled. The goal in this period is weaning from TPN while stabilizing enteral nutrition and oral intake. In patients requiring an elemental or low-residue diet, HEN can be started. In patients unable to be weaned from TPN, HPN can be started.

COMPLICATIONS IN NUTRITIONAL MANAGEMENT SBS patients require long-term nutritional management and careful attention must be paid to metabolic complications. Iron is mainly absorbed from the duodenum, so excess supplementation is not necessary. However, if iron absorption is decreased due to bleeding from marginal ulcers or duodenal mucosal injury, iron deficiency anaemia can develop. Malabsorption of bile acids necessary for absorption of fats and fat-soluble vitamins can lead to vitamin D deficiency, abnormal calcium metabolism, abnormalities in trace elements (e.g. zinc, manganese, copper) and bone disorders (osteomalacia and osteoporosis). Malabsorption of bile acids also diminishes the bile acid pool, with an increase in gallstone formation.

Mild liver dysfunction is a frequent complication in TPN patients. However, particular attention is required in SBS patients, because progressive intrahepatic cholestasis and hepatic fibrosis can become life-threatening. Periodic monitoring is also necessary so that patients do not become deficient in major nutrients such as amino acids or in vitamins or electrolytes.

End-stage cancer

INDICATIONS The use of TPN in palliative care for end-stage cancer is fairly common in Japan. In Japan, it is gradually being understood that palliative care should be introduced not only for end-stage cancer, but also during all cancer treatment. When TPN is considered in patients with recurrent cancer, oral intake has become difficult and malnutrition is either present or anticipated. Specific instances include: (i) malnutrition due to adverse events with cancer treatment (e.g. chemotherapy, radiotherapy, surgery); (ii) gastrointestinal obstruction due to cancer; (iii) gastrointestinal dysfunction associated with ascites and carcinomatous peritonitis; and (iv) cancer cachexia. In particular, for cancer cachexia, a global consensus has emerged that artificial feeding, including TPN, is not indicated. In Japan, nutrition is often managed as described in the following section.

CLINICAL COURSE IN END-STAGE CANCER PATIENTS (CACHEXIA) The European Society for Parenteral and Enteral Nutrition (ESPEN) in 2010 proposed that cachexia be classified in three stages: (i) pre-cachexia; (ii) cachexia; and (iii) refractory cachexia. The stage before cachexia when metabolic abnormalities are mild and no obvious cachectic symptoms are present is called 'pre-cachexia' (Muscaritoli *et al.*, 2010). Meanwhile, end-stage cachexia, when metabolic abnormalities are severe and nutritional status is unlikely to improve even with nutritional support, is called 'refractory cachexia' (Fearon *et al.*, 2011). Appropriate nutritional support is now considered important when there is little progression of cachexia; in other words, at a stage when metabolic abnormalities are mild (Arends *et al.*, 2006; Bozzetti *et al.*, 2009). With nutritional support started at this stage, development of malnutrition can be delayed, malnutrition due to other causes can be improved and tolerance to anticancer therapy can be increased.

In patients in Japan with recurrent or end-stage cancer, but not refractory cachexia, metabolic and nutritional management is basically similar to nutritional management in other patients. However, end-stage patients eventually develop irreversible metabolic changes, which then clearly result in reduced energy consumption (Fig. 7.1) (Higashiguchi, 2008). At this point in time, a down-shift in fluid and nutritional management is appropriate. Therefore, 'Guidelines for fluid and nutritional management in end-stage cancer patients' with a 'down-shift' based on whether refractory cachexia is present have been proposed (Higashiguchi *et al.*, 2004).

FLUID AND NUTRITIONAL MANAGEMENT IN CANCER PATIENTS *Pre-cachexia and cachexia.* Nutritional management in patients without refractory cachexia generally involves the supply of energy (calories) and nutrients that are neither excessive nor deficient. Oral intake should first be considered, with enteral and parenteral nutrition only when necessary.

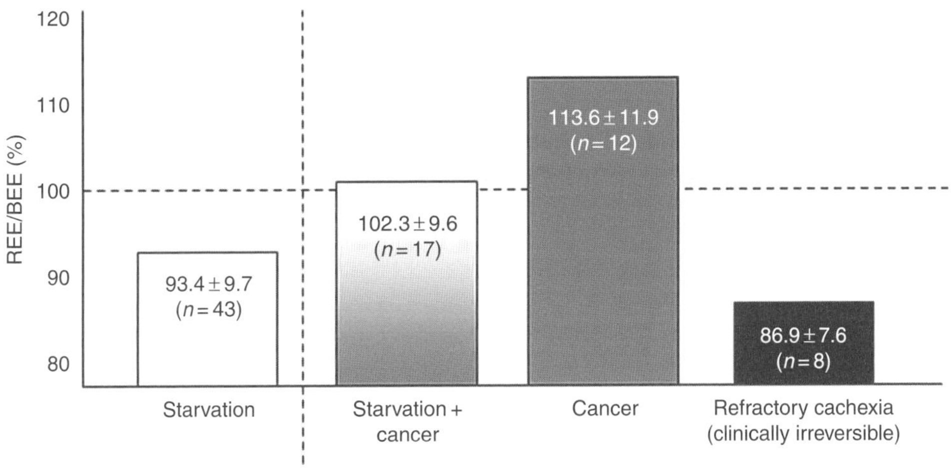

Fig. 7.1. Energy consumption and cancer progression (REE/BEE, resting energy expenditure/basal energy expenditure). (From Higashiguchi, 2008.)

1. Fluid administration: 30–40 ml/kg body weight/day (about 35 ml/day/kg body weight). Note, for end-stage patients: 25–35 ml/kg body weight/day (about 30 ml/day/kg body weight).
2. Required calories (kcal/day): basal energy expenditure (BEE) × activity factor (AF) × stress factor (SF). BEE (kcal/day) is calculated using the Harris–Benedict equation:

Males: 66 + (13.7 × weight in kg) + (5.0 × height in cm) – (6.8 × age in years).

Females: 655 + (9.6 × weight in kg) + (1.7 × height in cm) – (4.7 × age in years).

AF adjusts for the patient's physical activity. Physical activity is the component of energy expenditure under the control of the individual. For hospitalized patients, however, physical activity is limited, so a simple adjustment for activity is recommended in Japan (Long *et al.*, 1979): AF = 1.0 for bedridden patients and AF = 1.2 for ambulatory patients. SF adjusts for metabolic stress. Many hospitalized patients are hypermetabolic, so a simple adjustment for metabolic stress is recommended in Japan based on organ failure (SF = 1.2, 1.4 or 1.6 if one, two or three organs have failed), body temperature (37°C, SF = 1.2; 38°C, SF = 1.4; 39°C, SF = 1.6) and the presence of major burns (SF = 1.5–2.0).
3. Amount of amino acids (protein) (g/day): weight (kg) × stress factor (SF); including essential amino acids.
4. Amount of fats (g/day): 20–50% of required calories × 1/9 (0.5–1.0 g/kg body weight); including essential fatty acids. Rate of fat administration in parenteral nutrition is 0.1–0.2 g/kg body weight/h.
5. Amount of carbohydrates (g/day): required calories – (amount of amino acids) – (amount of fats). Non-protein calories/nitrogen (NPC/N) is 150–200 kcal/day; 300–500 kcal/day in patients with renal insufficiency.
6. Amount of vitamins and trace elements: daily required amounts.

Refractory cachexia. In patients with clinically apparent refractory cachexia, excessive fluids and energy (calories) should be reduced and the impact on remaining physical function should be controlled.

In Japan, patients able to maintain oral intake should be allowed to eat foods that they like and are able to eat. The following preparations are recommended with the understanding and consent of the patient: (i) vitamins and trace element preparations; (ii) high-fat high-protein nutrition in patients with lung metastases and respiratory insufficiency; (iii) glutamine, soluble fibre and oligosaccharides (GFO®) (Higashiguchi *et al.*, 2009) in patients with poor food intake, decreased immune function or who are receiving narcotics; and (iv) branched-chain amino acids in patients with muscle atrophy or limb weakness (Higashiguchi *et al.*, 2010).

In patients unable to tolerate oral intake, the wishes of the patient and family should be given first priority.

1. Fluid administration: 15–25 ml/kg body weight/day (about 20 ml/day/kg body weight; 500–1000 ml/day). Thirst (dry mouth) should be prevented not only by intravenous fluids, but also by oral care and green tea spray.

2. Required calories (kcal/day): 5–15 kcal/kg body weight/day (about 200–600 kcal/day).
3. Nutrients: (i) primarily carbohydrates; and (ii) amino acids (branched-chain amino acids), with small amounts of essential fatty acids when necessary.
4. Vitamins and trace elements: required daily amounts to prevent stomatitis and decubitus ulcers.

Fluid and nutritional management according to these standards can minimize suffering from end-stage symptoms, improve QoL and help patients to achieve a peaceful death.

Conclusion

The indications for HPN in Japan are generally the same as the indications for TPN in hospitalized patients. However, it is important for HPN that a patient's clinical symptoms and condition be stable and that nutrition be managed in a setting where the need for emergency measures will be unlikely. Careful evaluation during hospitalization and regular monitoring of the patient's clinical symptoms and condition when receiving HPN are therefore necessary.

Acknowledgement

The authors express their sincere gratitude to Professor Noriyasu Shirotani for his valuable guidance and encouragement throughout this work.

References

Arends, J., Bodoky, G., Bozzetti, F., Fearon, K., Muscaritoli, M., Selga, G., van Bokhorst-de van der Schueren, M.A., von Meyenfeldt, M.; DGEM (German Society for Nutritional Medicine), Zürcher, G., Fietkau, R., Aulbert, E., Frick, B., Holm, M., Kneba, M., Mestrom, H.J., Zander, A.; ESPEN (European Society for Parenteral and Enteral Nutrition) (2006) ESPEN Guidelines on Enteral Nutrition: non-surgical oncology. *Clinical Nutrition* 25, 245–259.

Bozzetti, F., Arends, J., Lundholm, K., Micklewright, A., Zurcher, G. and Muscaritoli, M.; ESPEN (2009) ESPEN Guidelines on Parenteral Nutrition: non-surgical oncology. *Clinical Nutrition* 28, 445–454.

Fearon, K., Strasser, F., Anker, S.D., Bosaeus, I., Bruera, E., Fainsinger, R.L., Jatoi, A., Loprinzi, C., MacDonald, N., Mantovani, G., Davis, M., Muscaritoli, M., Ottery, F., Radbruch, L., Ravasco, P., Walsh, D., Wilcock, A., Kaasa, S. and Baracos, V.E. (2011) Definition and classification of cancer cachexia: an international consensus. *Lancet Oncology* 12, 489–495.

Hatakeyama, K. (1993) Short bowel syndrome. In: Ogoshi, S. (ed.) *Manual for Fluid and Nutritional Management.* Igakusyoin, Tokyo, pp. 119–128.

Higashiguchi, T. (2008) Nutritional management for cancer cachexia. *Japanese Journal of Clinical Nutrition* 113, 602–607.

Higashiguchi, T. (2011) Where are we standing in all over the world, considering about the development of medical system for nutritional therapy. *Journal of Japanese Society for Parenteral and Enteral Nutrition* 26, 5–10.
Higashiguchi, T., Ito, A., Murai, M. and Iida, T. (2004) Nutritional management for terminally cancer patients. *The Japanese Journal of Medical Society* 132, 61–64.
Higashiguchi, T., Ito, A., Futamura, A., Kodama, Y., Sadamaoto, T., Murai, M., Shibata, K., Kaneko, T., Tomatsu, A., Chihara, T., Shinpo, H., Miki, S., Yamaguchi, M., Hino, K. and Kondo, Y. (2009) Effect of glutamine–fiber–oligosaccharide (GFO) on the pathological and functional changes in the intestinal mucosa associated with total parenteral nutrition in rats. *Japanese Journal of Surgical Metabolism and Nutrition* 43, 51–60.
Higashiguchi, T., Futamura, A. and Ito, A. (2010) Effect of a complementary nutrition diet for improving clinical condition and function in terminal cancer patients: a controlled clinical trial. *Japanese Journal of Surgical Metabolism and Nutrition* 44, 157–169.
Koyama, M., Hatakeyama, K. and Yamadera, Y. (1984) Metabolism and management after massive intestinal resection. *Surgical Therapy* 51, 43–50.
Long, C.L., Schaffel, N., Geiger, J.W., Schiller, W.R. and Blakemore, W.S. (1979) Metabolic response to injury and illness: estimation of energy and protein needs from indirect calorimetry and nitrogen balance. *JPEN Journal of Parenteral and Enteral Nutrition* 3, 452–456.
Muscaritoli, M., Anker, S.D., Argilés, J., Aversa, Z., Bauer, J.M., Biolo, G., Boirie, Y., Bosaeus, I., Cederholm, T., Costelli, P., Fearon, K.C., Laviano, A., Maggio, M., Rossi Fanelli, F., Schneider, S.M., Schols, A. and Sieber, C.C. (2010) Consensus definition of sarcopenia, cachexia and pre-cachexia: joint document elaborated by special interest groups (SIG) 'cachexia-anorexia in chronic wasting diseases' and 'nutrition in geriatrics'. *Clinical Nutrition* 29, 154–159.
Onodera, T. (2001) The guidelines for home parenteral nutrition. In: Prompting Institute of Total Health (ed.) *Prerequisites for Implementation, Indications, and Contraindications for Home Parenteral Nutrition.* Bunkodo, Tokyo, pp. 1–8 (in Japanese).
Shirotani, N. (2006) Home parenteral nutrition. In: Japanese Society for Parenteral and Enteral Nutrition (ed.) *Guideline of Parenteral and Enteral Nutrition.* Nankodo, Tokyo, pp. 25–28.
Takagi, Y. (2003) Home parenteral and enteral nutrition in Japan – present and future. *Japanese Journal of Gastroenterology* 100, 819–828.
Takagi, Y. and Okada, A. (1996) Short bowel syndrome. *Clinical Digestive Medicine* 11, 495–502.

II Clinical Conditions

8 Transition from Acute to Chronic Intestinal Failure

Simon Lal* and Jon Shaffer

Intestinal Failure Unit, Salford Royal NHS Foundation Trust, Salford, UK

Key Points

- Intestinal failure is defined as a reduction in the functioning gut mass below the minimal amount necessary for adequate digestion and absorption of food.
- There are three types of intestinal failure depending on the potential reversibility and the duration of the intestinal failure.
- Type 3 is chronic intestinal failure requiring long-term nutritional support, usually home parenteral nutrition and transplantation.

Introduction

The term 'intestinal failure' (IF) was originally defined as 'a reduction in the functioning gut mass below the minimal amount necessary for adequate digestion and absorption of food' (Fleming and Remington, 1981). In order to reflect its varied disease aetiology, an international consensus group proposed that intestinal failure should be defined as resulting 'from obstruction, dysmotility, surgical resection, congenital defect or disease-associated loss of absorption and is characterized by the inability to maintain protein–energy, fluid, electrolyte, or micronutrient balance' (O'Keefe *et al.*, 2006). While this definition is all-encompassing, it may not necessarily reflect the varied duration and severity of intestinal failure that is commonly seen in day-to-day practice. Indeed, although chronic (or permanent) intestinal failure is relatively rare, acute (reversible within 6 months) intestinal failure occurs relatively frequently in the post-operative period (Lal *et al.*, 2006).

*E-mail: simon.lal@srft.nhs.uk

(eds F. Bozzetti, M. Staun and A. Van Gossum)

Types of Intestinal Failure

Intestinal failure can be divided into three practical types:

1. Type 1 IF is self-limiting intestinal failure that occurs following abdominal surgery, whereby patients require fluid, electrolyte, enteral and/or parenteral nutritional support for a limited period of time, before making a full recovery without complication.
2. Type 2 IF occurs in severely ill patients, who develop septic, metabolic and nutritional complications following gastrointestinal surgery. These patients need multidisciplinary input and nutritional support to permit recovery.
3. Type 3 IF is chronic intestinal failure requiring long-term nutritional support, usually home parenteral nutrition (HPN) and transplantation.

Type 1 IF is the most common, with the majority of patients being managed in non-specialist units. The recent National Confidential Enquiry into Patient Outcome and Death (NCEPOD) evaluated the care of hospital patients receiving parenteral nutrition (PN) support in the UK and identified that 93% of patients in hospitals throughout the UK received PN for <30 days, with the majority of these patients needing nutritional support as a result of post-surgical complications (NCEPOD, 2010). By contrast, and fortunately, the more severe type 2 IF and type 3 IF are less common. While the incidence of type 3 IF is readily available from a variety of national registries (Smith *et al.*, 2011), the true incidence of type 2 IF is less well known.

A significant proportion of patients will develop type 3 IF *de novo* without pre-existing type 2 IF; for example, patients with dysmotility (e.g. systemic sclerosis) or radiation enteritis, who have not undergone previous intestinal surgery, may become dependent on HPN after a prolonged period of nutritional impairment that cannot be managed via the enteral route. The remaining patients will have developed type 3 IF after in-patient management of their acute (type 2) illness by a multidisciplinary team of specialist nurses, physicians, surgeons, dieticians, pharmacists, radiologists and, where necessary, psychologists (Lal *et al.*, 2006). This will involve achieving control of intra-abdominal sepsis through radiological or surgical drainage, optimizing the patient's nutritional and metabolic status, and defining the residual intestinal anatomy before considering surgical repair of persistent fistulas or considering restoration of intestinal continuity in patients who have previously undergone an intestinal diversion procedure. It may take several months for sepsis resolution and nutritional repletion to be achieved before definitive surgery can be contemplated. Indeed, about 50% of patients with type 2 IF will be discharged from hospital necessitating a prolonged period of home nutritional support before being deemed fit for surgical intervention; this will typically be via the parenteral route, but a small proportion of selected patients may receive adequate nutrition via the enteral (e.g. fistuloclysis) (Teubner *et al.*, 2004) route.

There are currently only a few dedicated multidisciplinary intestinal failure units and the initial evidence suggests that they not only produce better survival figures for the management of acute conditions such as high-output enterocutaneous fistula, but also lower rates of complications associated with type 3 IF such as catheter sepsis. Such units are labour intensive and expensive to set up but will justify their costs by producing better results.

A percentage of patients with type 2 IF may ultimately become nutritionally autonomous following restoration of intestinal continuity; the remainder will develop chronic, type 3 IF and remain on HPN.

Following resolution of their acute intestinal failure, those patients who require HPN will need to be trained to manage their PN just like any other HPN patient.

Summary

There are three types of intestinal failure depending on the potential reversibility and the duration of such condition. HPN is used in type 3 IF which includes that arising after severe and persistent surgical complications or, more rarely, after radiotherapy or in primitive intestinal diseases that compromise the gut motility.

References

Fleming, C.R. and Remington, M. (1981) Intestinal failure. In: Hill, G.L. (ed.) *Nutrition and the Surgical Patient*. Churchill Livingstone, Edinburgh, pp. 219–235.

Lal, S., Teubner, A. and Shaffer, J.L. (2006) Intestinal failure a review. *Alimentary Pharmacology & Therapeutics* 24, 19–31.

O'Keefe, S.J.D., Buchman, A.L., Fishbein, T.M., Jeejeebhoy, K.N., Jeppesen, P.B. and Shaffer, J. (2006) Short bowel syndrome and intestinal failure: consensus definitions and overview. *Clinical Gastroenterology and Hepatology* 4, 6–10.

National Confidential Enquiry into Patient Outcome and Death (2010) Parenteral nutrition: a mixed bag. Available at: http://www.ncepod.org.uk/2010pn.htm (accessed 7 July 2014).

Smith, T., Micklewright, A., Hirst, A., Jones, B. and Baxter, J. (2011) Annual BANS Report, 2011. Artificial Nutrition Support in the UK 2000–2010. Available at: http://www.bapen.org.uk/pdfs/bans_reports/bans_report_11.pdf (accessed 7 July 2014).

Teubner, A., Morrison, K., Ravishankar, H.R., Anderson, I.D., Scott, N.A. and Carlson, G.L. (2004) Fistuloclysis can successfully replace parenteral feeding in the nutritional support of patients with enterocutaneous fistula. *British Journal of Surgery* 91, 625–631.

9 Short Bowel Syndrome

Alastair Forbes*

Norwich Medical School, University of East Anglia, Norwich, UK

Key Points

- Short bowel syndrome is an important form of intestinal failure.
- It usually follows major intestinal resection.
- Requirements for fluid and electrolytes as well as nutrition must be considered.
- Oral fluid restriction is often the key to optimal management.
- Generous amounts of sodium and magnesium are often required.
- Pharmacological options are of value but currently of limited efficacy.

Introduction

Short bowel syndrome (SBS) is an important form of intestinal failure. The latter can be defined from the absence of sufficient functional intestine; accordingly health can no longer be sustained by ordinary food and drink (O'Keefe *et al.*, 2006). SBS usually follows extensive small bowel resection and may emerge or be exacerbated when a sub-critically shortened intestine is further compromised by severe inflammation or motility disorders as may occur in Crohn's disease or radiation enteritis. SBS is relatively rare; the prevalence is about 2 per 100,000 in most evaluated populations and the annual incidence is usually found to be no more than about 0.1 per 100,000.

The underlying aetiology varies according to the reporting centre but in most countries at least 40% of cases follow resection for intestinal ischaemia and a further 20% or so can be attributed to unexpected complications of abdominal surgery. Historically Crohn's disease accounted for up to a third of long-term cases in

*E-mail: alastair.forbes@uea.ac.uk

the UK, but this figure was never so high in most other countries and is generally falling, a phenomenon attributed to better medical therapy and to less radical surgery. In infants SBS is most often the result of birth defects such as gastroschisis or from necrotizing enterocolitis. Intestinal volvulus is an important additional cause in older children (Duro *et al.*, 2008).

SBS poses several challenges for the patient and for his or her physician. Most patients will have problems with fluid and electrolyte balance as well as nutritional failure. It is easier to consider these two aspects separately from a pedagogic viewpoint but it should be recognized that in clinical practice both elements should be considered concurrently. SBS is of course best managed when it is anticipated and when steps are taken before the patient is severely dehydrated, malnourished and with major derangements of electrolytes. Preventive action should be embarked upon in the patient with less than 150 cm of small bowel in continuity with the colon and in those with an ileostomy/jejunostomy and less than 200 cm of small bowel proximal to the stoma. However it is often the case that the surgical team will have assiduously recorded how much has been removed with less indication of how much small bowel remains; in such cases we can suspect SBS in anyone with an output from the bowel (from the anus, a stoma or a fistula) of greater than 1.5 l/day.

Fluid Balance and the Intestine

Although reference texts apportion different relative volumes to the various gastrointestinal secretions and the consequent normal luminal fluid volume, a total in the region of 8 l in 24 h is reasonably consistent (Table 9.1). Secretion is however predominantly proximal and net fluid absorption is predominantly distal. We can hypothesize for clarity that intake and secretion are mainly jejunal and that fluid absorption is mainly ileal. As a consequence, in most clinical scenarios where the ileum has been lost, the gastrointestinal output volume is indirectly proportional to the overall small bowel length, with normal, positive fluid balance requiring about 100 cm.

The colon takes on special significance in the patient with SBS if he or she has been sufficiently fortunate to retain some, or all, of the colon in continuity with the residual small intestine. In health the colon has limited nutritional impact (delivery of short-chain fatty acids to the colonocyte) and acts mainly to reabsorb

Table 9.1. An example of normal gastrointestinal volumes over a 24 h period.

Food and drink	1500 ml
Saliva	750 ml
Gastric secretion	1250 ml
Biliary secretion	1000 ml
Pancreatic secretion	1000 ml
Jejunal secretion	2500 ml
Total	8000 ml
Stool liquid	~125 ml

water and electrolytes. This capacity becomes more critical in SBS and may equate to about 50 cm of small intestine. Fluid balance can thus be managed with significantly less than the 100 cm needed in the patient whose small intestine terminates in a stoma (Nightingale *et al.*, 1992). There may also be nutritional value from fermentation of non-absorbed carbohydrates by the colonic bacteria.

Thus it can be appreciated that the effluent from a proximal stoma or fistula in a patient with SBS may be substantial and can easily exceed 5 l/day. This almost inevitably results in negative fluid balance and consequent thirst. This leads to the central paradox of management of this condition.

Most patients with clinically important SBS are 'net secretors'. The response of the proximal small bowel is a secretory one, driven mainly by the sodium gradient and the linked osmolarity of the luminal content. Only when the luminal sodium concentration reaches 90–100 mmol/l does net absorption begin (Powell-Tuck *et al.*, 2010). Because of the virtual absence of sodium in ordinary drinks the immediate consequence of drinking is the secretion of fluid into the lumen. This is no less true in the dehydrated, thirsty patient. In the normal individual this shift is readily compensated more distally where the sodium concentration has re-equilibrated and where the active reabsorption of sodium and water is favoured (ileum and colon). The sodium/water deficit is remedied, and if excess is imbibed this can be excreted in the urine. The patient with SBS also has the proximal secretory response, but lacks some, or all, of the distal bowel where absorption occurs. The inevitable response to thirst and drinking is therefore an increase in output, which is often even greater than the additional input. Understanding this paradox is vital to the correct management of SBS and education (of staff and patients) as to its importance is critical to safe and effective care.

Diagnosis, Investigation and Assessment

The diagnosis of SBS may be self-evident in a patient in whom there has been a major ischaemic catastrophe in the superior mesenteric vascular territory leaving less than 50 cm of viable small intestine. It is not so obvious in the patient in whom a lesser resection has taken place, where the surgeon has not measured the residual intestine, or when anatomically there is more intestine but its function is questionable (as in the patient with Crohn's disease affecting multiple sites). It will often be inappropriate to investigate for bowel length in the peri-operative period and in any case our objective is an assessment of function. Nutritional adequacy (protein–energy balance) is difficult to assess and is to some extent a medium- to long-term issue of observation and repeated clinical judgements, but fluid and electrolyte balance are of immediate concern.

Inexpert clinicians will examine the serum electrolytes, and perhaps the plasma osmolarity, serum urea or creatinine and full blood count. These are of course abnormal in dehydration and decompensated SBS, but they are not sensitive investigations. Prior evidence of an impending problem can be ascertained from serial body weight estimations and careful fluid balance records. However, it is really only in the critical care unit that the latter can be relied upon and there it is generally difficult to weigh the patient. The key to unlock the problem of assessment is the urine sodium concentration.

In SBS, as in other states of relative dehydration, the urine sodium is reduced because of the kidney's avidity for sodium, and therefore water, to maintain an effective circulating volume. Levels below 20 mmol/l indicate impending hypovolaemic renal failure and a need for action (Powell-Tuck *et al.*, 2010). The test is simple (only a random untimed sample is required) and reliable. Apparently reassuring, but misleading, levels over 20 mmol/l occur only in established renal failure, where the kidneys are no longer able to concentrate the urine and retain sodium, and in the patient ill-advisedly placed on diuretics (which are almost always contraindicated in SBS).

Low serum magnesium is common in SBS as there is substantial loss in diarrhoeal fluids and hypomagnesaemia is the usual cause of tetany in these patients. Low serum calcium in SBS is generally the result of uncorrected low serum magnesium. Hypokalaemia is surprisingly unusual.

Management of SBS

The principal aims of management are to:

- minimize sodium-poor fluid intake;
- increase sodium intake;
- reduce gut secretion;
- reduce the speed of intestinal transit; and
- overcome nutritional deficiencies.

It will be noted that fluid and electrolyte balance requires a different – if usually complementary – approach from the optimization of nutritional status in patients with SBS. It is therefore convenient to have a mental picture of two simple algorithms (Fig. 9.1).

Most patients with established SBS require fluids, electrolytes and nutrients, but some who are nutritionally independent still need daily intravenous fluid, sodium and magnesium. Occasionally patients are truly dependent on systemic fluids but at only low volumes, and some have a specific but isolated need for parenteral magnesium. It is unusual for a patient with SBS to need intravenous nutrients without additional fluids, which marks an important distinction from those with other forms of intestinal failure (such as from the motility disorders) who can sometimes be managed with low-volume parenteral nutrition (PN) on a less than daily basis (see Chapter 11 in this volume).

At the time of initial presentation and when there are acute crises, it will often be necessary to resuscitate the patient with a sodium-based intravenous preparation. Balanced electrolyte solutions such as Hartman's or Ringer's are almost always preferable to so-called normal (0.9%; 154 mmol/l) saline. These limit the administration of chloride ions, which are less needed (other than in uncontrolled vomiting), promote hyperchloraemic acidosis and are disproportionally difficult for the sick patient to excrete (Yunos *et al.*, 2012).

Disturbed fluid/electrolyte balance	**Protein/energy malnutrition**
⇓	⇓
Restriction of free fluids	Encourage hyperphagia
⇓	⇓
Addition of oral rehydration solution	Oral nutritional supplements
⇓	⇓
Overnight ORS by tube usually by PEG	Overnight tube feeding usually by PEG
⇓	⇓
Subcutaneous fluids/electrolytes for low volume/mmol requirement	Parenteral nutrition (not daily) at home
⇓	⇓
Long-term home intravenous fluids almost always daily	Long-term daily home parenteral nutrition

Fig. 9.1. Scheme for consideration of management in short bowel syndrome. ORS, oral rehydration solution; PEG, percutaneous endoscopic gastrostomy.

Intravenous sodium (and fluid) administration should be combined with a reduction in the oral intake of fluid – typically to no more than 500 ml of 'free' fluids every 24 h. Concurrently the oral sodium intake should be increased and appropriate high-salt dietary measures instituted. Rigorous attention to this regimen can be expected to reduce the gastrointestinal efflux by as much as 50% or by about 2 l, whichever is less. However in patients with very high outputs, this is generally the single most valuable intervention.

Oral rehydration solution (ORS) is needed in patients whose fluid and sodium balance remains negative despite the above measures. It is important that patients and staff understand that it is not expected to reduce effluent volumes, but to render them less hazardous. With astute use of ORS the influx and efflux of sodium become more nearly equal. It will be recalled that the sodium concentration must reach 90–100 mmol/l in the proximal small bowel in order for its net absorption to commence. However many proprietary ORS preparations are low in sodium, and none contains more than 60 mmol/l. The original WHO solution contained sodium at 90 mmol/l, but had unnecessary amounts of potassium and was adapted, with a gain in palatability, to produce the St Mark's formula (Table 9.2). The choice between bicarbonate and citrate may be the patient's decision based on taste preference. Solutions can be flavoured with (very) small amounts of fruit squash concentrate or lemon juice, and are better tolerated if served straight from the refrigerator (or kept cold in a vacuum flask). Large amounts of flavouring should not be used, as these will change the sodium/glucose ratio, which has been selected to take full advantage of their coupled transport. If ice is used it should be made from the ORS itself.

Proprietary ORS mixes reconstituted with half the normal quantity of water can also be very useful. It might seem counterproductive to aim for the unnecessarily high sodium content of 120 mmol/l, as these drinks are inevitably less palatable. However their use introduces some greater latitude into the overall fluid allowance, and it becomes possible to have a drink of choice (e.g. tea or coffee) and yet maintain an average sodium concentration near 90 mmol/l across the day. Additionally, some patients benefit from overnight enteral tube delivery of these solutions.

In general patients who have recurring hypomagnesaemia will prove to be dependent on parenteral fluids. This is because it is logistically difficult to obtain suitable preparations for oral use (the data are best for the unlicensed magnesium oxide) and because doses at even a low therapeutic level tend to have a counterproductive osmotic laxative effect.

Enteral nutrition – food

Regular intake of food should be encouraged in the great majority of patients with SBS. It is contraindicated only in those in the very acute post-operative phase in whom there is a risk of provoking peritonitis. In the more 'established' patient with high output from stoma or fistula it is to be expected that the osmotic effect of the food will increase the resting output. However this should be a stimulus to the introduction of other measures to reduce the volume (see above and below). Only when these fail and stoma/fistula management has become impossible should one consider reverting to a nil-by-mouth approach.

Table 9.2. ORS for patients with SBS (the St Mark's solution).

In 1 l of water (not necessarily sterile):
20 g glucose
3.5 g sodium chloride
2.5 g sodium bicarbonate (or sodium citrate)
Yields sodium 90 mmol/l

There may be only modest nutritional gain in patients with especially short small intestine and in those with persisting disease in the bowel remnant, but the pleasure and psychological advantages to be obtained from eating and its social connotations should not be underestimated.

Eating 'little and often' is usually best, and most patients find that intestinal losses are less if solid food is separated from liquid. There will almost inevitably be idiosyncratic 'problem foods' that they will need to avoid, but these vary a great deal from person to person and are difficult to anticipate. In the first place it is wise to advocate an energy-rich diet. Advice on enteral fat intake should reflect the presence or absence of the colon. In patients with no colon, a high fat intake is useful because it is rich in energy and generally should cause no problems. In those with a colon, however, a tendency to the unpleasant phenomenon of steatorrhoea may limit fat tolerance. Additionally, the use of energy sources biased towards fat diminishes the relative availability of unabsorbed carbohydrate in the colon. Although this carbohydrate is metabolized by intestinal microorganisms for their own purposes (bacterial fermentation), significant amounts of nutrients become available to the patient. It has been estimated that some patients may assimilate as much as 500 kcal/day by this mechanism.

Enteral nutrition – formula feeds

When the combined effects of hyperphagia (spontaneous and facilitated) and optimized fluid balance have failed to achieve nutritional stability, enteral feeds may be considered. Their use is primarily to increase nutrient assimilation outside meal times and in general they offer convenience rather than any special advantage over snack foods. Oral nutritional supplements should not be elemental in patients with SBS: the high osmolarity and volume, low energy density and poorer palatability of such feeds render them almost comprehensively ill suited. Indeed polymeric feeds are not obviously inferior to semi-digested formulations, and there are no data to support the use of modified/supplemented feeds such as those containing extra glutamine or nucleotides.

The choice between regular (1 kcal/ml) and high-energy (≥1.5 kcal/ml) preparations will be prompted by the patient's needs, but it is often the case that the greater osmolarity of high-energy feeds aggravates the tendency to negative fluid balance in SBS without nutritional gain.

Commercial feeds are intentionally low in sodium content and it will therefore usually be necessary to introduce additional salt in patients with SBS. Ordinary table salt can be used, but it is difficult to achieve full dissolution at room temperature, and it is often more practical to employ vials of strong NaCl (e.g. 5% = 830 mmol/l) otherwise intended for intravenous use.

Overnight tube feeding can be helpful in increasing the number of absorptive hours in borderline patients and in those who cannot tolerate the formulae orally, but its efficacy is not assured given its tendency to increase lower gastrointestinal losses and hence a need to empty stoma appliances overnight. It is therefore always wise to conduct a trial with a nasogastric tube before proceeding to gastrostomy insertion. Jejunal feeding is generally inappropriate in patients with SBS.

Pharmacological measures

SBS patients are prescribed a so-called antisecretory regimen, but much of the impact of this is not antisecretory as the main action of the opioid component (acting via μ receptors) is to delay transit. However the proton pump inhibitor does usefully reduce the intraluminal volume, as the majority of the normal gastric secretion is of acid. There is some dispute in intestinal failure circles as to whether this benefit is sustained for more than 6 months or so. In the author's centre it is normally continued in the longer term.

The quantity of opioids used in SBS often gives rise to comment and concern as it is almost universally the case that doses will exceed those described in standard product information. Patients with SBS need much larger amounts because the combination of short intestine and rapid transit greatly reduces their effect. It is common to need doses of loperamide of more than 100 mg/day. This is not hazardous. In the relatively unlikely event of excessive administration, patients notice abdominal discomfort and/or distension, and they should be cautioned about this as the dose is titrated upwards against the gastrointestinal output. Loperamide is less likely to cross the blood–brain barrier and to be responsible for any central effects, and is therefore preferred to codeine phosphate, but it should be noted that many patients find that a combination of the two drugs suits better than a regimen based on equivalent doses of one alone.

Determined use of a regimen based on opioids and high-dose proton pump inhibitor, in combination with strict restriction of sodium-free fluids, can be expected to reduce the gastrointestinal efflux by a further 20% (or 500–1000 ml/day) over and above the reduction achieved by fluid and salt strategies alone (Table 9.3). These effects are admittedly modest, but may be sufficient to allow an undisturbed night's sleep and can secure a meaningful improvement in quality of life.

Anticholinergic agents (and their fixed-dose combinations with opioids) are occasionally useful, but the common side-effect of a dry mouth is a limiting factor not least since it causes confusion in respect of the patient's hydration.

Hormonal manipulation with somatostatin and its longer-acting derivatives such as octreotide has proved less effective than might have been expected. Gastrointestinal output is reduced by about 500 ml/day in trials, but this is relatively seldom replicated in clinical practice. Given the inconvenience of injections (and the significant cost) it has become conventional to perform a 3- to 5-day trial of octreotide at a dose of 300 μg/day. If this is measurably and clinically effective, it is logical to introduce maintenance therapy with one of the longer-acting

Table 9.3. Enteral therapy in short bowel syndrome.

Limit free fluid intake to 500 ml/day
Oral rehydration solution with sodium ≥ 90 mmol/l *ad libitum*
'Antisecretory' regimen, with high-dose opioids and proton pump inhibitors
Encourage oral feeding
Consider low-osmolarity formula feed
Consider enteral tube delivery of feed and/or ORS
Additional magnesium and specific micronutrients as required

formulations. If however there is no obvious response, the entire drug group can be abandoned; this has proved to be the case in more than 95% of the present author's patients.

Several trials have considered the use of human growth hormone with or without other potentially active agents. The literature weakly favours the use of low-dose growth hormone monotherapy, which reduces stomal losses and promotes an anabolic state (Seguy *et al.*, 2003). The modest effect, uncertain long-term risks and cost have combined to militate against its routine use.

The glucagon-like peptide, GLP-2, and its derivative teduglutide, is associated with an increasingly impressive research portfolio and its use is considered in detail elsewhere in this volume (Chapter 37).

Parenteral therapy

Inevitably some intestinal failure patients will require parenteral support, and in most of those with a substantially shortened intestine this will entail both fluids and nutrients. Nonetheless, fluid restriction (and to a lesser extent enteral therapy) should be continued, as it is only by this approach that the patient will be maximally stable from the perspective of fluid shifts across critical cell membranes. All the components of the regimen described above should therefore be continued, but it is reasonable, in aiming to optimize quality of life, to apply them less rigidly, with (for example) the omission of ORS.

In borderline patients with modest fluid, sodium and/or magnesium deficits in whom the parenteral fluid requirement is less than 1 l/day it is worth considering a regular prescription of subcutaneous fluids. The patient or carer can easily and safely be taught to place a subcutaneous cannula each night. An infusion time of 6–10 h will usually permit the administration of at least 500 ml of fluid, which can readily accommodate 75 mmol of sodium and at least 4 mmol of magnesium. The patient should be warned that a swelling may develop during the infusion time; this acts as a 'depot', diminishing over the following few hours.

The intravenous catheter

When PN or intravenous fluids are necessary in patients with SBS it is almost inevitable that this will be a long-term consideration with concomitant importance of the security of the venous access. A subcutaneous tunnel and strict aseptic technique will normally be employed and in some patients an implanted port will be appropriate. These issues are addressed in more detail elsewhere (for further details about venous access, please refer to Chapter 19 of this volume).

The intravenous regimen

PN formulations used in patients with SBS are similar to those used in post-operative and intensive care practice, but the quantities of sodium and magnesium and the volume of fluid required will be greater. It is key to provide full quotas of water- and fat-soluble vitamins, and proportionately more important than in the short-term patient to ensure that the trace elements are included. It will be noted that the intravenous multivitamin preparations do not contain vitamin K. Many patients will need anticoagulation because of their underlying condition, but where this is not the case the risk of vitamin K deficiency should be borne in mind. Monitoring the trace elements and adjusting their provision is a challenge as many are available only in fixed-dose combinations. SBS patients are particularly prone to deficits in zinc and selenium, as well as to potentially toxic accumulation of manganese and perhaps copper (Wardle *et al.*, 1999). Glutamine has been shown to be ineffective and need not be added (Culkin *et al.*, 2008).

Excessive use of lipid emulsions, and particularly the 'first generation' emulsions based entirely on soybean oil, has been strongly linked to the cholestasis of long-term intravenous nutrition. This is not an issue in the early days after the surgical insult when the patient is often malnourished, but becomes more important in the recovery phase. It is therefore recommended that from about 4 weeks into therapy the lipid administration is limited to no more than 3 g/kg body weight/week (or a maximum of no more than 1 l of 20% lipid emulsion per week). It is possible that the dangers can be overcome by the (partial) substitution of soy-derived *n*-6 long-chain fatty acids by *n*-9 or *n*-3 fats (Cavicchi *et al.*, 2000).

It is sometimes forgotten that the great majority of patients with SBS can, and indeed should, eat, even when intravenous nutrition has become necessary. This can lead to inadvertent hyperalimentation, especially once the processes of intestinal adaptation (including compensatory hyperphagia) have occurred. Although recovery will usually be incomplete there can be substantial nutrient absorption. It is difficult to measure this and for practical purposes this process is judged by long-term monitoring of body weight. A recent analysis of the author's patients indicated that the mean energy provision/requirement was only 55% of the daily estimate. However it is less than certain that satisfactory weight reflects normal body composition and attention should always be given to nitrogen balance and micronutrient status, difficult though these are to assess. In any event, the term 'total' PN is inappropriate and should be avoided in discussion of these patients' management.

Prediction of the need for intravenous nutrition

The need for long-term intravenous nutrition for patients with SBS is to quite a large extent predictable and is (for example) almost certain to be required in those with a very short bowel syndrome where less than 80 cm terminates in stoma or a fistula, or when less than 50 cm is partly salvaged by anastomosis to the colon. The probability is also high in any patient in whom the output (diarrhoea, stoma or fistula volume) is >1.5 l/day, and becomes certain when such a high output persists despite the full set of measures outlined above.

A need for long-term PN can also be predicted with confidence in patients with a low circulating citrulline concentration. Several groups around the world have confirmed the original data from Paris and, although the precise prognostic threshold varies a little from centre to centre, a patient with a fasting level of less than 20 μmol/l is almost certain to need long-term parenteral support (Crenn *et al.*, 2000).

Alternatives to PN

The future for patients with SBS is looking a little more encouraging as several other contributions to this volume illustrate. Hormonal manipulation with teduglutide, bowel lengthening surgical procedures, intestinal transplantation and creation of a tissue-engineered artificial intestine are all showing considerable promise for a range of patients who until recently were inevitably subject to lifelong PN.

Summary

SBS is usually the result of major surgical resection. Its optimal management is greatly influenced by the remaining anatomical status, being easier if there is colon in continuity and more difficult if there is a proximal stoma or fistula. Normal proximal secretory responses of the intestine frequently make the patient with SBS a net secretor, such that additional low-sodium oral fluids worsen their fluid balance. Apparently paradoxical, fluid restriction may be essential. Pharmacological agents act mainly to delay transit; high doses of opioids may be necessary but also are safe. Long-term PN will include large-volume regimens with high levels of sodium and magnesium, but with limitations on soy-based lipids and with care needed in respect of the trace elements. Newer hormonal therapies look promising, but surgical reconstruction and transplantation are also options for some patients.

References

Cavicchi, M., Beau, P., Crenn, P. and Messing, B. (2000) Prevalence of liver disease and contributing factors in patients receiving home parenteral nutrition for permanent intestinal failure. *Annals of Internal Medicine* 132, 525–532.

Crenn, P., Coudray-Lucas, C., Thuillier, F., Cynober, L. and Messing, B. (2000) Postabsorptive plasma citrulline concentration is a marker of absorptive enterocyte mass and intestinal failure in humans. *Gastroenterology* 119, 1496–1505.

Culkin, A., Gabe, S., Bjarnason, I., Grimble, G., Madden, A. and Forbes, A. (2008) A double blind, randomized, controlled crossover trial of glutamine supplementation in home parenteral nutrition. *European Journal of Clinical Nutrition* 62, 575–583.

Duro, D., Kamin, D. and Duggan, C. (2008) Overview of pediatric short bowel syndrome. *Journal of Pediatric Gastroenterology and Nutrition* 47(Suppl. 1), S33–S36.

Nightingale, J.M., Lennard-Jones, J.E., Gertner, D.J., Wood, S.R. and Bartram, C.I. (1992) Colonic preservation reduces need for parenteral therapy, increases incidence of renal stones, but does not change high prevalence of gall stones in patients with a short bowel. *Gut* 33, 1493–1497.

O'Keefe, S.J., Buchman, A.L., Fishbein, T.M., Jeejeebhoy, K.N., Jeppesen, P.B. and Schaffer, J. (2006) Short bowel syndrome and intestinal failure: consensus definitions and overview. *Clinical Gastroenterology and Hepatology* 4, 6–10.

Powell-Tuck, J., Gosling, P., Lobo, D.N., Allison, S.P., Carlson, G.L., Gore, M., Lewington, A.J., Pearse, R.M. and Mythen, M.G. (2010) British consensus guidelines on intravenous fluid therapy for adult surgical patients: GIFTASUP. Available at: http://www.bapen.org.uk/professionals/education-research-and-science/bapen-principles-of-good-nutritional-practice/giftasup?showall=&limitstart= (accessed 28 July 2014).

Seguy, D., Vahedi, K., Kapel, N., Souberbielle, J.C. and Messing, B. (2003) Low-dose growth hormone in adult home parenteral nutrition-dependent short bowel syndrome patients: a positive study. *Gastroenterology* 124, 293–302.

Wardle, C.A., Forbes, A., Roberts, N.B., Jawhari, A.V. and Shenkin, A. (1999) Hypermanganesemia in long-term intravenous nutrition and chronic liver disease. *JPEN Journal of Parenteral and Enteral Nutrition* 23, 350–355.

Yunos, N.M., Bellomo, R., Hegarty, C., Story, D., Ho, L. and Bailey, M. (2012) Association between a chloride-liberal vs chloride-restrictive intravenous fluid administration strategy and kidney injury in critically ill adults. *Journal of the American Medical Association* 308, 1566–1572.

10 Gastrointestinal Fistulae

Geert Wanten[1*] and Jon Shaffer[2]

[1]Radboud University Nijmegen Medical Centre, Nijmegen, The Netherlands;
[2]Intestinal Failure Unit, Salford Royal NHS Foundation Trust, Salford, UK

Key Points

- Fistulae are a complication of, e.g. Crohn's disease, cancer or diverticular disease, or may appear secondary to gastrointestinal surgery or trauma.
- Initial treatment should focus on correction of fluid and electrolyte balances and control of fistula output.
- The importance of sepsis identification and management cannot be overemphasized.
- The current mainstay of therapy for closure of fistulae is parenteral nutrition and giving the patient (nearly) nil by mouth, although evidence that this practice increases the rate of fistula closure is lacking.
- Home parenteral nutrition for patients with fistulae may be instigated for a number of months, but only in order to achieve appropriate conditions for definitive surgery, which generally should not be performed any earlier than 3–6 months after a fistula has developed.

Introduction

A gastrointestinal fistula, i.e. an abnormal communication from the gastrointestinal tract to an adjacent organ (bladder, vagina, skin or more distal bowel), can lead to severe malnutrition and fluid deficiencies, depending on its anatomical origin and output. Thus, a proximal jejunal enterocutaneous fistula associated with underlying sepsis will result in devastating fluid and nutrient losses which, untreated, can lead to a mortality rate of 50% (Soeters *et al*., 1979; Dudrick *et al*., 1999) (see also Table 10.1). Patients with gastric or colonic fistulae have a milder

*E-mail: geert.wanten@radboudumc.nl

Table 10.1. Electrolyte composition (in mEq/l) of gastrointestinal secretions. (From Fenves and Emmett, 1996; Bleier and Hedrick, 2010; Polk and Schwab, 2012.)

	Volume (ml)	Na^+	K^+	H^+	Cl^-	HCO_3^-
Chyme (gastric)	2000	40–65	10	90	100–140	–
Pancreatic fluid	1000	135–155	5		55–75	70–90
Bile	1000	135–155	5		80–110	35–50
Succus (small bowel)	3500	120–130	10		50–60	50–70
Stool (colon)	1000–4000	25–50	35–60		20–40	30–45

clinical course than those with duodenal or small bowel fistulae (Polk and Schwab, 2012). So far, mortality of fistula patients has remained disproportionately high (6–33%) in comparison with other surgical conditions and is mainly caused by sepsis (Lloyd *et al.*, 2006). By contrast a rectovaginal fistula, while having an important impact on a patient's quality of life, has little effect on mortality or nutritional status. The management of oesophageal, rectal and anal fistulas are different and will not be considered in this discussion.

Enteroatmospheric fistulae are defined as communications or connections between the lumen of the bowel or other hollow viscus and the atmosphere (open abdomen or chest) and these may be deep, with drainage into the peritoneal cavity, or superficial, with drainage through granulation tissue near the bowel (Lundy and Fisher, 2010; Polk and Schwab, 2012).

Primary, spontaneous fistulae are a complication of an underlying disease process, e.g. Crohn's disease, cancer or diverticular disease. More than 75% of all fistulae however are secondary, i.e. they develop shortly after gastrointestinal surgery or trauma (Haffejee, 2004). In a specialist intestinal failure unit, fistulae account for between 44 and 80% of referrals (Scott *et al.*, 1991; A. Teubner, personal communication, 2005). Approximately 75–85% of fistulae that develop after an operation are due to bowel injury, inadvertent enterotomy or anastomotic leakage (Berry and Fischer, 1996). These fistulae are almost always associated with local sepsis and it is the management of the sepsis that dominates the therapeutic approach (Visschers *et al.*, 2008). While sepsis in this setting may be characterized by pyrexia, leucocytosis, thrombocytosis and raised inflammatory markers such as C-reactive protein, it may also develop more insidiously with disturbed liver function tests, hyponatraemia and hypoalbuminaemia (Carlson, 2003). Whereas mildly disturbed liver function test are common in patients with intestinal failure and may be related to the use of drugs (especially antibiotics), biliary disease, cholestasis and overfeeding, overt jaundice is often related to sepsis and requires further investigation (Gardiner, 2011). It should be emphasized that well-powered controlled trials on the management of gastrointestinal fistulae are lacking and that current concepts of treatment lean heavily on expert opinion.

Up to 60% of post-operative fistulae will heal spontaneously with appropriate nursing and nutritional care within 6 weeks. Factors associated with failure to heal include (Reber *et al.*, 1978; Levy *et al.*, 1989; Schein and Decker, 1990; Campos *et al.*, 1996; Tassiopoulos *et al.*, 1996; Lloyd *et al.*, 2006; Visschers *et al.*, 2008; Polk and Schwab, 2012):

- persistent sepsis;
- mucocutaneous continuity;
- extra-colonic and high-output (>500 ml/day) fistulae;
- presence of an open abdomen;
- local disease, e.g. Crohn's or malignancy, causing fistulation;
- distal obstruction to the fistula;
- wide discontinuity of bowel;
- multiple, complex fistulae;
- untreated undernutrition; and
- unstable metabolic disease.

Recurrence of Enterocutaneous Fistulae after Surgical Repair

Martinez *et al.* recently reported on their experience in 71 patients (Martinez *et al.*, 2012). In line with available literature, these authors found a 31% recurrence rate; this was increased in high-output and small bowel enteroatmospheric fistulae and in those with a history of open abdomen treatment, whereas it was lowered for colonic fistulae.

Care of the Patient with a Gastrointestinal Fistula

General principles of care are: (i) control and drainage of sepsis; (ii) the provision of adequate nutritional support to prevent the development of malnutrition and maintain fluid and electrolyte balances; (iii) medical therapy; (iv) expert nursing and stoma care; (v) identification of anatomical structures; and (vi) definitive surgery.

Nutritional support

There are no specific differences in the nutritional requirements of patients with gastrointestinal fistulae from others, although those with a proximal fistula and high output will become volume-depleted and develop disturbed fluid, acid–base and electrolyte balances that need resuscitation and correction by intravenous supplementation (see also Tables 10.1 and 10.2). Similar to short bowel syndrome, treatment starts with a restriction of hypo-osmolar fluids that are low in sodium, whereas the use of rehydration solutions high in sodium and glucose is encouraged. Before the advent of parenteral nutrition in the late 1960s, patients with proximal fistulae developed malnutrition in up to 75% of cases and this contributed significantly to the high mortality of about 50% for this condition in those days (Edmunds *et al.*, 1960). Experts advocate starting total parenteral nutrition with adequate supplementation of vitamins and trace elements early, i.e. within 24–48 h after the appearance of a fistula, also because the use of parenteral nutrition has been identified as an independent predictor for spontaneous fistula closure. On the other hand, spontaneous fistula closure is not likely to occur after more than 7–8 weeks (Lloyd *et al.*, 2006; Visschers *et al.*, 2008). There

Table 10.2. An indication of nutritional requirements of fistula patients. (From Bleier and Hedrick, 2010.)

Baseline: carbohydrate and fat, 20 kcal/kg body weight/day; protein, 0.8–1 g/kg body weight/day; ≤30% of total calories as lipid
Low-output fistulae (<200 ml/day): carbohydrate and fat, 25–30 kcal/kg body weight/day; protein, 1.5–2 g/kg body weight/day
High-output fistulae (>500 ml/day): up to 2× normal caloric requirement and 2–2.5× normal protein requirement

is no unequivocal evidence to show that oral restriction leads to fistula closure, but it is generally agreed that oral intake should be limited to nil by mouth (if tolerated) or to the limited use of clear fluids (up to 500 ml/day) (Lloyd *et al.*, 2006; Visschers *et al.*, 2008). Those patients for whom it is known that spontaneous healing will not take place may eat and drink freely as long as fistula output does not compromise wound care or lead to uncontrollable fluid losses. Although there is debate as to whether fistula output determines spontaneous closure, successful limitation of fistula output to minimize fluid and electrolyte losses enables some patients to wean off parenteral support. The practice of intubating the distal limb of a fistula (if accessible) allows a number of patients to be enterally fed who would otherwise require parenteral nutrition. For instance, this practice of fistuloclysis with feeding of polymeric feeds and without re-feeding of secretions enabled Teubner *et al.* to discontinue parenteral nutrition in 11 out 12 patients with a small bowel fistula who were awaiting reconstructive surgery (Teubner *et al.*, 2004). This approach was also favourable from the economic perspective since treatment cost was reduced at least fourfold, and it can also be managed successfully in the home setting.

Long-term parenteral nutrition in the home setting (HPN)

Although experts agree that the primary role of nutritional support in the setting of a patient with a gastrointestinal fistula is the prevention of malnutrition with its sequelae, the discussion on the optimal route of nutrition, i.e. enteral versus parenteral, is not closed and benefits and risks of each treatment strategy have to be balanced (Lloyd *et al.*, 2006). Home parenteral nutrition (HPN) has been used in the management of fistulae for many years (Byrne *et al.*, 1979; Mughal and Irving, 1986), partly as a means of providing for prolonged spontaneous closure but also as a means to allow timing for definitive surgery. The evidence for a critical role for parenteral nutrition in fistula healing is lacking despite the fact that 'bowel rest' reduces gastrointestinal secretion volumes by nearly 50% (Lloyd *et al.*, 2006). The percentage of HPN patients with fistulae as their underlying problem is relatively small – currently the Acute Intestinal Failure Unit at Hope Hospital, Salford, UK admits approximately 60 new patients per year – and nearly 50% of these patients have a fistula but only four or five will go home on HPN. This is always for a number of months and only to allow appropriate conditions for definitive surgery. Some of these patients may require long-term HPN, but this is mostly because they have short bowel syndrome. This compares with the figures of 6% and 7% reported in the two surveys by the Home Artificial Nutrition working group of the European Society for Parenteral and Enteral Nutrition (ESPEN-HAN) (Van Gossum *et al.*, 1996, 1999). Of note, most of these patients had either Crohn's disease or gastrointestinal cancer as their underlying diagnosis.

Medical therapy

This comprises antisecretory (histamine-2 receptor antagonists, proton pump inhibitors, somatostatin/octreotide) and antimotility (loperamide, codeine, sucralfate) agents, digestive supplements (pancreatic enzymes) and bulking agents (dietary fibre).

In the case that stoma losses cannot be controlled by fluid management, the next step is to reduce gastric secretions (which may approach 1–2 l/day) by means of H2 receptor antagonists or proton pump inhibitors (e.g. ranitidine 300 mg twice daily or omeprazole 40 mg twice daily). In addition, high-dose antimotility agents such as loperamide (up to 32 mg four times daily) or codeine (up to 60 mg four times daily) help to slow down bowel transit. Sucralfate is an agent that not only decreases gastric acidity, but also has constipation as a possibly helpful side-effect (Polk and Schwab, 2012). Loperamide is also available in liquid form, but this has the drawbacks of poor palatability and a high osmolarity. The use of codeine in high doses is limited by its sedative effect. Addition of pancreatic enzymes may promote fat and protein absorption, while dietary fibre can help to thicken enteric contents.

Octreotide is a synthetic analogue of the hormone somatostatin that has an inhibitory effect on gastrointestinal secretions (gastric, pancreatic) and which reduces splanchnic blood flow, gastric emptying and gallbladder contractions (Lloyd *et al.*, 2006). Octreotide, due to its longer plasma half-life compared with somatostatin, can be given by subcutaneous injection and a long-acting formulation for intramuscular administration once monthly is available. Octreotide non-specifically reduces stoma output by approximately 1 l/day. The recommended dose is 25–100 μg two or three times daily and treatment can be continued quite safely in the long term although side-effects, mainly in the form of nausea/vomiting, diarrhoea or constipation, gallstones and disturbed glucose metabolism, occur in >10% of patients. While studies comparing the effects of somatostatin and octreotide on top of standard treatment are small and differ in design, the overall impression is that somatostatin infusion, but possibly not octreotide injection, reduces fistula output and decreases the time to fistula closure, whereas none of these agents seems to increase spontaneous fistula closure (Sitges-Serra *et al.*, 1993; Hesse *et al.*, 2001; Jamil *et al.*, 2004; Lloyd *et al.*, 2006).

Infliximab, a monoclonal antibody against tumour necrosis factor-α that is used to treat immune-mediated diseases, is helpful in controlling active Crohn's disease and has a role in the management of peri-anal fistulae, but has little effect on internal or enterocutaneous fistulae (Miehsler *et al.*, 2004; Parsi *et al.*, 2004). Experimental therapies to treat fistulae include vacuum sealing of the fistula tract (Medeiros *et al.*, 2004) and the use of adipose mesenchymal stem cells

(Garcia-Olmo *et al.*, 2005). The potential therapeutic benefits of hormonal agents that have been implicated in intestinal mucosal atrophy, such as glucagon-like peptide-2, have not been characterized.

Nursing/stoma care

Skin damage due to leakage of aggressive intestinal fluids precludes wound healing and therefore expert stoma care is of key importance, including the use of adequate wound-managing systems. As such, multiple/complex fistulae therefore require multidisciplinary care and these constitute a considerable challenge in the maintenance of skin, fluids, wound and psychological care.

Delineating anatomy: creation of the 'roadmap'

Patients with resistant fistulae require radiological contrast studies, including fistulography, to delineate the accurate length, quality, relationships and connections of remaining bowel and to rule out stenosis. Patients with less than 120 cm of usable small bowel are at risk for small bowel syndrome and at least 75 cm is required for successful enteral feeding (Polk and Schwab, 2012). An assessment of citrulline can be helpful to provide an estimation of functional residual bowel length, since a serum level <20 μmol/l has a high sensitivity and specificity for the presence of permanent intestinal failure (Williams *et al.*, 2010). Ultrasound, computed tomography (CT) – and, if necessary, magnetic resonance imaging and white cell scans – are mandatory in identifying any underlying sepsis. This can be prominent on scanning even though the patient may not be systemically ill or the usual inflammatory markers are not markedly elevated.

Sepsis control

Here a crucial step forward was the introduction in the final decades of the previous century of high-resolution radiological techniques (CT, ultrasound) that enable precise drainage of fluid collections without a need for extensive surgical exploration (Johnson *et al.*, 1981). Still, radiological drainage of abscesses and collections of infection may need to be performed repeatedly in order to be successful. In complex cases drains should be inserted to allow repeated washouts of septic areas and to prevent re-accumulation of material. If it is clear that sepsis management cannot be obtained by this method, a defunctioning stoma proximal to the site of the (first) fistula may be required.

Definitive surgery

In general, expert centres have adopted a more defensive surgical strategy over time with the advent of radiological drainage techniques and materials, such as absorbable meshes, that enable temporary abdominal wall closure (Visschers *et al.*, 2008). The importance of avoiding fistula resection in the presence of sepsis is reiterated. A serum albumin >30 g/l is a reasonable target, but may not be achievable for many weeks. The presence of widespread sepsis after multiple attempts at surgery may lead to obliteration of the peritoneal cavity and a very demanding surgical environment. HPN for a number of months (on average, 6 months) can provide this interval and allow the patient to return to home, often after many months in hospital (Carlson, 2003; Evans *et al.*, 2003). Reconstruction is then possible in a non-septic, controlled environment. It is generally agreed that patients should not undergo restorative surgery within 3–6 months after the development of a gastrointestinal fistula (Carlson, 2003; Evenson and Fisher, 2006; Lloyd *et al.*, 2006).

Recent evidence to guide treatment comes from a retrospective analysis of 135 patients with enterocutaneous fistulae who were treated at a Dutch referral centre between 1990 and 2005 (Visschers *et al.*, 2008). Multiple logistic regression analysis revealed that the major negative prognostic factor for spontaneous fistula closure was the presence of an abdominal wall defect whereas a lowered pre-operative albumin level (<25 g/l) had a significant negative impact on surgical closure and mortality rates, with ongoing sepsis being the most important cause of death. Importantly, all these patients were treated according to a standardized management protocol called 'SOWATS' that is based on the outcome of a large retrospective study (Soeters *et al.*, 1979) from the same centre and which encompasses controlling of Sepsis, Optimization of nutrition state, Wound care, Assessment of fistula anatomy, Timing of surgery and Surgical strategy. This protocol resembles the structured approach called 'SNAP' (Skin care, Nutrition, Anatomy definition and Planned procedure) that was introduced by the group from Salford Royal NHS Trust in the UK (Kaushal and Carlson, 2004) and is part of the principles for managing patients with acute intestinal failure as described by the national surgical society from the UK, and which is named 'SLOW STUFF' (Sepsis, Liver dysfunction, Obstruction, Wound, Stoma, Talking, Undernutrition, Fluids and electrolytes) (Association of Surgeons of Great Britain and Ireland, 2010). Using the SOWATS protocol, the authors managed to achieve a success rate for restorative operations that were performed after a median of 53 days with fistula closure in 97 out of 107 patients (91%), at the cost of a mortality rate of 10%. This latter finding is in line with the notion that mortality rates of over 50% have fallen to 20% or less with the greater the delay in surgical repair of the fistula (Carlson, 2003; Lynch *et al.*, 2004; Olaison *et al.*, 2005).

Several expert surgical principles have been described (Lloyd *et al.*, 2006; Shetty *et al.*, 2006; Visschers *et al.*, 2008), including: (i) a complete dissection of the bowel tract should be performed to ensure passage and allow mobilization of the abdominal wall; (ii) the number of anastomoses should be limited to the minimum; (iii) anastomoses should be covered by healthy tissue and positioned away from sutures of the abdominal wall; (iv) the use of non-absorbable meshes should be prevented because of the associated infection risk and to reduce fistula recurrence; and (v) if necessary, defunctioning proximal double-barrelled enterostomies can be created in order to protect critical distal anastomoses.

Outcome

The prognosis is mainly dependent on the recognition and management of sepsis, but also the underlying disease. Thus, Crohn's disease as the cause of the fistula requires HPN prior to surgery, while cancer fistulae usually involve HPN only as a terminal treatment.

Summary

The management of gastrointestinal fistulae is both supportive and dependent on the underlying disease. Persistent post-operative fistulae are usually associated with sepsis, malnutrition and fluid and electrolyte losses. In complex fistulae or patients in whom surgery is best delayed as long as possible, HPN for a number of months can play a useful role. In those patients with cancer as the cause of the fistula, HPN can provide helpful palliation.

References

Association of Surgeons of Great Britain and Ireland (2010) The surgical management of patients with acute intestinal failure. Available at: http://www.asgbi.org.uk/en/publications/issues_in_professional_practice.cfm (accessed September 2010).

Berry, S.M. and Fischer, J.E. (1996) Classification and pathophysiology of enterocutaneous fistulas. *Surgical Clinics of North America* 76, 1009–1018.

Bleier, J.I. and Hedrick, T. (2010) Metabolic support of the enterocutaneous fistula patient. *Clinics in Colon and Rectal Surgery* 23, 142–148.

Byrne, W.J., Burke, M., Fonkalsrud, E.W. and Ament, M.E. (1979) Home parenteral nutrition: an alternative approach to the management of complicated gastrointestinal fistulas not responding to conventional medical or surgical therapy. *JPEN Journal of Parenteral and Enteral Nutrition* 3, 355–359.

Campos, A.C., Meguid, M.M. and Coelho, J.C. (1996) Factors influencing outcome in patients with gastrointestinal fistula. *Surgical Clinics of North America* 76, 1191–1198.

Carlson, G.L. (2003) Surgical management of intestinal failure. *Proceedings of the Nutrition Society* 62, 711–718.

Dudrick, S.J., Maharaj, A.R. and McKelvey, A.A. (1999) Artificial nutrition support in patients with gastrointestinal fistulas. *World Journal of Surgery* 23, 570–576.

Edmunds, L.H. Jr, Williams, G.M. and Welch, C.E. (1960) External fistulas arising from the gastro-intestinal tract. *Annals of Surgery* 152, 445–471.

Evans, J.P., Steinhart, A.H., Cohen, Z. and McLeod, R.S. (2003) Home total parenteral nutrition: an alternative to early surgery for complicated inflammatory bowel disease. *Journal of Gastrointestinal Surgery* 7, 562–566.

Evenson, A.R. and Fisher, J.E. (2006) Current management of enterocutaneous fistuale. *Journal of Gastrointestinal Surgery* 10, 455–464.

Fenves, A.Z. and Emmett, M. (1996) Fluid and electrolytes. In: O'Leary, J.P. (ed.) *The Physiologic Basis of Surgery*, 2nd edn. Williams and Willams, Baltimore, Maryland.

Garcia-Olmo, D., Garcia-Arranz, M., Herreros, D., Pascual, I., Peiro, C. and Rodriguez-Montes, J.A. (2005) A phase I clinical trial of the treatment of Crohn's fistula by adipose mesenchymal stem cell transplantation. *Diseases of the Colon and Rectum* 48, 1416–1423.

Gardiner, K.R. (2011) Home parenteral nutrition and intestinal failure clinical network (HIFNET) and parenteral nutrition management of acute intestinal failure. *Proceedings of Nutrition Society* 70, 321–328.
Haffejee, A.A. (2004) Surgical management of high output enterocutaneous fistulae: a 24-year experience. *Current Opinion in Clinical Nutrition and Metabolism Care* 7, 309–316.
Hesse, U., Ysebaert, D. and de Hemptinne, B. (2001) Role of somatostatin-14 and its analogues in the management of gastrointestinal fistulae: clinical data. *Gut* 49(Suppl. 4), iv11–iv21.
Jamil, M., Ahmed, U. and Sobia, H. (2004) Role of somatostatin analogues in the management of enterocutaneous fistulae. *Journal of the College of Physicians and Surgeons of Pakistan* 14, 237–240.
Johnson, W.C., Gerzof, S.G. and Robbins, A.H. (1981) Treatment of abdominal abscesses: comparative evaluation of operative drainage versus percutaneous catheter drainage guided by computed tomography or ultrasound. *Annals of Surgery* 194, 510–520.
Martinez, J.L., Luque-de-León, E., Ballinas-Oseguera, G., Mendez, J.D., Juárez-Oropeza, M.A. and Román-Ramos, R. (2012) Factors predictive of recurrence and mortality after surgical repair of enterocutaneous fistula. *Journal of Gastrointestinal Surgery* 16, 156–164.
Kaushal, M. and Carlson, G.L. (2004) Management of enterocutaneous fistulas. *Clinics in Colon and Rectal Surgery* 17, 79–88.
Levy, E., Frileux, P. and Cugnenc, P.H. (1989) High-output external fistulae of the small bowel: management with continuous enteral nutrition. *British Journal of Surgery* 76, 676–679.
Lloyd, D.A., Gabe, S.M. and Windsor, A.C. (2006) Nutrition and management of enterocutaneous fistula. *British Journal of Surgery* 93, 1045–1055.
Lundy, J.B. and Fisher, J.E. (2010) Historical perspectives in the care of patients with enterocutaneous fistula. *Clinics in Colon and Rectal Surgery* 23, 133–141.
Lynch, A.C., Delaney, C.P., Senagore, A.J., Connor, J.T., Remzi, F.H. and Fazio, V.W. (2004) Clinical outcome and factors predictive of recurrence after enterocutaneous fistula surgery. *Annals of Surgery* 240, 825–831.
Medeiros, A.C., Aires-Neto, T., Marchini, J.S., Brandao-Neto, J., Valenca, D.M. and Egito, E.S. (2004) Treatment of post-operative enterocutaneous fistulas by high-pressure vacuum with a normal oral diet. *Digestive Surgery* 21, 401–405.
Miehsler, W., Reinisch, W., Kazemi-Shirazi, L., Dejaco, C., Novacek, G., Ferenci, P., Herbst, F., Karner, J., Telcky, B., Scfhober, E. and Vogelsang, H. (2004) Infliximab: lack of efficacy on perforating complications in Crohn's disease. *Inflammatory Bowel Diseases* 10, 36–40.
Mughal, M. and Irving, M. (1986) Home parenteral nutrition in the United Kingdom and Ireland. *Lancet* 2, 383–387.
Olaison, G., Runstrom, B., Hallbrook, O., Nystrom, P.O. and Sjodahl, R. (2005) Enterocutaneous fistulas – persisting conditions but the healing capacity can be surgically restored. Current treatment and surgical skills reduce the mortality. *Lakartidningen* 102, 861–865.
Parsi, M.A., Lashner, B.A., Achkar, J.P., Connor, J.T. and Brzezinski, A. (2004) Type of fistula determines responses to infliximab in patients with fistulous Crohn's disease. *American Journal of Gastroenterology* 99, 445–449.
Polk, T.M. and Schwab, C.W. (2012) Metabolic and nutritional support of the enterocutaneous fistula patient: a three-phase approach. *World Journal of Surgery* 36, 524–533.
Reber, H.A., Roberts, C., Way, L.W. and Dunphy, J.E. (1978) Management of external gastrointestinal fistulas. *Annals of Surgery* 188, 460–467.
Schein, M. and Decker, G.A. (1990) Gastrointestinal fistulas associated with large abdominal wall defects: experience with 43 patients. *British Journal of Surgery* 77, 97–100.
Scott, N.A., Leinhardt, D.J., O'Hanrahan, T., Finnegan, S., Shaffer, J.L. and Irving, M.H. (1991) Spectrum of intestinal failure in a specialised unit. *Lancet* 337, 471–473.

Shetty, V., Teubner, A., Morrison, K. and Scott, N.A. (2006) Proximal loop jejunostomy is a useful adjunct in the management of multiple intestinal suture lines in the septic abdomen. *British Journal of Surgery* 93, 1247–1250.

Sitges-Serra, A., Guiro, X., Pereira, J.A. and Nubiola, P. (1993) Treatment of gastrointestinal fistulas with sandostatin. *Digestion* 54(Suppl. 1), 38–40.

Soeters, P.B., Ebeid, A.M. and Fischer, J.E. (1979) Review of 404 patients with gastrointestinal fistulas. Impact of parenteral nutrition. *Annals of Surgery* 190, 189–202.

Tassiopoulos, A.K., Baum, G. and Halverson, J.D. (1996) Small bowel fistulas. *Surgical Clinics of North America* 76, 1175–1181.

Teubner, A., Morrison, K., Ravishankar, H.R., Anderson, I.D. and Carlson, G.L. (2004) Fistuloclysis can successfully replace parenteral feeding in the nutritional support of patients with enterocutaneous fistula. *British Journal of Surgery* 91, 625–631.

Van Gossum, A., Bakker, H., De Francesco, A., Ladefoged, K., Leon-Sanz, M., Messing, B., Pironi, L., Pertkiewicz, M., Shaffer, J., Thul, P. and Wood, S. (1996) Home parenteral nutrition in adults: a multicentre survey in Europe in 1993. *Clinical Nutrition* 15, 53–59.

Van Gossum, A., Bakker, H., Bozetti, F., Staun, M., Leon-Sanz, M., Hebuterne, X., Pertkiewicz, M., Shaffer, J. and Thul, P. (1999) Home parenteral nutrition in adults: a European multicentre survey in 1997. *Clinical Nutrition* 18, 135–140.

Visschers, R.G., Olde Damink, S.W., Winkens, B., Soeters, P.B. and van Gemert, W. (2008) Treatment strategies in 135 consecutive patients with enterocutaneous fistulas. *World Journal of Surgery* 32, 445–453.

Williams, L.J., Zolfaghari, S. and Boushey, R.P. (2010) Complications of enterocutaneous fistulas and their management. *Clinics in Colon and Rectal Surgery* 23, 209–220.

11 Chronic Intestinal Pseudo-obstruction

Francisca Joly[1,2*], Vanessa Bon Djemah[1], Sabrina Layec[3], Olivier Corcos[1] and Yoram Bouhnik[1]

[1]*Department of Gastroenterology and Nutrition Support, Beaujon Hospital, Assistance Publique – Hôpitaux de Paris, Université Paris VII, Clichy, France;* [2]*Gastrointestinal and Metabolic Dysfunctions in Nutritional Pathologies, Inserm UMR 1149, Centre de Recherche sur l'Inflammation Paris Montmartre – UFR de Médecine Paris Diderot, Paris, France;* [3]*Intestinal Rehabilitation, Clinique Saint-Yves, Rennes, France*

Key Points

- Chronic intestinal pseudo-obstruction (CIPO) is defined as a rare, severe, disabling disorder characterized by chronic and/or recurrent symptoms suggesting bowel obstruction, in the absence of fixed lumen-occluding lesions.
- CIPO is classified as either idiopathic (most common in children) or secondary (most common in the adult population).
- Recurrent episodes of obstruction are the most frequent clinical presentation, together with malabsorption and diarrhoea.
- Diagnosis is based on the clinical presentation, with long-standing symptoms and the absence of mechanical obstruction and – in some cases – a family history.
- Prokinetic drugs are systematically used in CIPO but their effectiveness is generally poor.
- Nutritional support is of great importance and home parenteral nutrition is required in 60–80% of infants and 20–50% of adults.
- Surgery, explorative or with resection, may be an option, or alternatively decompressive or feeding stomas.
- Long-term outcome is characterized by a 10–25% infant mortality rate. In adults, the clinical course, long-term outcome and prognostic factors are less well known because of the limited data on the small numbers of patients with heterogeneous onset and severity of the disease.

*E-mail: francisca.joly@gmail.com

Introduction

Chronic intestinal pseudo-obstruction (CIPO) is today an important indication for home parenteral nutrition (HPN) in both adults and children. CIPO refers to a heterogeneous group of disorders (Table 11.1) characterized by symptoms of intestinal obstruction in the absence of mechanical evidence of obstruction. It is caused by ineffective intestinal contractions. CIPO may be classified as either a primary disease, which is usually limited to the hollow viscera, or a secondary disease, associated with an existing systemic disorder. CIPO may predominate as a 'total' gut disease from oesophagus to anal sphincter or as a 'localized' disease that is gastric and intestinal or intestinal alone; segmental gut disease is not the rule with the exception of an isolated megaduodenum. Recurrent episodes of obstruction are the usual clinical fate with, most frequently, malabsorptive diarrhoea. CIPO may also be the case; i.e. malabsorptive diarrhoea without obvious obstruction. Besides nutritional support, the symptomatic treatment usually consists of prokinetic drugs, such as low doses of octreotide and erythromycin. In case of a systemic disease causing CIPO, specific treatments are also cornerstone such as, for example, in systemic lupus erythematosus. The most severe forms may require a stoma for nutrition and/or decompression. Generally, other surgical procedures are not recommended except in cases of a CIPO complication such as peritonitis due to perforation (with or without diverticula) or bowel ischaemia. Severe CIPO patients with an intestinal 'functional' insufficiency, especially those affected by the diffuse forms of disease, may need long-term HPN. In the latter case, when there is a failure of HPN, alternative treatment such as extensive

Table 11.1. Principal aetiology of CIPO.

Idiopathic CIPO
MNGIE (mitochondrial neurogastrointestinal encephalomyopathy) and other mitochondrial cytopathies
Intestinal neuronal dysplasia
Hirschsprung disease and diffuse aganglionosis
Multiple endocrine neoplasia type IIb
Neurofibromatosis type 1
Others
Secondary CIPO
Smooth muscle disorders (connective tissue disease, amyloidosis, diffuse lymphoid infiltration of the small intestine, muscular dystrophies)
Diseases of the central nervous system (Parkinson's disease, other cause of dysautonomia)
Visceral sporadic neuropathies (paraneoplastic syndrome, post-infectious syndrome such as Chagas disease, Epstein–Barr virus, cytomegalovirus, varicella zoster virus, rotavirus)
Drug-related toxicity (isoniazide, anthraquinone, adriamycin, calcium channel inhibitors, anticholinergic drugs)
Metabolic disorders (hypothyroidism, acute intermittent porphyria, Fabry's disease, hyperparathyroidism)
Miscellaneous (coeliac refractory sprue, radiation enteritis, Crohn's disease, post-surgical disorders)

resection or intestinal transplantation should be discussed case by case in an intestinal tertiary care centre.

Definition and Classification of CIPO

According to a consensus working group in the 1980s, CIPO is defined as a rare, severe, disabling disorder characterized by chronic and/or recurrent symptoms suggesting bowel obstruction, including radiographic documentation of dilated bowel with air/fluid levels, in the absence of a fixed lumen-occluding lesion (Rudolph *et al.*, 1997). More largely, CIPO corresponds to a wide and heterogeneous group of gastrointestinal nerve and muscle disorders. Although familial forms with autosomal dominant, autosomal recessive or X-linked modes of inheritance have been reported, CIPO is a sporadic disease (De Giorgio *et al.*, 2004; Stanghellini *et al.*, 2007; Di Nardo *et al.*, 2008). Usually, CIPO is classified either as idiopathic or secondary. Idiopathic CIPO is the most prominent paediatric cause and occurs in 40% of adult CIPO patients (De Giorgio *et al.*, 2004). It usually refers to hollow visceral disorder (Table 11.1). Secondary forms of CIPO occur in 60% of adult patients and rarely in children. The list of potential causes of CIPO is not exhaustive (Table 11.1). The most common causes are metabolic disorders (diabetes mellitus, hypothyroidism), neuropathic drug-related injuries (vincristine, anticholinergic drugs), paraneoplastic and post-infectious syndromes and amyloidosis (Rudolph *et al.*, 1997; Schuffler *et al.*, 1981; Connor and Di Lorenzo, 2006; Joly *et al.*, 2006). Recent data have focused on the role of neurotropic viruses like herpes and JC virus, a polyomavirus (Selgrad *et al.*, 2009; De Giorgio *et al.*, 2010).

Some patients with apparently idiopathic CIPO may have primary defects of the mitochondrial oxidative phosphorylation pathway. Disorders often involve many organs with most frequent dysfunctions of the nervous system and ocular muscles. CIPO is rarely the main clinical problem but this occurs with mitochondrial neurogastrointestinal encephalopathy (MNGIE), an autosomal recessive syndrome resulting in the loss of thymidine phosphorylase activity. In a series of 80 CIPO patients, mitochondrial defects were identified in 19% of the study cohort (Amiot *et al.*, 2009).

In parallel to aetiological classification, histopathological classification has been made, considering abnormal pathological and manometric findings (Stanghellini *et al.*, 1987; Wood, 2002). Digestive motility is a highly coordinated process of mixing, absorption and propulsion of ingesta throughout the gastrointestinal tract, eventually leading to expulsion of residues. Many actors are involved in digestive motility, from the central neural network, through the enteric nervous system to digestive smooth muscle (Goyal and Hirano, 1998). Digestive motility is also regulated by a pacemaker activity evoked by the interstitial cells of Cajal (ICCs), which generate slow waves of phasic changes in intraluminal pressure (Thomsen *et al.*, 1998; Lee *et al.*, 1999). Loss of ICCs in the digestive tract has been associated with the idiopathic form of CIPO (Isozaki *et al.*, 1997; Feldstein *et al.*, 2003). Thus CIPO can be classified into three different entities: (i) mesenchymopathies; (ii) visceral neuropathies; and (iii) visceral myopathies (De Giorgio *et al.*,

2004). Combined forms may also coexist in the same tissue specimens from the same patient. Neuropathic CIPO can be distinguished into two major forms: (i) degenerative neuropathy characterized by a picture of neural degeneration in the absence of an evident inflammatory response; and (ii) inflammatory neuropathy in which a significant inflammatory/immune response can be identified within the glia and/or the enteric nerve processes (Krishnamurthy and Schuffler, 1987; Di Nardo *et al.*, 2008). Inflammatory neuropathies are characterized by $CD3^+$ T lymphocytes. Patients with lymphocytic myenteric ganglionitis may develop a humoral response characterized by antinuclear neuronal antibodies (ANNA-1/anti-Hu). Other types of inflammatory neuropathies are characterized by either eosinophils or mast cells, but the number of reported patients is limited. As for neuropathies, enteric myopathies can also be classified into inflammatory and degenerative forms. Inflammatory myopathies are characterized by immune infiltrate, mainly composed by $CD4^+$ and $CD8^+$ lymphocytes. A structured classification of gastrointestinal neuromuscular pathologies including CIPO was presented in 2009 by an international working group (London Classification of gastrointestinal neuromuscular pathology), based on histopathological criteria (Knowles *et al.*, 2010). This classification describes main histopathological abnormalities for each of the three entities (neuropathies, myopathies and mesenchymopathies). Histopathological phenotypes for congenital and acquired intestinal pseudo-obstruction as described in the London Classification are reported in Table 11.2.

Diagnosis

CIPO remains a challenge to diagnose because of the non-specific symptoms, rarity of the disease, insidious onset and, most of the time, the lack of laboratory and morphological tests. Frequently, between the symptoms onset and the time of diagnosis, CIPO history is characterized by multiple non-contributive laparotomies or non-indicated bowel resection (Hanks and Weber, 1981; Mann *et al.*, 1997). This fact leads one to consider two most important fates before considering

Table 11.2. Histopathological phenotypes from the London Classification. (From Knowles and Martin, 2011.)

Congenital CIPO
Aetiological: aganglionosis, hypoganglionosis ± intraneural nuclear inclusions, degenerative neuropathy, muscularis propria malformations and degenerative leiomyopathy
Morphological: abnormal neurochemical coding, neural immaturity, abnormal ICC networks
Acquired CIPO
Aetiological: hypoganglionosis ± degenerative neuropathy ± lymphocytic or eosinophilic ganglionitis ± abnormal neurochemical coding, degenerative leiomyopathy ± lymphocytic or eosinophilic leiomyositis
Morphological: increased glia, abnormal ICC network, filament protein abnormalities and polyglucosan inclusion bodies

a CIPO diagnosis: (i) a high degree of suspicion; and (ii) exclusion, with certainty, of a mechanical bowel obstruction (Rudolph *et al.*, 1997; Di Lorenzo, 1999). Stable, intermittent or long-standing symptoms of incomplete bowel obstruction are often present years before diagnosis. In two retrospective studies, mean time between symptoms onset and diagnosis ranged from 5.8 to 8 years (Mann *et al.*, 1997; Stanghellini *et al.*, 2005). A positive family history background of such disorder and presence of extra-intestinal symptoms should also alert the physician. Manometry plays a role by providing some information regarding the pathophysiological mechanism (neuropathy or myopathy), but because of its lack of specificity, the diagnosis of CIPO cannot rely only on it (Stanghellini *et al.*, 2007). Indications of full-thickness biopsies must be discussed because in clinical experience surgery may worsen the underlying disease (directly by as yet unknown mechanism or by increasing the presence of adhesions) (De Giorgio *et al.*, 2004) and the number of patients for whom specific therapy can be guided by histopathology is limited. However, with the advancement provided by minimally invasive surgery and a wide array of tests to analyse gut tissues, a histopathological diagnosis can provide valuable insight into the aetiology, pathogenesis and prognosis of some forms of gastrointestinal neuromuscular disorders (Knowles and Martin, 2011). When laparoscopy and full-thickness biopsy appears acceptable in terms of safety, it should be performed in a jejunal site to achieve a high diagnostic yield (Knowles *et al.*, 2008).

Laboratory (thyroid-stimulating hormone, autoantibodies) tests are useful to diagnose secondary forms of CIPO, with the search for ANNA-1/anti-Hu when a paraneoplastic syndrome is suspected. In the case of patients with MNGIE, lactic acid and thymidine phosphorylase should be measured and genetic testing performed.

Epidemiology

The heterogeneity of the disease and the lack of observatory study group are also factors of epidemiological uncertainty. Based on the registry of the American Pseudo-Obstruction and Hirschsprung's Society (now part of the international Foundation for Functional Gastrointestinal Disorders), prevalence in the USA is estimated to be 100 newborns per year (0.3 paediatric case per million births per year) (Di Lorenzo, 1999). These data only concern the neonatal form of CIPO. The French web registry of HPN collects data on patients with intestinal failure requiring HPN: in this database, CIPO accounts for 10% of adult and infant patients, equivalent to 0.3 patients per million per year.

Natural History

The paediatric form of CIPO is mainly present at birth or in early infancy (Vargas *et al.*, 1988; Faure *et al.*, 1999). The adult form occurs in young people (20–40 years), with more women than men (sex ratio of 2:3) (Hanks and Weber, 1981; Pitt *et al.*, 1985; Mann *et al.*, 1997; Stanghellini *et al.*, 2005; Amiot *et al.*, 2009).

Symptoms of CIPO are directly caused by ineffective propulsion and include classic signs of bowel obstruction, including nausea, vomiting, abdominal pain and/or distension, loss of weight and anorexia. Symptoms are often chronic and increase progressively with time. There seems to be no difference between symptoms at onset and at follow-up (Stanghellini *et al.*, 2005). Sometimes CIPO is revealed by an acute obstructive episode mimicking mechanical bowel obstruction, explaining futile surgery. In some cases, severe clinical forms of CIPO present with intolerance to oral intake, permanent obstruction, intractable pain and rapid loss of weight with protein–energy malnutrition and life-threatening deficiencies, requiring HPN.

Long-term outcome was generally poor despite surgical and medical therapies. Three types of complications are often reported during outcome of CIPO: (i) HPN-related complications (catheter-related sepsis, thrombosis, PN-related liver disease) (Howard and Ashley, 2003); (ii) associated disease complications (renal and urinary, cardiac, central and peripheral nervous systems); and (iii) specific complications of CIPO (dehydration, metabolic disturbances, bacterial translocation, peritonitis, gastro-oesophageal reflux disease with or without Barrett mucosa, inhaled pneumonia) (Joly *et al.*, 2006). In the literature, the rate of PN-related complications in CIPO patients does not seem to differ compared with other causes of intestinal failure. We can however expect that PN-related liver disease might develop more rapidly due to bacterial overgrowth and bacterial translocation.

HPN requirement occurs in 60–80% of infants and 20–50% of adults (Hanks and Weber, 1981; Mann *et al.*, 1997; Faure *et al.*, 1999; Mousa *et al.*, 2002; Stanghellini *et al.*, 2005). Considering infants, long-term outcome is characterized by a 10–25% mortality incidence before adulthood. In infants requiring HPN, survival and percentage of weaning are slightly better in patients with short bowel syndrome (SBS) than in patients with CIPO (Howard *et al.*, 1991; Mousa *et al.*, 2002; Colomb *et al.*, 2007; Diamanti *et al.*, 2008). Although part of the morbidity and mortality is attributable to complications of treatment, including surgery and PN, studies have revealed some factors influencing poor outcome in children and a low probability of reaching intestinal autonomy: short small bowel, exclusive PN with impossible enteral feeding, urinary tract involvement, neonatal form, acute onset of the disease, no migrating motor complex (MMC) on manometry findings and visceral myopathy (Vargas *et al.*, 1988; Faure *et al.*, 1999; Di Lorenzo and Youssef, 2010). Congenital CIPO has been also associated with increased morbidity and mortality compared with acquired forms (Huang *et al.*, 1995). In adults, clinical course, long-term outcome and prognostic factors are less known because data derive from clinical series reporting small numbers of patients with heterogeneous onset and severity of the disease. Initial reports showed a 25–30% mortality rate at early follow-up (Hanks and Weber, 1981; Vargas *et al.*, 1988). A recent review of the literature reported the survival of patients on HPN and showed that patients with SBS and CIPO have similar outcomes with a survival rate of 90% at 1 year, 70% at 5 years and 60% at 10 years (Pironi *et al.*, 2012). When considering primary disease, survival is not different except for inflammatory bowel diseases in which prognosis is better and for intestinal obstruction, associated with a decreased survival (Messing, 1995; Vantini *et al.*, 2004; Howard, 2006). The possible decrease in mortality rate achieved in the recent era probably results from improvement in overall management including nutritional support. Some prognostic factors of poor outcome have been identified: bursts, hypomotility, inadequate response to a meal on manometrical study and inability to restore oral feeding (Stanghellini *et al.*, 2007) (see Table 11.3). In a series of 51 CIPO patients, Amiot and colleagues confirmed the inability to restore oral feeding to be a negative prognostic factor, as is systemic sclerosis (Lloyd *et al.*, 2006; Brown *et al.*, 2008; Amiot *et al.*, 2009). On the contrary, age below 20 years at occurrence of symptoms was associated with better survival (Amiot *et al.*, 2009).

Nutritional Support and Overall Management

The main goals of management of CIPO are: (i) improvement of intestinal propulsion; and (ii) maintenance of adequate nutritional status including fluid and mineral balances. Indeed, as a consequence of chronic dysmotility, inadequate oral intake, increased losses (vomiting, diarrhoea) and malabsorption aggravated by chronic intestinal malfunction, malnutrition should be systematically evaluated. If treatment of bacterial overgrowth should be systematic, different modes of therapy are available according to the severity of the disease. Dietary education may be sufficient for patients with mild and moderate symptoms. If oral food intake becomes inadequate, nutritional support must be set up with enteral or parenteral nutrition.

Prokinetics

Whereas their effectiveness on clinical symptoms is poor, prokinetic drugs are systematically used in CIPO, probably because of their potential to improve digestive motility on manometry findings (Soudah *et al.*, 1991; Tack *et al.*, 1992; Quigley, 1999). Lack of effectiveness is possibly explained by the poor intestinal bioavailability of oral drugs. In some cases, combined use of prokinetics could improve

Table 11.3. Prognostic factors of poor outcome in infant and adult CIPO patients.

Absence of MMCs
Hypomotility
Bursts
Inadequate or absence of response to meal
Systemic sclerosis
Myopathy
Urinary involvement
Malrotation
Acute onset
SBS
Absence of oral feeding and need for total PN

digestive motility (Verne *et al.*, 1995). The latest to be evaluated is prucalopride, a highly specific serotonin receptor agonist with enterokinetic effects. To date, few data are available. It was recently tested in seven CIPO patients. For three of the four patients who completed the study, there was an improvement in pain but function was not changed substantially (Emmanuel *et al.*, 2012).

Bacterial overgrowth treatment

Intestinal bacterial overgrowth has often been described during digestive motility disorder (Parson *et al.*, 1969; Riordan *et al.*, 1996) and it has been shown that improvement of digestive motility reduces bacterial overgrowth (Soudah *et al.*, 1991). Sequential antibiotic therapy is very effective in treating intestinal bacterial overgrowth and to reduce malabsorption (Attar *et al.*, 1999). A correlation between bacterial translocation and absence of MMC activity has been demonstrated and can result in a worsening of digestive motility disorder (Nieuwenhuijs *et al.*, 1998). A potential life-threatening consequence of bacterial overgrowth relates to bacterial translocation (Berg, 1999; Madl and Druml, 2003). Although unabsorbable antibiotics, like rifaximin, should represent the treatment of choice, courses of other antibiotics such as metronidazole, ciprofloxacin and doxycycline may be introduced to decrease resistance (Stanghellini *et al.*, 2007).

Dietary measures

Dietary measures are influenced by disease phenotype and aim to achieve sufficient intakes of micro- and macronutrients orally (Scolapio *et al.*, 1999). Patients with gastroparesis usually have lowering of oral intake and early satiety whereas patients with predominantly small bowel involvement often suffer nausea, abdominal pain and diarrhoea. In people with decrease of gastric emptying, liquid or blended food is better tolerated than solid food (Camilleri and Phillips, 1991). Oral intake should also be fractionated and divided into five or six meals per day. Dietary measures also include the use of a low-lactose, low-fibre, low-fat diet in order to optimize gut motility and decrease the risk of bacterial overgrowth and gastric bezoar. Associated multivitamin and micronutrient supplementation is also needed (iron, folate, calcium and vitamins D, K and B_{12}) in order to prevent specific deficiencies (Smith *et al.*, 2003).

Enteral nutrition

Enteral feeding by ostomy is a potential effective method of nutritional support, which could be used despite oral feeding intolerance. However, it should be used carefully with iso-osmolar nutrients at a slow, continuous infusion rate to prevent poor tolerance and enteral nutrition-related pneumonia. If the trial period is positive, infusion rate and volume of infusion can be increased progressively. Ostomy could be also helpful for venting procedures.

Parenteral nutrition

HPN is necessary in severe CIPO patients in whom other supportive methods have failed (Messing and Joly, 2006). Because of higher cost, morbidity and mortality and the low probability of weaning off HPN, it should not be started before an oral and/or enteral nutrition trial (Smith *et al.*, 2003). Specificities of HPN in CIPO patients related to chronic bowel obstruction and lowering of oral intake are as follows:

- Higher fluid volume requirement to prevent dehydration, especially in the case of refractory vomiting or permanent suction ostomy. Fluid volume requirement must also be adapted in real time because of frequent and variable increased digestive losses (diarrhoea, vomiting). The same is true for hydroelectrolytic adaptation, especially for maintenance of sodium, potassium and magnesium balances.
- Higher number of weekly infusions, six or seven per week versus four or five for SBS (unpublished personal data).
- To prevent PN-related liver disease, especially in exclusive HPN (patients with intractable obstruction), lipid parenteral intake should be limited (e.g. minimal intake to prevent fatty acid deficiency).
- Micronutrient and vitamin supplements (selenium, vitamins B_1, B_6 and E) should be given and adapted during regular nutritional surveys.
- Necessity to maintain minimal oral feeding in order to: (i) reduce parenteral caloric needs; and (ii) prevent complications of exclusive HPN (bacterial translocation, liver disease, biliary complication and partial intestinal villi atrophy, especially induced by bacterial overgrowth).
- Mitochondrial cytopathies could require specific vitamin supplementation, e.g. coenzyme Q_{10}, ubiquinone or its synthetic variant, idebenone (Geromel *et al.*, 2002).

Surgical procedures

Surgical intervention often occurs before and/or during CIPO management with about three procedures per patient (Hanks and Weber, 1981; Mann *et al.*, 1997; Stanghellini *et al.*, 2005; Amiot *et al.*, 2009). Surgery cannot be curative, so it must be limited to the refractory presentation of CIPO with only selected indications. The most common and efficient surgical procedure consists of venting or feeding ostomy (Pitt *et al.*, 1985). Venting ostomies decrease the frequency of admission for acute obstructive symptoms and the frequency of vomiting, and also prevent abdominal pain and retching in patients who have undergone antireflux surgery. Besides, gastrointestinal motility may improve as the bowel becomes less dilated (Di Lorenzo, 1999). Furthermore, a combined nasogastric-nasojejunal tube is available that allows simultaneous gastric suction and jejunal infusion (Patrick *et al.*, 1997). Explorative laparotomy could be done for viscerolysis in cases of suspicion of mechanical bowel obstruction caused by previous laparotomy. In those cases, full-thickness biopsy or limited small bowel resection during the surgical procedure could be realized for full histopathological examination. Bowel resection or surgical bypass must be considered with great caution. Few patients with a documented isolated diseased segment can benefit from this kind of procedure (Murr *et al.*, 1995). On the contrary, extant CIPO disease does not benefit and patients often experience peri-operative complications. In a few cases, patients with CIPO non-responsive to maximal medical and surgical therapy, and with complications such as dehydration or severe intestinal translocation, benefit from subtotal bowel resection (Schuffler *et al.*, 1985; Mughal and Irving, 1988; Joly *et al.*, 2003; Lapointe, 2010) or intestinal transplantation (Buchman *et al.*, 2003; Masetti *et al.*, 2004; Blondon *et al.*, 2005; Grant *et al.*, 2005). In cases of subtotal resection, best results have been reported with jejunocolonic anastomosis whereas preservation of a small length of ileum seemed to expose the patient to post-operative recurrence of obstruction (Lapointe, 2010). Intestinal transplantation has become a life-saving procedure for patients with irreversible intestinal failure. The indications are defined as: (i) life-threatening complications of HPN; (ii) lack of venous access for HPN; (iii) chronic intestinal failure with a high risk of mortality; and (iv) primary disease-related poor quality of life despite optimal HPN. More than 1800 intestinal transplantations have been performed (40% in adult patients) in the last 10 years (Smith *et al.*, 2013). Thirteen per cent of adult patients suffering from intestinal failure due to CIPO were transplanted (Smith *et al.*, 2013). Because of the extent of the digestive malfunction, multivisceral transplantation may be indicated. Mangus *et al.* reported their experience of 100 multivisceral transplants between 2004 and 2010. In this work, indications of multivisceral transplantation included intestinal failure alone, intestinal failure with cirrhosis, complete portal mesenteric thrombosis, slow-growing central abdominal tumours, intestinal pseudo-obstruction and frozen abdomen. Multivisceral transplantations were often performed with a 1-year patient and graft survival (approximately 72% and 70%) relatively similar to that in isolated small bowel transplantation or combined liver and small bowel transplantation performed for other indications (intestinal failure due to short bowel) (Mangus *et al.*, 2013). In a series of 376 patients transplanted between 1990 and 2006, CIPO patients represented 15% of the indications for transplantation. Five-year survival rate was not different from that observed for other indications (Abu-Elmagd *et al.*, 2012). Multivisceral transplantation should be considered in adult patients suffering from CIPO and PN life-threatening complications.

Summary

CIPO is an important indication for HPN in both adults and children. CIPO refers to a heterogeneous group of disorders (Table 11.1) characterized by symptoms of intestinal obstruction in the absence of mechanical evidence of obstruction. It is caused by ineffective intestinal contractions. CIPO may be classified as either a primary disease, usually limited to the hollow viscera, or a secondary disease, associated with an existing systemic disorder. CIPO may predominate as a 'total' gut disease from oesophagus to anal sphincter or as a 'localized' disease, which is gastric and intestinal or intestinal alone; segmental gut disease is not the rule, with the exception of an isolated megaduodenum.

Recurrent episodes of obstruction follow the usual clinical presentation, together with malabsorptive diarrhoea; pseudo-CIPO may also be the case, i.e. malabsorptive diarrhoea without obvious obstruction.

Besides nutritional support, symptomatic treatment usually consists of prokinetic drugs, such as low doses of octreotide and erythromycin. In the case of a systemic disease causing CIPO, specific treatments are also the cornerstone here, such as, for example, in systemic lupus erythematosus.

The most severe forms may require ostomy for nutrition and/or decompression. Otherwise, surgery should be avoided with the exception of surgical complications associated with CIPO, such as peritonitis due to perforation (with or without diverticula) or bowel ischaemia. Patients severely affected by CIPO with an intestinal 'functional' insufficiency, especially those affected by diffuse forms of the disease, may need long-term HPN. In the latter case, when there is a failure of HPN, alternative treatment such as extensive resection or intestinal transplantation should be discussed case by case in an intestinal tertiary care centre.

References

Abu-Elmagd, K.M., Kosmach-Park, B., Costa, G., Zenati, M., Martin, L., Koritsky, D.A., Emerling, M., Murase, N., Bond, G.J., Soltys, K., Sogawa, H., Lunz, J., Al Samman, M., Shaefer, N., Sindhi, R. and Mazariegos, G.V. (2012) Long-term survival, nutritional autonomy, and quality of life after intestinal and multivisceral transplantation. *Annals of Surgery* 256, 494–508.

Amiot, A., Joly, F., Alves, A., Panis, Y., Bouhnik, Y. and Messing, B. (2009) Long-term outcome of chronic intestinal pseudo-obstruction adult patients requiring home parenteral nutrition. *American Journal of Gastroenterology* 104, 1262–1270.

Attar, A., Flourie, B., Rambaud, J.C., Franchisseur, C., Ruszniewski, P. and Bouhnik, Y. (1999) Antibiotic efficacy in small intestinal bacterial overgrowth-related chronic diarrhoea: a crossover, randomized trial. *Gastroenterology* 117, 794–797.

Berg, R.D. (1999) Bacterial translocation from the gastrointestinal tract. *Advances in Experimental Medicine and Biology* 473, 11–30.

Blondon, H., Polivka, M., Joly, F., Flourie, B., Mikol, J. and Messing, B. (2005) Digestive smooth muscle mitochondrial myopathy in patients with mitochondrial-neuro-gastro-intestinal encephalomyopthy (MNGIE). *Gastroentérologie Clinique et Biologique* 29, 773–778.

Brown, M., Teubner, A., Shaffer, J. and Herrick, A.L. (2008) Home parenteral nutrition – an effective and safe long-term therapy for systemic sclerosis-related intestinal failure. *Rheumatology (Oxford)* 47, 176–179.

Buchman, A.L., Scolapio, J. and Fryer, J. (2003) AGA technical review on short bowel syndrome and intestinal transplantation. *Gastroenterology* 124, 1111–1134.

Camilleri, M. and Phillips, S.F. (1991) Acute and chronic intestinal pseudo-obstruction. *Advances in Internal Medicine* 36, 287–306.

Colomb, V., Dabbas-Tyan, M., Taupin, P., Talbotec, C., Revillon, Y., Jan, D., De Potter, S., Gorski-Colin, A.M., Lamor, M., Herreman, K., Corriol, O., Landais, P., Ricour, C. and Goulet, O. (2007) Long-term outcome of children receiving home parenteral nutrition: a 20-year single-center experience in 302 patients. *Journal of Pediatric Gastroenterology and Nutrition* 44, 347–353.

Connor, F.L. and Di Lorenzo, C. (2006) Chronic intestinal pseudo-obstruction: assessment and management. *Gastroenterology* 130, 29–36.

De Giorgio, R., Sarnelli, G., Corinaldesi, R. and Stanghellini, V. (2004) Advances in our understanding of the pathology of chronic intestinal pseudo-obstruction. *Gut* 53, 1549–1552.

De Giorgio, R., Ricciardiello, L., Naponelli, V., Selgrad, M., Piazzi, G., Felicani, C., Serra, M., Fronzoni, L., Antonucci, A., Cogliandro, R.F., Tonini, M., Knowles, C.H. and Stanghellini, V. (2010) Chronic intestinal pseudo-obstruction related to viral infections. *Transplantation Proceedings* 42, 9–14.

Diamanti, A., Basso, M.S., Castro, M., Di Ciommo, V., Bracci, F., Ferretti, F., Pietrobattista, A. and Gambarara, M. (2008) Irreversible intestinal failure: prevalence and prognostic factors. *Journal of Pediatric Gastroenterology and Nutrition* 47, 450–457.

Di Lorenzo, C. (1999) Pseudo-obstruction: current approaches. *Gastroenterology* 116, 980–987.

Di Lorenzo, C. and Youssef, N.N. (2010) Diagnosis and management of intestinal motility disorders. *Seminars in Pediatric Surgery* 19, 50–58.

Di Nardo, G., Blandizzi, C., Volta, U., Colucci, R., Stanghellini, V., Barbara, G., Del Tacca, M., Tonini, M., Corinaldesi, R. and De Giorgio, R. (2008) Review article: molecular, pathological and therapeutic features of human enteric neuropathies. *Alimentary Pharmacology & Therapeutics* 28, 25–42.

Emmanuel, A.V., Kamm, M.A., Roy, A.J., Kerstens, R. and Vandeplassche, L. (2012) Randomised clinical trial: the efficacy of prucalopride in patients with chronic intestinal pseudo-obstruction – a double-blind, placebo-controlled, cross-over, multiple n=1 study. *Alimentary Pharmacology & Therapeutics* 35, 48–55.

Faure, C., Goulet, O., Ategbo, S., Brenton, A., Tounian, P., Ginies, J.L., Roquelaure, B., Despres, C., Scaillon, M., Maurage, C., Paquot, I., Hermier, M., De Napolis, S., Dabadie, A., Huet, F., Baudon, J.J., Larchet, M. and French-speaking Group of Pediatric Gastroenerology (1999) Chronic intestinal pseudo-obstruction syndrome: clinical analysis, outcome, and prognosis in 105 children. *Digestive Diseases and Sciences* 44, 953–959.

Feldstein, A.E., Miller, S.M., El-Youssef, M., Rodeberg, D., Lindor, N.M., Burgart, L.J., Szurszewski, J.H. and Farrugia, G. (2003) Chronic intestinal pseudo-obstruction associated with altered interstitial cells of Cajal networks. *Journal of Pediatric Gastroenterology and Nutrition* 36, 492–497.

Geromel, V., Darin, N., Chrétien, D., Bénit, P., DeLonlay, P., Rötig, A., Munnich, A. and Rustin, P. (2002) Coenzyme Q_{10} and idebenone in the therapy of respiratory chain diseases: rationale and comparative benefits. *Molecular Genetics and Metabolism* 77, 21–30.

Goyal, R.K. and Hirano, I. (1998) The enteric nervous system. *New England Journal of Medicine* 334, 1106–1115.

Grant, D., Abu-Elmagd, K., Reyes, J., Tzakis, A., Langnas, A., Fishbein, T., Goulet, O., Farmer, D. and on behalf of the Intestine Transplant Registry (2005) 2003 report of the intestine transplant registry: a new era has dawned. *Annals of Surgery* 241, 607–613.

Hanks, J.B. and Weber, W.B. (1981) Chronic primary intestinal pseudo-obstruction. *Surgery* 89, 175–182.

Howard, L. (2006) Home parenteral nutrition: survival, cost, and quality of life. *Gastroenterology* 130, 52–59.

Howard, L. and Ashley, C. (2003) Management of complications in patients receiving home parenteral nutrition. *Gastroenterology* 124, 1651–1661.

Howard, L., Heaphey, L., Fleming, C.R., Lininger, L. and Steiger, E. (1991) Four years of North American registry home parenteral nutrition outcome data and their implications for patient management. *JPEN Journal of Parenteral and Enteral Nutrition* 15, 384–393.

Huang, Y.C., Lee, H.C., Huang, F.Y., Kao, H.A., Yeh, M.L., Chang, P.Y., Sheu, J.C., Shih, S.L. and Chen, B.F. (1995) Neonatal onset of chronic intestinal pseudo-obstruction syndrome. *Clinical Pediatrics* 34, 241–247.

Isozaki, K., Hirota, S., Miyagawa, J., Taniguchi, M., Shinomura, Y. and Matsuzawa, Y. (1997) Deficiency of c-kit+ cells in patients with a myopathic form of chronic idiopathic intestinal pseudo-obstruction. *American Journal of Gastroenterology* 92, 332–334.

Joly, F., Zeballos, J., Benoist, S., Lavergne, A., Panis, Y., Mikol, J., Valleur, P. and Messing, B. (2003) Subtotal small bowel resection (SBR) in chronic intestinal pseudo-obstruction (CIPO) refractory to treatment. *Clinical Nutrition* 22, 56–57.

Joly, F., Amiot, A., Coffin, B., Lavergne-Slove, A., Messing, B. and Bouhnik, Y. (2006) Chronic intestinal pseudo-obstruction. *Gastroentérologie Clinique et Biologique* 30, 975–985.

Knowles, C.H. and Martin, J.E. (2011) Enteric neuromuscular pathology update. *Gastroenterology Clinics of North America* 40, 695–713.

Knowles, C.H., Veress, B., Tornblom, H., Wallace, S., Paraskeva, P., Darzi, A., Martin, J.E., Nyberg, B. and Lindberg, G. (2008) Safety and diagnostic yield of laparoscopically assisted full-thickness bowel biospy. *Neurogastroenterology and Motility* 20, 774–779.

Knowles, C.H., De Giorgio, R., Kapur, R.P., Bruder, E., Farrugia, G., Geboes, K., Lindberg, G., Martin, J.E., Meier-Ruge, W.A., Milla, P.J., *et al.* (2010) The London Classification of gastrointestinal neuromuscular pathology: report on behalf of the Gastro 2009 International Working Group. *Gut* 59, 882–887.

Krishnamurthy, S. and Schuffler, M.D. (1987) Pathology of neuromuscular disorders of the small intestine and colon. *Gastroenterology* 93, 610–639.

Lapointe, R. (2010) Chronic idiopathic intestinal pseudo-obstruction treated by near total small bowel resection: a 20-year experience. *Journal of Gastrointestinal Surgery* 14, 1937–1942.

Lee, J.C., Thuneberg, L., Berezin, I. and Huizinga, J.D. (1999) Generation of slow waves in membrane potential is an intrinsic property of interstitial cells of Cajal. *American Journal of Physiology* 277, 409–423.

Lloyd, D.A., Vega, R., Bassett, P., Forbes, A. and Gabe, S.M. (2006) Survival and dependence on home parenteral nutrition: experience over a 25-year period in a UK referral centre. *Alimentary Pharmacology & Therapeutics* 24, 1231–1240.

Madl, C. and Druml, W. (2003) Gastrointestinal disorders of the critically ill. Systemic consequences of ileus. *Best Practice & Research. Clinical Gastroenterology* 17, 445–456.

Mangus, R.S., Tector, A.J., Kubal, C.A., Fridell, J.A. and Vianna, R.M. (2013) Multivisceral transplantation: expanding indications and improving outcomes. *Journal of Gastrointestinal Surgery* 17, 179.

Mann, S.D., Debinski, H.S. and Kamm, M.A. (1997) Clinical characteristics of chronic idiopathic intestinal pseudo-obstruction in adults. *Gut* 41, 675–681.

Masetti, M., Di Benedetto, F., Cautero, N., Stangghellini, V., De Giorgio, R., Lauro, A., Begliomini, B., Siniscalchi, A., Pironi, L., Cogliandro, R. and Pinna, A.D. (2004) Intestinal transplantation for chronic intestinal pseudo-obstruction in adult patients. *American Journal of Transplantation* 4, 826–829.

Messing, B. (1995) Long-term outcome and quality of life of adult patients on home parenteral nutrition. *Clinical Nutrition* 14, 24–27.

Messing, B. and Joly, F. (2006) Guidelines for management of home parenteral adult chronic intestinal failure patients. *Gastroenterology* 130, 43–51.

Mousa, H., Hyman, P.E., Cocjin, J., Flores, A.F. and Di Lorenzo, C. (2002) Long-term outcome of congenital intestinal pseudo-obstruction. *Digestive Diseases and Sciences* 47, 2298–2305.

Mughal, M.M. and Irving, M.H. (1988) Treatment of end stage chronic intestinal pseudo-obstruction by subtotal enterectomy and home parenteral nutrition. *Gut* 29, 1613–1617.

Murr, M.M., Sarr, M.G. and Camilleri, M. (1995) The surgeon's role in the treatment of chronic intestinal pseudo-obstruction. *American Journal of Gastroenterology* 90, 2147–2151.

Nieuwenhuijs, V.B., Verheem, A., van Duijvenbode-Beumer, H., Visser, M.R., Verhoef, J., Gooszen, H.G. and Akkermans, L.M. (1998) The role of interdigestive small bowel motility in the regulation of gut microflora, bacterial overgrowth, and bacterial translocation in rats. *Annals of Surgery* 228, 188–193.

Parson, A.J., Brzechwa-Ajdukiewicz, A. and McCarthy, C.F. (1969) Intestinal pseudo-obstruction with bacterial overgrowth in the small intestine. *American Journal of Digestive Diseases* 14, 200–205.

Patrick, P.G., Marulendra, S., Kirby, D.F. and Delegge, M.H. (1997) Endoscopic naso-gastric-jejunal feeding tube placement in critically ill patients. *Gastrointestinal Endoscopy* 45, 72–76.

Pironi, L., Goulet, O., Buchman, A., Messing, B., Gabe, S., Candusso, M., Bond, G., Gupte, G., Pertkiewicz, M., Steiger, E., Forbes, A., Van Gossum, A. and Pinna, A.D. (2012) Outcome on home parenteral nutrition for benign intestinal failure: a review of the literature and benchmarking with the European prospective survey of ESPEN. *Clinical Nutrition* 31, 831–845.

Pitt, H.A., Mann, L.L., Berquist, W.E., Ament, M.E., Fonkalsrud, E.W. and DenBesten, L. (1985) Chronic intestinal pseudo-obstruction. Management with total parenteral nutrition and a venting enterostomy. *Archives of Surgery* 120, 614–618.

Quigley, E.M. (1999) Chronic intestinal pseudo-obstruction. *Current Treatment Options in Gastroenterology* 2, 239–250.

Riordan, S.M., McIver, C.J., Walker, B.M., Duncombe, V.M., Bolin, T.D. and Thomas, M.C. (1996) Bacteriological method for detecting small intestinal hypomotility. *American Journal of Gastroenterology* 91, 2399–2405.

Rudolph, C.D., Hyman, P.E., Altschuler, S.M., Christensen, J., Colletti, R.B., Cucchiara, S., Di Lorenzo, C., Flores, A.F., Hillemeier, A.C., McCallum, R.W. and Vanderhoof, J.A. (1997) Diagnosis and treatment of chronic intestinal pseudo-obstruction in children: report of consensus workshop. *Journal of Pediatric Gastroenterology and Nutrition* 24, 102–112.

Schuffler, M.D., Rohrmann, C.A., Chaffee, R.G., Brand, D.L., Delaney, J.H. and Young, J.H. (1981) Chronic intestinal pseudo-obstruction. A report of 27 cases and review of the literature. *Medicine (Baltimore)* 60, 173–196.

Schuffler, M.D., Leon, S.H. and Krishnamurthy, S. (1985) Intestinal pseudo-obstruction caused by a new form of visceral neuropathy: palliation by radical small bowel resection. *Gastroenterology* 89, 1152–1156.

Scolapio, J.S., Ukleja, A., Bouras, E.P. and Romano, M. (1999) Nutritional management of chronic intestinal pseudo-obstruction. *Journal of Clinical Gastroenterology* 28, 306–312.

Selgrad, M., De Giorgio, R., Fini, L., Cogliandro, R.F., Williams, S., Stanghellini, V., Barbara, G., Tonini, M., Corinaldesi, R., Genta, R.M., Domiati-Saad, R., Meyer, R., Goel, A., Boland, C.R. and Ricciardiello, L. (2009) JC virus infects the enteric glia of patients with chronic idiopathic intestinal pseudo-obstruction. *Gut* 58, 25–32.

Smith, D.S., Williams, C.S. and Ferris, C.D. (2003) Diagnosis and treatment of chronic gastroparesis and chronic intestinal pseudo-obstruction. *Gastroenterology Clinics of North America* 32, 619–658.

Smith, J.M., Skeans, M.A., Thompson, B., Horslen, SP., Edwards, E.B., Harper, A.M., Snyder, J.J., Israni, A.K. and Kasiske, B.L. (2013) OPTN/SRTR 2011 Annual Data Report: intestine. *American Journal of Transplantation* 13, 103–118.

Soudah, H.C., Hasler, W.L. and Owyang, C. (1991) Effect of octreotide on intestinal motility and bacterial overgrowth in scleroderma. *New England Journal of Medicine* 325, 1461–1467.

Stanghellini, V., Camilleri, M. and Malagelada, J.R. (1987) Chronic idiopathic intestinal pseudo-obstruction: clinical and intestinal manometric findings. *Gut* 28, 5–12.

Stanghellini, V., Cogliandro, R.F., De Giorgio, R., Barbara, G., Morselli-Labate, A.M., Cogliandro, L. and Corinaldesi, R. (2005) Natural history of chronic idiopathic intestinal pseudo-obstruction in adults: a single center study. *Clinical Gastroenterology and Hepatology* 3, 449–458.

Stanghellini, V., Cogliandro, R.F., De Giorgio, R., Barbara, G., Salvioli, B. and Corinaldesi, R. (2007) Chronic intestinal pseudo-obstruction: manifestations, natural history and management. *Neurogastroenterology and Motility* 19, 440–452.

Tack, J., Janssens, J., Vantrappen, G., Peeters, T., Annese, V., Depoortere, I., Muls, E. and Bouillon, R. (1992) Effect of erythromycin on gastric motility in controls and in diabetic gastroparesis. *Gastroenterology* 103, 72–79.

Thomsen, L., Robinson, T.L., Lee, J.C., Farraway, L.A., Hughes, M.J., Andrews, D.W. and Huizinga, J.D. (1998) Interstitial cells of Cajal generate a rhythmic pacemaker current. *Nature Medicine* 4, 848–851.

Vantini, I., Benini, L., Bonfante, F., Talamini, G., Sembenini, C., Chiarioni, G., Maragnolli, O., Benini, F. and Capra, F. (2004) Survival rate and prognostic factors in patients with intestinal failure. *Digestive and Liver Disease* 36, 46–55.

Vargas, J.H., Sachs, P. and Ament, M.E. (1988) Chronic intestinal pseudo-obstruction syndrome in paediatrics: results of a national survey by members of the North American Society of Gastroenterology and Nutrition. *Journal of Pediatric Gastroenterology and Nutrition* 7, 323–332.

Verne, G.N., Eaker, E.Y., Hardy, E. and Sninsky, C.A. (1995) Effect of octreotide and erythromycin on idiopathic and scleroderma-associated intestinal pseudo-obstruction. *Digestive Diseases and Sciences* 40, 1892–1901.

Wood, J.D. (2002) Neural and humoral regulation of gastrointestinal motility. In: Schuster, M.M., Crowell, M.D. and Koch, K.L. (eds) *Gastrointestinal Motility in Health and Disease.* BC Deckey, London, pp. 19–42.

12 Radiation Enteropathy

Federico Bozzetti*

Faculty of Medicine, University of Milan, Milan, Italy

Key Points

- Radiation enteropathy (RE) may require home parenteral nutrition (HPN) in subacute conditions since a prolonged period of bowel rest can allow a regression of the lesions and lead to an improvement of bowel function.
- In chronic RE, long-term HPN represents a life-saving procedure because of the irreversible intestinal failure due to either the disease or the consequences of surgical complications.
- The final outcome for patients on HPN for RE depends both on the potential complications of long-term parenteral nutrition and the progressive damage to other (neurological, urological, bony, etc.) structures included in the radiation field. Furthermore, the presence of occult tumour relapses within the peritoneum and retroperitoneum in patients undergoing multiple surgical procedures may be difficult to identify and can cause late cancer mortality.

Introduction

Within 2 years of Roentgen's discovery of ionizing radiation in 1895, the detrimental effects of radiation on the gastrointestinal tract were described (Walsh, 1897). The effect of photons is due to the interaction of the electromagnetic waves with normal tissues through the production of electrons, which combine with cell water and induce the formation of hydroxyl radicals. These radicals cause cell death through single or double DNA breaks and through interaction with the cell membrane. Cells are most vulnerable to the killing effect of radiation during the G2 and M phases and consequently rapidly proliferating tissues, such

*E-mail: federicobozzetti@gmail.com

as small intestine crypt cells, are particularly sensitive to radiation: they undergo apoptosis and are shed from the intestinal villus. Furthermore, ionizing radiation activates translation of the gene coding for transforming growth factor-β, a multifunctional peptide growth factor that acts as a potent fibrogenic and pro-inflammatory cytokine. Transforming growth factor-β promotes fibrosis by stimulating the expression of collagen and fibronectin genes and the chemotaxis of fibroblasts, and it also inhibits the degradation of the extracellular matrix. Chemotherapy increases the sensitivity of non-cancerous tissues to damage from radiotherapy.

Histopathologically, the damage from radiation enteropathy (RE) initially involves mucosa, which suffers cellular devitalization, and submucosa, which becomes oedematous, but subsequently is characterized by diffuse collagen deposition and progressive occlusive vasculitis. The fibrosis and vasculitis progress over time and result in narrowing of the intestinal loops with dilation of the bowel proximal to the stricture, which then thickens the affected segments of intestine and serosa. Severe stenosis, ulceration, necrosis and perforation of the intestinal wall may sometimes occur.

The clinical scenario of RE encompasses nausea, vomiting, abdominal cramps and watery, blood-tinged diarrhoea, which are all present in the acute phase of RE. They are also concurrent with the treatment and may last days or weeks, but usually reverse spontaneously after a few weeks to the more dramatic picture of the chronic and established RE. This appears several months, years or decades after the radiation therapy, and is characterized by intestinal obstruction, perforation and bleeding which require hospitalization and, sometimes, surgery. Between these two types of RE there is a subacute type that appears clinically within 3–18 months after completion of radiation therapy (Schier *et al.*, 1964), and it may progress for several years or even regress and/or exhibit long periods of quiescence. It is argued that the introduction of new chemotherapies, biological agents and more targeted radiotherapy techniques over the last two decades will diminish toxicity rates, but the long-term effects of these new cancer treatments are unknown. For instance, the experience with the technique of imaging modulated radiotherapy is still in its infancy and one possibility is that this technique changes only the timing and spectrum of toxicity.

The Radiation-Therapy Oncology Group and the European Organisation for Research and Treatment of Cancer (RTOG) proposed in 1991 (Trott and Herrmann, 1991) criteria for scoring the radiation morbidity of irradiation of the lower gastrointestinal tract and pelvis, which is reported in Table 12.1.

Whereas the prevalence of acute RE is difficult to estimate because of the large variety of radiation plans and chemotherapy schedules, the frequency of subacute and chronic RE is better known. However, the mildest types may escape the radiologist, whereas the later and more severe types occur years after the end of radiation therapy and patients may then be admitted to other institutions or undergo emergency surgery.

The prevalence of RE has increased in recent years because of the use of radiation as a part of a multi-disciplinary approach to cancer (Galland and Spencer, 1987). Usually quoted data vary between 0.5 and 16.9% of patients undergoing radiation therapy (Shamblin *et al.*, 1964; Poddar *et al.*, 1982; Harling and

Table 12.1. Radiation morbidity scoring criteria for the lower gastrointestinal tract including pelvis.

Score	Criteria
0	No change
1	Increased frequency or change in quality of bowel habits not requiring medication; rectal discomfort not requiring analgesics
2	Diarrhoea requiring parasympatholytic drugs (e.g. Lomotil); mucous discharge not necessitating sanitary pads; rectal or abdominal pain requiring analgesics
3	Diarrhoea requiring parenteral support; severe mucous or blood discharge necessitating sanitary pads; abdominal distension (flat-plate radiograph demonstrates distended bowel loops)
4	Acute or subacute obstruction, fistula or perforation; gastrointestinal bleeding requiring transfusion; abdominal pain or tenesmus requiring tube decompression or bowel diversion

Balslev, 1988). An investigation on the prevalence of severe ileitis, defined as a 'requiring surgery' complication, performed at the Institute of Radiological Sciences of the University of Milan (Cerrotta *et al.*, 1995) showed that such a complication occurred in 7.3% out of 191 patients within a mean period of 23 months (range 4–87 months) after receiving standard adjuvant post-operative radiation therapy following a radical resection of rectal cancer. A more recent paper that included 164 patients receiving adjuvant radiotherapy for cervical cancer reported that after a median follow-up of 60 months (range 38–119 months), 22 (13.4%) patients had developed an RTOG grade 2 radiation injury to the intestine, four had a grade 3 complication requiring surgery and three had died (Chen *et al.*, 2004).

Risk Factors

There are several factors that increase the risk of RE; they can be divided into patient-related and therapy-related (Table 12.2). The concurrent addition of chemotherapeutic agents to radiation therapy may also increase the rate of acute intestinal toxicity, although whether this may also lead to chronic radiation enteritis is still unclear. In a recent study (Gérard *et al.*, 2006) on 733 patients randomized to receive pre-operative radiotherapy or chemoradiotherapy using fluorouracil and leucovorin, the acute toxicity rate increased from 2.2% after radiotherapy alone to 13.5% after the addition of chemotherapy. Bosset *et al.* (2006) reported in 1011 patients with T3–4 resectable rectal cancer that pre-operative radiotherapy was associated with acute diarrhoea in 17.3% of patients and rose to 37.6% with concurrent use of fluorouracil without any increase in the late gastrointestinal toxicity. In keeping with these data a systematic review of trials comparing chemoradiation with radiation alone in patients with locally advanced cervical cancer concluded that, although combined treatment resulted in a twofold increase in acute gastrointestinal toxicity, this was not associated with an increase in late gastrointestinal adverse effects (Kirwan *et al.*, 2003).

Table 12.2. Risk factors associated with chronic RE.

Patient factors	Treatment factors
Reduced body mass index	Previous abdominal surgery
Smoking	Volume of small bowel in radiotherapy field
Co-morbidities (e.g. diabetes mellitus, hypertension, inflammatory bowel, collagen vascular disease)	Dose
	Fractioning
	Concurrent chemotherapy
	Radiotherapy technique

The type of chemotherapy used may affect the severity of small bowel toxicity. In patients with locally advanced cervical cancer treated with chemoradiation, the addition of mitomycin to fluorouracil alone increased late intestinal toxicity from 10 to 26% (Rakovitch *et al.*, 1997).

Preliminary data from phase I and II trials for advanced rectal cancer have shown that the addition of newer agents, such as oxaliplatin and irinotecan, to chemoradiotherapy with fluorouracil is associated with a higher frequency of acute diarrhoea; moreover, it would seem that late toxicity is increased with irinotecan (Mohiuddin *et al.*, 2006; Ryan *et al.*, 2006).

Natural History of RE and Frequency of HPN

The natural history of chronic RE is that of a progressive and relentless disease with further complications becoming apparent in about half of those surviving the initial lesion: 5% of patients finally require surgery (Galland and Spencer, 1987) and 10–25% die either as a direct result of the injury or as a result of complications from surgery to correct it (De Cosse *et al.*, 1969; Russell and Welch, 1979). Galland and Spencer (1985) followed 70 patients who presented to a surgical unit with RE appearing after an average interval of 2 years since radiation therapy; none of them received HPN, median survival was about 2.5 years and 5-year survival was 42%. It is noteworthy that RE accounted for 62% of the deaths, directly (1/3) or indirectly (2/3) as consequence of a surgical complication. A recent study has reported that moderate sustained acute (cumulative) toxicity might predict severe late effects better than peak reaction (Wedlake *et al.*, 2010).

HPN is never used in acute RE because these patients are parenterally fed in hospital for a few weeks, the time necessary for the acute phase to subside. In the past, however, patients were erroneously explored and resected to try and change a transient, reversible, acute condition and this resulted in chronic intestinal failure, which then required permanent HPN.

The first attempts to keep alive patients with intestinal failure due to RE, through HPN, date back to the pioneers of HPN (Broviac and Scribner, 1974). Results from this first small series of patients were published by the University of Washington in Seattle (Miller *et al.*, 1979) followed by the Cleveland Clinic (Lavery *et al.*, 1980).

Reports from databases or registers from different countries show that RE accounts for a percentage ranging from 4–6% in Canada (Detsky *et al.*, 1986), the USA (Howard *et al.*, 1991, 1995) and the UK (Mughal and Irving, 1986), to 13% and 21% in Europe (Messing *et al.*, 1989) and France (Messing *et al.*, 1988). The British Artificial Nutrition Survey has shown that chronic radiation enteritis accounts for 4.1% of all patients currently receiving HPN (Jones *et al.*, 2007). The multicentre survey in Europe in 1993 (Van Gossum *et al.*, 1996) reported that RE accounted for 8% of underlying diseases among patients receiving HPN, with Spain, France and Belgium registering the highest number of patients.

The percentage of new patients receiving HPN for RE appears to have decreased over the past several years (Howard, 1993), which is probably due to the improved radiation field delivery and improved surgical treatment.

Indications for HPN

Patients candidate for HPN are those affected by chronic sub-obstruction, pain caused by oral/enteral nutrition, long-standing wasting or, frequently, a combination of these factors. Moreover, a common indication is the intestinal failure consequent to extensive surgical resections that result in small bowel syndrome or are followed by severe post-operative complications. For these reasons, the potential indications for surgery, HPN or both in patients affected by RE should be considered and discussed together with the patient.

As a general rule, patients with acute RE should never be submitted to surgery; symptoms usually subside with time and intravenous fluids/nutrition can be provided for a limited period of bowel rest. On the contrary, patients affected by complicated chronic RE are almost always candidates for surgery because obstruction or stenoses are by this time irreversible and one cannot expect bleeding, perforation or obstruction to resolve spontaneously. However, if the injury to the gut is widespread or if an extensive small bowel resection is required, patients will usually need long-term HPN if they are to survive.

A more flexible approach is required for patients with a subacute RE. Every effort should be made to determine whether the RE is localized or diffuse while the patient is still receiving a short course of total parenteral nutrition (TPN). The diagnostic work-up includes a plain X-ray of the abdomen and a contrast X-ray study (if possible) of the small bowel, a colonoscopy and an abdominal computed tomography scan. A careful evaluation of patients' symptoms and their association with the oral intake of nutrients is also crucial for a proper assessment of the extent of the disease. Quite often the enteropathy is more diffuse than one expects.

If RE is limited (usually confined to distal ileum because loops of the small intestine are trapped in the pelvis during radiotherapy) and there is no improvement (or there is a rapid relapse) of symptoms after a short course of TPN and medical therapy, the patient is a candidate for resective or bypass surgery.

The problem is much more complex when RE involves long tracts of the small bowel or compromises the intestinal motility of a large part of the jejunum and ileum. Husebye *et al.* (1994) have shown that late RE is characterized by impaired fasting motility and attenuated postprandial motor response after a meal. This dysfunction of intestinal motility is typical of intestinal pseudo-obstruction, a condition characterized by the absence of structural luminal occlusion and due to the presence of adynamic intestinal segments acting as functional stenoses (Conklin and Anuras, 1981).

In such conditions one should persevere with TPN as long as possible because the only role of surgery is the removal of large parts of the gut to relieve a state of permanent obstruction with a high chance to finally have a short bowel associated or not with a stoma. Therefore if symptoms subside, one should consider a long period (several months) of HPN. Only if symptoms do not subside, or recur quickly when enteral nutrition is resumed after a long period of HPN, should surgery be considered. In fact, since the patient is already on HPN, the inability of surgery to solve the problem and the consequent need to maintain the patient indefinitely on HPN cannot be considered as a total failure. In such a case, the possibility of an ultimate need for permanent HPN (due to the unresolved obstruction or the need for an extensive small bowel resection) should be discussed with the patient and his/her family prior to the operation.

It is possible in the near future that the approach to surgery or PN or HPN will be partly modulated by the level of plasma citrulline. Citrulline, a nitrogen end product of small bowel enterocyte glutamine metabolism, is a potential plasma biomarker of intestinal failure. Lutgens and co-workers (Lutgens *et al.*, 2003, 2004; Lutgens and Lambin, 2007) found a correlation between plasma citrulline and the morphological end points of epithelial radiation damage, the dose received and the volume of small bowel in the radiation field.

Nutritional Regimen

There is no specific nutritional regimen for patients on HPN because of RE. Energy and nitrogen requirements follow the standard guidelines for intravenous nutrition of malnourished patients and administration is usually cyclic during the night. However, if patients have a short bowel remnant or a high-output stoma, water and electrolyte requirements can be extremely high and require long periods for HPN infusion, as occurs in patients with short bowel syndrome (SBS).

Outcome

The outcomes for patients on HPN for RE may be described in terms of survival, rehabilitation, discontinuation of HPN and resumption of full oral intake.

Survival

Data on survival are biased by the fact that one cannot be definitely sure that patients with RE do not harbour a residual tumour, and a high percentage of these patients succumb because of a recurrent cancer. Sometimes the nutritional response to TPN, which is much better in simply malnourished patients than in wasted cancer patients, may help us understand whether the patient has RE only, or both RE and a recurrent cancer.

Mortality due to cancer accounts for 13–33% of patients on HPN according to different series (Miller *et al.*, 1979; Lavery *et al.*, 1980; Silvain *et al.*, 1992; Scolapio *et al.*, 2002) and reflects a different selection of patients. RE per se represents the most frequent cause for mortality and only 1–2% of deaths are due to TPN/central venous catheter complications (Howard *et al.*, 1991; Silvain *et al.*, 1992; Scolapio *et al.*, 2002).

The overall survival of patients according to different series (Silvain *et al.*, 1992; Messing *et al.*, 1995, 1999; Howard and Malone, 1996; Scolapio *et al.*, 1999, 2002; Van Gossum *et al.*, 1999; Vantini *et al.*, 2004; Gavazzi *et al.*, 2006; Lloyd *et al.*, 2006) is the following at 1, 3, 5 and 10 years: 83% (range 58–100%), 78% (range 60–100%), 62% (range 36–90%) and 56% (range 41–90%), respectively. The database of the Italian Society for Parenteral and Enteral Nutrition reports a 15-year survival of 53%.

If one considers patients affected by severe RE, the prognosis is poorer: Silvain *et al.* (1992) reported that survival probability was 58% at 1 year and 36% at 5 years, while Girvent *et al.* (2000) reported that of the 15 patients referred with intestinal failure after surgery for complications of RE and actively treated, one-third died in hospital and a further third required institution of HPN.

Thus it appears that surgical complications and recurrence of tumour account for the high immediate and early mortality of patients on TPN for RE. A multivariate study showed that age >60 years, vascular disease and occurrence of an intestinal perforation or fistula portend a poor prognosis (Silvain *et al.*, 1992).

Rehabilitation

The rehabilitation of patients can also be a challenge because of the damage extending beyond the gut, such as radiation nephritis, myelopathy and neuritis. Approximately 50% of patients have been reported to be partially rehabilitated and to live lives of reasonable quality (Howard *et al.*, 1995) or somewhat more (Lavery *et al.*, 1980).

Resumption of oral intake

Baticci and Bozzetti (1982) first reported that HPN and bowel rest for some months can achieve a spontaneous resolution of intestinal obstruction and allow the resumption of oral alimentation without surgical intervention. A further report of one case appeared in 1983 (Selby *et al.*, 1983). Silvain *et al.* (1992) and Scolapio *et al.* (2002) showed that approximately one-third of patients were able to discontinue HPN and resume oral intake. Bozzetti *et al.* (1995) reported that five out of ten patients with subacute RE were able to achieve oral nutritional autonomy after 19 months (range 1–32 months) of TPN. A longer follow-up of the previous original study of the National Cancer Institute of Milan (Gavazzi *et al.*, 2006) including three additional patients confirmed that 54% of patients on HPN showed resolution of their intestinal obstruction without surgery and the overall 5-year survival was 90%.

Summary

Acute RE is frequently reversible and patients have to be treated in a conservative way with total bowel rest and TPN. In chronic RE, HPN may have a role when enteropathy involves large parts of the small bowel or in SBS due to previous resective surgery. In these patients, HPN may be required indefinitely. In subacute RE not amenable by surgery because of multiple scattered lesions or a picture of ill-localized pseudo-obstruction, HPN is recommended: it may allow resolution of the intestinal obstruction in about one-third to one-half of patients.

References

Baticci, F. and Bozzetti, F. (1982) L'enteropatia da raggi. *Argomenti di Oncologia* 3, 149–162.

Bosset, J.F., Collette, L., Calais, G., Mineur, L., Maingon, P., Radosevic-Jelic, L., Daban, A., Bardet, E., Beny, A., Ollier, J.C. and EORTC Radiotherapy Group Trial 22921 (2006) Chemotherapy with preoperative radiotherapy in rectal cancer. *New England Journal of Medicine* 355, 1114–1123.

Bozzetti, F., Cozzaglio, L., Gavazzi, C. and Gennari, L. (1995) Radiation enteropathy. *Tumori* 81(Suppl.), 117–121.

Broviac, J.W. and Scribner, B.H. (1974) Prolonged parenteral nutrition at home. *Surgery, Gynecology & Obstetrics* 139, 24–28.

Cerrotta, A., Cardani, G., Lozza, L., Kenda, R., Tana, S., Valvo, F. and Zucali, R. (1995) Occlusione ileale dopo trattamento radiochirurgico per neoplasia rettosigmoidea. *La Radiologia Medica* 89, 643–646.

Chen, S.W., Liang, J.A., Yang, S.N., Hung, Y.C., Yeh, L.S., Shiau, A.C. and Lin, F.J. (2004) Radiation injury to intestine following hysterectomy and adjuvant radiotherapy for cervical cancer. *Gynecologic Oncology* 95, 208–214.

Conklin, J.R. and Anuras, S. (1981) Radiation-induced recurrent intestinal pseudoobstruction. *American Journal of Gastroenterology* 75, 440–444.

De Cosse, J.J., Rhodes, R.S., Wentz, W.B., Regan, J.W., Dworken, H.J. and Holden, W.D. (1969) The natural history and management of radiation-induced injury of the gastrointestinal tract. *Annals of Surgery* 170, 369–373.

Detsky, A.S., McLaughlin, J.R., Abrams, H., Whittaker, J.S., Whitwell, J., L'Abbè, K. and Jeejeebhoy, K. (1986) A cost–utility analysis of HPN program at Toronto General Hospital: 1970–1982. *JPEN Journal of Parenteral and Enteral Nutrition* 10, 49–57.

Galland, R.B. and Spencer, J. (1985) Natural history of clinically established radiation enteritis. *Lancet* 1, 1257–1258.

Galland, R.B. and Spencer, J. (1987) Natural history and surgical management of radiation enteritis. *British Journal of Surgery* 74, 742–747.

Gavazzi, C., Bhoori, S., Lovullo, S., Cozzi, G. and Mariani, L. (2006) Role of home parenteral nutrition in chronic radiation enteritis. *American Journal of Gastroenterology* 101, 374–379.

Gérard, J.P., Conroy, T., Bonnetain, F., Bouché, O., Chapet, O., Closon-Dejardin, M.T., Untereiner, M., Leduc, B., Francois, E., Maurel, J., Seitz, J.F., Buecher, B., Mackiewicz, R.,

Ducreux, M. and Bedenne, L. (2006) Preoperative radiotherapy with or without concurrent fluorouracil and leucovorin in T3–4 rectal cancers: results of FFCD 9203. *Journal of Clinical Oncology* 24, 4620–4625.
Girvent, M., Carson, G.L., Anderson, I., Shaffer, J., Irving, M. and Scott, N.A. (2000) Intestinal failure after surgery for complicated radiation enteritis. *Annals of the Royal College of Surgeons of England* 82, 198–201.
Harling, H. and Balslev, I. (1988) Long-term prognosis of patients with severe radiation enteritis. *American Journal of Surgery* 155, 517–529.
Howard, L. (1993) Home parenteral and enteral nutrition in cancer patients. *Cancer* 72(Suppl. 11), 3531–3541.
Howard, L. and Malone, M. (1996) Current status of home parenteral nutrition in the United States. *Transplant Proceedings* 28, 2691–2695.
Howard, L., Heaphey, L., Fleming, C.R., Lininger, L. and Steiger, E. (1991) Four years of North American registry home parenteral nutrition outcome data and their implications for patient management. *JPEN Journal of Parenteral and Enteral Nutrition* 15, 384–393.
Howard, L., Ament, M. and Fleming, C.R. (1995) Current use and clinical outcome of home parenteral and enteral nutrition therapies in the United States. *Gastroenterology* 109, 355–365.
Husebye, E., Hauer-Jensen, M., Kjorstad, K. and Skar, V. (1994) Severe late radiation enteropathy is characterized by impaired motility of proximal small intestine. *Digestive Diseases and Sciences* 39, 2341–2349.
Jones, B., Holden, C., Stratton, R., Micklewright, A. and Dalzell, M. (2007) *Annual BANS Report 2007: Artificial Nutrition Support in the UK 2000–2006*. BAPEN, Redditch, UK.
Kirwan, J.M., Symonds, P., Green, J.A., Tierney, J., Collingwood, M. and Williams, C.J. (2003) A systematic review of acute and late toxicity of concomitant chemoradiation for cervical cancer. *Radiotherapy and Oncology* 68, 217–226.
Lavery, I.C., Stiger, E. and Fazio, V.W. (1980) Home parenteral nutrition in management of patients with severe radiation enteritis. *Diseases of the Colon and Rectum* 23, 91–93.
Lloyd, D.A., Vega, R., Bassett, P., Forbes, A. and Gabe, S.M. (2006) Survival and dependence on home parenteral nutrition: experience over a 25-year period in a UK referral centre. *Alimentary Pharmacology & Therapeutics* 24, 1231–1240.
Lutgens, L. and Lambin, P. (2007) Biomarkers for radiation-induced small bowel epithelial damage: an emerging role for plasma citrulline. *World Journal of Gastroenterology* 13, 3033–3042.
Lutgens, L.C., Deutz, N.E., Gueulette, J., Cleutjens, J.P., Berger, M.P., Wouters, B.G., von Meyenfeldt, M.F. and Lambin, P. (2003) Citrulline: a physiologic marker enabling quantitation and monitoring of epithelial radiation-induced small bowel damage. *International Journal of Radiation Oncology, Biology, Physics* 57, 1067–1074.
Lutgens, L.C., Deutz, N.E., Granzier-Peeters, M., Beets-Tan, R., De Ruysscher, D., Gueulette, J., Cleutjens, J., Berger, M., Wouters, B., von Meyenfeldt, M. and Lambin, P. (2004) Plasma citrulline concentration: a surrogate end point for radiation-induced mucosal atrophy of the small bowel. A feasibility study in 23 patients. *International Journal of Radiation Oncology, Biology, Physics* 60, 275–285.
Messing, B., Landais, P., Goldfarb, B., Lemann, M., Joeyeux, H., Gouttebel, R., Bouletrau, P., Matuchansky, P. and Beau, P. (1988) Nutrition parenterale a domicile chez l'adult: resultats d'une énquete multicentrique en France. *La Presse Médicale* 17, 845–849.
Messing, B., Landais, P., Goldfarb, B. and Irving, M.H. (1989) Home PN in adults: a multicentre survey in Europe. *Clinical Nutrition* 8, 3–9.
Messing, B., Lémann, M., Landais, P., Gouttebel, M.C., Gérard-Boncompain, M., Saudin, F., Van Gossum, A., Beau, P., Guédon, C., Barnoud, D., Beliah, M., Joyeux, H., Bouletreau, P., Robert, D., Matuchansky, C., Leverve, X., Lerebours, E., Carpentier, Y. and Rambaudet,

J.C. (1995) Prognosis of patients with nonmalignant chronic intestinal failure receiving long-term home parenteral nutrition. *Gastroenterology* 108, 1005–1010.

Messing, B., Crenn, P., Beau, P., Boutron-Ruault, M.C., Rambaud, J.C. and Matuchansky, C. (1999) Long-term survival and parenteral nutrition dependence in adult patients with the short bowel syndrome. *Gastroenterology* 117, 1043–1050.

Miller, D.G., Ivey, M. and Young, J. (1979) Home parenteral nutrition in the treatment of severe radiation enteritis. *Annals of Internal Medicine* 91, 858–860.

Mohiuddin, M., Winter, K., Mitchell, E., Hanna, N., Yuen, A., Nichols, C., Shane, R., Hayostek, C., Willett, C. and Radiation Therapy Oncology Group Trial 0012 (2006) Randomized phase II study of neoadjuvant combined-modality chemoradiation for distal rectal cancer: Radiation Therapy Oncology Group Trial 0012. *Journal of Clinical Oncology* 24, 650–655.

Mughal, M. and Irving, M.H. (1986) Home parenteral nutrition in the United Kingdom and Ireland. *The Lancet* 328, 383–386.

Poddar, P.K., Bauer, J.J., Gelerent, I., Salky, B. and Kreel, I. (1982) Radiation injury to the small intestine. *Mount Sinai Medical Journal of Medicine* 49, 144–149.

Rakovitch, E., Fyles, A.W., Pintilie, M. and Leung, P.M. (1997) Role of mitomycin C in the development of late bowel toxicity following chemoradiation for locally advanced carcinoma of the cervix. *International Journal of Radiation Oncology, Biology, Physics* 38, 979–987.

Russell, J.C. and Welch, J.P. (1979) Operative management of radiation injuries of the intestinal tract. *American Journal of Surgery* 137, 433–437.

Ryan, D.P., Niedzwiecki, D., Hollis, D., Mediema, B.E., Wadler, S., Tepper, J.E., Goldberg, R.M. and Mayer, R.J., Cancer and Leukemia Group B 89901 (2006) Phase I/II study of preoperative oxaliplatin, fluorouracil, and external-beam radiation therapy in patients with locally advanced rectal cancer. *Journal of Clinical Oncology* 24, 2557–2562.

Schier, J., Symmonds, R.E. and Dahlin, D.C. (1964) Clinicopathologic aspects of actinic enteritis. *Surgery, Gynecology & Obstetrics* 119, 1019–1025.

Scolapio, J.S., Fleming, C.R., Kelly, D.G., Wick, D.M. and Zinsmeister, A.R. (1999) Survival of home parenteral nutrition-treated patients: 20 years of experience at the Mayo Clinic. *Mayo Clinic Proceedings* 74, 217–222.

Scolapio, J.S., Ukleja, A., Burnes, J.U. and Kelly, D.G. (2002) Outcome of patients with radiation enteritis treated with home parenteral nutrition. *American Journal of Gastroenterology* 97, 662–666.

Selby, R.R., Mertz, G.H. and Gilsford, L. (1983) Spontaneous resolution of intestinal obstruction while receiving home parenteral nutrition. *American Journal of Surgery* 146, 742–745.

Shamblin, J.R., Symmonds, R.E., Sauer, W.G. and Childs, D.S. Jr (1964) Bowel obstruction after pelvic and abdominal radiation: factitial enteritis or recurrent malignancy? *Annals of Surgery* 160, 81–89.

Silvain, C., Besson, I., Ingrand, P., Beau, P., Fort, E., Matuchansky, C., Carretier, M. and Morichau-Beauchant, M. (1992) Long-term outcome of severe radiation enteritis treated by total parenteral nutrition. *Digestive Diseases and Sciences* 37, 1065–1071.

Trott, K.R. and Herrmann, T. (1991) Radiation effects on abdominal organs. In: Scherer, E., Streffer, C. and Trott, K.R. (eds) *Radiopathology of Organs and Tissues*. Springer, Berlin, pp. 313–346.

Van Gossum, A., Bakker, A., De Francesco, A., Ladefoged, K., Leon-Sanz, M., Messing, M., Pironi, L., Pertkiewicz, M., Shaffer, J., Thul, P. and Wood, S. (1996) Home parenteral nutrition in adults: a multicentre survey in Europe in 1993. *Clinical Nutrition* 15, 53–59.

Van Gossum, A., Peeters, I. and Lievin, V. (1999) Home parenteral nutrition in adults: the current use of an experienced method. *Acta Gastroenterologica Belgica* 62, 201–209.

Vantini, I., Benini, L., Bonfante, F., Talamini, G., Sembenini, C., Chiarioni, G., Maragnolli, O., Benini, F. and Capra, F. (2004) Survival rate and prognostic factors in patients with intestinal failure. *Digestive and Liver Disease* 36, 46–55.

Walsh, D. (1897) Deep tissue traumatism from roentgen rays exposure. *British Medical Journal* 2, 272–274.

Wedlake, L.J., Thomas, K., Lalji, A., Blake, P., Khoo, V.S., Tait, D. and Andreyev, H.J. (2010) Predicting late effects of pelvic radiotherapy: is there a better approach? *International Journal of Radiation Oncology, Biology, Physics* 78, 1163–1170.

13 Home Parenteral Nutrition in Cancer Patients

Federico Bozzetti*

Faculty of Medicine, University of Milan, Milan, Italy

Key Points

- Patients candidate for home parenteral nutrition (HPN) should not be terminal even if they are incurable.
- Incurable cancer patients may enter an HPN programme if they have a life expectancy due to the tumour of longer than 3 months, symptoms are controlled and they are aware of the limitations of the treatment.
- The suggested regimen should include about 30 kcal/kg body weight/day (1:1 glucose/fat ratio, amino acid 1–1.5 g/kg body weight/day, 1 mEq Na/kg body weight/day) in a total fluid volume ≤30 ml/kg body weight/day.
- Median survival of these patients usually exceeds that allowed by a total macronutrient starvation in most series.
- Maintenance of quality of life for a short period of time is more common than a true improvement.
- Crucial issues include: (i) the estimate of the life expectancy; (ii) the communication with the patient and his/her family for balancing their expectations with the realistic benefits of HPN; and (iii) definition of the criteria for withholding and withdrawing the nutritional support.

Introduction

Indications for nutritional support of the cancer patient that are commonly accepted by the scientific community include: (i) treatment of malnourished patients if this allows them to receive the planned programme of oncological therapy; and (ii) treatment of patients suffering from severe iatrogenic complications or chronic sequelae following chemotherapy, radiation therapy or surgery.

*E-mail: federicobozzetti@gmail.com

On the contrary, indications for HPN in incurable cancer patients represent a continuous source of debate and controversy not only among different specialists, but even among physicians working in the same field.

There are two main reasons for this. On one hand, there is the clear awareness among clinicians that current medical care has evolved to such a point, by transforming previously lethal diseases into chronic conditions, that malnutrition and inability to feed may finally represent – in some patients – the main determinant for length of survival, even in malignant diseases. On the other hand, all physicians involved in HPN practice know perfectly well that patients with benign intestinal failure survive 'thanks' to HPN whereas cancer patients finally die 'despite' nutritional support.

Besides these two pivotal points, there are a number of psychological, cultural and economic factors that can affect the options of the caregiver, patient and his/her relatives. The decision whether or not to start and whether or not to withdraw an incurable cancer patient from an HPN programme is always difficult (Weiss *et al.*, 1982).

Areas of Controversy

The incurable versus the terminal cancer patient

When discussing with different specialists (surgeons, oncologists, palliativists, nutritionists, etc.) involved in the care of cancer patients generically defined as 'terminal' and who are potentially candidates for an HPN programme, it is important to be sure that they refer to the same type of patient.

It should be clear that while all terminal cancer patients are 'oncologically' incurable, not all incurable cancer patients are 'biologically' terminal. On the other side there are cancer patients who are 'biologically' but not 'oncologically' terminal; for instance, those affected by an overwhelming sepsis following a biliary drainage for a small obstructing cancer of the papilla of Vater. The oncological definition of 'terminal' often means that no oncological therapy is available for the patient, whose survival may range from a few days to several months (Murray *et al.*, 2005). However, in common parlance, 'terminal' refers to patients in a state of agony or pre-agony where palliation of symptoms and not nutritional support is the absolute priority.

In order to avoid any ambiguity in defining the severity of the state of patients and their potential candidacy for HPN, it is better to adopt the term 'incurable' to focus on cancer patients who have exhausted all available oncological therapies and might sometimes require a nutritional support if aphagic and not agonizing (Bozzetti, 2003).

Nutritional support: a therapy versus a basic human care

This question is not merely academic. Many state laws and professional groups consider artificial nutrition as a form of medical therapy (Capron, 1991; Dyer,

1993; MacFie, 1996; Huang and Ahronheim, 2000), a point of view that is not universally shared (Hodges *et al.*, 1994).

A therapy needs to be validated through randomized clinical trials in order to be accepted as an evidence-based medicine, and in such a trial one arm may receive no treatment or merely the standard treatment. However, in aphagic/obstructed cancer patients it would be impermissible to have a randomized no-treatment arm, which means progressive undernutrition until death, as the standard treatment simply does not exist.

Emphasizing the cultural and symbolic value of nourishment, which is traditionally viewed as an expression of love and care for both the living and the dying, Miles (1989) made the important distinction that while physicians tend to see 'nourishment' as a medical treatment aimed at achieving physiological objectives, families see 'feeding as an act of community'. Cultural and religious representations play a major role in determining the importance of nutrition in daily life and medical care, and influence the decision not only of the patient.

Nutritional support might be considered by patients and their families a basic need that not only sustains life but provides comfort as well and is associated with respect for human dignity. The influence of these cultural and religious differences may affect the therapeutic decisions of both the patient and the physician.

It is common experience that anorexia and hypophagia of a dying cancer patient represent a major concern for both the patient and their family members (Holden, 1991; McClement *et al.*, 2003; Orrevall *et al.*, 2004). A study on the specific nutritional situation prior to the introduction of HPN from the perspective of patients with advanced cancer and their family members, conducted in order to understand factors contributing to the decision to accept HPN, has been published (Orreval *et al.*, 2004). Patients reported wanting and trying to eat, but being unable to do so; family members experienced powerlessness and frustration, as they could not enable the patient to eat. This desperate and chaotic nutritional situation in the family influenced the patient's willingness to accept HPN. A further study from the same group reported that the interviewed patients with advanced cancer and their family members experienced physical, social and psychological benefits from HPN treatment (Orrevall *et al.*, 2005).

The point that nutrition cannot be completely equated to a therapy is clearly recognized in the Guidelines for the Use of Parenteral and Enteral Nutrition in Adult and Pediatric Patients of the American Society for Parenteral and Enteral Nutrition (A.S.P.E.N.), where the A.S.P.E.N. Board of Directors and the Clinical Guideline Task Force (2002) writes:

> A major distinction between therapeutic trial of efficacy of a drug or a procedure and the feeding of nutrients known to be essential to maintenance of human health and survival must be made. Withholding a drug or invasive procedure will not produce disease in otherwise healthy humans, whereas essential nutrients must be provided to both healthy and ill people.

In the introduction to the clinical practice guidelines of the European Society for Parenteral and Enteral Nutrition (ESPEN), Bozzetti and Forbes (2009) have synthesized the potential ambiguity (see Table 13.1).

Table 13.1. Potential implications of the misconception of (H)PN as therapy versus support.

HPN as a therapy	HPN just a support
A drug is any chemical agent that affects living processes	Also 'natural' nutrition affects living processes (paradoxically, all humans got intrauterine PN)
Physicians prescribe PN	Patients and relatives may call for PN and in some countries dieticians can prescribe HPN
Physicians and medical societies consider PN as a therapy	Nourishment is viewed by relatives as an act of love and care
PN is a medical therapy for ill people	Nutrition is essential to both ill and healthy people
It has to be validated by randomized clinical trial	It is ethically impossible to have a no-PN arm and hence a grade A recommendation

The above-mentioned considerations lead to the final conclusion that the value of HPN in incurable cancer patients has to be assessed regardless of the absence of randomized clinical trials and keeping in mind that absence of evidence is not evidence of absence (Altman and Bland, 1995).

In this context it is appropriate to report the position of the Roman Catholic Church (United States Conference of Catholic Bishops, 2009) on the use of artificial nutrition and hydration near the end of life: 'there should be a presumption in favour of providing nutrition and hydration to all patients who require medically-assisted nutrition and hydration' and this approach should be warranted as long as 'there is sufficient benefit to outweigh the burdens involved in the patient'.

Natural History of the Incurable Cancer Patient and Prevalence of HPN

Cancer cachexia occurs during the terminal course of disease in approximately 70% of patients with cancer and it is recognized as the cause of death in 5–23% (Warren, 1932; Klastersky *et al.*, 1972; Inagaki *et al.*, 1974; Ambrus *et al.*, 1975) of terminal cancer patients.

Anorexia, hypophagia and continuing negative energy balance are prominent features of cachexia. Hypermetabolism and weight loss are significant predictors of decreased survival (Bosaeus *et al.*, 2002). These factors may explain why cancer patients account for a high percentage – sometimes even the majority – of the subjects enrolled in HPN programmes.

Registers of HPN patients in various countries report the following figures: Italy, 57% (De Francesco *et al.*, 1995); the USA, 46% (Howard *et al.*, 1991, 1995); France, 18% (Messing *et al.*, 1988); and Japan, 12% (T. Ito, 2013, personal communication). In a European survey of 500 patients receiving HPN in 1997 (Van Gossum *et al.*, 1999), it was found that cancer patients accounted for 60%, 39%, 27%, 23%, 8% and 5% in The Netherlands, Spain, France, Belgium, Denmark and the UK, respectively.

A quite recent analysis reported that the prevalence of HPN in adults in Italy is 22.3 per million inhabitants and cancer patients account for 60.9% of the overall series with an incidence of 1.3 per million inhabitants (L. Pironi, 2013, personal communication).

Indications for HPN

The clinical status

The incurable cancer patient who is the ideal candidate for HPN has the following characteristics: he/she is aphagic because of malignant obstruction (or subobstruction), without severe or untreatable symptoms and without an important functional impairment of organs/apparatus. Hence he/she has relatively good performance status (>50 by the Karnofsky–Burchenal index), with no (or minimal) involvement of vital organs such as the liver or the lung. Notably, the life expectancy of this patient is likely to depend more on starvation and the continuing deterioration of his/her nutritional status than on tumour progression.

In clinical practice, peritoneal carcinomatosis, especially that occurring in slow-growing tumours (some ovarian carcinomas, some retroperitoneal tumours, some relatively indolent gastrointestinal tumours, some intra-abdominal recurrences), is the condition with the most appropriate indication. The worst candidate (indeed, a non-candidate) is a heavily symptomatic elderly patient in poor condition, with altered function of many organs and in need of intensive palliative care.

Life expectancy and its predictability

The most crucial point is the assessment of life expectancy, which is extremely important for a proper indication to undergo HPN. There is in fact no rationale for feeding intravenously a subject who is going to succumb from cancer rather than from starvation/undernutrition.

In healthy adult subjects, a nitrogen loss critical for survival occurs after a loss of 33–37% of the usual/ideal body weight (Kotler *et al.*, 1989), i.e. after 60–75 days of starvation, as demonstrated by the tragic experiences of the Leningrad siege, the Warsaw ghetto and the Irish hunger strike (Brozek *et al.*, 1946; Fliederbaum, 1979; Winick, 1979). From a careful scrutiny of the literature, we found that the survival of hospitalized patients with malignant obstruction usually does not exceed 2 months if patients are not supported by parenteral nutrition (PN) (Tunca *et al.*, 1981; Piver *et al.*, 1982; Krebs and Goplerud, 1983; Baines *et al.*, 1985; Gemlo *et al.*, 1986; Rubin *et al.*, 1989; Mercadante, 1995; Hardy *et al.*, 1998; Laval *et al.*, 2000; Mercadante *et al.*, 2000; Mystakidou *et al.*, 2000; Ripamonti *et al.*, 2000), and survival is reduced again to less than 2 months (Porzio *et al.*, 2011) or to only 19 days if patients are followed at home (Mercadante, 1995) (Table 13.2). However, prediction of length of survival has proved to be poor in several studies (Parkes, 1972; Yates *et al.*, 1980; Mor *et al.*, 1984; Evans and McCarthy, 1985; Rueben *et al.*, 1988; Addington-Hall *et al.*, 1990; Bruera *et al.*, 1992; Viganò *et al.*, 2000) with just a few exceptions (Maltoni *et al.*, 1999; Pirovano *et al.*, 1999; Caraceni *et al.*, 2000).

Table 13.2. Survival of patients with inoperable malignant obstruction.

Study	No. of patients	Survival (days, mean)
Tunca *et al.* (1981)[a]	27	33
Piver *et al.* (1982)[a]	11	60
Krebs and Goplerud (1983)[a]	14	<30
Baines *et al.* (1985)	40	87
Gemlo *et al.* (1986)	27	60
Rubin *et al.* (1989)[a]	11	54
Hardy *et al.* (1998)[b]	39	75
Laval *et al.* (2000)[b]	58	41
Ripamonti *et al.* (2000)[b]	17	11
Mercadante *et al.* (2000)[b]	18	2–37
Mystakidou *et al.* (2002)[b]	68	7–61

[a]Patients with ovarian cancer.
[b]Patients in palliative care units receiving symptomatic agents.

In a report Caraceni *et al.* (2000) have shown that patients with a favourable palliative score (<5.5) have >70% probability of surviving 2 or 3 months depending on the presence or absence of delirium. However, in a prospective investigation (Cristakis and Lamont, 2000) in which 343 physicians were asked to estimate the length of survival of 468 patients (with a median survival of 24 days), there was an overestimation of survival by a factor of 5.3. Overall, only 20% of the predictions were accurate, i.e. within 33% of the number of days that the patient actually survived; 63% were optimistic and 17% were pessimistic.

This tendency to overestimate the survival time has long been recognized (Foster and Lynn, 1988; Pearlman, 1988; Schonwetter *et al.*, 1990; Llobera *et al.*, 2000). It is interesting to note that physicians in the upper quartile of practical experience were the most accurate, which leads to the supposition that the senior director of care may be the best judge (Cristakis and Lamont, 2000).

Unfortunately, accuracy is generally higher when predicting short-term survival, delirium being a strong indicator of short-term survival (Morita *et al.*, 1999; Caraceni *et al.*, 2000); it is definitely worse when considering patients who are not actually dying.

However, it may be difficult to apply these scores to patients who are potential candidates for HPN because some of these indices include variables, such as dysphagia or weight loss, that are responsible per se for nutritional deterioration – apart from reflecting the severity of the disease – and that could be partially reversed through nutritional support. Therefore, a judicious use of HPN in this setting requires careful clinical assessment on a patient-by-patient basis (Hoda *et al.*, 2004). Few studies (and none prospectively) have reported that Karnofsky performance status (Cozzaglio *et al.*, 1997; Pironi *et al.*, 1997; Pasanisi *et al.*, 2002; Santarpia *et al.*, 2006; Soo and Gramlich, 2008; Chermesh *et al.*, 2011), serum albumin level (Pasanisi *et al.*, 2002) and serum cholinesterase level (Santarpia *et al.*, 2006) were prognostically significant; however, these data proved unsuitable to guide the clinician in the recommendation of HPN. As consequence, also the European (Bozzetti *et al.*, 2009) and American (A.S.P.E.N. Board of

Directors and the Clinical Guideline Task Force, 2002) guidelines on PN are quite vague on this issue.

Symptom palliation

HPN should not be provided on the presumption of preventing hunger or thirst. These symptoms are rarely experienced by terminally ill cancer patients (McCann *et al.*, 1994) and even in less advanced conditions: patients are usually anorectic. Thirst, if present, is not always a consequence of dehydration and may be managed with assiduous mouth care. These points should be clarified with the patient and the family.

Nutritional Regimen

Many cancer patients on HPN have requirements for macronutrients and micronutrients quite comparable to those of other patients receiving intravenous nutrition, provided they do not have short bowel syndrome.

However, since patients with peritoneal carcinomatosis are frequently represented in many series of HPN, this suggests the use of a 'modified' diet with reference to the content of water and sodium and the composition of energy. Such a diet, even if not strictly specific for cancer patients, may be accepted as a prudent diet.

Water

A restriction in water administration is advised for several reasons:

1. Cachexia is often associated with the expansion of the extracellular fluid volume.
2. If patients have peritoneal carcinomatosis an overzealous administration of water, glucose and sodium can sharply precipitate an impending ascitis. Gamble first demonstrated in 1946 that glucose reduces renal sodium excretion (Gamble, 1989) and, for the same reasons, the loss of extracellular fluid, and Bloom (1962) suggested that this effect was mediated by insulin through an increased sympathetic activity. The effects of a glucose-based PN on positive water and sodium balance have been demonstrated by Rudman *et al.* (1975) and subsequently described in oncologic patients by Fan *et al.* (1988), Bozzetti *et al.* (1990) and Gray and Meguid (1990).
3. In cancer patients there may be excessive production of antidiuretic hormone (ADH) due to the tumour (Moses and Streeten, 1967), the presence of nausea, which frequently occurs in advanced stages of disease, or the administration of morphine. Furthermore, the wasting syndrome is associated with loss of intracellular water and solutes which affects the hypothalamic osmoreceptor cells by stimulating ADH release at levels that maintain serum osmolality sodium at

subnormal levels (Steiner and Bruera, 1998). In consequence, the clearance of free water is decreased, also because the urea load presented to the kidney is reduced secondary to protein undernutrition, whereas the synthesis of endogenous water is maintained by the oxidation of carbohydrates and fats (Kerndt *et al.*, 1982) and insensible water loss drops due to reduced physical activity (Bruera *et al.*, 1996).

The total volume of fluid and sodium should not exceed 30 ml/kg body weight/day and 1 mmol/kg body weight/day, respectively.

Energy

Many investigators have reported that cancer patients may be hypometabolic, normometabolic or hypermetabolic. When energy expenditure is expressed by unit of body cell mass, a consistent percentage of patients are shown to be hypermetabolic. However, if we consider the total energy expenditure (TEE), which includes the resting energy expenditure plus the physical activity energy expenditure, this value may appear decreased in advanced cancer patients compared with values predicted for healthy individuals (Gibney *et al.*, 1997; Moses *et al.*, 2004) mainly because of a reduction in physical activity.

Recent data (Cereda *et al.*, 2007; Bencini *et al.*, 2008) obtained with the use of a wearable device, the Sense-Wear ARMBAND (Sensormedics Italia Srl), indicate that the TEE of weight-stable leukaemic patients and weight-losing bedridden patients with gastrointestinal tumours is about 24 and 28 kcal/kg body weight/day, respectively.

Since there is also evidence in human cancer that the host uses fat while the preferred fuel for cancer cells is glucose, a high ratio of lipid calories to glucose calories (i.e. 50:50) is desirable.

Nitrogen

Finally, a supply of 1–1.5 g amino acids/kg body weight/day or more should be recommended in most cases.

Outcome

Survival

Survival of cancer patients on HPN depends on the severity of basic disease, i.e. type of tumour and stage. Unfortunately, many series pool together patients with simple iatrogenic complications of the oncological therapy (radiation enteropathy or chronic surgical sequelae), patients with active cancer receiving chemotherapy or radiation therapy and patients with advanced incurable cancer. Therefore, disparity in the composition of the series and indications for HPN can account for different survival rates in different reports. Main series reporting the number of patients and outcome are summarized in Tables 13.3–13.5.

Looking at the experience described in the literature it appears that:

- in large series from national databases or registries on long-term HPN in cancer (Northern American Home Parenteral and Enteral Nutrition Registry, 1987–1994; Elia *et al.*, 2000), 19–50% of patients survive at 6 months, even if we cannot be sure that these figures apply to incurable cancer patients (Table 13.3);

Table 13.3. Database and registry data on HPN outcome.

Study	No. of patients	Outcome and survival
Howard *et al.* (1991)	777	50% at 6 months, 25% at 1 year
Howard (1992)	1362	50% at 6–9 months, 25% at 1 year
Howard *et al.* (1995)	2122	37% at 1 year
Messing *et al.* (1998a,b)	524	19% at 6 months
Van Gossum *et al.* (1999)	200	26% at 6–12 months
SINPE Register (2004, unpublished results)	1103	20% at 1 year, median 6 months

Table 13.4. HPN outcome data from selected retrospective series.

Study	No. of patients	Outcome and median survival
Weiss *et al.* (1982)	9	67% ≥6 months (15–578 days)
Hurley *et al.* (1990)	9	13.6 months (mean)
August *et al.* (1991)[a]	17	53 days (range 5–208 days), 88% felt HPN beneficial
King *et al.* (1993)[b]	61	60 days (range 82–780 days), 23% ≥30 days
Mercadante (1995)	13	3–121 days (23% ≥30 days)
Cozzaglio *et al.* (1997)	75	121 days (range 30–456 days)
Pasanisi *et al.* (2001)	76	74 days (range 6–301 days), 85% ≥30 days
Duersken *et al.* (2004)	9	26–433 days (2% >1 year)
Hoda *et al.* (2004)	52	152 days (range 30–4620 days), 31% ≥1 year
Brard *et al.* (2006)	28	72 days
Santarpia *et al.* (2006)	152	45 days (range 6–1269 days), 11% ≥90 days
Fan (2007)	115	6.5 months
Chermesh *et al.* (2011)	38	140 days (range 20–783 days)

[a]33% fistulas, 22% radiation enteropathy.
[b]18% small bowel syndrome/radiation enteropathy.

Table 13.5. HPN outcome data from prospective studies.

Study	No. of patients	Outcome and survival
Pironi *et al.* (1997)	29	85 days (mean), acceptable compliance in 90%
Bozzetti *et al.* (2002)	69	122 days (median) (range 30–426 days)
Violante *et al.* (2006)	140	81 days (mean)

- in retrospective analyses on more limited series which however include probably incurable patients, the median survival (when reported) is about 100 days, but there are long survivors (Table 13.4); and
- in the few prospective studies, the mean survival is 85–122 days (Table 13.5).

The survival of incurable cancer patients according to a recent multi-centre European study (Bozzetti *et al.*, 2014) is shown in Fig. 13.1.

Quality of life

Before attempting to clarify the effects of HPN on the quality of life of the patient, it should be noted that if anxiety, depression, shortness of breath and sense of well-being are the major determinants of the will to live, as pointed out by Chochinov *et al.* (1999), then a lack of control over these symptoms will have a major impact on the response to HPN.

Data on quality of life are sparse. Some retrospective analyses (King *et al.*, 1993; Cozzaglio *et al.*, 1997; Scolapio *et al.*, 1999) would suggest a limited benefit in cancer patients on HPN: the Karnofsky performance index increased in 7% of patients after 1 month (Pironi *et al.*, 1999) and in 68% of patients surviving longer than 3 months (Cozzaglio *et al.*, 1997); the ability to sustain daily activities and oral alimentation in 27% of patients (Torelli *et al.*, 1999). According to the data of the North American Home Parenteral and Enteral Nutrition Registry (Howard, 2000), 29% of patients appeared to be fully rehabilitated at the 1-year mark.

Bozzetti *et al.* (2002) undertook a prospective study on 69 advanced cancer patients enrolled in an HPN programme in six different Italian centres. The main end points of the study were: (i) the change in nutritional status and determination of the length of survival; and (ii) the evaluation of the impact of HPN on quality of life measured through the Rotterdam Symptom Checklist questionnaire. These parameters were collected at the start of HPN and then at monthly intervals. These patients were severely malnourished, almost aphagic, and beyond any chance of oncological cure. The median survival was 4 months (range 1–14 months), one-third of patients survived longer than 7 months and nutritional

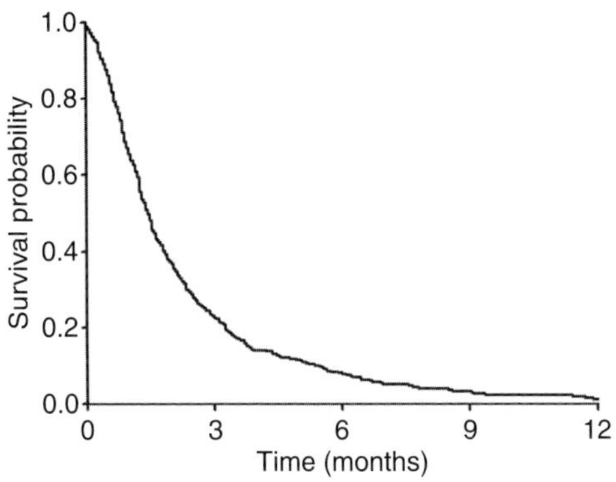

Fig. 13.1. Survival of incurable cancer patients (n=414) on HPN. (From Bozzetti *et al.*, 2014.)

status was stable until death. Indices of quality of life remained stable until 2–3 months before death.

The authors concluded that HPN may benefit a limited fraction of patients who may survive longer than the time allowed by a condition of depletion and starvation. This time is probably less than 2 months and half the time of expected survival of healthy subjects undergoing voluntary or forced starvation (Brozek *et al.*, 1946) or a hunger strike. Provided that patients survived more than 3 months, there was some evidence that quality of life remained stable and acceptable for further months.

Conclusions

The traditional goals of medicine are cure sometimes, relief occasionally and comfort always.

We should realize that although we are no longer dealing with the 'curative' dimension of treatment, there is nevertheless a constant danger that decisions in this field may become expressions of futility and therapeutic obstinacy or of palliative extremism, unless they are rationalized and shared by physicians, patients and/or their families.

In addition, it is common that some ethical and emotional problems can be 'pre-empted' by discussing them with the patient, his/her family and the healthcare team from the onset.

Therefore we think that the approaches to the potential enrolment of an incurable cancer patient in an HPN programme should follow three subsequent steps: (i) communicating; (ii) differentiating between effects and benefits; and (iii) the trial-and-error approach.

Communicating

The worst experience for any patient is to believe that there is no consistency among the options of care proposed by different specialists, i.e. the surgeon, medical oncologist, palliativist, nutritionist and other caregivers, and that these options fluctuate from day to day. Therefore, the physician should discuss the specific treatment options with patients only after having made a decision regarding the treatment goals.

At this point there is the delicate problem of the patient's awareness and consent. In southern Europe, only 25–38% of patients are aware of the diagnosis when their disease is at an advanced stage (Mosconi *et al.*, 1991; Pronzato *et al.*, 1992; Centeno-Cortes and Nunez-Olarte, 1994; Grassi *et al.*, 2000) and less than half of these wanted to be given more information. A 1999 survey of 2088 patients with metastatic disease found that 39% believed it to be 'difficult to cure' and 47% considered their disease 'severe' (IGEO, 1999). In Spain only 11.5% of patients with a fatal prognosis knew about their short-term inexorable future (Espinosa *et al.*, 1993). Relatives may sometimes be responsible for patients' ignorance about their diagnosis and prognosis because in almost 73–84% of cases they want to avoid patients being informed in a straightforward manner about the state of disease advancement (Espinosa *et al.*, 1993; Grassi *et al.*, 2000). More importantly, according to one investigation (Lo *et al.*, 1986), only 12% of cancer patients wanted to personally discuss the matter of life-sustaining treatments.

We have to respect the right of patients 'not to know': the Council of Europe in Chapter III, Article 10, paragraph 2 of the Convention of Human Rights and Biomedicine, which came into force on 10 September 1996, states that 'everyone is entitled to know any information collected about his or her health. However, the wish of an individual not to be so informed shall be observed.' In fact, one-third of physicians believe that patients never want to know the truth (Grassi *et al.*, 2000) and an equal percentage believe that informed consent is necessary to respect patient autonomy (Ordine dei Medici, 2001).

While adequate information should always be given to patients when actively or implicitly requested, there is much uncertainty about the true comprehension of the communication. Indeed, the ability of the patient to actively negotiate a decision with the caregiver requires four intact cognitive functions: (i) the ability to clearly understand the information relevant to the decision; (ii) the ability to fully appreciate the situation and the consequences of alternative approaches; (iii) the ability to elaborate and weigh the information rationally in the context of a coherent set of values and goals; and (iv) the ability to communicate or transfer choices to the physician regarding care.

It is noteworthy that a study carried out in an important Canadian palliative care centre has reported the presence of cognitive deficit in 44% of patients at the moment of hospitalization and in 55% at time of death or upon hospital discharge (Pereira *et al.*, 1997).

If diagnosis and especially prognosis are not disclosed to the patient, the physician and/or relatives should try to take a decision according to the presumed will of the patient. This is quite a difficult task (Rosenfeld *et al.*, 2000).

In fact, a self-report measure of the desire for death distributed to 92 terminally ill cancer patients with a life expectancy of less than 6 months demonstrated substantial fluctuations in will-to-live score within various intervals of time (12–24 h, 7 days, 1 month) (Chochinov *et al.*, 1999). Therefore, the assessment of a patient's will to live should be repeated several times and only if the answers are consistent should this information be utilized to determine whether to initiate or withdraw a life-sustaining treatment.

Asking for informed consent by anticipating some situations before they actually occur is also fraught with difficulties. Coppola *et al.* (1999) showed in 2536 patients that there was no constancy in the choices of preferences regarding live-saving treatments expressed in advance, both verbally and in writing. Specifically, the desire to undergo artificial nutrition as a life-sustaining procedure ranged from a very low percentage of subjects by Coppola *et al.* (1999) to about 70% of patients by Pearlman (1988).

In Italy, for instance, the Italian National Bioethics Committee issued a document on advanced directives which accepts such practice and yet states that advanced directives may not be mandatory for the physician, and thus were called 'advanced declaration of treatment' (Comitato Nazionale per la Bioetica, 2003).

Differentiating between effects and benefits

The goals to be attained through an HPN approach should be discussed realistically with the patient and the family. The metabolic effects of short-term PN (Bozzetti, 1989) and HPN (Bosaeus *et al.*, 2002) in cancer patients are reported in the literature. Do these effects translate into a clinical benefit for the patient?

If the goal of HPN is simply to blunt progressive nutritional deterioration and to ensure a longer survival for the patient while he/she remains within the family home, the answer is probably 'yes', at least for a certain number of patients who are considered good candidates.

If the goal of HPN is to improve the patient's quality of life, the answer is quite uncertain. This is because the quality of life of the patient is not only a strictly individual matter, but may be related more to the symptoms of the primary disease and the previous oncological treatment than to intestinal failure or malnutrition.

A predefinition of the goals of HPN and the chances of success is essential not only to avoid over-optimistic expectations such as 'my husband was condemned to die because he could not eat . . . now HPN will avoid it!', but also because if HPN will not be able to attain those end points, to withdraw it will be less traumatic for the family and ethically acceptable for the physician.

The trial-and-error approach

Since the discrimination between good candidates and bad candidates will select/exclude only a small percentage of patients, for the majority of them the benefit of HPN is unpredictable and its indication very uncertain. Especially in this group of patients it is worthwhile to adopt the trial-and-error approach. That is, one can initiate HPN and withdraw it if it is found to be inappropriate or not beneficial on a subsequent reassessment. This was also the final conclusion of the Consensus Meeting launched by the European Association for Palliative Care in 1996 (Bozzetti *et al.*, 1996).

Summary

The use of HPN in incurable cancer patients is still controversial because this type of support may be considered a life-saving procedure in aphagic patients and consequently not suitable for a randomized comparison with a 'no intravenous feeding' approach.

Moreover, patients and relatives do not understand that, even if able to prevent a starvation-dependent death, HPN will not be able to prevent a cancer-dependent death.

HPN may be recommended in aphagic patients if they are not going to die from tumour progression prior to starvation (that could occur in about 2 months).

Furthermore, asymptomatic patients, with a good performance status, could maintain an acceptable quality of life during HPN.

Our ability to recommend or withhold an HPN programme is very limited and many series report that only 30–50% of the patients have a prolongation of the presumed survival through HPN. For this reason patients and relatives should be actively involved in the decision process about HPN.

There is some empirical knowledge that patients with a good Karnofsky index, who are aphagic because of gastrointestinal obstruction/subobstruction, relatively asymptomatic and with tumours confined to non-vital organs (usually the peritoneum) are probably the best candidates.

The nutritional regimen should be water- and salt-restricted (especially in patients with an impending ascitis), with a glucose/fat calorie ratio of about 1:1 and an energy provision of about 30 kcal/kg body weight/day.

Future clinical research should focus on investigating which patient-dependent or tumour-dependent factors can predict the response to HPN in terms of nutritional benefit, longer survival and maintenance and/or improvement of quality of life.

References

Addington-Hall, J.M., MacDonald, L.D. and Anderson, H.R. (1990) Can the Spitzer Quality of Life Index help to reduce prognostic uncertainty in terminal care? *British Journal of Cancer* 62, 695–699.

Altman, D.G. and Bland, J.M. (1995) Absence of evidence is not evidence of absence. *British Medical Journal* 311, 485.

Ambrus, J.L., Ambrus, C.M., Mink, I.B. and Pikren, J.W. (1975) Causes of death in cancer patients. *Journal of Medicine* 6, 61–64.

A.S.P.E.N. Board of Directors and the Clinical Guideline Task Force (2002) Guidelines for the use of parenteral and enteral nutrition in adult and pediatric patients. *JPEN Journal of Parenteral and Enteral Nutrition* 26(1 Suppl.), 1SA–138SA.

August, D.A., Thorn, D., Fisher, R.I. and Welchek, C.M. (1991) Home parenteral nutrition for patients with inoperable malignant bowel obstruction. *JPEN Journal of Parenteral and Enteral Nutrition* 15, 323–327.

Baines, M., Oliver, D.J. and Carter, R.L. (1985) Medical management of intestinal obstruction in patients with advanced malignant disease. *The Lancet* 2, 990–994.

Bencini, L., Di Leo, A., Pozzessere, D. and Bozzetti, F. (2008) Total energy expenditure in patients with advanced solid tumours: a preliminary report. *Nutritional Therapy & Metabolism* 26, 45–47.

Bloom, W.L. (1962) Inhibition of salt excretion by carbohydrate. *Archives of Internal Medicine* 109, 26–32.

Bosaeus, I., Daneryd, P. and Lundholm, K. (2002) Dietary intake, resting energy expenditure, weight loss and survival in cancer patients. *Journal of Nutrition* 132(11 Suppl.), 3465S–3466S.

Bozzetti, F. (1989) Effects of artificial nutrition on nutritional status of cancer patients. *JPEN Journal of Parenteral and Enteral Nutrition* 13, 406–420.

Bozzetti, F. (2003) Home total parenteral nutrition in incurable cancer patients: a therapy, a basic humane care or something in between? *Clinical Nutrition* 22, 109–111.

Bozzetti, F. and Forbes, A. (2009) The ESPEN clinical practice Guidelines on Parenteral Nutrition: present status and perspectives for future research. *Clinical Nutrition* 28, 359–364.

Bozzetti, F., Ammatuna, M., Migliavacca, S., Facchetti, G., Cozzaglio, L. and Morabito, A. (1990) Comparison of glucose versus fat solutions in cancer patients: a controlled cross-over study. *Clinical Nutrition* 9, 325–330.

Bozzetti, F., Amadori, D., Bruera, E., Cozzaglio, L., Corlì, O., Filiberti, A., Rapin, C.H., Neuenschwander, H., Aoun, M., Basso Ricci, S., De Conno, F., Doci, R., Garrone, M., Gentilini, M., Lery, N., Mantell, M., Sheldon-Collins, R. and Trompino, G. (1996) Guidelines on artificial nutrition versus hydration in terminal cancer patients. *Nutrition* 12, 163–167.

Bozzetti, F., Cozzaglio, L., Biganzoli, E., Chiavenna, G., De Cicco, M., Donati, D., Gilli, G., Percolla, S. and Pironi, L. (2002) Quality of life and length of survival in advanced cancer patients on home parenteral nutrition. *Clinical Nutrition* 21, 281–288.

Bozzetti, F., Arends, J., Lundholm, K., Micklewright, A., Zurcher, G. and Muscaritoli, M. (2009) ESPEN Guidelines on Parenteral Nutrition: non-surgical oncology. *Clinical Nutrition* 28, 445–454.

Bozzetti, F., Santarpia, L., Pironi, L., Thul, P., Klek, S., Gavazzi, C., Tinivella, M., Joly, F., Jonkers, C., Baxter, J., Gramlich, L., Chicharro, L., Staun, M., Van Gossum, A., Lo Vullo, S. and Mariani, L. (2014) The prognosis of incurable cachectic cancer patients on home parenteral nutrition: a multi-centre observational study with prospective follow-up of 414 patients. *Annals of Oncology* 25, 487–493.

Brard, L., Weitzen, S., Strubel-Lagan, S.L., Swamy, N., Gordinier, M.E., Moore, R.G. and Granai, C.O. (2006) The effect of total parenteral nutrition on the survival of terminally ill ovarian cancer patients. *Gynecologic Oncology* 103, 176–180.

Brozek, J., Well, S. and Keys, A. (1946) Medical aspects of semistarvation in Leningrad siege (1941–1942). *American Review of Soviet Medicine* 4, 70–86.

Bruera, E., Miller, M.J., Kuehn, N., MacEachern, T. and Hanson, J. (1992) Estimate of survival of patients admitted to a palliative care unit: a prospective study. *Journal of Pain and Symptoms Management* 7, 82–86.

Bruera, E., Belzile, M., Watanabe, S. and Fainsinger, R.L. (1996) Volume of hydration in terminal cancer patients. *Supportive Care in Cancer* 4, 147–150.

Capron, A.M. (1991) The implications of the Cruzan decision for clinical nutrition teams. *Nutrition in Clinical Practice* 6, 89–94.

Caraceni, A., Nanni, O., Maltoni, M., Piva, L., Indelli, M., Arnoldi, E., Monti, M., Montanari, L., Amadori, D. and De Conno, F.; Italian Multicenter Study Group on Palliative Care (2000) Impact of delirium on the short term prognosis of advanced cancer patients. *Cancer* 89, 1145–1149.

Centeno-Cortes, C. and Nunez-Olarte, J.M. (1994) Questioning diagnosis disclosure in terminal cancer patients: a prospective study evaluating patients' responses. *Palliative Medicine* 8, 39–44.

Cereda, E., Turrini, M., Ciapanna, D., Marbello, L., Pietrobelli, A. and Corradi, E. (2007) Assessing energy expenditure in cancer patients: a pilot validation of a new wearable device. *JPEN Journal of Parenteral and Enteral Nutrition* 31, 502–507.

Chermesh, I., Mashiach, T., Amit, A., Haim, N., Papier, I., Efergan, R., Lachter, J. and Eliakim, R. (2011) Home parenteral nutrition (HTPN) for incurable patients with cancer with gastrointestinal obstruction: do the benefits outweigh the risks? *Medical Oncology* 28, 83–88.

Chochinov, H.M., Tataryn, D., Clinch, J.J. and Dudgeon, D. (1999) Will to live in the terminally ill. *Lancet* 354, 816–819.

Comitato Nazionale per la Bioetica (2003) *Dichiarazioni anticipate di trattamento.* Presidenza del Consiglio dei Ministri, Dipartimento per l'Informazione e l'Editoria, Rome.

Coppola, K.M., Bookwala, J., Ditto, P.H., Lockhart, L.K., Danks, J.H. and Smucker, W.D. (1999) Elderly adults' preference for life-sustaining treatments: the role of impairment, prognosis and pain. *Death Studies* 23, 617–634.

Cozzaglio, L., Balzola, F., Cosentino, F., De Cicco, M., Fellagara, M., Gaggiotti, G., Gallitelli, L., Giacosa, A., Orban, A., Fadda, M., Gavazzi, C., Pirovano, F. and Bozzetti, F. (1997) Outcome of cancer patients receiving home parenteral nutrition. *JPEN Journal of Parenteral and Enteral Nutrition* 21, 339–342.

Cristakis, N.A. and Lamont, E.B. (2000) Extent and determinants of error in doctors' prognosis in terminally ill patients: prospective cohort study. *British Medical Journal* 320, 469–473.

De Francesco, A., Fadda, M. and Malfi, G. (1995) Home parenteral nutrition in Italy: data from the Italian National Register. *Clinical Nutrition* 14, 6–9.

Duersken, R., Ting, E., Thomson, P., McCurdy, K., Linscer, J., Larsen-Celhar, S. and Brennenstuhl, E. (2004) Is there a role for TPN in terminally ill patients with bowel obstruction? *Nutrition* 20, 760–763.

Dyer, C. (1993) Law Lords rule that Tony Bland does not create precedent. *British Medical Journal* 306, 413–414.

Elia, M., Russell, C.A. and Stratton, R.G. (2000) *Trends in Home Artificial Nutrition Support in the UK during 1996–1999. A Report by the British Artificial Nutrition Survey (BANS).* BAPEN, Redditch, UK.

Espinosa, E., Gonzalez Baron, M., Poveda, J., Ordonez, S. and Zamora, P. (1993) The information given to the terminal patient with cancer. *European Journal of Cancer* 29, 1795–1798.

Evans, C. and McCarthy, M. (1985) Prognostic uncertainty in terminal care: can the Karnofsky index help? *The Lancet* 1, 1204–1206.

Fan, B.G. (2007) Parenteral nutrition prolongs the survival of patients associated with malignant gastrointestinal obstruction. *JPEN Journal of Parenteral and Enteral Nutrition* 31, 508–510.

Fan, S.T., Lau, W.Y., Wong, K.K. and Chan, P.M. (1988) Preoperative parenteral nutrition in esophageal cancer: a prospective randomized clinical trial. *Clinical Nutrition* 8, 23–27.

Fliederbaum, J. (1979) Clinical aspects of hunger disease in adults. In: Winick, M. (ed.) *Hunger Disease.* Wiley, New York, pp. 11–43.

Foster, L.E. and Lynn, J. (1988) Predicting life span for applicant to inpatient hospital. *Archives of Internal Medicine* 48, 2540–2543.

Gamble, J.L. (1989) The Harvey Lectures, Series XLIII, 1946–1947: Physiological information gained from studies on the life raft ration. *Nutrition Reviews* 47(7), 199–201.

Gemlo, B., Rayner, A.A., Lewis, B., Wong, A., Viele, C.S., Ungaretti, J.R., DeLorimier, A.A. and Hohn, D.C. (1986) Home support of patients with end-stage malignant bowel obstruction using hydration and venting gastrostomy. *American Journal of Surgery* 152, 100–104.

Gibney, E., Elia, M., Jebb, S.A., Murgatroyd, P. and Jennings, G. (1997) Total energy expenditure in patients with small-cell lung cancer: results of a validated study using the bicarbonate-urea method. *Metabolism* 46, 1412–1417.

Grassi, L., Giraldi, T., Messina, E.G., Magnai, V., Valle, E. and Cartei, G. (2000) Physicians' attitude to and problems with truth-telling to cancer patients. *Supportive Care in Cancer* 8, 40–45.

Gray, G.E. and Meguid, M.M. (1990) Can total parenteral nutrition reverse hypoalbuminemia in oncology patients? *Nutrition* 6, 225–228.

Hardy, J., Ling, J., Mansi, J., Isaacs, R., Bliss, J., A'Hern, R., Blake, P., Gore, M., Shepherd, J. and Hanks, G. (1998) Pitfalls in placebo-controlled trials in palliative care: desamethasone for the palliation of malignant bowel obstruction. *Palliative Medicine* 12, 437–442.

Hoda, D., Jatoi, A., Burnes, J., Loprinzi, C. and Kelly, D. (2004) Should patients with advanced, incurable cancers ever be sent home with total parenteral nutrition? *Cancer* 103, 863–868.

Hodges, M.O., Tolle, S.W., Stocking, C. and Cassell, C.K. (1994) Tube feeding: internists' attitudes regarding ethical obligations. *Archives of Internal Medicine* 154, 1013–1020.

Holden, C.M. (1991) Anorexia in terminally ill cancer patient: the emotional impact on the patient and the family. *Hospice Journal* 7, 73–84.

Howard, L. (1992) Home parenteral nutrition in patients with a cancer diagnosis. *JPEN Journal of Parenteral and Enteral Nutrition* 16(6 Suppl.), 93S–99S.

Howard, L. (2000) A global prospective of home parenteral and enteral nutrition. *Nutrition* 16, 625–628.

Howard, L., Heaphey, L., Fleming, C.R., Lininger, L. and Steiger, E. (1991) Four years of North America Registry home parenteral nutrition outcome data and their implication for patient management. *JPEN Journal of Parenteral and Enteral Nutrition* 15, 384–393.

Howard, L., Ament, U., Fleming, C.R., Shike, M. and Steiger, E. (1995) Current use and clinical outcome of home parenteral and enteral nutrition therapies in the United States. *Gastroenterology* 109, 355–365.

Huang, Z.B. and Ahronheim, J.C. (2000) Nutrition and hydration in terminally ill patients. *Clinics in Geriatric Medicine* 16, 313–325.

Hurley, R.S., Campbell, S.M. and Mirtallo, J.M. (1990) Outcome of cancer and noncancer patients on HPN. *Nutrition in Clinical Practice* 5, 59–62.

IGEO (Italian Group for the Evaluation of Outcome in Oncology) (1999) Awareness of disease among Italian cancer patients: is there a need for further improvement in patient information? *Annals of Oncology* 10, 1095–1100.

Inagaki, J., Rodriguez, V. and Bodey, G.P. (1974) Causes of death in cancer patients. *Cancer* 33, 568–573.

Kerndt, P.R., Naughton, J.L., Driscoll, C.E. and Loxterkamp, D.A. (1982) Fasting: the history, pathophysiology and complications. *Western Journal of Medicine* 137, 379–399.

King, L.A., Carson, L.F., Costantinides, N., House, M.S., Adcock, L.L., Prem, K.A., Twiggs, L.B. and Cerra, F.B. (1993) Outcome assessment of home parenteral nutrition in patients with gynaecologic malignancies: what have we learnt in a decade of experience? *Gynecologic Oncology* 51, 377–382.

Klastersky, J., Daneau, D. and Verhest, A. (1972) Causes of death in patients with cancer. *European Journal of Cancer* 8, 149–154.

Kotler, D.P., Tierney, A.R., Wang, J. and Pierson, R.N. Jr (1989) Magnitude of body-cell-mass depletion and the timing of death from wasting in AIDS. *American Journal of Clinical Nutrition* 50, 444–447.

Krebs, H.B. and Goplerud, D.R. (1983) Surgical management of bowel obstruction in advanced ovarian cancer. *Obstetrics and Gynecology* 61, 327–335.

Laval, G., Girardier, J., Lassaunière, J.M., Leduc, B., Haond, C. and Schaerer, R. (2000) The use of steroids in the management of inoperable intestinal obstruction in terminal patients: do they remove the obstruction? *Palliative Medicine* 14, 3–10.

Llobera, J., Estevam, M., Rifà, J., Benito, E., Terrasa, J., Rojas, C., Pons, O., Catalàn, G. and Avellà, A. (2000) Terminal cancer: duration and prediction of survival time. *European Journal of Cancer* 36, 2036–2043.

Lo, B., McLeod, G.A. and Saika, G. (1986) Patient attitudes to discussing life-sustaining treatment. *Archives of Internal Medicine* 146, 1613–1615.

MacFie, J. (1996) Ethical implications of recognizing nutritional support as a medical therapy. *British Journal of Surgery* 83, 1567–1568.

Maltoni, M., Nanni, O., Pirovano, M., Scarpi, E., Indelli, M., Martini, C., Monti, M., Arnoldi, E., Piva, L. and Amadori, D. for the Italian Multicentric Study Group on Palliative Care (1999) Successful validation of the palliative prognostic score in terminally ill cancer patients. *Journal of Pain and Symptoms Management* 17, 240–247.

McCann, R.M., Hall, W.J. and Groth-Juncker, A. (1994) Comfort care for terminally ill patients. The appropriate use of nutrition and hydration. *Journal of the American Medical Association* 272, 1263–1266.

McClement, S.E., Degner, F. and Harlos, M.S. (2003) Family behavior regarding the nutritional care of a terminally ill relative: a qualitative study. *Journal of Palliative Medicine* 6, 737–748.

Mercadante, S. (1995) Bowel obstruction in home-care cancer patients: 4 years experience. *Supportive Care in Cancer* 3, 190–193.

Mercadante, S., Ripamonti, C., Casuccio, A., Zecca, E. and Groff, L. (2000) Comparison of octreotide and hyoscine butylbromide in controlling gastrointestinal symptoms due to malignant inoperable bowel obstruction. *Supportive Care in Cancer* 8, 188–191.

Messing, B., Landais, P., Goldfarb, B., Lemann, M., Joyeux, H., Gouttebel, M.C., Robert, D., Bouletreau, P., Matuchansky, C. and Beau, P. (1988) Home parenteral nutrition for adults. Results of a multicenter survey in France. *La Presse Médicale* 17, 845–849.

Messing, B., Barnoud, D., Beau, P., Bornet, J.L., Chambrier, C., Constanzo, J.D., Gerard-Boncompain, M., Guedon, C., Hebuterne, X., Heresbach, D., de Ledinghen, V., Lescut, D., Reimund, J.M., Senesse, P., Beliah, M., Bouletreau, P., Bretagne, J.F., Descos, L., Duclos, B., Kerjean, A., Lerebours, E., Leverve, X., Morichau-Beauchant, M., Paris, J.C. and Rampal, P. (1998a) Données épidémiologiques 1993–1995 de la nutrition parentérale à domicile en centres agréés chez l'adulte en France. *Gastroenterology Clinique et Biologique* 22, 413–418.

Messing, B., Landais, P., Golfarb, B., Lemann, M., Joyeux, H., Gouttebel, M.C., Robert, D., Bouletreau, P., Beau, P., Colin, R. and Lerebours, E. (1998b) Nutrition parenterale a domicile chez l'adult: resultats d'une enquete multicentrique en France. *La Presse Médicale* 17, 845–849.

Miles, S.H. (1989) Futile tube feeding at the end of life: families, virtues and treatment decisions. *Theoretical Medicine* 8, 293–302.

Mor, V., Laliberte, L., Morris, L., Morris, J. and Wiemann, M. (1984) The Karnofsky performance status scale. An examination of its reliability and validity in a research setting. *Cancer* 53, 2002–2007.

Morita, T., Tsunoda, J., Inoue, S. and Chihara, S. (1999) Perceptions and decision-making on rehydration of terminally ill cancer patients and family members. *American Journal of Hospital Palliative Care* 16, 509–516.

Mosconi, P., Meyerowitz, B.E., Liberati, M.C. and Liberati, A. (1991) Disclosure of breast cancer diagnosis: patient and physician reports. *Annals of Oncology* 2, 273–280.

Moses, A.M. and Streeten, D.H. (1967) Differentiation of polyuric states by measurement of responses to changes in plasma osmolality induced by hypertonic saline infusions. *American Journal of Medicine* 42, 368–377.

Moses, A.W., Slater, C., Preston, T., Barber, M.D. and Fearon, K.C. (2004) Reduced total energy expenditure and physical activity in cachectic patients with pancreatic cancer can be modulated by an energy and protein dense oral supplement enriched with *n*-3 fatty acids. *British Journal of Cancer* 90, 996–1002.

Murray, S.S., Kendall, M., Boyd, K. and Sheikh, A. (2005) Illness trajectories and palliative care. *British Medical Journal* 330, 1007–1011.

Mystakidou, K., Tsilika, E., Kalaidopoulou, O., Chondros, K., Georgaki, S. and Papadimitriou, L. (2002) Comparison of octreotide administration vs conservative treatment in the management of inoperable bowel obstruction in patients with far advanced cancer: a randomised, double-blind, controlled clinical trial. *Anticancer Research* 22, 1187–1192.

Northern American Home Parenteral and Enteral Nutrition Registry (1987–1994) *Annual Report 1985–1992*. Oley Foundation, Albany, New York.

Ordine dei Medici (2001) Consenso informato e accanimento terapeutico. Atti del Congresso, Turin, Italy, November–December 2001.

Orrevall, Y., Tishelman, C., Herrington, M.K. and Permert, J. (2004) The path from oral nutrition to home parenteral nutrition: a qualitative interview study of the experiences of advanced cancer patients and their families. *Clinical Nutrition* 23, 1280–1287.

Orrevall, Y., Tishelman, C. and Permert, J. (2005) Home parenteral nutrition: a qualitative interview of the experiences of advanced cancer patients and their families. *Clinical Nutrition* 24, 961–970.

Parkes, C.M. (1972) Accuracy of predictions of survival in later stages of cancer. *British Medical Journal* 2, 29–31.

Pasanisi, F., Orban, A., Scalfi, L., Alfonsi, L., Santarpia, L., Zurlo, E., Celona, A., Potenza, A. and Contaldo, F. (2002) Predictors of survival in terminal cancer patients with irreversible bowel obstruction receiving home parenteral nutrition. *Nutrition* 17, 581–584.

Pearlman, R.A. (1988) Inaccurate predictions of life expectancy. Dilemmas and opportunities. *Archives of Internal Medicine* 148, 2537–2538.

Pereira, J., Hanson, J. and Bruera, E. (1997) The frequency and clinical course of cognitive impairment in patients with terminal cancer. *Cancer* 79, 835–842.

Pironi, L., Ruggeri, E., Tanneberger, S., Giordani, S., Pannuti, F. and Miglioli, M. (1997) Home artificial nutrition in advanced cancer. *Journal of the Royal Society of Medicine* 90, 597–603.

Pironi, L., Ruggeri, E., Paganelli, F., Pannuti, F. and Miglioli, M. (1999) Impact of home parenteral nutrition on performance status in advanced cancer patients. *Clinical Nutrition* 18(1), 52.

Pirovano, M., Maltoni, M., Nanni, O., Marinari, M., Indelli, M., Zaninetta, G., Petrella, V., Barni, S., Zecca, E., Leporini, G., La Bianca, R. and Amadori, D. (1999) A new palliative prognostic score: a first step for staging of terminally ill cancer patients. *Journal of Pain and Symptoms Management* 17, 231–239.

Piver, M.S., Barlow, J.J., Lele, S.B. and Frank, A. (1982) The management of ovarian cancer induced by intestinal obstruction. *Gynecological Oncology* 13, 44–49.

Porzio, G., Aielli, F., Verna, L., Galletti, B., Shoja, E., Razavi, G. and Ficorella, C. (2011) Can malignant bowel obstruction in advanced cancer patients be treated at home? *Supportive Care in Cancer* 19, 431–433.

Pronzato, P., Bertelli, G., Losardo, P. and Landucci, M. (1992) What do the advanced cancer patients know about their disease? A report from Italy. *Supportive Care in Cancer* 2, 242–244.

Ripamonti, C., Mercadante, S., Groff, L., Zecca, E., De Conno, F. and Casuccio, A. (2000) Role of octreotide, scopolamine butylbromide, and hydration in symptom control of patients with inoperable bowel obstruction and nasogastric tubes: a prospective randomised trial. *Journal of Pain and Symptoms Management* 19, 23–34.

Rosenfeld, B., Breitbart, W., Galietta, M., Kaim, M., Funesti-Esch, J., Pessin, H., Nelson, C.J. and Brescia, R. (2000) The schedule of attitudes towards hastened death measuring desire for death in terminally ill cancer patients. *Cancer* 88, 2868–2875.

Rubin, S.C., Hoskins, W.J., Benjamin, I. and Lewis, J.L. (1989) Palliative surgery for intestinal obstruction in advanced ovarian cancer. *Gynecological Oncology* 34, 16–19.

Rudman, D., Millikan, W.J., Richardson, T.J., Bixler, T.J. 2nd, Stackhouse, J. and McGarrity, W.C. (1975) Elemental balances during intravenous hyperalimentation of underweight adult subjects. *Journal of Clinical Investigation* 55, 94–104.

Rueben, D.B., Mor, V. and Hiris, J. (1988) Clinical symptoms and length of survival in patients with terminal cancer. *Archives of Internal Medicine* 148, 1586–1591.

Santarpia, L., Alfonsi, L., Pasanisi, F., De Caprio, C., Scalfi, L. and Contaldo, F. (2006) Predictive factors of survival in patients with peritoneal carcinomatosis on home parenteral nutrition. *Nutrition* 22, 355–360.

Schonwetter, R.S., Teasdale, T.A., Storey, P. and Luchi, R.J. (1990) Estimation of survival time in terminal cancer patients: an impedance to hospice admissions? *Hospice Journal* 6, 65–79.

Scolapio, J.S., Fleming, C.R., Kelly, D.G., Wick, D.M. and Zinsmeister, D.C. (1999) Survival of home parenteral nutrition-treated patients: 20 years of experience at the Mayo Clinic. *Mayo Clinic Proceedings* 74, 217–222.

Soo, I. and Gramlich, L. (2008) Use of parenteral nutrition in patients with advanced cancer. *Applied Physiology, Nutrition, and Metabolism* 33, 102–106.

Steiner, N. and Bruera, E. (1998) Methods of hydration in palliative care patients. *Journal of Palliative Care* 14(2), 6–13.

Torelli, G.F., Campos, A.C. and Meguid, M.M. (1999) Use of TPN in terminally ill cancer patients. *Nutrition* 15, 665–667.

Tunca, J.C., Buchler, D.A., Mack, E.A., Ruzicka, F.F., Crowley, J.J. and Carr, W.F. (1981) The management of ovarian-cancer-caused bowel obstruction. *Gynecologic Oncology* 12, 186–192.

United States Conference of Catholic Bishops (2009) *Ethical and Religious Directives for Catholic Health Care Services, Fifth Edition. Issued by USCCB, November 17, 2009.* United States Conference of Catholic Bishops, Washington, DC.

Van Gossum, A., Bakker, H., Bozzetti, F., Staun, M., Leon-Sanz, M., Hebuterne, X., Pertkiewicz, M., Shaffer, J. and Thul, P. (1999) Home parenteral nutrition in adults: a European multicentre survey in 1997. ESPEN Home Artificial Nutrition Working Group. *Clinical Nutrition* 18, 135–140.

Viganò, A., Dorgan, M., Buckingham, J., Bruera, E. and Suarez-Almazor, M.E. (2000) Survival prediction in terminal cancer patients: a systematic review of the medical literature. *Palliative Medicine* 14, 363–374.

Violante, G., Alfonsi, L., Santarpia, L., Cillis, M.C., Negro, G., De Caprio, C., Russo, N., Contaldo, F. and Pasanisi, F. (2006) Adult home parenteral nutrition: a clinical evaluation after a 3-year experience in a Southern European centre. *European Journal of Clinical Nutrition* 60, 58–61.

Warren, S. (1932) The immediate cause of death in patients with cancer. *American Journal of Medical Sciences* 8, 610–615.

Weiss, S.M., Worthington, P.H., Prioleau, M. and Rosato, F.E. (1982) Home total parenteral nutrition in cancer patients. *Cancer* 50, 1210–1213.

Winick, M. (1979) *Hunger Disease: Studies by the Jewish Physicians in the Warsaw Ghetto.* Wiley, New York.

Yates, J., Chalmer, B. and McKegney, P. (1980) Evaluation of patients with advanced cancer using the Karnofky performance status. *Cancer* 45, 2220–2224.

14 Rare Underlying Diseases and Indications

André Van Gossum[1*], Marianna Arvanitakis[1] and Ezra Steiger[2]

[1]*Clinic of Intestinal Diseases and Clinical Nutrition, Hôpital Erasme, Free University of Brussels, Brussels, Belgium;* [2]*Center for Human Nutrition, The Cleveland Clinic, Cleveland, Ohio, USA*

Key Points

- Home parenteral nutrition (HPN) is used in patients with chronic intestinal failure due to benign or malignant disease.
- In the case of advanced cancer, intestinal obstruction related to diffuse carcinomatosis is the most frequent indication.
- Considering benign diseases, Crohn's disease, mesenteric infarction (with short bowel), radiation enteritis and motility disorder such a chronic pseudo-obstruction are the main underlying diseases. In this case, short bowel is the indication in 80% of the patients.
- Besides common indications and underlying diseases, HPN may successfully be used for unusual indications including systemic sclerosis, amyotrophic lateral sclerosis, early or late post-bariatric surgery complications, intra-abdominal desmoid tumour and amyloidosis.

Introduction

Home parenteral nutrition (HPN) is a life-saving technique in patients presenting a chronic intestinal failure. According to the guidelines of the European Society for Parenteral and Enteral Nutrition (ESPEN), HPN support should be used in patients who cannot meet their nutritional requirements by enteral intake and who are able to receive therapy outside an acute care setting (Staun *et al.*, 2009). When considering HPN it is mandatory to differentiate between underlying diseases and the indication itself. HPN may be used in patients with benign underlying diseases or cancer diseases.

*E-mail: andre.vangossum@erasme.ulb.ac.be

For adult patients the most frequent underlying diseases are Crohn's disease, mesenteric infarction, radiation enteritis, diffuse villous atrophy, intestinal motility disorder and post-surgical conditions (Pironi *et al.*, 2011).

In the case of benign diseases, short bowel is the most frequent indication for parenteral nutrition (50–80%) followed by intestinal fistula, malabsorption, obstruction and severe malnutrition. Considering the British Artificial Nutrition Survey (BANS) Registry, the percentage of patients requiring HPN for Crohn's disease is decreasing progressively (Smith *et al.*, 2010). In France, Elriz *et al.* (2011) reported that chronic intestinal failure requiring HPN is rare during Crohn's disease but the incidence has remained stable over time. Surgical procedures play a minor role in the occurrence of severe chronic intestinal failure compared with Crohn's disease severity.

For cancer patients, the main indication is bowel obstruction related to carcinomatosis.

All of the classical underlying diseases and indications are detailed in other chapters. In this chapter, we focus on some rare clinical situations that require HPN.

Systemic Sclerosis

A retrospective review of systemic sclerosis (SSc) patients on HPN followed at the University Health Network, Toronto, Canada, was published recently (Jaw *et al.*, 2012). At initiation of HPN, the mean age of 12 patients was 48 ± 3 years and the median body mass index (BMI) was 16.8 kg/m^2. This increased significantly to 18.3 kg/m^2 at 6 months and 19.7 kg/m^2 at 12 months. The mean Karnofsky score at baseline was 58 ± 3 and the score at 12 months of 39 ± 13 did not change significantly. So, HPN improved the nutritional status but not the functional status of patients with SSc. Brown *et al.* (2008) also reported a series of eight patients with SSc who developed bacterial overgrowth not responding to antibiotics and who benefited from HPN.

Amyotrophic Lateral Sclerosis

Abdelnour-Mallet *et al.* (2011) reviewed the case records of patients from French amyotrophic lateral sclerosis (ALS) centres treated with HPN by an implantable port between January 2005 and October 2009. Seventy-three patients received HPN for a total of 11,908 catheter-days. The incidence of catheter-related sepsis was 3.11/1000 catheter-days. Metabolic complications were frequent but without serious consequences on mortality. The authors concluded that HPN is an alternative procedure to percutaneous endoscopic gastrostomy in advanced ALS patients.

Post-bariatric Surgery

The use of bariatric surgery (also named 'metabolic surgery') for treating obesity and diabetes is growing around the world. Although the different procedures are considered to be safe, about 3–5% of patients may experience post-surgical complications such as fistula, leakage and abscess. In these patients, enteral feeding may be extremely difficult or badly tolerated.

Hamilton *et al.* (2011) reported a series of 23 patients with an average study length of 1.5 months. They received hypocaloric HPN for an anastomotic leak/fistula or bowel obstruction. Patients received an average of 1.2 g of protein and a median of 13.6 kcal per kilogram actual body weight per day. BMI decreased by 7.1% ± 5.2% and serum albumin increased by 12.5%, from 2.8 ± 0.5 to 3.2 ± 0.6 g/dl. Readmissions occurred in 52.2% of patients with 40% of complications related to HPN.

The use of HPN for patients with complications related to post-bariatric surgery is increasing in several countries. In clinical practice, HPN may be indicated in patients who experience early post-operative complications or in patients who develop late nutritional deficiencies as is observed in patients with short bowel syndrome. When enteral nutrition support is inadequate the use of hypocaloric feeding in these patients can allow for continued weight loss while improving visceral proteins.

Intra-abdominal Desmoid Tumours

Fistulae, small bowel obstruction and malabsorption are complications of intra-abdominal desmoid tumours (IADs) that may require HPN. The Cleveland Clinic Nutrition Team reviewed a series of 1615 HPN patients between 1990 and 2008 (Shatnawei *et al.*, 2010, 2013). Eighteen of 1615 patients had an IAD. In comparison with controls, who required HPN because of fistulae, small bowel obstruction and malabsorption, IAD patients had a longer duration of HPN, were younger and were more likely to receive HPN for malabsorption. HPN for IAD patients maintained BMI but did not increase serum albumin levels despite receiving more protein than controls.

Gastrointestinal Amyloidosis

Immunoglobulin light-chain (AL) amyloidosis is a rare disease that can affect several organs including the gut. Madsen *et al.* (2009) reported a series of 11 patients with gastrointestinal amyloidosis. The most prominent symptom was weight loss ($n = 10$), followed by diarrhoea ($n = 5$). At presentation, nine patients had hypoalbuminaemia and six patients had anaemia. Three patients were treated with HPN. Despite conventional chemotherapy and supportive nutrition, the prognosis is severe.

The use of HPN has also been described in patients with severe anorexia nervosa (Latzery *et al.*, 2000), sclerosing encapsulating peritonitis (Fragkos *et al.*, 2011), mucosal diseases such as in patients with complex immune deficiency and intestinal atrophy (Vafa *et al.*, 2009) or unexplained nausea and vomiting (Abdalian *et al.*, 2012).

Summary

Intestinal malabsorption or obstruction is a common complication of several unusual diseases that require HPN to sustain life. The approach to HPN fluid formulations may have to be individualized as for the obese patient post bypass who would benefit from hypocaloric feeding. A multidisciplinary evaluation of the patient's underlying disease, indications for HPN, specific nutritional needs, expected outcomes of therapy including quality of life and the patient's wishes will help to formulate an optimal plan for managing HPN in these rare circumstances.

References

Abdalian, R., Fernandes, G., Duerksen, D., Jeejeebhoy, K.N., Whittaker, S., Gramlich, L. and Allard, J.P. (2012) Prescription of trace elements in adults on home parenteral nutrition: current practice based on the Canadian Home Parenteral Nutrition Registry. *JPEN Journal of Parenteral and Enteral Nutrition* 37, 410–415.

Abdelnour-Mallet, M., Verschueren, A., Guy, N., Soriani, M.H., Chalbi, M., Gordon, P., Salachas, F., Bruneteau, G., le Forestier, N., Lenglet, T., Desnuelle, C., Clavelou, P., Pouget, J., Meininger, V. and Pradat, P.F. (2011) Safety of home parenteral nutrition in patients with amyotrophic lateral sclerosis: a French national survey. *Amyotrophic Lateral Sclerosis* 12, 178–184.

Brown, M., Teubner, A., Shaffer, J. and Herrick, A.L. (2008) Home parenteral nutrition – an effective and safe long-term therapy for systemic sclerosis-related intestinal failure. *Rheumatology (Oxford)* 47, 176–179.

Elriz, K., Palascak-Juif, V., Joly, F., Seguy, D., Beau, P., Chambrier, C., Boncompain, M., Fontaine, E., Laharie, D., Savoye, G. and Lerebours, E. (2011) Crohn's disease patients with chronic intestinal failure receiving long-term parenteral nutrition: a cross-national adult study. *Alimentary Pharmacology & Therapeutics* 34, 931–940.

Fragkos, K.C., Al-Sulttan, F.M., Mookerjee, R.P., Winstanley, A. and Forbes, A. (2011) Review of the literature and description of a case of sclerosing encapsulating peritonitis requiring home parenteral nutrition. *Zeitschrift für Gastroenterologie* 49, 1543–1548.

Hamilton, C., Dasari, V., Shatnawei, A., Lopez, R., Steiger, E. and Seidner, D. (2011) Hypocaloric home parenteral nutrition and nutrition parameters in patients following bariatric surgery. *Nutrition in Clinical Practice* 26, 577–582.

Jaw, H., Fernandes, G., Saqui, O. and Allard, J.P. (2012) Home parenteral nutrition in patients with systemic sclerosis: a retrospective review of 12 cases. *Journal of Rheumatology* 39, 1004–1007.

Latzer, Y., Eysen-Eylat, D. and Tabenkin, H. (2000) A case report: treatment of severe anorexia nervosa with home total parenteral hyperalimentation. *International Journal of Eating Disorders* 27, 115–118.

Madsen, L.G., Gimsing, P. and Schiødt, F.V. (2009) Primary (AL) amyloidosis with gastrointestinal involvement. *Scandinavian Journal of Gastroenterology* 44, 708–711.

Pironi, L., Joly, F., Forbes, A., Colomb, V., Lyszkowska, M., Baxter, J., Gabe, S., Hébuterne, X., Gambarara, M., Gottrand, F., Cuerda, C., Thul, P., Messing, B., Goulet, O., Staun, M. and Van Gossum, A. (2011) Long-term follow-up of patients on home parenteral nutrition in Europe: implications for intestinal transplantation. *Gut* 60, 17–25.

Shatnawei, A., Hamilon, C., Quintini, C., Steiger, E. and Kirby, D.F. (2010) Use of home parenteral nutrition in patients with intra-abdominal desmoid tumors. *Nutrition in Clinical Practice* 25, 290–295.

Shatnawei, A., Habib, M., Hamilton, C., Steiger, E., Kirby, D.F., Speerhas, R. and Quintini, C. (2013) The association between home parenteral nutrition and patients with FAP-associated intra-abdominal desmoids: a retrospective study. *JPEN Journal of Parenteral and Enteral Nutrition* 37, 683–688.

Smith, T., Mickelwright, A., Hirst, A., Gowan, H. and Baxter, J. (2010) *Annual BANS Report, 2010. Artificial Nutrition Support in the UK 2000–2009.* BAPEN, Redditch, UK.

Staun, M., Pironi, L., Bozzetti, F., Baxter, J., Forbes, A., Joly, F., Jeppesen, P., Moreno, J., Hebuterne, X., Pertkiewicx, M., Muhllebach, S., Shenkin A. and Van Gossum, A. (2009) ESPEN guidelines on parenteral nutrition: home parenteral nutrition (HPN) in adult patients. *Clinical Nutrition* 28, 467–479.

Vafa, H., Ballarin, A., Arvanitakis, M., Vereecken, S., Dutat, F., Lagasse, C., Lievin, V. and Van Gossum, A. (2010) Lessons from 20 year experience of Home Parenteral Nutrition in adult patients. *Acta Gastroenterologica Belgica* 73, 451–456.

15 Home Parenteral Nutrition in the Elderly

Xavier Hébuterne* and Stéphane M. Schneider

Gastroenterology and Clinical and Nutrition Department, Archet Hospital, University Hospital of Nice, Nice, France

Key Points

- Patients over the age of 60 years probably account for more than half of the patients receiving home parenteral nutrition (HPN).
- Ischaemic bowel disease and radiation enteritis are the most frequent diagnostic entities.
- Mortality is higher and rehabilitation and quality of life are lower for elderly HPN patients.
- Even though cardiac tolerance is lower and glucose intolerance more frequent, the complication rate is not more frequent in elderly HPN patients compared with younger ones.
- There is an age-related resistance to re-feeding.
- Social considerations are more important in this group of patients, with less self-care.
- Age per se should not contraindicate HPN use.

Introduction

Home parenteral nutrition (HPN) was first proposed for young patients with short bowel syndrome (SBS) and severe malabsorption, but due to the ageing of the general population and the progress of medical care, elderly patients are more and more likely candidates for HPN. In this chapter we discuss the specific points of HPN in the elderly patient.

*E-mail: xavier.hebuterne@unice.fr

Prevalence of Elderly in HPN Programmes

A 1987 report by the US Office of Technology Assessment on Life-Sustaining Technologies and the Elderly discussed the then current utilization of total parenteral nutrition (TPN) for elderly people and the related issues of patient access to treatment, decision-making practices and quality of care. It was shown that about 40% of all patients receiving parenteral nutrition (PN) were over 65 years of age. Data from commercial home nutrition services and small registries indicated that about 20% of people on HPN were over 65 (Maslow, 1988).

In another study, the use of home parenteral therapy in geriatric patients and the effect of ageing on the clinical outcome of HPN therapy were assessed between 1985 and 1992. Data were obtained from Medicare parenteral and enteral nutrition workload statistics, Blue Cross and Blue Shield of South Carolina, and the North American Home Parenteral and Enteral Nutrition (HPEN) Patient Registry. On the basis of these data it was estimated that in 1992 there were 40,000 HPN patients in the USA. One-quarter to one-third of the HPN group was aged ≥65 years, depending on the underlying diagnosis (Howard and Malone, 1997).

The percentages of geriatric patients starting HPN within the major diagnostic groups are presented in Table 15.1. As expected, the proportion of the elderly on HPN was highest in the radiation enteritis and ischaemic bowel disease groups.

In the survey of the Home Artificial Nutrition (HAN) working group of the European Society for Parenteral and Enteral Nutrition (ESPEN) conducted in 1993, 14% of patients were between 61 and 70 years of age and 9% were >70 years old (Van Gossum *et al.*, 1996). In the second survey conducted by the same group in 1997 the proportion of elderly was higher, with 18% of patients aged 61–70 years and 10% aged >70 years (Van Gossum *et al.*, 1999). Between 1993 and 1995, a 3-year epidemiological survey of HPN was conducted in French adult HPN centres; 17% of patients started HPN between 61 and 70 years of age, and 12% when over 70 years of age (Messing *et al.*, 1998).

The lack of recent epidemiological studies does not allow us to update these data. However, we can safely guess that more and more elderly patients are currently treated with HPN. The more recent experience from an Italian centre reports a median age of 60 years in HPN patients, the oldest one being 93 years old (Violante *et al.*, 2006). Also, for patients with SBS, there is no indication of small bowel transplantation after the age of 65 years.

Table 15.1. Proportion of geriatric patients starting HPN within the major diagnostic groups. (From Howard and Malone, 1997.)

Diagnosis	Number of patients	Number of patients aged ≥65 years (%)
Cancer	2122	470 (22)
Crohn's disease	562	45 (8)
Ischaemic bowel disease	331	95 (29)
Motility disorders	299	63 (21)
Radiation enteritis	145	53 (37)

The proportion of HPN patients with malignant diseases varies between countries: in North America, 40% of patients receiving HPN had malignant diseases (1985–1991) compared with 5% in the UK (1977–1991) (Elia, 1995). The proportion of patients is also relatively low in Denmark, intermediate in France and Belgium, and high in Italy and The Netherlands (Van Gossum *et al.*, 1996, 1999). These differences contribute to the wide variation in the age distribution of HPN patients. In the future, HPN will be used more and more in patients with malignant disease, which will increase the age of patients treated.

Prognosis and Rehabilitation of Elderly Patients on HPN

In a study conducted in 1997, Howard and Malone (1997) evaluated the outcome of geriatric patients receiving HPN in the USA. They selected patients with Crohn's disease, ischaemic bowel disease and motility disorders, and compared patients over 65 years old with middle-aged patients (aged 35–55 years). As expected, the 12-month survival rate was lower in the elderly (71%) compared with the middle-aged patients (92%). However, the complication rate was similar in the two patient groups. The number of hospital admissions for HPN-related complications was 0.9 per patient-year in the two groups of patients and the number of hospital admissions for non-HPN-related complications was 0.7 per patient-year in elderly patients and 0.9 per patient-year in middle-aged patients. The 12-month rehabilitation status in the two groups of patients is represented in Fig. 15.1.

A more recent study of 268 patients with SBS did not show an association between age and HPN dependency (Amiot *et al.*, 2013); in this study, age was, expectedly, associated with a higher mortality risk on follow-up. A prospective

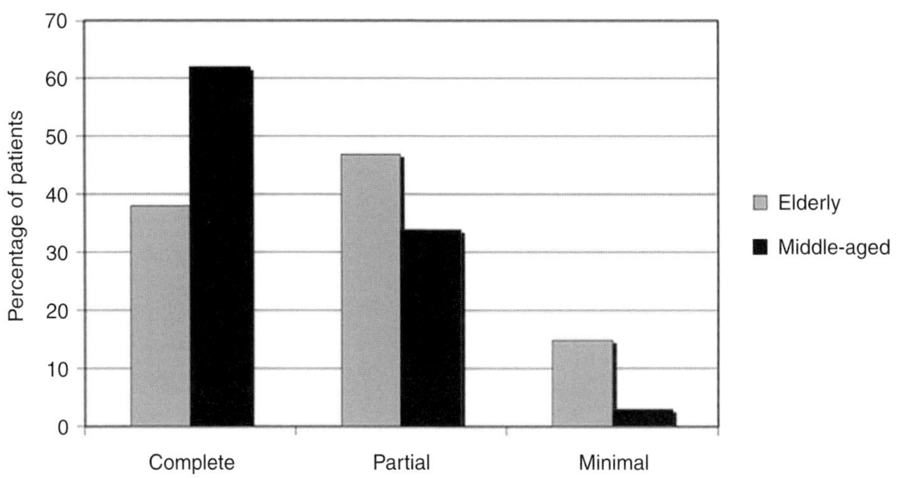

Fig. 15.1. Rehabilitation status at 12 months of elderly (≥65 years) and middle-aged patients (35–55 years) receiving HPN. (From Howard and Malone, 1997.)

study of catheter-related complications in 254 cancer patients (36% over the age of 70 years) totalling more than 51,000 catheter-days did not report age as a risk factor for such complications (Cotogni *et al.*, 2013). On the other hand, another prospective study of 1499 patients (2992 catheters) showed older age to be associated with a higher risk of central catheter vascular erosion (Walshe *et al.*, 2007).

Figure 15.2 presents the gradual way in which age influences rehabilitation in HPN-treated patients with Crohn's disease. These results clearly show that age negatively influences rehabilitation in HPN patients. They also suggest that illness leading to HPN therapy has more devastating effects in geriatric patients than in middle-aged patients. Quality of life has become an increasingly important outcome in elderly patients; an age older than 55 or 60 years may alter quality of life negatively in HPN patients (Richards *et al.*, 1997; Oz *et al.*, 2008). However, age per se should not disqualify geriatric subjects for HPN therapy, and ESPEN does not advise against HPN in these patients (Staun *et al.*, 2009).

Specificities of PN in the Elderly

Tolerance

Cardiac and renal functions are more likely to be impaired in older persons. Therefore fluid and sodium intake should be limited, and especially so during periods of mobilization of extracellular water that has accumulated due to inflammatory processes or during an earlier stage of re-feeding (Sobotka *et al.*, 2009).

A study by Volpi *et al.* (2000) suggested that the anabolic response to a mixed glucose/amino acid meal was reduced in older men. This study suggests that insulin resistance occurs even in healthy elderly volunteers. This, and most importantly the increased prevalence of diabetes mellitus with age, should lead to systematic glycaemia monitoring in the elderly (Morley, 2002).

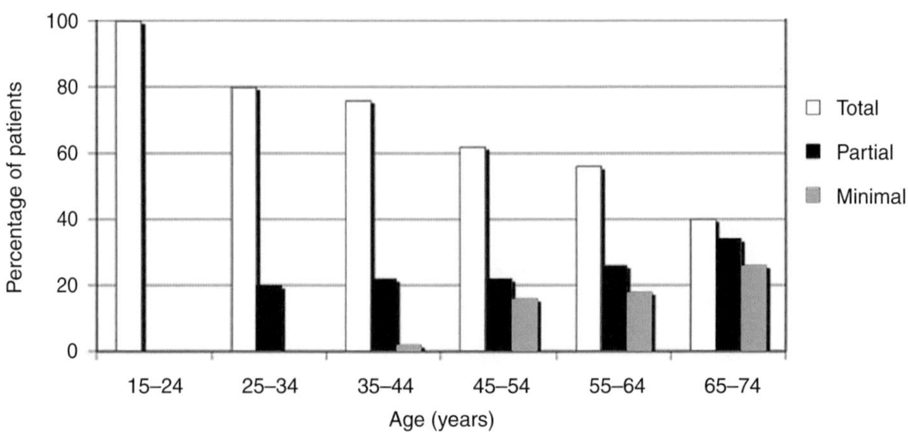

Fig. 15.2. Influence of age on the degree of rehabilitation in patients with Crohn's disease receiving HPN. (From Howard and Malone, 1997.)

Efficacy

In malnourished elderly patients, dietary supplementation increases protein synthesis and induces a gain in fat-free mass (Bos *et al.*, 2000). However, many clinical observations suggest that the repair of a malnourished state is more difficult in the elderly than in younger patients. The energy excess requirement for 1 kg of weight gain in young females with anorexia nervosa was shown to be about 7500 kcal/kg (Walker *et al.*, 1979); in contrast, the energy excess requirement was shown to be between 8856 and 22,620 kcal/kg in malnourished nursing home patients (Hébuterne *et al.*, 2001). The comparison of thc efficacy of cyclic enteral nutrition in 51 young patients (mean age 45 ± 15 years) with 46 elderly patients (mean age 77 ± 6 years) suggested that the repair of a malnourished state is more difficult in the elderly than in young people (Hébuterne *et al.*, 1995). For similar energy intakes during a mean 27 days of enteral nutrition, the weight gain was 6.3 kg in patients less than 65 years old and only 4.7 kg in elderly patients, and some biological nutritional parameters increased more in the young patients than in the elderly. In particular, the gain in nutritional proteins (albumin, transferrin, transthyretin) was much lower in the elderly than in younger patients, whereas inflammatory status was similar in the two groups. However, in this study, the duration of re-feeding was not standardized and body composition was not measured. We therefore conducted another study of 3-week enteral re-feeding to compare the effects of cyclic enteral nutrition on the nutritional assessment parameters and body composition in middle-aged and elderly patients, in order to determine if age alone could affect the nutritional effects of tube feeding (Hébuterne *et al.*, 1997). This study clearly demonstrated a reduced efficacy of re-nutrition in the elderly, and the gain of body cell mass was lower in the elderly (1.6 kg) than in the young patients (2.7 kg). This result was not due to differences in patients' condition, and nutrient absorption was satisfactory and similar in the two groups of patients. During PN, Shizgal *et al.* (1992) evaluated the effect of age on the response to TPN in 325 patients by measuring body composition by multiple-isotope dilution at the onset and at 2-week intervals during the course of TPN. With advancing age, more energy was required to maintain the body cell mass of malnourished patients (Fig. 15.3).

Substrate oxidation

A study conducted in patients treated by TPN for intestinal failure demonstrated important metabolic differences between elderly and middle-aged patients (Al-Jaouni *et al.*, 2002). For similar energy supplies, elderly patients oxidized more fat and less glucose than middle-aged patients. Twelve elderly patients (eight females, four males; mean age 72 ± 5 years) and 12 middle-aged patients (nine females, three males; mean age 39 ± 13 years) who were on cyclic TPN for intestinal failure were investigated in stable condition after at least 15 days of TPN. In the fasting state, resting energy expenditure was significantly higher in the elderly patients than in the middle-aged patients. During TPN, lipid oxidation was significantly higher in the elderly patients than in the middle-aged patients (Fig. 15.4) and

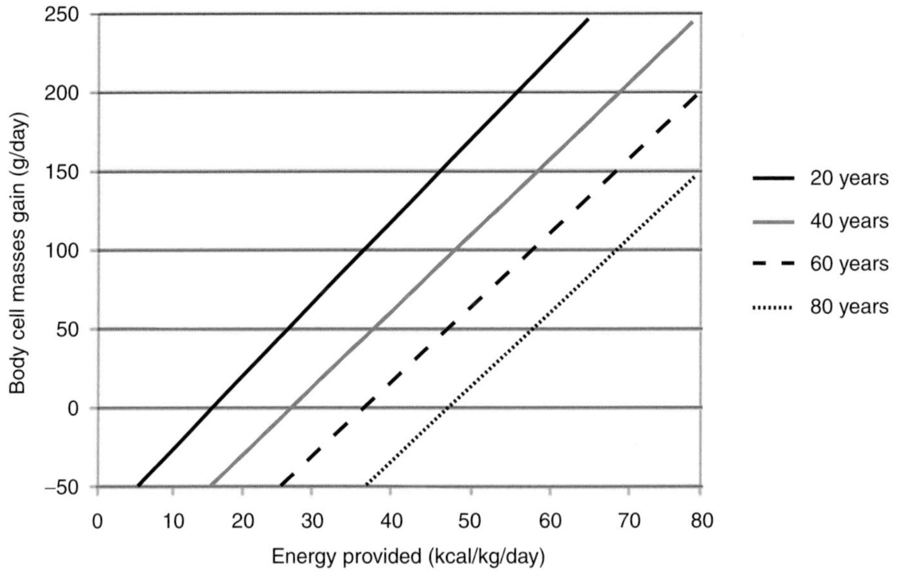

Fig. 15.3. Influence of age on the relationship between the daily changes in body cell mass and energy intake. (From Shizgal *et al.*, 1992.)

glucose oxidation was significantly lower in elderly than in middle-aged patients. Areas under the curves of glucose and free fatty acids were significantly higher in the elderly patients whereas area under the curve of insulin was lower, suggesting insulin resistance in the elderly (Fig. 15.5). The reduction of glucose oxidation during TPN may affect treatment tolerance. Therefore, knowing the importance of glucose control in critically ill patients (Van den Berghe *et al.*, 2001), glucose control of elderly patients on TPN is an important issue. A study in 20 healthy volunteers submitted to a hypertriglyceridaemic clamp showed a similar capacity in young and older subjects to oxidize a high intravenous triglyceride load (Aberg *et al.*, 2006).

In the study by Al Jaouni *et al.*, we failed to observe any effect of age on the thermogenic response to TPN. Previously published results concerning the effect of age on thermogenic response are contradictory. In some studies, glucose-induced thermogenesis was apparently decreased in elderly subjects compared with young subjects (Golay *et al.*, 1983; Bloesch *et al.*, 1988). In other investigations, the thermogenic response after ingestion of a liquid mixed meal was found to be decreased in elderly men (Thorne and Wahren, 1990; Visser *et al.*, 1995) but not in elderly women (Visser *et al.*, 1995). Other authors reported a similar thermogenic response to a protein load in elderly and young subjects (Tuttle *et al.*, 1954). However, none of these studies concerned malnourished patients fed by TPN. We observed a thermogenic effect of TPN of between 9.8 and 13.6% of the energy infused; a finding consistent with studies on young subjects in whom the thermogenic effect of TPN varies between 5 and 17% (Lindmark *et al.*, 1986; Vernet *et al.*, 1986; Sobotka *et al.*, 1991).

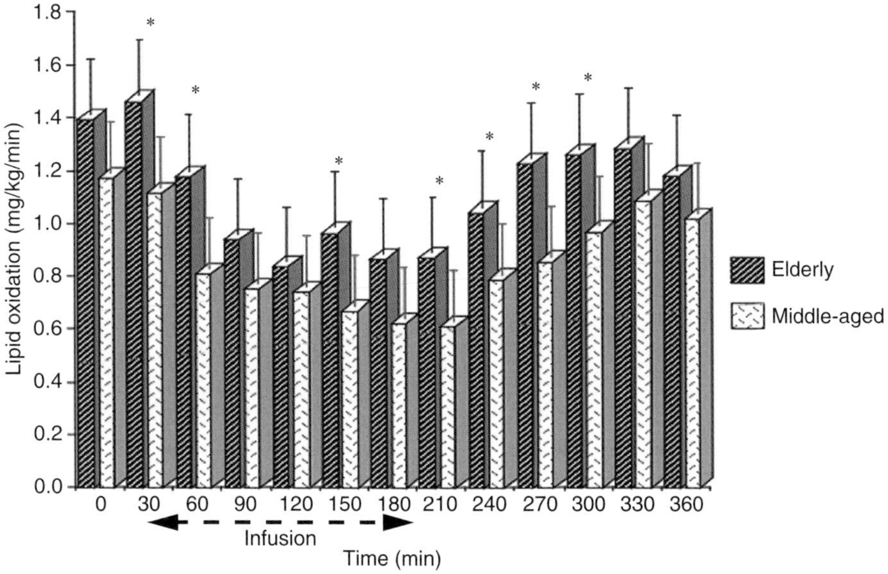

Fig. 15.4. Fat oxidation in elderly and younger patients during TPN. (From Al-Jaouni *et al.*, 2002.)

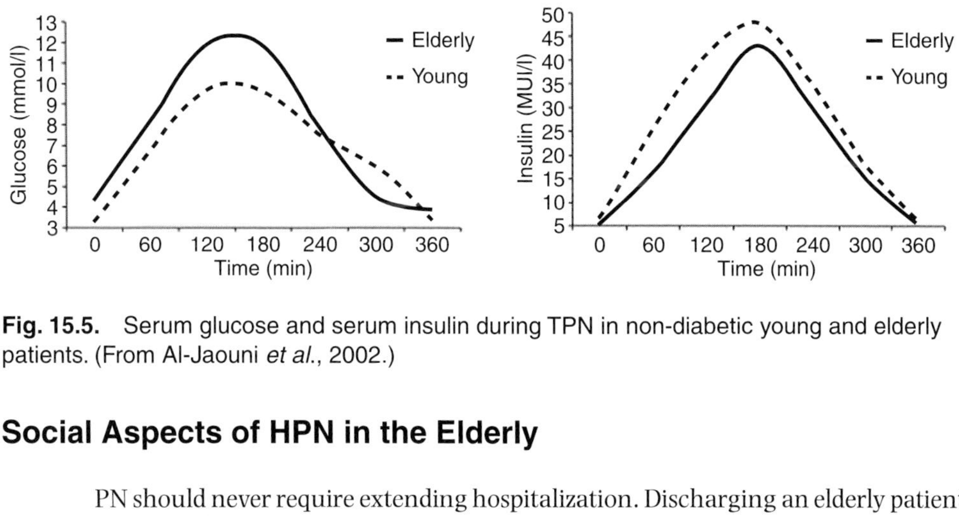

Fig. 15.5. Serum glucose and serum insulin during TPN in non-diabetic young and elderly patients. (From Al-Jaouni *et al.*, 2002.)

Social Aspects of HPN in the Elderly

PN should never require extending hospitalization. Discharging an elderly patient from the hospital to his/her home or to an institution to pursue HPN therapy requires a good deal of advanced planning. HPN is 65% more cost-effective than in-hospital TPN but has potentially life-threatening complications, and requires close cooperation and the effective organization provided by a multidisciplinary team of healthcare professionals. Training elderly patients for self-administration of HPN proves difficult, due to neurological and rheumatic disorders (including cognitive disorders) and sometimes difficulties in grasping the importance of strict asepsis, and most patients will require the intervention of a carer (Jones *et al.*, 2005). Patients and/or their family still need to be trained to address emergency situations such as hyperthermia. HPN should not be performed in elderly patients living alone. Instructions should be provided to nurses working in the community or in institutions to deal with most emergent situations. At all times, a reference HPN centre may be reached in case of an HPN-related complication. As dependency levels of HPN patients are rising, this makes care from remote centres more difficult (Freshwater *et al.*, 2005). Of course, pharmacological sedation or physical restraining of the patient to make HPN possible is not justified (Sobotka *et al.*, 2009).

Conclusion

More than 50% of HPN patients may be over 60 years of age. As the most recent epidemiological data to be published are more than 15 years old, new surveys are mandatory. Because of the ageing of the general population and medical progress, the prevalence of elderly patients treated with HPN will increase in the future. Specific metabolic features suggest that PN formulas and/or flow rates should be specifically adapted for the elderly and glucose tolerance of PN should be carefully monitored. Transferring a geriatric patient from the hospital to home or an institution may be sometimes difficult and a referring HPN centre should always be available.

References

Aberg, W., Thorne, A., Olivecrona, T. and Nordenstrom, J. (2006) Fat oxidation and plasma removal capacity of an intravenous fat emulsion in elderly and young men. *Nutrition* 22, 738–743.

Al-Jaouni, R., Schneider, S.M., Rampal, P. and Hébuterne, X. (2002) Effect of age on substrate oxidation during total parenteral nutrition. *Nutrition* 18, 20–25.

Amiot, A., Messing, B., Corcos, O., Panis, Y. and Joly, F. (2013) Determinants of home parenteral nutrition dependence and survival of 268 patients with non-malignant short bowel syndrome. *Clinical Nutrition* 32, 368–374.

Bloesch, D., Schutz, Y., Breitenstein, E., Jequier, E. and Felber, J.P. (1988) Thermogenic response to an oral glucose load in man: comparison between young and elderly subjects. *Journal of the American College of Nutrition* 7, 471–483.

Bos, C., Benamouzig, R., Bruhat, A., Roux, C., Mahe, S., Valensi, P., Gaudichon, C., Ferriere, F., Rautureau, J. and Tome, D. (2000) Short-term protein and energy supplementation activates nitrogen kinetics and accretion in poorly nourished elderly subjects. *American Journal of Clinical Nutrition* 71, 1129–1137.

Cotogni, P., Pittiruti, M., Barbero, C., Monge, T., Palmo, A. and Boggio Bertinet, D. (2013) Catheter-related complications in cancer patients on home parenteral nutrition: a prospective study of over 51,000 catheter days. *JPEN Journal of Parenteral and Enteral Nutrition* 37, 375–383.

Elia, M. (1995) An international perspective on artificial nutritional support in the community. *The Lancet* 345, 1345–1349.

Freshwater, D.A., Saadeddin, A., Deel-Smith, P., Digger, T. and Jones, B.J. (2005) Can home parenteral nutrition be provided by non-specialised centres? 2300 weeks of experience at a district general hospital in the United Kingdom. *Clinical Nutrition* 24, 229–235.

Golay, A., Schutz, Y., Broquet, C., Moeri, R., Felber, J. and Jequier, E. (1983) Decreased thermogenic response to an oral glucose load in older subjects. *Journal of the American Geriatric Society* 31, 144–148.

Hébuterne, X., Broussard, J.F. and Rampal, P. (1995) Acute renutrition by cyclic enteral nutrition in elderly and younger patients. *Journal of the American Medical Association* 273, 638–648.

Hébuterne, X., Péroux, J., Schneider, S. and Rampal, P. (1997) Effects of refeeding by cyclic enteral nutrition on body composition: comparative study of elderly and younger patients. *Clinical Nutrition* 16, 283–289.

Hébuterne, X., Bermon, S. and Schneider, S.M. (2001) Ageing and muscle: the effects of malnutrition, re-nutrition, and physical exercise. *Current Opinion in Clinical Nutrition and Metabolic Care* 4, 295–300.

Howard, L. and Malone, M. (1997) Clinical outcome of geriatric patients in the United States receiving home parenteral and enteral nutrition. *American Journal of Clinical Nutrition* 66, 1364–1370.

Jones, B., Holden, C., Dalzell, M., Micklewright, A. and Glencorse, C. (2005) *Annual BANS Report. Artificial Nutrition Support in the UK 2005.* BAPEN, Redditch, UK.

Lindmark, L., Bennegard, K., Eden, E., Svaninger, G., Ternell, M. and Lundholm, K. (1986) Thermic effect and substrate oxidation in response to intravenous nutrition in cancer patients who lose weight. *Annals of Surgery* 204, 628–636.

Maslow, K. (1988) Total parenteral nutrition and tube feeding for elderly patients: findings of an OTA study. *JPEN Journal of Parenteral and Enteral Nutrition* 12, 425–432.

Messing, B., Barnoud, D., Beau, P., Bornet, J.L., Chambrier, C., Constanzo, J.D., Gerard-Boncompain, M., Guedon, C., Hébuterne, X., Heresbach, D., de Ledinghen, V., Lescut, D., Reimund, J.M., Senesse, P., Beliah, M., Bouletreau, P., Bretagne, J.F., Descos, L., Duclos, B., Kerjean, A., Lerebours, E., Leverve, X., Morichau-Beauchant, M., Paris, J.C. and Rampal, P. (1998) A 1993–1995 epidemiological survey of home parenteral nutrition in approved centers for adults in France. *Gastroentérologie Clinique et Biologique* 22, 413–418.

Morley, J.E. (2002) Nutrition in the elderly. *Current Opinion in Gastroenterology* 18, 240–245.

Oz, V., Theilla, M. and Singer, P. (2008) Eating habits and quality of life of patients receiving home parenteral nutrition in Israel. *Clinical Nutrition* 27, 95–99.

Richards, D.M., Deeks, J.J., Sheldon, T.A. and Shaffer, J.L. (1997) Home parenteral nutrition: a systematic review. *Health Technology Assessment* 1, 1–59.

Shizgal, H., Martin, M. and Gimmon, Z. (1992) The effect of age on the caloric requirement of malnourished individuals. *American Journal of Clinical Nutrition* 55, 783–789.

Sobotka, L., Zadak, Z., Bures, J. and Pidrman, V. (1991) Influence of rapid amino acid and lipid emulsion administration on gas exchange and resting energy expenditure. *Nutrition* 7, 200–203.

Sobotka, L., Schneider, S.M., Berner, Y.N., Cederholm, T., Krznaric, Z., Shenkin, A., Stanga, Z., Toigo, G., Vandewoude, M. and Volkert, D. (2009) ESPEN guidelines on parenteral nutrition: geriatrics. *Clinical Nutrition* 28, 461–466.

Staun, M., Pironi, L., Bozzetti, F., Baxter, J., Forbes, A., Joly, F., Jeppesen, P., Moreno, J., Hébuterne, X., Pertkiewicz, M., Muhlebach, S., Shenkin, A. and Van Gossum, A. (2009) ESPEN guidelines on parenteral nutrition: home parenteral nutrition (HPN) in adult patients. *Clinical Nutrition* 28, 467–479.

Thorne, A. and Wahren, J. (1990) Diminished meal-induced thermogenesis in elderly man. *Clinical Physiology* 10, 427–437.

Tuttle, W., Horvath, S., Presson, L. and Daum, K. (1954) Specific dynamic action of protein in men past 60 years of age. *Journal of Applied Physiology* 5, 631–634.

Van den Berghe, G., Wouters, P., Weekers, F., Verwaest, C., Bruyninckx, F., Schetz, M., Vlasselaers, D., Ferdinande, P., Lauwers, P. and Bouillon, R. (2001) Intensive insulin therapy in the critically ill patients. *New England Journal of Medicine* 345, 1359–1367.

Van Gossum, A., Bakker, H., De Francesco, A., Ladefoged, K., Leon-Sanz, M., Messing, B., Pironi, L., Pertkiewicz, M., Shaffer, J., Thul, P. and Wood, S. (1996) Home parenteral nutrition in adults: a multicentre survey in Europe in 1993. *Clinical Nutrition* 15, 53–59.

Van Gossum, A., Bakker, H., Bozzetti, F., Staun, M., Leon-Sanz, M., Hébuterne, X., Pertkiewicz, M., Shaffer, J. and Thul, P. (1999) Home parenteral nutrition in adults: a European multicentre survey in 1997. ESPEN-Home Artificial Nutrition Working Group. *Clinical Nutrition* 18, 135–140.

Vernet, O., Christin, L., Schutz, Y., Danforth, E. Jr and Jequier, E. (1986) Enteral versus parenteral nutrition: comparison of energy metabolism in healthy subjects. *American Journal of Physiology* 250, E47–E54.

Violante, G., Alfonsi, L., Santarpia, L., Cillis, M.C., Negro, G., De Caprio, C., Russo, N., Contaldo, F. and Pasanisi, F. (2006) Adult home parenteral nutrition: a clinical evaluation after a 3-year experience in a Southern European centre. *European Journal of Clinical Nutrition* 60, 58–61.

Visser, M., Deurenberg, P., van Staveren, W.A. and Hautvast, J.G. (1995) Resting metabolic rate and diet-induced thermogenesis in young and elderly subjects: relationship with body composition, fat distribution, and physical activity level. *American Journal of Clinical Nutrition* 61, 772–778.

Volpi, E., Mittendorfer, B., Rasmusen, B. and Wolfe, R.R. (2000) The response of muscle protein anabolism to combined hyperaminoacidemia and glucose-induced hyperinsulinemia is impaired in the elderly. *Journal of Clinical Endocrinology and Metabolism* 85, 4481–4490.

Walker, J., Roberts, S., Halmi, K. and Goldberg, S. (1979) Caloric requirements for weight gain in anorexia nervosa. *American Journal of Clinical Nutrition* 32, 1396–1400.

Walshe, C., Phelan, D., Bourke, J. and Buggy, D. (2007) Vascular erosion by central venous catheters used for total parenteral nutrition. *Intensive Care Medicine* 33, 534–537.

III Complications

16 Home Parenteral Nutrition-associated Liver Disease

Vanessa Bon Djemah[1*], Virginie Colomb[2], Olivier Corcos[1], Bernard Messing[1] and Francisca Joly[1,3]

[1]Department of Gastroenterology and Nutrition Support Department, Intestinal Failure Rehabilitation Centre – University of Paris Diderot, France; [2]French Association against Cystic Fibrosis 'Vaincre la mucoviscidose', Paris, France; [3]INSERM, U773, UFR de Médecine Paris 7 – Paris, France

Key Points

- Home parenteral nutrition (HPN)-associated liver disease is related to both the HPN regimen and underlying disease.
- Risk factors include: (i) a ratio of long-chain triacylglycerols (LCT)/glucose >40% or more than 1 g LCT/kg body weight/day; (ii) presence of short bowel, no remnant ileum or <150 cm and colon exclusion; (iii) infection; (iv) hyperalimentation; (v) glucose administration >7 mg/kg body weight/min; and (vi) continuous versus cyclic HPN.
- Prevention (absence of chronic cholestasis) is of the utmost importance.
- Therapy includes, besides optimization of the nutritional regimen: (i) the use of ursodeoxycholic acid, taurine and α-tocopherol supplementation; (ii) short-term antibiotic cover; (iii) re-establishment of colon continuity; and (iv) implementation of enteral feeding.

Introduction

Home parenteral nutrition (HPN)-related liver disease would be better termed HPN-associated liver disease (HPNALD) because not only the HPN regimen (quantity, quality and rhythm of administration) plays a role but also the underlying disease, leading to a varying duration of HPN (1 month to long-term or indefinite HPN). Optimization of HPN delivery over the last 35 years has now delineated favourable conditions avoiding, in the majority of cases, the occurrence of jaundice, i.e. intrahepatic cholestasis, the most frequent clinically encountered situation of HPNALD (Howard and Ashley, 2003). This improvement has uncovered

*E-mail: vanessabondjemah@gmail.com

the importance of steatosis associated with HPN. This histological lesion is increasingly considered responsible for fibrosis and cirrhosis in short bowel syndrome (SBS), as in the general population. However, this progress is hampered by the huge increase in the use of industrial nutritive mixtures in HPN patients (Van Gossum *et al.*, 2001), mixtures that should be considered 'non suitable' for the specific intravenous (IV) nutrition needs of any HPN patient, child or adult (Cavicchi *et al.*, 2000). Therefore, a specific tailored nutritive mixture ('all-in-one' container) must remain the rule rather than the exception for HPN patients, especially for those who are expected to be long-term HPN patients; i.e. those with benign but chronic – permanent – intestinal failure, in whom alternative treatments to long-term HPN are endeavoured, namely the potential HPN candidates for reconstructive surgery or intestinal transplantation (Chan *et al.*, 1999; Buchman *et al.*, 2003; Grant *et al.*, 2005). This approach is of primary importance considering that in the past two decades HPNALD led to liver failure in one of every five patients on long-term HPN (Messing *et al.*, 1995), resulting in either death or being put on a waiting list for combined liver–intestinal transplantation (Buchman *et al.*, 2003). Prevention of HPNALD is therefore of crucial importance from the first days of parenteral nutrition (PN), and the first months of the PN regimen have to be managed carefully in order to avoid chronic cholestasis; i.e. a duration of ≥6 months. This supports that the management of these patients should lie in the hands of expert centres covering the full spectrum of intestinal failure therapy (Buchman *et al.*, 2003).

Prevalence

Chronic abnormalities in liver function tests are reported to occur during HPN in both children and adults, with a wide frequency ranging from 15 to 85% in several series (Bowyer *et al.*, 1985; Stanko *et al.*, 1987; Clarke *et al.*, 1991; Ito and Shils, 1991; Messing *et al.*, 1992; Quigley *et al.*, 1993). In a prospective cohort study of 90 long-term HPN patients enrolled between 1985 and 1996 in two approved HPN centres, actuarial occurrence of severe liver disease (SLD) (bilirubin level > 60 μmol/l, factor V < 50%, portal hypertension, encephalopathy, ascites, gastrointestinal bleeding, histologically proven extensive fibrosis or cirrhosis) was determined by the Kaplan–Meier method: 58 patients (65%) developed chronic cholestasis and 37 (42%) developed SLD after 6 (range: 3–132) months and 17 (range: 2–155) months, respectively. Among these patients, 22 showed histologically proven extensive fibrosis ($n = 17$) or cirrhosis ($n = 5$) after 27 (range: 2–148) months. The prevalence of SLD was 26 ± 9% and 50 ± 13% at 2 and 6 years, respectively. Liver disease was responsible for the death of 7% of patients (22% of the deaths). In these HPN patients with intestinal failure, mean non-protein calorie intake was 88 ± 13% of their resting energy expenditure (REE) (glucose: 4.0 ± 1.2 g/kg body weight/day, soy-based long-chain triacylglycerol (LCT) – or standard 20% lipid – emulsion: 0.64 ± 0.20 g/kg body weight/day), thus intending to avoid the deleterious effect of 'hyperalimentation' (Cavicchi *et al.*, 2000). This long-term HPN regimen included however a wide range of LCT/glucose ratio: 8–40% (cf. below). Indeed, after 2 years of HPN, glucose-based HPN was associated with macrovacuolar steatohepatitis and SLD in less than 25% of patients (Bowyer *et al.*, 1985) whereas lipid-based HPN, i.e. ternary mixtures including standard LCT emulsions of more than 1 g/kg body weight/day, was associated with portal inflammation, ductular abnormalities, microvacuolar steatosis and cholestatic SLD in 50% of patients (Cavicchi *et al.*, 2000).

Diagnosis

Mild increases in liver function tests, mainly indicative of cholestasis (total alkaline phosphatase (ALP) and γ-glutamyltransferase) with a lesser increase in the levels of aspartate aminotransferase/alanine aminotransferase enzymes, are usually seen, with an increase in conjugated bilirubin in 50% of cases. Intrahepatic cholestasis implies non-obstructed and non-dilated bile ducts, a fact that should be verified with liver imaging (Nanji and Anderson 1985; Burnes *et al.*, 1992). If HPNALD persists, severe histological changes consisting of extensive portal fibrosis and/or cirrhosis have been reported which lead, over months to years, to liver failure and death (Stanko *et al.*, 1987; Clarke *et al.*, 1991; Ito and Shils, 1991; Burnes *et al.*, 1992). Chronic cholestasis could be defined as a value at least 1.5-fold the upper limit of normal on two of three liver function measures persisting for at least 6 months, and is associated with a five times higher risk of liver disease (Cavicchi *et al.*, 2000). When liver function tests become abnormal, the occurrence of extensive fibrosis and liver failure can be seen within months in the case of a high degree of PN dependence, i.e. poor oral intake and ongoing IV hyperalimentation (Stanko *et al.*, 1987; Messing *et al.*, 1992). On the other hand, at least in adults, optimized HPN is compatible with long-standing (≥5 years) non-complicated HPNALD cirrhosis (personal unpublished observations). Peculiar clinical findings are: (i) the absence of pruritus despite 'bronze' jaundice, this is probably due to the disrupted enterohepatic cycle of bile acids in patients with short gut and no remnant ileum; (ii) portal hypertension, although less pronounced due to the decreased portal blood flow following intestinal resection, may present in enterostomy patients with stoma blood losses, either overt or occult, and this calls for stoma care; and (iii) in HPN patients, jaundice with increased conjugated and unconjugated bilirubin, splenomegaly and thrombocytopenia (but not hepatomegaly, anaemia or leucopenia) can be significantly associated with noticeable sea-blue histiocytes ($CD68^+$ activated macrophages) infiltration of bone marrow without haemophagocytosis (Stanko *et al.*, 1987; Messing *et al.*, 1992; Bigorgne *et al.*, 1996, 1998). This latter fate means there is an accumulation of polyunsaturated fatty acids (PUFAs), coming from an overly high long-term standard lipid delivery through ternary mixtures, in the reticuloendothelial cells (Stanko *et al.*, 1987; Messing *et al.*, 1992; Bigorgne *et al.*, 1996, 1998). This sea-blue histiocyte syndrome might be present in adults as a chronic one (Silverstein *et al.*, 1970) or, especially in children, as a flare up revealed by underlying infection (Colomb *et al.*, 2000). Phytosterolaemia has been described in HPNALD in children and in preliminary adult studies as a biological marker of IV fat infusion (Moss and Amii, 1999). Unfortunately, there is no diagnostic criterion other than liver biopsy. Indeed, neither ultrasound nor computed tomography scan or

FibroScan has proved its efficiency in the detection of liver disease. However, these diagnostic tests can help exclude other causes of cholestasis.

After having excluded bile duct stone(s) by imaging, positive HPNALD diagnosis relies on liver biopsy: histological elemental lesions are composed of micro/macrovacuolar steatosis, portal inflammation and ductular abnormalities, and hepatocyte necrosis; these lesions, despite being non-specific, form a suggestive pattern. They can be of very early occurrence, ≥30 days of PN (Levecq *et al.*, 1988), and when chronic cholestasis is seen, extensive or bridging fibrosis and cirrhosis are respectively documented in 35% and 11% of cases after a median duration of 2 and 3 years (Cavicchi *et al.*, 2000).

Indeed, in a study looking at the natural history of HPNALD, the probability of developing either abnormalities in liver function tests or histological HPNALD were very close and non-significantly different during the mean 5-year follow-up (Cavicchi *et al.*, 2000). Microvacuolar steatosis, phospholipidosis (Degott *et al.*, 1988), accumulation of phospholipids, polyunsaturated triglycerides within hepatocytes and hyperplasia of macrophages, i.e. Kupffer cells in and around sinusoids or in and around portal areas (Levecq *et al.*, 1988; Imamura *et al.*, 2005), need special staining to be revealed (Oil Red O and OTAN–Baker+), and are especially seen when ternary nutritive mixtures are used. This fate explains why microsteatosis was not described with the use of IV fat infusions whereas hepatocyte macrosteatosis was easily demonstrated, for instance with high glucose infusions (Messing *et al.*, 1977, 1979).

Pathophysiology

HPNALD is multifactorial and recent reviews have listed implicated variables (Buchman *et al.*, 1993). We favour pragmatic – but yet incomplete – pathophysiology, best delineated between nutrition- and patient-related variables, because this allows practical management (prophylaxis and curative treatment) of such a complication. Indeed, pathogenesis of HPNALD, if intricate and multifactorial, involves patient-dependent factors, especially SBS (Stanko *et al.*, 1987; Clarke *et al.*, 1991; Ito and Shils 1991; Cavicchi *et al.*, 2000), and nutrition factors, especially 'intravenous hyperalimentation' (Luman and Shaffer, 2002) or soy-rich PUFA triacylglycerol emulsion (more than 1 g/kg body weight/day) even without hyperalimentation (Stanko *et al.*, 1987; Bigorgne *et al.*, 1996; Cavicchi *et al.*, 2000).

Patient-related variables

Lack of enteral feeding seems to be associated with HPNALD. A few studies have demonstrated the negative effect of large ileum resection. In univariate analysis, ileum resection (Messing *et al.*, 1994) and in multivariate analysis, short bowel either less than 150 cm (Luman and Shaffer, 2002) (odds ratio (OR) = 3.2, 95% confidence interval (CI) 1.5–5.3) or less than 50 cm (OR = 2.1, 95% CI 1.2–3.7) (Cavicchi *et al.*, 2000) and colon exclusion (OR = 3.9, 95% CI 1.7–5.6) (Messing *et al.*, 1994) were related to the development of chronic cholestasis during HPN. In the former study, chronic cholestasis was associated with the development of SLD (OR = 4.8, 95% CI 1.6–13.7) (Cavicchi *et al.*, 2000).

In very short bowel, especially if enteral protein absorption is less than 25% of total needs in children (Geggel *et al.*, 1985), the systemic taurine pool is depleted (plasma, platelet and lymphocyte levels are significantly lower than controls) (Kopple *et al.*, 1990; Iglicki *et al.*, 1996). Indeed, in nine HPN-dependent SBS patients receiving taurine-free HPN, taurine turnover was one-third less than reference values (A.M. Badran *et al.*, personal unpublished data). In addition, despite normalization of plasma taurine levels in SBS patients using long-term taurine-enriched (300 mg/day) amino acid solutions, a huge persistent depletion of taurine- versus glycine-conjugated bile salts, irrespective of the length of the remnant jejunum, was documented. This indirect evaluation of the enterohepatic bile salt pool through dosage of plasma bile salts suggests that huge bile salt losses due to the ruptured enterohepatic cycle (Ferezou *et al.*, 1993) are not easily corrected with IV provision of taurine (Kopple *et al.*, 1990).

Other factors implicated in the occurrence of HPNALD are intestinal bacterial overgrowth and translocation (Chazouilleres *et al.*, 1987) and/or disruption of the enterohepatic bile acid pool with the occurrence of tertiary deconjugated 'toxic' bile acids (Fouin-Fortunet *et al.*, 1982). Then colon exclusion of several months' duration, with morphopolynuclear inflammation of the mucosa (Harig *et al.*, 1989) and changes in the bacterial flora (Neut *et al.*, 1989), induces translocation with ensuing cholestasis. In the same line of evidence, sepsis – either systemic or gut-induced – is a factor increasing the occurrence of cholestasis in children or adults receiving PN (Messing *et al.*, 1992; Matsui *et al.*, 1993; Beau *et al.*, 1994a). Indeed, it has been postulated that PN-associated chronic cholestasis could be exacerbated by sepsis and that Kupffer cell dysfunction may participate in its pathogenesis (Scott-Conner and Grogan, 1994; Cavicchi *et al.*, 2000; Pironi *et al.*, 2003a).

Nutrition-related variables

When short-term ternary hyperalimentation was used (45–60 kcal/kg body weight/day), cholestasis was more frequent (ALP: 25–60%, bilirubin: 12–30%) than with lower ternary PN levels (30–40 kcal/kg body weight/day) (ALP: 15–25%, bilirubin: 5–10%) (Allardyce *et al.*, 1978; Bengoa *et al.*, 1985; Messing, *et al.*, 1992). Malnourished patients are more prone to liver injury provoked by a load of excess macronutrients (Lerebours *et al.*, 1986; Braxton and Lowry, 1995), focusing again on the importance of an appropriate IV infusion when a diagnosis of intestinal failure is made. Glucose infusion of more than 7 mg/kg body weight/min is associated with a respiratory quotient of more than one, meaning *de novo* lipid synthesis in the liver with saturated triglyceride depots in hepatocytes (Wolfe *et al.*, 1988; Just *et al.*, 1990). A parallel increase in blood triglycerides can be observed (Messing *et al.*, 1977). Essential fatty acid deficiency or choline deficiency decreases lower extrusion of liver triglycerides, leading to higher macrosteatosis (Fleming *et al.*, 1976; Jeejeebhoy *et al.*, 1976; Reif *et al.*, 1991;

Demetriou, 1992; Buchman *et al.*, 1995; Reimund *et al.*, 2001; Howard and Ashley, 2003).

A factor contributing to fatty liver development is bacterial translocation (Neut *et al.*, 1989; Moss and Amii, 1999). It is therefore logical to foresee steatohepatitis under the above-mentioned conditions. A great amount of the lipid infusion is not oxidized and thus is stored, especially if simultaneous infusion of glucose is realized with ternary mixtures (Just *et al.*, 1991). These depots are loaded within reticuloendothelial cells, especially in the spleen and liver (Degott *et al.*, 1988; Levecq *et al.*, 1988; Zoli *et al.*, 1998; Reimund *et al.*, 2001).

Lipoprotein X (LPX) is made of an equimolecular amount of cholesterol and phospholipids, the former being taken up from cell membranes. LPX is a marker of the abnormal metabolism of lipid infusion: its blood level increase with the triacylglycerol IV load but its production is greater with the 10% versus the 20% lipid emulsion due to a twofold higher phospholipids/triacylglycerols ratio (Messing *et al.*, 1990). LPX, like PUFA lipids, are deposited in Kupffer cells and hepatoctes, thus explaining microsteatosis (cf. above).

It was observed that liver function test abnormalities were more frequent ($P<0.02$) in ternary 'all-in-one' mixtures ($n=48$; 54%) than when lipids were infused separately ($n=58$; 29%) (Beau *et al.*, 1988). Stability of ternary mixtures was one possible explanation for this fact (Gerard-Boncompain *et al.*, 1992). In multivariate analysis, an IV lipid input (20% soy emulsions, rich in PUFAs) of more than 1 g/kg body weight/day was clearly associated during PN with both chronic cholestasis (OR = 2.3, 95% CI 1.6–5.9) and SLD (OR = 3.4, 95% CI 1.6–6.8) (Cavicchi *et al.*, 2000). This fate was linked only to IV lipid intake and observed without hypercaloric feeding (cf. above). The probability of being free of SLD after 2 years of HPN was only 50% when a dose of soy-based lipid exceeding 1 g/kg body weight/day was used, compared with >80% when less than 1 g/kg body weight/day was given. In the latter situation, less than 25% of cases developed SLD after 6 years of HPN for intestinal failure (Cavicchi *et al.*, 2000). Therefore standard 20% lipid emulsions (soy-rich PUFAs) are dramatically deleterious for the liver when used at a dosage rate of more than 1 g/kg body weight/day.

In general, blood essential fatty acid (EFA) profiles in HPN patients indicate normal arachidonic acid levels, even with low amounts of IV PUFAs, i.e. 5–10% of calorie load, but decreased docosahexaenoic acid, even with large amounts of IV PUFAs (up to 50% of calorie load). Thus, a relative unbalance/deficit of *n*-3 lipids is observed, with a further specific negative effect of a very short bowel (Chambrier *et al.*, 2002). The use of medium-chain triacylglycerol (MCT)/LCT solution – 50 g per infusion – for 4 months did not change most of the EFA profiles (Chambrier *et al.*, 2004). These observations suggest that pro-inflammatory leucotrienes and cytokines might be increased with ternary mixtures (Reimund *et al.*, 2004a).

Lipoperoxidation induced by acute IV lipid infusion is a well-known phenomenon (Lemoyne *et al.*, 1988; Van Gossum *et al.*, 1988) and it is further increased with: (i) the HPN duration; (ii) the soy PUFA load (1 g/kg body weight/day); and (iii) a lower vitamin E status (Pironi *et al.*, 1998). Effectively, the ratio vitamin E (α-tocopherol)/g of PUFAs that induces the lowest lipid peroxidation was estimated to be ≅0.6, depending on the degree of unsaturation (Valk and Hornstra, 2000; MacDonald *et al.*, 2001), a ratio that is hardly found in most lipid emulsions; i.e. total tocopherols/g of PUFAs is usually 0.33 (range: 0.15–3.3). Furthermore, tocopherols are considered to be poorly available in lipid emulsion and competition exists between the α- and more abundant but less active forms, whereas exchange is very active at the time of chylomicron metabolism (Kelly and Sutton, 1989; Steephen *et al.*, 1991). In the short term (10 days), 3.4 g of α-tocopherol/g of PUFAs (MCT/LCT enriched in vitamin E) reduced the peroxidation versus LCT controls (ratio of 0.2) in ternary mixture PN (Jonas *et al.*, 2000; Manuel-y-Keenoy *et al.*, 2002).

In addition, storage of all-in-one mixtures may induce the following: (i) degradation/losses of vitamins E, C, etc. in ethylvinyl acetate bags (Gomis Munoz *et al.*, 1996; Silvers *et al.*, 2001; Pironi *et al.*, 2003b), (ii) light-induced peroxidation that may require darkened storage/delivery conditions; and (iii) an increased amount of oversized fat globules in some all-in-one mixtures (Allwood and Martin, 2000; Driscoll *et al.*, 2001, 2003). The latter fate induces enhanced fat trapping in the reticuloendothelial system and peroxidation.

Liver tolerance of new or semi-recent lipid emulsions (mixed MCT/LCT, olive oil-based, enriched *n*-3, etc.) have been poorly studied during HPN (Chambrier *et al.*, 2004; Reimund *et al.*, 2004b, 2005) and a clear-cut conclusion cannot be made at this point. In contrast, during the last decade many case reports and open studies have shown that the use of injectable lipid emulsions (ELIs) based on fish oils rich in *n*-3 PUFAs seems beneficial in patients with intestinal failure. Decrease of icteric cholestasis in 4–12 weeks has been noted with such emulsions (Koletzko and Goulet, 2010). It is however important to note in these observations that a strong dose of ELI soy was replaced by 1 g fish oil/kg and the decrease in liver abnormalities after the switch to fish oil was equivalent to the decrease after a stop of ELI. Decreased choleresis is a contributing factor of HPNALD: no food intake (i.e. exclusive PN), continuous instead cyclic PN delivery, excess or unbalanced amino acid infusion (deficit in taurine or *S*-adenosyl donors) were associated with cholestasis in few clinical (Messing *et al.*, 1982) but in many experimental studies (Belli *et al.*, 1987; De Bandt *et al.*, 1999).

Lastly, excess contaminants such as aluminium, manganese and copper in nutritive mixtures (Quigley *et al.*, 1993; Reynolds *et al.*, 1998; Van Gossum and Neve, 1998; Blaszyk *et al.*, 2005), or iron delivery, or deficit in antioxidants such as selenium, glutathione and vitamin C may also facilitate peroxidation of macronutrients; ensuing inflammatory liver fibrosis secondary to excess iron deposits (or other metals) is not treatable through antioxidant supplementation.

To summarize, the last decades have proved the implication of the type of lipid emulsion in HPNALD. Mechanisms involved are: (i) impairment of biliary secretion; (ii) liver toxicity of phytosterols present in soy oil; (iii) reticuloendothelium system overload; and (iv) excess of PUFAs, responsible for lipid peroxidation, conversion to arachidonic acid and overproduction of pro-inflammatory cytokines.

Treatment: Preventive and Curative

Patient-related

After a case report of efficient sequential ursodeoxycholic acid (UDCA) treatment (Lindor and Burnes, 1991), it was shown that UDCA given orally (15 mg/kg body weight/day) can improve HPN-associated cholestasis in both children ($n=7$) and adults ($n=9$) (Geggel *et al.*, 1985; Beau *et al.*, 1994b; Spagnuolo *et al.*, 1996). Biological improvement could be achieved in 2–8 weeks (Beau *et al.*, 1994b; Spagnuolo *et al.*, 1996). At 30 mg/kg body weight/day, even in SBS, incorporation at a level of 40% in the bile salt pool was demonstrated (Iglicki *et al.*, 1996). UDCA decreases the reduced choleresis, protects hepatocytes from overproduction of cytotoxic biliary acids (Poupon and Poupon, 1995) and reduces HLA class I antigen overexpression on hepatocytes (Innes *et al.*, 1988; Calmus *et al.*, 1990).

Taurine parenteral supplementation has been reported to ameliorate PN-associated cholestasis through promoted bile flow (Guertin *et al.*, 1991, 1993) and to prevent lithocholic acid-induced cholestasis in guinea pigs (Guertin *et al.*, 1991). In children, it has been proposed to include taurine in parenteral nutrition solutions (Cooke *et al.*, 1984; Howard and Thompson, 1992; Helms *et al.*, 1999). Taurine may be beneficial by increasing hydrophilic tauro-conjugated bile acids and preventing cell membrane changes caused by oxidative stress (Guertin *et al.*, 1991; Redmond *et al.*, 1998). Taurine has been also shown to reduce pro-inflammatory cytokine production in Kupffer cells and to ameliorate defective phagocytic and pro-inflammatory cell microbicidal capacities (Redmond *et al.*, 1998). In 15 patients with portal fibrosis at baseline who received UDCA with ($n=6$) or without ($n=9$) taurine, we found ten responders with a better response to both treatments and in those with the shortest HPN duration. Our policy is to treat intestinal failure due to very short bowel with taurine-enriched amino acid solution (Hardison, 1978) and to instigate oral UDCA as early as we can in the course of the disease. Multicentre trials are necessary to confirm whether the association of UDCA and taurine could prevent SLD in long-term HPN.

Short-term courses of oral or IV antibiotic treatments were shown to reduce cholestasis of (H)PN patients (Beau *et al.*, 1994a). Our policy is to give oral sequential antibiotic treatment oriented against Gram-negative or anaerobic bacteria, especially when patients have dysmotile bowel or incomplete bowel stenoses. Re-establishment of colon continuity instead of diversion is associated with a lower risk of cholestasis during HPN (Messing *et al.*, 1994). Meanwhile, our policy is to nourish the excluded segment with short-chain fatty acid enemas (Gerard-Boncompain *et al.*, 1992).

Nutritionally related

Drastic reduction, just sufficient to prevent essential fatty acid deficiency, or suppression of soy lipid emulsion for several months was demonstrated to reduce chronic cholestasis and lipid thesaurismosis in both children and adults (Gerard-Boncompain *et al.*, 1992; Colomb *et al.*, 2000). Our policy is to give cyclic nocturnal PN with no more energy than 1.2 times the REE, with less than 1 g/kg body weight/day or no more than 33% of total calories as 20% lipid emulsion (Cavicchi *et al.*, 2000). Replacement of standard soy emulsions with LCT/MCT or oleic acid-based and/or fish oil-based emulsions might represent an advantage (Reimund *et al.*, 2004b; Thomas-Gibson *et al.*, 2004), but should be tested through large multicentre trials. Reducing as much as possible the HPN regimen, i.e. the number of cycles per week and the quantity of each cycle (Messing *et al.*, 1999), implies maximal use of enteral feeding and optimal treatment of the underlying disease having led to intestinal failure. For SBS, dietetic advice and optimization of absorption now include, beside the usual gastroenterological medications, indications for recombinant human growth hormone administration and bowel reconstruction (see Chapter 37 in the current volume). In most cases, HPN is just complementary, but complete, individualized feeding avoiding both excess and deficits of minerals and micronutrients. Supplements of α-tocopherol according to IV PUFAs (cf. above) and reduction of trace metals when cholestasis is present (Howard and Ashley, 2003) should not be omitted. Adjustment to both IV supply and remnant gut absorption according the aetiology of the intestinal failure is beyond the scope of this chapter. However, it can be stated that there is no documented carnitine deficiency during long-term HPN (Bowyer *et al.*, 1988, 1989; Messing *et al.*, 1999) and therefore no obvious benefit of using MCT-enriched IV lipids for increasing their oxidation during HPN in unstressed, stable patients – with some exceptions due to the underlying disease (e.g. chronic intestinal pseudo-obstruction due to mitochondrial cytopathies, severe renal insufficiency, cirrhosis) (Goulet *et al.*, 1992; Richelle *et al.*, 1993).

Future Developments

The natural history of HPNALD (Cavicchi *et al.*, 2000) and the main contributing factors, related to both nutrition and the patient, have been described. These suggested factors act more as combined than as isolated factors. Controlled intervention studies, at a multicentre level, need to be performed to confirm the primary prophylaxis of HPNALD through choleretic treatment associated with new IV fat sources at an appropriate level plus antiperoxidative treatment such as α-tocopherol and other supplements. These long-term therapeutic trials, though difficult to set up, have to be settled as soon as possible through an expert consensus meeting in order to implement such studies at an international level in centres managing all the facets of intestinal failure treatment (Buchman *et al.*, 2003). The main goal is to reduce SLD to a minimum; SLD still remains too frequent as illustrated by the high number of combined liver–intestinal transplants depicted in the last report of the international transplant registry, i.e. 50% and 51% in children and adults, respectively (Grant *et al.*, 2005).

Summary

HPNALD can be reduced to less than 20% after 5 years of HPN for intestinal failure (Cavicchi *et al.*, 2000). HPN needs to be tailored, from the early days of PN, for each single patient deemed to depend on HPN for more than 6 months. Presently, industrial nutritive mixtures do not fulfil the goal, mainly because their IV lipid loads are too high. To prevent HPNALD, optimized HPN and optimized disease treatment are two facets of a single coin, because minimal PN dependency is one way to avoid excess delivery of IV macronutrient infusion of each complete PN cycle. It is also necessary to focus on perfect nursing care to obtain complete autonomy of patients in managing the PN infusion cycle; indeed, reducing the rate of line sepsis can be achieved through patient's autonomy (Nahon *et al.*, 1997). It is therefore a pity that a European survey (Van Gossum *et al.*, 2001) indicates that complete education of patients is less accomplished now than in the past (Messing *et al.*, 1988). Indeed, line sepsis control is just as important as other physiopathological factors contributing to HPNALD.

References

Allardyce, D.B., Salvian, A.J. and Quenville, N.F. (1978) Cholestatic jaundice during total parenteral nutrition. *Canadian Journal of Surgery* 21, 332–339.

Allwood, M.C. and Martin, H.J. (2000) The photodegradation of vitamins A and E in parenteral nutrition mixtures during infusion. *Clinical Nutrition* 19, 329–342.

Beau, P., Chammartin, F. and Matuchansky, C. (1988) Biological hepatic abnormalities, cholestatic jaundice and hospital artificial nutrition. A comparative study in adults with cyclic total parenteral nutrition and enteral nutrition. *Gastroentérologie Clinique et Biologique* 12, 326–331.

Beau, P., Barrioz, T. and Ingrand, P. (1994a) Total parenteral nutrition-related cholestatic hepatopathy, is it an infectious disease? *Gastroentérologie Clinique et Biologique* 18, 63–67.

Beau, P., Labat-Labourdette, J., Ingrand, P. and Beachant, M. (1994b) Is ursodeoxycholic acid an effective therapy for total parenteral nutrition-related liver disease? *Journal of Hepatology* 20, 240–244.

Belli, D.C., Fournier, L.A., Lepage, G., Youssef, I., Weber, A., Tuchweber, B. and Roy, C. (1987) Total parenteral nutrition-associated cholestasis in rats: comparison of different amino acid mixtures. *JPEN Journal of Parenteral and Enteral Nutrition* 11, 67–73.

Bengoa, J.M., Hanauer, S.B., Sitrin, M., Baker, A. and Rosenberg, I. (1985) Pattern and prognosis of liver function test abnormalities during parenteral nutrition in inflammatory bowel disease. *Hepatology* 5, 79–84.

Bigorgne, C., Le Tourneau, A., Vahedi, K., Rio, B., Messing, B., Molina, T., Audouin, J. and Diebold, J. (1996) Sea-blue histiocyte syndrome in bone marrow secondary to total parenteral nutrition including fat-emulsion sources: a clinicopathologic study of seven cases. *British Journal of Haematology* 95, 258–262.

Bigorgne, C., Le Tourneau, A., Vahedi, K., Rio, B., Messing, B., Molina, T., Audouin, J. and Diebold, J. (1998) Sea-blue histiocyte syndrome in bone marrow secondary to total parenteral nutrition. *Leukemia and Lymphoma* 28, 523–529.

Blaszyk, H., Wild, P.J., Oliveira, A., Kelly, D.G. and Burgart, L.J. (2005) Hepatic copper in patients receiving long-term total parenteral nutrition. *Journal of Clinical Gastroenterology* 39, 318–320.

Bowyer, B.A., Fleming, C.R., Ludwig, J., Petz, J. and McGill, D.B. (1985) Does long-term home parenteral nutrition in adult patients cause chronic liver disease? *JPEN Journal of Parenteral and Enteral Nutrition* 9, 11–17.

Bowyer, B.A., Miles, J.M., Haymond, M.W. and Fleming, C.R. (1988) L-Carnitine therapy in home parenteral nutrition patients with abnormal liver tests and low plasma carnitine concentrations. *Gastroenterology* 94, 434–438.

Bowyer, B.A., Fleming, C.R., Haymond, M.W. and Miles, J. (1989) L-Carnitine: effect of intravenous administration on fuel homeostasis in normal subjects and home-parenteral-nutrition patients with low plasma carnitine concentrations. *American Journal of Clinical Nutrition* 49, 618–623.

Braxton, C. and Lowry, S.F. (1995) Parenteral nutrition and liver dysfunction: new insight? *JPEN Journal of Parenteral and Enteral Nutrition* 19, 3–4.

Buchman, A.L., Moukarzel, A., Jenden, D.J., Roch, M., Rice, K. and Ament, M.E. (1993) Low plasma free choline is prevalent in patients receiving long term parenteral nutrition and is associated with hepatic aminotransferase abnormalities. *Clinical Nutrition* 12, 33–37.

Buchman, A.L., Dubin, M.D., Moukarzel, A.A., Jenden, D.J., Roch, M., Rice, K.M., Gornbein, J. and Ament, M.E. (1995) Choline deficiency: a cause of hepatic steatosis during parenteral nutrition that can be reversed with intravenous choline supplementation. *Hepatology* 22, 1399–1403.

Buchman, A.L., Scolapio, J. and Fryer, J. (2003) AGA technical review on short bowel syndrome and intestinal transplantation. *Gastroenterology* 124, 1111–1134.

Burnes, J.U., O'Keefe, S.J., Fleming, C.R., Devine, R.M., Berkner, S. and Herrick, L. (1992) Home parenteral nutrition – a 3-year analysis of clinical and laboratory monitoring. *JPEN Journal of Parenteral and Enteral Nutrition* 16, 327–332.

Calmus, Y., Gane, P., Rouger, P. and Poupon, R. (1990) Hepatic expression of class I and class II major histocompatibility complex molecules in primary biliary cirrhosis: effect of ursodeoxycholic acid. *Hepatology* 11, 12–15.

Cavicchi, M., Beau, P., Crenn, P., Degott, C. and Messing, B. (2000) Prevalence of liver disease and contributing factors in patients receiving home parenteral nutrition for permanent intestinal failure. *Annals of Internal Medicine* 132, 525–532.

Chambrier, C., Garcia, I., Bannier, E., Gerard-Boncompain, M. and Bouletreau, P. (2002) Specific changes in *n*-6 fatty acid metabolism in patients with chronic intestinal failure. *Clinical Nutrition* 21, 67–72.

Chambrier, C., Bannier, E., Lauverjat, M., Drai, J., Bryssine, S. and Bouletreau, P. (2004) Replacement of long-chain triglyceride with medium-chain triglyceride/long-chain triglyceride lipid emulsion in patients receiving long-term parenteral nutrition: effects on essential fatty acid status and plasma vitamin K_1 levels. *JPEN Journal of Parenteral and Enteral Nutrition* 28, 7–12.

Chan, S., McCowen, K.C., Bistrian, B.R., Thibault, A., Keane-Ellison, M., Forse, R.A., Babineau, T. and Burke, P. (1999) Incidence, prognosis, and etiology of end-stage liver disease in patients receiving home total parenteral nutrition. *Surgery* 126, 28–34.

Chazouilleres, O., Rautureau, M., Ink, O., Bisalli, A., Colombel, J.F. and Messing, B. (1987) Is chronic bacterial contamination of the small intestine associated with cholestasis in total parenteral feeding? *Gastroentérologie Clinique et Biologique* 11, 98–99.

Clarke, P.J., Ball, M.J. and Kettlewell, M.G. (1991) Liver function tests in patients receiving parenteral nutrition. *JPEN Journal of Parenteral and Enteral Nutrition* 15, 54–59.

Colomb, V., Jobert-Giraud, A., Lacaille, F., Goulet, O., Fournet, J.C. and Ricour, C. (2000) Role of lipid emulsions in cholestasis associated with long-term parenteral nutrition in children. *JPEN Journal of Parenteral and Enteral Nutrition* 24, 345–350.

Cooke, R.J., Whitington, P.F. and Kelts, D. (1984) Effect of taurine supplementation on hepatic function during short-term parenteral nutrition in the premature infant. *Journal of Pediatric Gastroenterology and Nutrition* 3, 234–238.

De Bandt, J.P., Lasnier, E., Rey, C., Coudray-Lucas, C., Poupon, R., Giboudeau, J. and Cynober, L.A. (1999) Effects of amino acids on bile acid-dependent and independent bile flow in the isolated perfused rat liver. *Journal of Hepatology* 30, 843–849.

Degott, C., Messing, B., Moreau, D., Chazouilleres, O., Paris, R., Colombel, J.F., Lebrec, D., Potet, F., Feldmann, G. and Benhamou, J.P. (1988) Liver phospholipidosis induced by parenteral nutrition: histologic, histochemical, and ultrastructural investigations. *Gastroenterology* 95, 183–191.

Demetriou, A.A. (1992) Lecithin increases plasma-free choline and decreases hepatic steatosis in long-term total parenteral nutrition patients. *JPEN Journal of Parenteral and Enteral Nutrition* 16, 487–488.

Driscoll, D.F., Giampietro, K., Wichelhaus, D.P., Peterss, H., Nehne, J., Niemann, W. and Bistrian, B.R. (2001) Physicochemical stability assessments of lipid emulsions of varying oil composition. *Clinical Nutrition* 20, 151–157.

Driscoll, D.F., Nehne, J., Peterss, H., Klutsch, K., Bistrian, B.R. and Niemann, W. (2003) Physicochemical stability of intravenous lipid emulsions as all-in-one admixtures intended for the very young. *Clinical Nutrition* 22, 489–495.

Ferezou, J., Beau, P., Parquet, M., Champarnaud, G., Lutton, C. and Matuchansky, C. (1993) Cholesterol and bile acid biodynamics after total small bowel resection and bile diversion in humans. *Gastroenterology* 104, 1786–1795.

Fleming, C.R., Smith, L.M. and Hodges, R.E. (1976) Essential fatty acid deficiency in adults receiving total parenteral nutrition. *American Journal of Clinical Nutrition* 29, 976–983.

Fouin-Fortunet, H., Le Quernec, L., Erlinger, S., Lerebours, E. and Colin, R. (1982) Hepatic alterations during total parenteral nutrition in patients with inflammatory bowel disease: a possible consequence of lithocholate toxicity. *Gastroenterology* 82, 932–937.

Geggel, H.S., Ament, M.E., Heckenlively, J.R., Martin, D.A. and Kopple, J.D. (1985) Nutritional requirement for taurine in patients receiving long-term parenteral nutrition. *New England Journal of Medicine* 312, 142–146.

Gerard-Boncompain, M., Claudel, J.P., Gaussorgues, P., Salord, F., Sirodot, M., Chevallier, M. and Robert, D. (1992) Hepatic cytolytic and cholestatic changes related to a change of lipid emulsions in four long-term parenteral nutrition patients with short bowel. *JPEN Journal of Parenteral and Enteral Nutrition* 16, 78–83.

Gomis Munoz, P., Miguelez Sanchez, S., Navarro Gonzalvez, J.A., Estenoz Alfaro, J., Alegre del Rey, E., Moreno Villares, J.M., Valero Zannuy, M.A. and Leon Sanz, M. (1996) Stability of vitamins in parenteral nutrition: a comparison of multi-layer and uni-layer bags. *Nutrición Hospitalaria* 11, 259–264.

Goulet, O., Postaire, M., De Potter, S., Boya, I., Jouniaux, A.M., Bereziat, G. and Ricour, C. (1992) Medium-chain triglycerides and long-term parenteral nutrition in children. *Nutrition* 8, 333–337.

Grant, D., Abu-Elmagd, K., Reyes, J., Tzakis, A., Langnas, A., Fishbein, T., Goulet, O. and Farmer, D. on behalf of the Intestine Transplant Registry (2005) 2003 report of the intestine transplant registry: a new era has dawned. *Annals of Surgery* 241, 607–613.

Guertin, F., Roy, C.C., Lepage, G., Perea, A., Giguere, R., Yousef, I. and Tuchweber, B. (1991) Effect of taurine on total parenteral nutrition-associated cholestasis. *JPEN Journal of Parenteral and Enteral Nutrition* 15, 247–251.

Guertin, F., Roy, C.C., Lepage, G., Yousef, I. and Tuchweber, B. (1993) Liver membrane composition after short-term parenteral nutrition with and without taurine in guinea pigs: the effect of taurine. *Proceedings of the Society of Experimental Biology and Medicine* 203, 418–423.

Hardison, W.G. (1978) Hepatic taurine concentration and dietary taurine as regulators of bile acid conjugation with taurine. *Gastroenterology* 75, 71–75.

Harig, J.M., Soergel, K.H., Komorowski, R.A. and Wood, C.M. (1989) Treatment of diversion colitis with short-chain-fatty acid irrigation. *New England Journal of Medicine* 320, 23–28.

Helms, R.A., Storm, M.C., Christensen, M.L., Hak, E.B. and Chesney, R.W. (1999) Cysteine supplementation results in normalization of plasma taurine concentrations in children receiving home parenteral nutrition. *Journal of Pediatrics* 134, 358–361.

Howard, L. and Ashley, C. (2003) Management of complications in patients receiving home parenteral nutrition. *Gastroenterology* 124, 1651–1661.

Howard, D. and Thompson, D.F. (1992) Taurine: an essential amino acid to prevent cholestasis in neonates? *Annals of Pharmacotherapy* 26, 1390–1392.

Iglicki, F., Crenn, P. and Messing, B. (1996) Plasma tauroconjugated bile acid levels in short bowel patients undergoing home parenteral nutrition. *Clinical Nutrition* 15, 4A.

Imamura, M., Ogawa, T., Sasaguri, Y., Chayama, K. and Ueno, H. (2005) Suppression of macrophage infiltration inhibits activation of hepatic stellate cells and liver fibrogenesis in rats. *Gastroenterology* 128, 138–146.

Innes, G.K., Nagafuchi, Y., Fuller, B.J. and Hobbs, K.E. (1988) Increased expression of major histocompatibility antigens in the liver as a result of cholestasis. *Transplantation* 45, 749–752.

Ito, Y. and Shils, M.E. (1991) Liver dysfunction associated with long-term total parenteral nutrition in patients with massive bowel resection. *JPEN Journal of Parenteral and Enteral Nutrition* 15, 271–276.

Jeejeebhoy, K.N., Langer, B., Tsallas, G., Chu, R.C., Kuksis, A. and Anderson, G.H. (1976) Total parenteral nutrition at home: studies in patients surviving 4 months to 5 years. *Gastroenterology* 71, 943–953.

Jonas, C.R., Puckett, A.B., Jones, D.P., Griffith, D.P., Szeszycki, E.E., Bergman, G.F., Furr, C.E., Tyre, C., Carlson, J.L., Galloway, J.R., Blumberg, J.B. and Ziegler, T.R. (2000) Plasma antioxidant status after high-dose chemotherapy: a randomized trial of parenteral nutrition in bone marrow transplantation patients. *American Journal of Clinical Nutrition* 72, 181–189.

Just, B., Messing, B., Darmaun, D., Rongier, M. and Camillo, E. (1990) Comparison of substrate utilization by indirect calorimetry during cyclic and continuous total parenteral nutrition. *American Journal of Clinical Nutrition* 51, 107–111.

Just, B., Messing, B. and Darmaun, D. (1991) Oral nutrition in patients receiving home cyclic parenteral nutrition: pattern of substrate utilization. *American Journal of Clinical Nutrition* 54, 560–564.

Kelly, F.J. and Sutton, G.L. (1989) Plasma and red blood cell vitamin E status of patients on total parenteral nutrition. *JPEN Journal of Parenteral and Enteral Nutrition* 13, 510–515.

Koletzko, B. and Goulet, O. (2010) Fish oil containing intravenous lipid emulsions in parenteral nutrition-associated cholestatic liver disease. *Current Opinion in Clinical Nutrition and Metabolic Care* 13, 321–326

Kopple, J.D., Vinton, N.E., Laidlaw, S.A. and Ament, M.E. (1990) Effect of intravenous taurine supplementation on plasma, blood cell, and urine taurine concentrations in adults undergoing long-term parenteral nutrition. *American Journal of Clinical Nutrition* 52, 846–853.

Lemoyne, M., Van Gossum, A., Kurian, R. and Jeejeebhoy, K.N. (1988) Plasma vitamin E and selenium and breath pentane in home parenteral nutrition patients. *American Journal of Clinical Nutrition* 48, 1310–1315.

Lerebours, E., Messing, B., Chevalier, B., Bories, C., Colin, R. and Bernier, J.J. (1986) An evaluation of total parenteral nutrition in the management of steroid-dependent and steroid-resistant patients with Crohn's disease. *JPEN Journal of Parenteral and Enteral Nutrition* 10, 274–278.

Levecq, H., Lageron, A., Gotheil, C., Callard, P. and Beaugrand, M. (1988) Hepatic lipid overload in 2 cases of cholestasis associated with parenteral feeding. *Gastroentérologie Clinique et Biologique* 12, 691–696.

Lindor, K.D. and Burnes, J. (1991) Ursodeoxycholic acid for the treatment of home parenteral nutrition-associated cholestasis. A case report. *Gastroenterology* 101, 250–253.

Luman, W. and Shaffer, J.L. (2002) Prevalence, outcome and associated factors of deranged liver function tests in patients on home parenteral nutrition. *Clinical Nutrition* 21, 337–343.

MacDonald, G.A., Bridle, K.R., Ward, P.J., Walker, N.I., Houglum, K., George, D.K., Smith, J.L., Powell, L.W., Crawford, D.H. and Ramm, G.A. (2001) Lipid peroxidation in hepatic steatosis in humans is associated with hepatic fibrosis and occurs predominantly in acinar zone 3. *Journal of Gastroenterology and Hepatology* 16, 599–606.

Manuel-y-Keenoy, B., Nonneman, L., De Bosscher, H., Vertommen, J., Schrans, S., Klutsch, K. and De Leeuw, I. (2002) Effects of intravenous supplementation with α-tocopherol in patients receiving total parenteral nutrition containing medium- and long-chain triglycerides. *European Journal of Clinical Nutrition* 56, 121–128.

Matsui, J., Cameron, R.G., Kurian, R., Kuo, G.C. and Jeejeebhoy, K.N. (1993) Nutritional, hepatic, and metabolic effects of cachectin/tumour necrosis factor in rats receiving total parenteral nutrition. *Gastroenterology* 104, 235–243.

Messing, B., Bitoun, A., Galian, A., Mary, J.Y., Goll, A. and Bernier, J.J. (1977) Does parenteral nutrition-induced fatty liver depend on the amount of glucose supplied? (author's translation) *Gastroentérologie Clinique et Biologique* 1, 1015–1025.

Messing, B., Latrive, J.P., Bitoun, A., Galian, A. and Bernier, J.J. (1979) Is fatty liver during total parenteral nutrition due to the amount of fat emulsion energy source? (author's translation) *Gastroentérologie Clinique et Biologique* 3, 719–724.

Messing, B., de Oliveira, F.J., Galian, A. and Bernier, J.J. (1982) Cholestasis during total parenteral nutrition: demonstration of facilitating factors; association with gallbladder lithiasis. *Gastroentérologie Clinique et Biologique* 6, 740–747.

Messing, B., Landais, P., Goldfarb, B., Lemann, M., Joyeux, H., Gouttebel, M.C., Robert, D., Bouletreau, P., Matuchansky, C., Beau, P., *et al.* (1988) Home parenteral nutrition for adults. Results of a multicentre survey in France. *La Presse Médicale* 17, 845–849.

Messing, B., Peynet, J., Poupon, J., Pfeiffer, A., Thuillier, F., Chazouilleres, O. and Legrand, A. (1990) Effect of fat-emulsion phospholipids on serum lipoprotein profile during 1 mo of cyclic total parenteral nutrition. *American Journal of Clinical Nutrition* 52, 1094–1100.

Messing, B., Colombel, J.F., Heresbach, D., Chazouilleres, O. and Galian, A. (1992) Chronic cholestasis and macronutrient excess in patients treated with prolonged parenteral nutrition. *Nutrition* 8, 30–36.

Messing, B., Zarka, Y., Lemann, M., Iglicki, F., Coffin, B. and Rambaud, J. (1994) Chronic cholestasis associated with long-term parenteral nutrition. *Transplantation Proceedings* 26, 1438–1439.

Messing, B., Lemann, M., Landais, P., Gouttebel, M.C., Gerard-Boncompain, M., Saudin, F., Vangossum, A., Beau, P., Guedon, C., Barnoud, D., *et al.* (1995) Prognosis of patients with nonmalignant chronic intestinal failure receiving long-term home parenteral nutrition. *Gastroenterology* 108, 1005–1010.

Messing, B., Crenn, P., Beau, P., Boutron-Ruault, M.C., Rambaud, J.C. and Matuchansky, C. (1999) Long-term survival and parenteral nutrition dependence in adult patients with the short bowel syndrome. *Gastroenterology* 117, 1043–1050.

Moss, R.L. and Amii, L.A. (1999) New approaches to understanding the etiology and treatment of total parenteral nutrition-associated cholestasis. *Seminars in Pediatric Surgery* 8, 140–147.

Nahon, S., Crenn, P. and Messing, B. (1997) Evaluation des complications infectieuses liées à la voie d'abord veineuse chez les patients en nutrition parentérale à domicile de 1993 à 1995. *Gastroentérologie Clinique et Biologique* 21, A185.

Nanji, A.A. and Anderson, F.H. (1985) Sensitivity and specificity of liver function tests in the detection of parenteral nutrition-associated cholestasis. *JPEN Journal of Parenteral and Enteral Nutrition* 9, 307–308.

Neut, C., Colombel, J.F., Guillemot, F., Cortot, A., Gower, P., Quandalle, P., Ribet, M., Romond, C. and Paris, J.C. (1989) Impaired bacterial flora in human excluded colon. *Gut* 30, 1094–1098.

Pironi, L., Ruggeri, E., Zolezzi, C., Savarino, L., Incasa, E., Belluzzi, A., Munarini, A., Piazzi, S., Tolomelli, M., Pizzoferrato, A. and Miglioli, M. (1998) Lipid peroxidation and antioxidant status in adults receiving lipid-based home parenteral nutrition. *American Journal of Clinical Nutrition* 68, 888–893.

Pironi, L., Paganelli, F., Labate, A.M., Merli, C., Guidetti, C., Spinucci, G. and Miglioli, M. (2003a) Safety and efficacy of home parenteral nutrition for chronic intestinal failure: a 16-year experience at a single centre. *Digestive and Liver Disease* 35, 314–324.

Pironi, L., Guidetti, M., Zolezzi, C., Fasano, M.C., Paganelli, F., Merli, C., Bersani, G., Pizzoferrato, A. and Miglioli, M. (2003b) Peroxidation potential of lipid emulsions after compounding in all-in-one solutions. *Nutrition* 19, 784–788.

Poupon, R. and Poupon, R.E. (1995) Ursodeoxycholic acid therapy of chronic cholestatic conditions in adults and children. *Pharmacology & Therapeutics* 66, 1–15.

Quigley, E.M., Marsh, M.N., Shaffer, J.L. and Markin, R.S. (1993) Hepatobiliary complications of total parenteral nutrition. *Gastroenterology* 104, 286–301.

Redmond, H.P., Stapleton, P.P., Neary, P. and Bouchier-Hayes, D. (1998) Immunonutrition: the role of taurine. *Nutrition* 14, 599–604.

Reif, S., Tano, M., Oliverio, R., Young, C. and Rossi, T. (1991) Total parenteral nutrition-induced steatosis: reversal by parenteral lipid infusion. *JPEN Journal of Parenteral and Enteral Nutrition* 15, 102–104.

Reimund, J.M., Duclos, B., Arondel, Y. and Baumann, R. (2001) Persistent inflammation and immune activation contribute to cholestasis in patients receiving home parenteral nutrition. *Nutrition* 17, 300–304.

Reimund, J.M., Scheer, O., Pinna, G., Duclos, B. and Baumann, R. (2004a) *In vitro* modulation of inflammatory cytokine production by three lipid emulsions with different fatty acid compositions. *Clinical Nutrition* 23, 1324–1332.

Reimund, J.M., Arondel, Y., Joly, F., Messing, B., Duclos, B. and Baumann, R. (2004b) Potential usefulness of olive oil-based lipid emulsions in selected situations of home parenteral nutrition-associated liver disease. *Clinical Nutrition* 23, 1418–1425.

Reimund, J.M., Rahmi, G., Escalin, G., Pinna, G., Finck, G., Muller, C.D., Duclos, B. and Baumann, R. (2005) Efficacy and safety of an olive oil-based intravenous fat emulsion in adult patients on home parenteral nutrition. *Alimentary Pharmacology & Therapeutics* 21, 445–454.

Reynolds, N., Blumsohn, A., Baxter, J.P., Houston, G. and Pennington, C.R. (1998) Manganese requirement and toxicity in patients on home parenteral nutrition. *Clinical Nutrition* 17, 227–230.

Richelle, M., Rubin, M., Kulapongse, S., Deckelbaum, R.J., Elwyn, D.H. and Carpentier, Y.A. (1993) Plasma lipoprotein pattern during long-term home parenteral nutrition with two lipid emulsions. *JPEN Journal of Parenteral and Enteral Nutrition* 17, 432–437.

Scott-Conner, C.E. and Grogan, J.B. (1994) The pathophysiology of biliary obstruction and its effect on phagocytic and immune function. *Journal of Surgery Research* 57, 316–336.

Silvers, K.M., Sluis, K.B., Darlow, B.A., McGill, F., Stocker, R. and Winterbourn, C.C. (2001) Limiting light-induced lipid peroxidation and vitamin loss in infant parenteral nutrition by adding multivitamin preparations to Intralipid. *Acta Paediatrica* 90, 242–249.

Silverstein, M.N., Ellefson, R.D. and Ahern, E.J. (1970) The syndrome of the sea-blue histiocyte. *New England Journal of Medicine* 282, 1–4.

Spagnuolo, M.I., Iorio, R., Vegnente, A. and Guarino, A. (1996) Ursodeoxycholic acid for treatment of cholestasis in children on long-term total parenteral nutrition: a pilot study. *Gastroenterology* 111, 716–719.

Stanko, R.T., Nathan, G., Mendelow, H. and Adibi, S.A. (1987) Development of hepatic cholestasis and fibrosis in patients with massive loss of intestine supported by prolonged parenteral nutrition. *Gastroenterology* 92, 197–202.

Steephen, A.C., Traber, M.G., Ito, Y., Lewis, L.H., Kayden, H.J. and Shike, M. (1991) Vitamin E status of patients receiving long-term parenteral nutrition: is vitamin E supplementation adequate? *JPEN Journal of Parenteral and Enteral Nutrition* 15, 647–652.

Thomas-Gibson, S., Jawhari, A., Atlan, P., Brun, A.L., Farthing, M. and Forbes, A. (2004) Safe and efficacious prolonged use of an olive oil-based lipid emulsion (ClinOleic) in chronic intestinal failure. *Clinical Nutrition* 23, 697–703.

Valk, E.E. and Hornstra, G. (2000) Relationship between vitamin E requirement and polyunsaturated fatty acid intake in man: a review. *International Journal for Vitamin and Nutrition Research* 70, 31–42.

Van Gossum, A. and Neve, J. (1998) Trace element deficiency and toxicity. *Current Opinion in Clinical Nutrition and Metabolic Care* 1, 499–507.

Van Gossum, A., Shariff, R., Lemoyne, M., Kurian, R. and Jeejeebhoy, K. (1988) Increased lipid peroxidation after lipid infusion as measured by breath pentane output. *American Journal of Clinical Nutrition* 48, 1394–1399.

Van Gossum, A., Vahdi, K., Abdel-Malik, Staun, M., Pertkiewicz, M., Shaffer, J., Hébuterne, X., Beau, P., Guedon, C., Schmit, A., Tjellesen, L., Messing, B., Forbes, A. and ESPEN-HAN Working Group (2001) Clinical, social and rehabilitation status of long-term home parenteral nutrition patients: results of a European multi-centre survey. *Clinical Nutrition* 20, 205–210.

Wolfe, B.M., Walker, B.K., Shaul, D.B., Wong, L. and Ruebner, B.H. (1988) Effect of total parenteral nutrition on hepatic histology. *Archives of Surgery* 123, 1084–1090.

Zoli, G., Corazza, G.R., Wood, S., Bartoli, R., Gasbarrini, G. and Farthing, M.J. (1998) Impaired splenic function and tuftsin deficiency in patients with intestinal failure on long-term intravenous nutrition. *Gut* 43, 759–762.

17 Metabolic Bone Disease in Long-term Home Parenteral Nutrition in Adults

Loris Pironi* and Federica Agostini

Center for Chronic Intestinal Failure, Department of Medical and Surgical Science, University of Bologna, Bologna, Italy

Key Points

- Almost all patients on home parenteral nutrition (HPN) for benign intestinal failure may develop metabolic bone disease characterized by osteopenia, osteoporosis or osteomalacia.
- The pathogenesis is multifactorial. General factors, like ageing and postmenopausal status, factors related to the patient's underlying illness, as well as factors due to the HPN may be involved.
- Epidemiological studies show that general factors and factors related to the underlying disease play the major pathogenetic role and that long-term HPN is not necessarily associated with a worsening of bone health; in some cases, an improvement occurs.
- Diagnosis and monitoring rely on bone mineral density assessment and the measurement of: (i) serum concentrations and urinary excretion of minerals; (ii) serum concentrations of vitamin D and parathyroid hormone; and (iii) biochemical markers of bone turnover.
- Prevention and treatment are based on lifestyle and dietary recommendations, treatment of the underlying disease related-factors and on optimization of vitamin D nutritional status and the parenteral solution. Intravenous bisphosphonates may prevent further bone demineralization. Data on treatment with other drugs are anecdotal.

Introduction

Patients on long-term home parenteral nutrition (HPN) often have a metabolic bone disease (MBD) that may present as osteomalacia, osteopenia or osteoporosis

E-mail: loris.pironi@unibo.it

(Seidner and Licata, 2000; Pironi *et al*., 2002; Staun *et al*., 2009). Osteomalacia is characterized by defective mineralization and increased osteoid, which is the unmineralized bone matrix. Osteoporosis is characterized by a loss of bone mass due to an equal reduction in bone mineral and bone matrix. Osteopenia is a state of low bone mass due to a decrease in bone mineralization that precedes the state of osteoporosis. The adult skeleton is composed of trabecular or cancellous bone and cortical bone. Trabecular bone appears as lace-like strands that make up the inner framework of the bones and gives bone its compressive strength. Cortical bone is located around the circumference of the bone shaft and is made of thick, densely packed layers of mineralized collagen. It is responsible for giving bone its rigidity. On an annual basis, about 4% of cortical bone and 28% of trabecular bone undergo remodelling (or bone turnover), which is required to repair and reinforce bone to compensate for the mechanical stress placed on the skeleton. Remodelling consists of the balanced activity of skeletal destruction (or bone resorption) by osteoclasts and skeletal reconstruction (or bone formation) by osteoblasts. Skeletal remodelling is regulated by numerous factors, including parathyroid hormone (PTH), vitamin D and serum calcium, magnesium and phosphorus concentrations (Seidner and Licata, 2000; Kanis, 2002; Ferrone and Geraci, 2007).

In most cases, MBD in HPN patients is due to general factors, like ageing and postmenopausal status, or to factors related to the patient's underlying disease (HPN-associated MBD). However, accelerated bone loss has been reported during the HPN, raising the question of a specific role of HPN-related factors (HPN-related MBD) (Foldes *et al*., 1990; Klein and Coburn, 1991; Verhage *et al*., 1995).

Epidemiology

Studies of bone histology or bone mineral density (BMD) showed the presence of MBD in 40–100% of patients (Shike *et al*., 1980, 1986; de Vernejoul *et al*., 1985; Lipkin *et al*., 1987, 1990; Saitta *et al*., 1993; Goodman *et al*., 2000; Pironi *et al*., 2002; Raman *et al*., 2006).

A European multicentre survey (Pironi *et al*., 2002) evaluated the prevalence of MBD by dual-energy X-ray absorptiometry (DEXA) at the lumbar spine and femoral neck. Osteopenia was observed in 43% and osteoporosis in 41%. Cross-sectional studies reported associations between BMD and age at diagnosis of intestinal failure (lower BMD in younger patients), body mass index (BMI) (higher BMD with higher BMI) (Cohen-Solal *et al*., 2003) and age at starting HPN (lower BMD in younger patients) (Pironi *et al*., 2004). Only one study reported a significant negative association between BMD and duration of HPN (Raman *et al*., 2006).

The incidence of MBD during HPN is unknown, because it may be already present before patients enter the HPN programme (Haderslev *et al*., 2003). Longitudinal studies showed that long-term HPN is not necessarily associated with a worsening of bone health and in some cases an improvement occurs (Foldes *et al*., 1990; Klein and Coburn, 1991; Saitta *et al*., 1993; Cohen-Solal *et al*., 2003; Haderslev *et al*., 2004; Pironi *et al*., 2004). The results suggest that a considerable part of the MBD variations during HPN is related to the patient's sex and age at starting HPN or at starting intestinal failure, as well as to factors related to the underlying disease (Cohen-Solal *et al.*, 2003; Haderslev *et al.*, 2004; Pironi *et al.*, 2004). These results do not rule out the risk of BMD decrease primarily due to HPN in the single patient.

Clinical Feature

MBD in long-term HPN may be characterized by asymptomatic osteopenia, bone pain localized mainly at the spine and lower joints or by bone fractures that occur with no or minimal trauma. A prevalence study (Pironi *et al.*, 2002) showed bone pain in 35% of patients (mainly at the spine, knee, hip, ankle, foot and hand) and bone fractures in 10% (spine, rib and hip), which were associated with the lowest values of BMD. MBD may have a negative impact on the patient's rehabilitation status (Van Gossum *et al.*, 2001; Pironi *et al.*, 2003).

Histology

Histomorphometric studies showed the presence of either osteomalacia (Klein *et al.*, 1980; Shike *et al.*, 1980; Lipkin *et al.*, 1987; Saitta *et al.*, 1993; Goodman *et al.*, 2000) or osteoporosis (de Vernejoul *et al.*, 1985; Shike *et al.*, 1986; Lipkin *et al.*, 1987; Saitta *et al.*, 1993; Goodman *et al.*, 2000). Analysis of the dynamic histomorphometric indices showed a low bone formation rate in most of the patients (Klein *et al.*, 1980; Shike *et al.*, 1980; de Vernejoul *et al.*, 1985; Lipkin *et al.*, 1987; Saitta *et al.*, 1993; Goodman *et al.*, 2000; Kanis, 2002). Increased bone turnover (Shike *et al.*, 1986; Lipkin *et al.*, 1987) or defective mineralization (Shike *et al.*, 1980) was also reported. Low bone turnover seems characteristic of HPN-associated MBD. In the only follow-up observation performed by bone histology, histomorphometry showed in most patients a feature of hyperkinetic bone turnover at the first assessment that evolved 6–12 months later to a feature of low bone formation rate (Shike *et al.*, 1980). An observation using serum osteocalcin and urinary pyridinium cross-links, as markers of bone turnover, reported data consistent with the early results by bone histomorphometry (Pironi *et al.*, 2000).

Pathogenesis

The pathogenesis of the MBD associated with HPN is multifactorial (Seidner and Licata, 2000). General factors and lifestyle-related factors such as age, menopause, reduced physical activity, low sunlight exposure, and alcohol and tobacco abuse may be involved. Underlying disease-related factors may be malnutrition, intestinal malabsorption of calcium, magnesium and vitamin D, calcium losses in the gut lumen, chronic inflammation (increased bone resorption by tumour necrosis factor-α (TNF-α), interleukin-1, interleukin-6 (IL-6) and prostaglandin E_2; decreased bone formation by TNF-α and IL-6) and drugs, such as corticosteroids, immunosuppressives, loop diuretics and long-term anticoagulation with heparin or warfarin. Patients with a short bowel may develop a metabolic acidosis due to the diarrhoea-induced losses of bicarbonate. Some patients may have a D-lactic acidosis due to bacterial overgrowth syndrome. Chronic metabolic acidosis can impair the metabolism of vitamin D, leading to osteomalacia, and can directly affect the bone buffering systems causing calcium and phosphorus resorption, leading to osteoporosis.

Several hypotheses have been advanced about the HPN-related factors. Aluminium overload was observed in the 1970s, when the amino acid solutions derived from caseine hydrolysis were highly contaminated with aluminium (Klein, 1995). High serum concentration and urinary excretion of aluminium were associated with osteomalcia, positive aluminium staining in bone, hypercalciuria and low serum concentrations of PTH and 1,25-dihydroxyvitamin D (Klein *et al.*, 1980; Ott *et al.*, 1983). This feature was reversible by replacing casein hydrolysate with crystalline amino acid solutions, which contain negligible quantities of the metal (Vargas *et al.*, 1988). Aluminium accumulates at the mineralization zone of bone, thus impairing bone mineralization, and reduces the secretion of PTH, thus impairing its physiological activity of stimulating bone formation. Aluminium also blocks the enzymatic conversion of 25-hydroxyvitamin D to 1,25-dihydroxyvitamin D by the specific renal enzyme and may directly inhibit proliferation of osteoblasts (Klein, 1995). Nowadays caseine hydrolysate solutions are no longer produced, but other nutrient solutions still may be contaminated with aluminium, such as phosphate salts, calcium gluconate, vitamins and trace metals (Klein, 1995). Mild increase of serum aluminium concentrations may still be observed without being associated with positive aluminium staining in bone histology (de Vernejoul *et al.*, 1985).

Either vitamin D deficiency or toxicity may occur. Vitamin D increases intestinal calcium and phosphorus absorption, and enhances renal tubular calcium resorption. At the bone level, vitamin D induces osteoclast formation and bone resorption and indirectly promotes bone mineralization via maintenance of extracellular calcium and phosphorus concentrations in a supersaturated state. Vitamin D deficiency results in osteomalacia in adults and rickets in children. Furthermore, vitamin D plays a significant role in the development of the giant osteoclast and in the regulation of both the immune system and several cell functions (DeLuca, 2009). Vitamin D insufficiency or deficiency (serum concentration of 25-hydroxyvitamin D <30 or <20 ng/ml, respectively) has been reported in most (77–100%) adult patients on HPN who were receiving intravenous (IV) multivitamin supplementation that included for each infusion day the recommended amount of 5 μg (200 IU) vitamin D_3 (cholecalciferol) (Compher *et al.*, 2007; Corey *et al.*, 2009; Thomson and Duerksen, 2011). Those patients who did not receive HPN daily were at higher risk of deficiency (Thompson and Duerksen, 2011), and an increased risk during transition from HPN to enteral nutrition has been observed (Yang *et al.*, 2011). In patients with short bowel syndrome (SBS), high doses of oral vitamin D failed to achieve appropriate serum levels of 25-hydroxyvitamin D whether they were receiving HPN (Kumar *et al.*, 2012) or not (Haderslev *et al.*, 2003). The hypothesis of vitamin D-poisoning has been advanced on the basis of a few studies from the same research group. It was suggested that the daily IV infusion of 25-hydroxyvitamin D amounts equal to the Recommended Daily Allowance for adult healthy people may impair PTH secretion. Consequently there would be a lack of its physiological actions like bone mineralization and 1,25-dihydroxyvitamin D synthesis, despite normal serum 25-hydroxyvitamin D concentrations. After vitamin D withdrawal, an increase of BMD was observed together with the normalization of PTH and 1,25-dihydroxyvitamin D (Shike *et al.*, 1981; Verhage *et al.*, 1995). No reports in the last decade have confirmed these findings.

High urinary calcium excretion is a frequent finding in patients on HPN (Klein *et al.*, 1980; Shike *et al.*, 1980, 1986; de Vernejoul *et al.*, 1985; Lipkin *et al.*, 1987; Saitta *et al.*, 1993). Boncompain-Gérard *et al.* (2000) measured urinary excretion of electrolytes before (diurnal, 12 h) and during (nocturnal, 12 h) parenteral nutrition in 16 patients. Urine volume and excretion of urea, creatinine, sodium, magnesium and phosphate, but not potassium, increased significantly in nocturnal urine compared with diurnal urine. On the basis on 24 h calciuria, seven patients were normocalciuric whereas nine were hypercalciuric. Both had excessive nocturnal calciuria, but only the hypercalciuric had diurnal hypercalciuria, the calcium supply being identical. BMD was slightly, although not significantly, higher in the normocalciuric group, but in all patients BMD correlated significantly with calciuria. Several cross-sectional studies have shown a positive correlation between renal calcium loss and the amount of amino acids, glucose, sodium and calcium infused with the parenteral solution (Klein and Coburn, 1991). On the contrary, urinary calcium was negatively correlated with IV phosphate load, which appears to enhance calcium reabsorption by the renal tubules independently of PTH (Sloan *et al.*, 1983; Wood *et al.*, 1986; Berkelhammer *et al.*, 1998). Metabolic acidosis, due to titratable acids produced by the metabolism of neutral and sulfur-containing amino acids, can induce bone calcium reabsorption (Klein and Coburn, 1991; Seidner and Licata, 2000). Finally, one study reported a greater calciuria with cyclic infusion than with continuous infusion (Wood *et al.*, 1985). Both increased glomerular filtration rate (IV fluids, amino acids, calcium and sodium, metabolic acidosis) and decreased reabsorption by the renal tubules (excessive IV amino acids, glucose and calcium and low IV phosphate) (Klein and Coburn, 1991) can be responsible for hypercalciuria during HPN. Some human studies (Lipkin *et al.*, 1988) and an investigation on a non-human primate model (Lipkin, 1998) suggested that during HPN, adaptation might occur allowing a reduction of renal calcium losses.

It has been also hypothesized that parenteral nutrition might alter the balance of the effect of PTH on bone between resorption and formation in the direction of resorption (Jeejeebhoy, 1998). Goodman *et al.* (2000) observed that long-term HPN would increase the regularity of PTH secretion together with moderate but persistent elevations in serum PTH concentrations. These might lower the PTH–PTH-related peptide receptor expression and diminish the response to physiological blood concentrations of PTH in target tissues. This would imply a reduced bone formation and turnover and a reduced renal calcium resorption.

Deficiency or toxicity of micronutrients known to interfere with bone metabolism has also been hypothesized to play a role in the development of HPN-related MBD (Shike *et al.*, 1986; Lipkin *et al.*, 1987; Seidner and Licata, 2000). Boulétreau *et al.* (2006) observed a positive correlation between serum fluoride concentrations and lumbar BMD but no correlation with femoral neck BMD in patients with SBS receiving HPN. The data were in agreement with the action of this electrolyte on trabecular bone formation, which increases cancellous bone density, but has no effect on cortical bone density. However, the risk of fluoride toxicity must also be considered, as in some studies high amounts of fluoride in drinking water have been associated with an increased risk for bone fractures. Osteocalcin, matrix Gla protein and protein S are vitamin K-dependent proteins involved in bone formation. In HPN patients supplemented with vitamin K, Aljarallah *et al.* (2012) observed a trend towards better hip BMD compared with no supplementation. So far, no studies to investigate the role of boron, silicon and copper deficiency in MBD of patients on HPN have been carried out (Nielsen, 2009), nor has potential toxicity from other micronutrients, like vitamin A, cadmium, strontium and vanadium, been investigated.

Finally, a limited number of human studies and a large number of animal investigations suggest that HPN administration may be associated with a chronic inflammatory condition characterized by increased circulating concentrations of pro-inflammatory cytokines, such as TNF-α and IL-6, that stimulate osteoclast activity resulting in low BMD. This chronic inflammation could be due to the lack of significant small intestinal mass (as in SBS) or the absence of small intestine stimulation (as in dysmotility syndromes), as well as to components within the parenteral solution, like lipid emulsions rich in *n*-6 fatty acids. It is also possible that the immune system interacts with the catheter as a foreign body and responds with inflammation (Hise *et al.*, 2008).

Diagnosis and Follow-up

Diagnosis of MBD relies on DEXA, for the definition of the degree of bone demineralization at starting HPN and its evolution during the treatment, and on biochemical parameters, for the assessment of bone turnover and the investigation of the potential pathogenetic mechanism (Table 17.1). DEXA assessment is usually made at the lumbar spine and/or hip and the result is expressed as a number of standard deviations from the mean BMD value of a young adult reference (T-score) and of age- and sex-matched healthy subjects (Z-score). The World Health Organization Study Group (WHO, 1994) defined the severity of MBD as osteopenia or osteoporosis on the basis of the T-score value. The relative risk of any fracture has been estimated to be 1.4–1.6 for every decrease in BMD of 1 SD below the BMD Z-score (Kanis, 2002). The predictive value of BMD for the assessment of fracture risk has been suggested in HPN patients too (Pironi *et al.*, 2002). DEXA measures BMD, independently of the presence of osteomalacia or osteoporosis. When a differential diagnosis is needed, bone histology is mandatory.

Biochemical assessment of MBD requires the measurement every 4 months of serum concentrations and 24 h urinary excretion of minerals (calcium, phosphorus, magnesium) and the annual assessment of serum PTH and 25-hydroxyvitamin D.

Table 17.1. Instrumental and biochemical parameters for the diagnosis and follow-up of MBD.

Parameter	Frequency of measurement
BMD by DEXA:	At starting HPN, then annually
at lumbar spine (trabecular bone)	
at femoral neck (cortical bone)	
Diagnosis (WHO diagnostic criteria):	
T-score (no. of SD below mean BMD of young subjects)	
>–1 = normal	
between –1 and –2.5 = osteopenia	
≤–2.5 = osteoporosis	
Follow-up:	
Z-score (no. of SD from normal BMD values corrected for sex and age)	
>–1 = normal	
between –1 and –2.0 = reduced	
≤–2.0 = severely reduced	
Serum and 24 h urinary excretion of calcium, magnesium and phosphorus	Stable patient: every 4 months Additional measurements as for markers of bone turnover
Serum 25-hydroxyvitamin D	Stable patient: annually
Plasma intact PTH (PTH 1–84)	Additional measurement in cases of:
Markers of bone turnover	• bone pain appearance
Formation: serum osteocalcin	• change of the metabolic and clinical feature
Resorption: serum cross-laps or urinary cross-links of bone collagen	• treatment with bone-damaging drugs
1,25-Dihydroxyvitamin D	When a vitamin D toxicity is hypothesized
Bone biopsy after double tetracycline labelling	In cases of doubtful diagnosis between osteomalacia and osteoporosis
Serum aluminium	In case of pathologic BMD T-score
Other nutrients potentially involved in MBD in HPN patients	Measurements according to the clinical suspicion

Prevention and Treatment

Prevention and treatment depend on the potential pathogenetic mechanisms (Table 17.2).

General and underlying disease-related factors must be searched and treated. Prevention of MBD related to HPN factors is based on the optimization of the parenteral solution. Aluminium contamination should be less than 25 μg/l (Klein, 1995). The amounts of minerals should aim to maintain the normal serum concentrations and 24 h urinary excretions. Attention must be paid to the Ca/P ratio in the solution even though the optimal ratio cannot be always achieved because of problems of stability in the solution. Sloan *et al.* (1983) observed that supplying at least 15 mEq of calcium and 15 mmol of phosphorus on a daily basis could promote retention of these elements. Others reported a positive calcium balance

Table 17.2. Prevention and treatment of MBD in patients on long-term HPN.

Intervention	Comments
General and lifestyle	
Encourage regular exercise (home-based, low-impact exercise programme)	
Encourage regular and adequate sunlight exposure	UVB radiation from a tanning bed or other device emitting UVB might be considered
Maintain normal protein–calorie nutritional status	
Diet rich in dairy food	If not contraindicated by the underlying intestinal functions
Avoid cigarette smoking and limit alcohol intake	
Oestrogen replacement therapy in perimenopausal and postmenopausal period	No study in HPN
Underlying disease factors	
Treat inflammatory conditions	
Use lowest possible dosage of bone-damaging drugs	Oral calcium and vitamin D supplementation may counteract corticosteroid effects
Maintain acid–base balance	Oral sodium bicarbonate supplementation in chronic diarrhoea Prevention of D-lactic acidosis (bacterial overgrowth)
Oral calcium supplementation	500–1000 mg twice daily
Oral magnesium supplementation	Magnesium oxide 12–24 mmol daily
Nutrients in the parenteral solution	
Fluids and sodium	Na: amounts not greater than losses, in order to avoid Na-induced hypercalciuria Fluids: as required to maintain balance Infusion rate: in some patients slowing the infusion rate may reduce hypercalciuria
Minerals	Daily amounts to maintain balance in adult patients are within wide ranges: Mg = 4–12 mmol Ca = 4.5–11 mmol P = 15–30 mmol Ca/P ratio = 1 mEq of Ca to 1 or 2 mmol of P (beware: risk of formation of calcium phosphate crystals in the solution)
Acetate	As required to avoid acidosis and to maintain serum bicarbonate in the normal range (160 mmol/day is appropriate in most patients)
Amino acids	Not exceeding the patient's needs, in order to avoid Na-induced hypercalciuria (1.5 g/kg body weight/day is appropriate in most patients)
Glucose and glucose/lipid ratio	No data in HPN

Table 17.2. *Continued.*

Intervention	Comments
Vitamin D	Recommended daily infusion for adults: 5 µg/day (200 IU/day) HPN infusion <1 per day: oral or IM vitamin D supplementation (as well as increased sunlight exposure) to maintain normal serum 25-hydroxyvitamin D concentrations Excess vitamin D: risk of bone demineralization Patients with low BMD, low serum PTH and 1,25-dihydroxyvitamin D concentrations associated with normal 25-hydroxyvitamin D: consider vitamin D withdrawal
Vitamin K supplementation	As required to maintain normal prothrombin time If required: 1 mg/day including that found in lipid emulsion
Aluminium	< 25 µg/l
Drugs	
Bisphosphonates	Clodronate: 1500 mg IV every 3 months (one randomized controlled trail) Pamidronate: 30–60 mg IM per month or 90 mg IV every 3–6 months
PTH analogue (teriparatide)	One case report in HPN
h-GH	One case series in HPN
GLP-2 analogue (teduglutide)	One case series in HPN
Calcitonin, testosterone, anabolic steroids, fluoride supplementation	No study in HPN (only anecdotal)

giving 12 mEq of calcium and 45 mmol (Berkelhammer *et al.*, 1998) or 33–42 mmol of phosphate (Wood *et al.*, 1986). Thus, a Ca/P ratio ranging from 1 mEq of calcium to 1 or 2 mmol of phosphate seems required to achieve a positive calcium balance. However, it should be noted that chronic excess of phosphorus could lead to bone loss as a result of secondary hyperparathyroidism. Amino acids and sodium should not be added in amounts greater than losses (Klein and Coburn, 1991). The recommended IV vitamin D for adults is 5 µg/day (200 IU/day) (Seidner and Licata, 2000). In some patients, slowing the infusion rate may reduce hypercalciuria (Klein and Coburn, 1991).

A recent position paper of the American Society for Parenteral and Enteral Nutrition has expressed concern as to whether the daily dose of 5 µg/day (200 IU/day) in current parenteral nutrition products is adequate to maintain normal serum concentrations of 25-hydroxyvitamin D in most patients who require long-term HPN (Vanek *et al.*, 2012). Oral or intramuscular (IM) vitamin D supplementation, as well as exposure to sunlight or a device emitting ultraviolet-B (UVB) radiation, could be required (Koutkia *et al.*, 2001; DeLuca, 2009).

To date, only one randomized controlled study and a few prospective observations have been carried out on bisphosphonates in patients on HPN. IV clodronate was able to decrease the urinary excretion of markers of bone resorption and to maintain BMD at the lumbar spine in patients on HPN after 12 months, but no significant increase of BMD was observed (Haderslev *et al.*, 2002a). Also, IV pamidronate showed trends towards improvement of BMD at both the spine and hip (D'Aoust *et al.*, 2002; Raman *et al.*, 2006).

A case report documented that the subcutaneous administration of the recombinant PTH, teriparatide, in a patient on HPN for SBS and having osteoporosis, normalized BMD after 18 months of treatment (Pazianas *et al.*, 2006). Case series suggested that human growth hormone (h-GH) and glucagon-like peptide-2 (GLP-2), intestinotrophic drugs that stimulate intestinal adaptation in SBS patients on HPN, also improve BMD (Haderslev *et al.*, 2002b; Tangpricha *et al.*, 2006).

Future Developments

MBD in HPN patients is a challenging issue for the clinician. Many aspects of both the pathogenesis and the treatment still need to be clarified. Future studies should investigate the impact of long-term HPN on bone-regulating hormones as well as the optimal dosage of vitamin D and minerals. Further studies are required also to assess the efficacy of bisphosphonates and the potential role of recombinant PTH, teriparatide, for the treatment of MBD in these particular patients.

Summary

Patients on long-term HPN are at high risk of developing an MBD like osteoporosis or osteomalacia. The MBD is often asymptomatic. Bone pain, mainly at the spine and lower joints, has been reported in one-third of patients and bone fractures in one-tenth. In most of the cases, the MBD is due to general factors, like ageing and postmenopausal status, or to causes related to the patient's underlying illness (HPN-associated MBD) that are already present before starting the HPN programme.

Follow-up studies indicate that long-term HPN is not necessarily associated with a worsening of bone health and in some cases an improvement occurs. Nevertheless, accelerated bone loss may occur during the HPN therapy, raising the question of a specific role of HPN in the pathogenesis of MBD (HPN-related MBD).

Hypercalciuria due to IV nutrient loads and vitamin D deficiency seem to play a major role. Micronutrient deficiency or toxicity, HPN-induced impaired PTH secretion/function and/or secretion of pro-inflammatory cytokines are also suggested HPN-related pathogenetic factors.

Diagnosis and monitoring rely on BMD assessment by bone densitometry (annually), evaluation of mineral balance (every 4 months) and evaluation of vitamin D nutritional status and biochemical markers of bone turnover (annually). Prevention and treatment are based on lifestyle and dietary recommendations, treatment of the underlying disease related-factors and on optimization of vitamin D nutritional status and of the parenteral solution. IV bisphosphonates may be useful to prevent further bone demineralization. Studies with other drugs for osteoporosis are anecdotal.

References

Aljarallah, B., Fernandes, G., Jeejeebhoy, K.N., Gramlich, L.M., Whittaker, J.S., Armstrong, D., Duerksen, D.R. and Allard, J.P. (2012) The Canadian home total parenteral nutrition (HTPN) registry: vitamin K supplementation and bone mineral density. *JPEN Journal of Parenteral and Enteral Nutrition* 36, 415–420.

Berkelhammer, C., Wood, R.J. and Sitrin, M. (1998) Inorganic phosphorus reduces hypercalciuria during total parenteral nutrition by enhancing renal tubular calcium absorption. *JPEN Journal of Parenteral and Enteral Nutrition* 22, 142–146.

Boncompain-Gérard, M., Robert, D., Fouque, D. and Hadj-Aïssa, A. (2000) Renal function and urinary excretion of electrolytes in patients receiving cyclic parenteral nutrition. *JPEN Journal of Parenteral and Enteral Nutrition* 24, 234–239.

Boulétreau, P.H., Bost, M., Fontanges, E., Lauverjat, M., Gutknecht, C., Ecochard, R., Delmas, P.D. and Chambrier, C. (2006) Fluoride exposure and bone status in patients with chronic intestinal failure who are receiving home parenteral nutrition. *American Journal of Clinical Nutrition* 83, 1429–1437.

Cohen-Solal, M., Baudoin, C., Joly, F., Vahedi, K., D'Aoust, L., De Vernejoul, M.C. and Messing, B. (2003) Osteoporosis in patients on long-term home parenteral nutrition: a longitudinal study. *Journal of Bone and Mineral Research* 18, 1989–1994.

Compher, C., Pazianas, M., Benedict, S., Brown, J.C., Kinosian, B.P. and Hise, M. (2007) Systemic inflammatory mediators and bone homeostasis in intestinal failure. *JPEN Journal of Parenteral and Enteral Nutrition* 31, 142–147.

Corey, B., Ackerman, K., Allen, P., Sceery, N. and Rafoth, C. (2009) Vitamin D status of New England home TPN patients – a snapshot of practice. *Nutrition in Clinical Practice* 24, 110.

D'Aoust, L., Baudoin, C., Joly, F., Vahedi, K., Cohen-Solal, M. and Messing, B. (2002) Osteoporosis in patients under long term home parenteral nutrition: results of iv biphosphonate treatment. *Clinical Nutrition* 21(Suppl. 1), 492–496.

DeLuca, H.F. (2009) Vitamin D and the parenteral nutrition patient. *Gastroenterology* 137, 79–91.

de Vernejoul, M.C., Messing, B., Modrowski, D., Bielakoff, J., Buisine, A. and Miravet, L. (1985) Multifactorial low remodelling bone disease during cyclic total parenteral nutrition. *Journal of Clinical and Endocrinology Metabolism* 60, 109–113.

Ferrone, M. and Geraci, M. (2007) A review of the relationship between parenteral nutrition and metabolic bone disease. *Nutrition in Clinical Practice* 22, 329–339.

Foldes, J., Rimon, B., Muggia-Sullam, M., Gimmon, Z., Leitcher, I., Steinberg, R., Menczel, J. and Freund, H.R. (1990) Progressive bone loss during long-term home total parenteral nutrition. *JPEN Journal of Parenteral and Enteral Nutrition* 14, 139–142.

Goodman, W.G., Misra, S., Veldhuis, J.D., Portale, A.A., Wang, H.J., Ament, M.E. and Salusky, I.B. (2000) Altered diurnal regulation of blood ionized calcium and serum parathyroid hormone concentrations during parenteral nutrition. *American Journal of Clinical Nutrition* 71, 560–568.

Haderslev, K.V., Tjellesen, L., Sorensen, H.A. and Staun, M. (2002a) Effect of cyclical intravenous clodronate therapy on bone mineral density and markers of bone turnover in patients receiving home parenteral nutrition. *American Journal of Clinical Nutrition* 76, 482–488.

Haderslev, K.V., Jeppesen, P.B., Hartmann, B., Thulesen, J., Sorensen, H.A., Graff, J., Hansen, B.S., Tofteng, F., Poulsen, S.S., Madsen, J.L., Holst, J.J., Staun, M. and Mortensen, P.B.

(2002b) Short-term administration of glucagon-like peptide-2. Effects on bone mineral density and markers of bone turnover in short-bowel patients with no colon. *Scandinavian Journal of Gastroenterology* 37, 392–398.

Haderslev, K.V., Jeppesen, P.B., Sorensen, H.A., Mortensen, P.B. and Staun, M. (2003) Vitamin D status and measurements of markers of bone metabolism in patients with small intestinal resection. *Gut* 52, 653–658.

Haderslev, K.V., Tjellesen, L., Haderslev, P.H. and Staun, M. (2004) Assessment of the longitudinal changes in bone mineral density in patients receiving home parenteral nutrition. *JPEN Journal of Parenteral and Enteral Nutrition* 28, 289–294.

Hise, M., Compher, C. and Brown, J. (2008) Inflammatory mediators and home parenteral nutrition. *Nutrition in Clinical Practice* 23, 42–48.

Jeejeebhoy, K.N. (1998) Metabolic bone disease and total parenteral nutrition: a progress report. *American Journal of Clinical Nutrition* 67, 186–187.

Kanis, J.A. (2002) Diagnosis of osteoporosis and assessment of fracture risk. *The Lancet* 359, 1929–1936.

Klein, G.L. (1995) Aluminum in parenteral solutions revisited – again. *American Journal of Clinical Nutrition* 61, 449–456.

Klein, G.L. and Coburn, J.W. (1991) Parenteral nutrition: effect on bone and mineral homeostasis. *Annual Review of Nutrition* 11, 93–119.

Klein, G.L., Ament, M.E., Bluestone, R., Targoff, C.M., Sherrard, D.J., Young, J.H., Norman, A.W. and Coburn, J. (1980) Bone disease associated with total parenteral nutrition. *The Lancet* 2, 1041–1044.

Koutkia, P., Lu, Z., Chen, T.C. and Holick, M.F. (2001) Treatment of vitamin D deficiency due to Crohn's disease with tanning bed ultraviolet B radiation. *Gastroenterology* 121, 1485–1488.

Kumar, P.R., Fenton, T.R., Shaheen, A.A. and Raman, M. (2012) Prevalence of vitamin D deficiency and response to oral vitamin D supplementation in patients receiving home parenteral nutrition. *JPEN Journal of Parenteral and Enteral Nutrition* 36, 463–469.

Lipkin, E.W. (1998) A longitudinal study of calcium regulation in a nonhuman primate model of parenteral nutrition. *American Journal of Clinical Nutrition* 67, 246–254.

Lipkin, E.W., Ott, S.M. and Klein, G.L. (1987) Heterogeneity of bone histology in parenteral nutrition patients. *American Journal of Clinical Nutrition* 146, 673–680.

Lipkin, E.W., Ott, S.M., Klein, G.L. and Deftos, L.J. (1990) Serum markers of bone formation in parenteral nutrition patients. *Calcified Tissue International* 47, 75–81.

Nielsen, F.H. (2009) Micronutrients in parenteral nutrition: boron, silicon, and fluoride. *Gastroenterology* 137, 55–60.

Ott, S.M., Maloney, N.A., Klein, G.L., Alfrey, C.A., Ament, M.E., Coburn, J.W. and Sherrard, D.J. (1983) Aluminum is associated with low bone formation in patients receiving chronic parenteral nutrition. *Annals of Internal Medicine* 98, 910–904.

Pazianas, M., Compher, C., Schiavone-Gatto, P. and Kinosian, B.P. (2006) Intestinal failure-associated metabolic bone diseases and response to teriparatide. *Nutrition in Clinical Practice* 21, 605–609.

Pironi, L., Zolezzi, C., Ruggeri, E., Paganelli, F., Pizzoferrato, A. and Miglioli, M. (2000) Bone turnover in short-term and long-term home parenteral nutrition for benign disease. *Nutrition* 16, 272–277.

Pironi, L., Labate, A.M., Pertkiewicz, M., Przedlacki, J., Tjellesen, L., Staun, M., De Francesco, A., Gallenca, P., Guglielmi, F.W., Van Gossum, A., Orlandoni, P., Contaldo, F. and Moreno Villares, J.M. (2002) Prevalence of bone disease in patients on home parenteral nutrition. *Clinical Nutrition* 21, 289–296.

Pironi, L., Paganelli, F., Labate, A.M., Merli, C., Guidetti, C., Spinucci, G. and Miglioli, M. (2003) Safety and efficacy of home parenteral nutrition for chronic intestinal failure: a 16-year experience at a single centre. *Digestive and Liver Disease* 5, 314–324.

Pironi, L., Tjellesen, L., De Francesco, A., Pertkiewicz, M., Morselli Labate, A.M., Staun, M., Przedlacki, J., Lezo, A., Orlandoni, P. and Pasanisi, F. (2004) ESPEN-Home Artificial Nutrition Working Group. Bone mineral density in patients on home parenteral nutrition: a follow-up study. *Clinical Nutrition* 23, 1288–1302.
Raman, M., Aghdassi, E., Baun, M., Yeung, M., Fairholm, L., Saqui, O. and Allard, J.P. (2006) Metabolic bone disease in patients receiving home parenteral nutrition: a Canadian study and review. *JPEN Journal of Parenteral and Enteral Nutrition* 30, 492–496.
Saitta, J.C., Ott, S.M., Sherrard, D.J., Walden, C.E. and Lipken, E.W. (1993) Metabolic bone disease in adults receiving long-term parenteral nutrition: longitudinal study with regional densitometry and bone biopsy. *JPEN Journal of Parenteral and Enteral Nutrition* 17, 214–219.
Seidner, D.L. and Licata, A. (2000) Parenteral nutrition-associated bone disease. Pathophysiology, evaluation and treatment. *Nutrition in Clinical Practice* 15, 163–170.
Shike, M., Harrison, J.E. and Sturtridge, W.C. (1980) Metabolic bone disease in patients receiving long-term total parenteral nutrition. *Annals of Internal Medicine* 92, 343–350.
Shike, M., Sturtridge, W.C., Tam, C.S., Harrison, J.E., Jones, G., Murray, T.M., Husdan, H., Whitwell, J., Wilson, D.R. and Jeejeebhoy, K.N. (1981) A possible role of vitamin D in genesis of parenteral-nutrition-induced metabolic bone disease. *Annals of Internal Medicine* 95, 560–568.
Shike, M., Shils, M.E., Heller, A., Alcock, N., Vigorita, V., Brockman, R., Holick, M.F., Lane, J. and Flombaum, C. (1986) Bone disease in prolonged parenteral nutrition: osteopenia without mineralization defect. *American Journal of Clinical Nutrition* 44, 89–98.
Sloan, G.M., White, D.E., Murray, M.S. and Brennan, F. (1983) Calcium and phosphorus metabolism during total parenteral nutrition. *Annals of Surgery* 197, 1–6.
Staun, M., Pironi, L., Bozzetti, F., Baxter, J., Forbes, A., Joly, F., Jeppesen, P., Moreno, J., Hébuterne, X., Pertkiewicz, M., Mühlebach, S., Shenkin, A. and Van Gossum, A. (2009) ESPEN guidelines on parenteral nutrition: home parenteral nutrition (HPN) in adult patients. *Clinical Nutrition* 28, 467–479.
Tangpricha, V., Luo, M., Fernández-Estívariz, C., Gu, L.H., Bazargan, N., Klapproth, J.M., Sitaraman, S.V., Galloway, J.R., Leader, L.M. and Ziegler, T.R. (2006) Growth hormone favourably affects bone turnover and bone mineral density in patients with short bowel syndrome undergoing intestinal rehabilitation. *JPEN Journal of Parenteral and Enteral Nutrition* 30, 480–486.
Thomson, P. and Duerksen, D.R. (2011) Vitamin D deficiency in patients receiving home parenteral nutrition. *JPEN Journal of Parenteral and Enteral Nutrition* 35, 499–504.
Vanek, V.W., Borum, P., Buchman, A., Fessler, T.A., Howard, L., Jeejeebhoy, K., Kochevar, M., Shenkin, A. and Valentine, C.J. (2012) A.S.P.E.N. position paper: recommendations for changes in commercially available parenteral multivitamin and multi-trace element products. *Nutrition in Clinical Practice* 27, 440–491.
Van Gossum, A., Vahedi, K., Abdel-Malik, Staun, M., Pertkiewicz, M., Shaffer, J., Hebuterne, X., Beau, P., Guedon, C., Schmit, A., Tjellesen, L., Messing, B. and Forbes, A.; ESPEN-HAN Working Group (2001) Clinical, social and rehabilitation status of long-term home parenteral nutrition patients: results of a European multicentre survey. *Clinical Nutrition* 20, 205–210.
Vargas, J.H., Klein, G.L., Ament, M.E., Ott, S.M., Sherrard, D.J., Horst, R.L., Berquist, W.E., Alfrey, A.C., Slatopolsky, E. and Coburn, J.W. (1988) Metabolic bone disease of total parenteral nutrition: course after changing from casein to amino acids in parenteral solution with reduced aluminium content. *American Journal of Clinical Nutrition* 48, 1070–1078.
Verhage, A.H., Cheong, W.K., Allard, J.P. and Jeejeebhoy, K.N. (1995) Increase in lumbar spine bone mineral content in patients on long-term parenteral nutrition without vitamin D supplementation. *JPEN Journal of Parenteral and Enteral Nutrition* 19, 431–436.

WHO (1994) *Assessment of Osteoporotic Fracture Risk and Its Role in Screening for Postmenopausal Osteoporosis. Report of a WHO Study Group. WHO Technical Report Series No. 843.* World Health Organization, Geneva, Switzerland.
Wood, R.J., Bengoa, J.M., Sitrin, M.D. and Rosenberg, I.H. (1985) Calciuretic effect of cyclic versus continuous total parenteral nutrition. *American Journal of Clinical Nutrition* 41, 614–619.
Wood, R.J., Sitrin, M.D., Cusson, G.J. and Rosenberg, I.H. (1986) Reduction of total parenteral nutrition-induced urinary calcium loss by increasing the phosphorus in the total parenteral nutrition prescription. *JPEN Journal of Parenteral and Enteral Nutrition* 10, 188–190.
Yang, C.J., Duro, D., Zurakowski, D., Lee Jaksic, T. and Duggan, C. (2011) High prevalence of multiple micronutrient deficiencies in children with intestinal failure: a longitudinal study. *Journal of Pediatrics* 159, 39–44.

18 Metabolic and Other Rare Complications of Home Parenteral Nutrition

ALAN L. BUCHMAN*

Glencoe, Illinois, USA

Key Points

- Rare complications are reviewed, including: (i) renal dysfunction; (ii) chromium toxicity and deficiency; (iii) aluminium toxicity; and (iv) manganese toxicity.
- The acceptable level for aluminium is <4–5 μg/kg body weight/day.
- Pathogenesis of hyperoxaluria is discussed and the suggested dose of ascorbic acid was set at 100–200 mg/day.
- Cardiopulmonary complications from precipitated crystals are considered.

Introduction

The administration of home parenteral nutrition (HPN) has long been known to carry the risk for potential side-effects or complications. Metabolic bone disease, hepatobiliary dysfunction and catheter-related complications are by far the more commonly seen unfortunate consequences of HPN. A body of literature does exist reporting less frequently seen complications that can still be equally damaging, particularly when not recognized. This chapter reviews these more rare complications of HPN, including renal and other metabolic derangements that are known to occur.

Renal Dysfunction

Although bone and liver disease are frequently cited complications of long-term HPN therapy, renal dysfunction associated with HPN also presents a challenging

*Email: a.buchman@hotmail.com

problem. HPN-associated nephropathy has been one of the more recently described phenomena seen in patients on longer-term HPN, although progression to end-stage renal disease has not been clearly established. Indeed, in one study the change in glomerular filtration rate (GFR), measured as creatinine clearance (CrCl), of 33 long-term HPN patients was evaluated prospectively (Buchman *et al.*, 1993). Among the 33 patients, CrCl declined by 3.5%±6.3% per year ($P=0.004$), greater than would be expected from increasing age alone.

Furthermore, tubular function, measured by tubular reabsorption of phosphate, was shown in the same study to be abnormal in 52% of the subjects (Buchman *et al.*, 1993). This finding, however, was not corroborated by a similar later study in children (Moukarzel *et al.*, 1991). Buchman *et al.* went on to note that the nephropathy associated with total parenteral nutrition (TPN) in the adult study was not explained fully by increasing patient age, change in nutritional status, HPN duration, use of nephrotoxic medications, number of bacteraemia/fungaemia episodes, infection rate or intravenous protein load (Buchman *et al.*, 1993). Another study assessed renal function, measured by multiple parameters including GFR and excretion of various electrolytes, during the periods before and during nocturnal administration of parenteral nutrition (PN) in 16 patients with short bowel syndrome. Nine patients had decreased GFR. While a statistically significantly increased level of urinary volume and electrolyte excretion occurred during the nocturnal phase of PN, some patients demonstrated hypercalciuria. This study, however, did not elucidate the mechanism by which renal impairment occurs in these patients (Boncompain-Gerard *et al.*, 2000). Indeed, the exact aetiology for the decline in CrCl and tubular function is still not fully understood, but appears largely related to chronic dehydration from excessive fluid losses (Lauverjat *et al.*, 2006), with other components yet to be identified. Chromium toxicity may also play a role in both glomerular and tubular damage. Moukarzel *et al.* showed that decreased GFR in children was associated with increased chromium intake as well as increased serum chromium concentration (Moukarzel *et al.*, 1992) (see section on heavy metal toxicity below). When supplemental chromium was removed from HPN solutions, GFR failed to improve. This could indicate irreversible damage or even that contaminant chromium concentration is of concern. Buchman *et al.* showed in an animal model of long-term PN that chromium deposited in the kidneys of rats and was associated with histological tubular damage (Buchman *et al.*, 2001).

The critically ill patient requiring continuous renal replacement therapy (CRRT) presents a particular challenge. While arguments for 'overfeeding' versus 'underfeeding' the acutely critically ill patient continue, it is clear that determination of the nutritional needs for critically ill CRRT patients can be more difficult than initially thought. CRRT adds another variable into an already complicated equation for estimating a patient's caloric needs; dialysis has no ability to continually adjust the ability to filter, concentrate, dilute and absorb. Scheinkestel *et al.* showed that patients who required continuous renal replacement therapy might exhibit markedly abnormal amino acid profiles (Scheinkestel *et al.*, 2003). These investigators found that when such patients were provided protein loads <2.5 g/kg body weight/day, their amino acid profiles remained markedly abnormal. These profiles subsequently normalized with an increase of protein loads to at least

2.5 g/kg body weight/day, and nitrogen balances became positive at even higher protein loads. Increased protein intake, however, has been associated with hypercalciuria, which may increase the risk for development of metabolic bone disease (Bengoa *et al.*, 1983).

Toxicities from Heavy Metals, Vitamins and Minerals

Among other potential factors in HPN-associated nephropathy include the possible role of heavy metal contamination of HPN solutions. Theoretically, heavy metals found in HPN solutions could deposit in various organs, including the liver, brain and kidneys. In a rat TPN model, significant chromium deposition occurred in the kidney and histological abnormalities were also noted (Buchman *et al.*, 2001). These findings appeared to confirm prior investigations which suggested the intravenously administered chromium was deposited primarily in the kidneys and liver (Tsapakos *et al.*, 1983). Autopsy data from eight patients who had received HPN for a mean of 14 years (range 2–21 years) also showed chromium accumulation in these organs (Howard *et al.*, 2007).

Despite correlation between the level of contamination and histological abnormalities, there was no clear relationship with changes in creatinine. Measurements of changes in serum creatinine alone, however, may not be a sensitive indicator for changes in renal function. Although one prior study did not show that excessive chromium infusion in adults was associated with diminished renal function (Buchman *et al.*, 1992, 1993), other studies in children have shown a significant negative relationship between the amount of chromium infusion, serum chromium concentration and a decline in GFR. Furthermore, these findings may be irreversible, as GFR did not improve when supplemental chromium was removed from the PN after a year, although serum chromium concentrations remained elevated (Moukarzel *et al.*, 1992).

Chromium is found primarily in a trivalent or hexavalent form, and these are the two forms most likely to be associated with histological derangements of the kidney or liver (Baines, 1965; Tandon *et al.*, 1978). During chromium toxicity, the proximal tubules and glomeruli are most commonly damaged and the degree of injury appears to be proportional to the level of chromium deposition (Buchman *et al.*, 2001). Indeed, prior investigations have shown significantly elevated serum chromium concentrations in patients found to have long-term HPN-associated nephropathy (Moukarzel *et al.*, 1991, 1992). The possibility of chromium deficiency during long-term TPN has also been raised. Several case reports describe neurological deficits confirmed by nerve conduction studies that appeared to be associated with chromium deficiency and resolved with chromium supplementation (Jeejeebhoy *et al.*, 1977). Another case report described similar neurological deficits in the setting of long-term HPN as well as glucose intolerance. This patient had normal serum chromium concentrations, but he experienced normalization of his symptoms following a 2-week course of daily infusions of 250 μg of trivalent chromium (Verhage *et al.*, 1996).

Chromium may play a significant role in the maintenance of euglycaemia, particularly in diabetic patients (Morris *et al.*, 1999). Normal insulin function depends, in part, on the trivalent form of chromium. Additionally, it has been shown that high serum glucose levels can lead to increased urinary chromium excretion (Ravina *et al.*, 1999). Wongseelashote *et al.* recently reported a small case series of patients with normal renal function receiving HPN as their sole nutrition who all required >20 units of insulin to maintain euglycaemia. They found that insulin requirements could be reduced in some patients by chromium supplementation (Wongseelashote *et al.*, 2004). The requirement of chromium in HPN, however, has not clearly been established.

Aluminium carries potential toxic risks when accumulated at abnormally high levels during long-term HPN use. Particularly at risk are infants and patients with abnormal renal function. The primary sequela of aluminium toxicity associated with HPN appears to be osteomalacia. The mechanisms of bone toxicity relate primarily to impaired calcium bone fixation or altered conversion of 25-hydroxyvitamin D to 1,25-dihydroxyvitamin D (Vargas *et al.*, 1988). Other derangements that can occur include encephalopathy, motor abnormalities affecting speech, seizures, dementia, myoclonus and pathological fractures. Indeed, increased aluminium levels in the brain have been found in HPN-treated premature infants (Bishop *et al.*, 1989). Renal insufficiency may also predispose patients to developing aluminium toxicity, as the kidneys act as the main route of excretion.

Aluminium is generally found as a contaminant in intravenous products, and the US Food and Drug Administration (FDA) has investigated this phenomenon in order to determine safe levels. This ultimately led the FDA in 2004 (FDA, 1998) to issue a report outlining standards for acceptable levels of aluminium in large and small volume parenterals (FDA, 2013). In this report, the FDA determined that the 'acceptable' level of aluminium intake for parenteral administration is approximately <4–5 μg/kg body weight/day. New labelling regulations have been published. These include labelling requirements for the package inserts of intravenous products, cautioning that the product contains aluminium at concentrations <25 μg/l. In addition, the FDA mandated that producers of large and small volume parenterals must demonstrate they use validated assay methods for measurement of aluminium contamination in their parenterals.

Manganese is another trace element that, in patients on long-term HPN, may accumulate to levels causing toxic side-effects. Acting both as an important coenzyme as well as playing a significant role in bone, cartilage and connective tissue formation, manganese is excreted normally in the biliary system. Toxic effects were first described in 1837 in Chilean manganese miners who developed *locura manganica*, or manganese madness. It is thought that patients who suffer from cholestatic liver disease or biliary obstruction may be most vulnerable to developing toxicity due to impaired clearance (Hambridge *et al.*, 1989). Elevated serum manganese concentration, however, does not necessarily correlate with toxicity (Siepler *et al.*, 2003). Wardle *et al.* demonstrated that compared with chronic liver disease or control subjects, patients who received HPN had elevated serum and whole blood manganese concentrations. Brain manganese concentration also increases (Bertinet *et al.*, 2000). None of these HPN patients, however, demonstrated any signs of manganese toxicity (Wardle *et al.*, 1999).

Manganese toxicity most commonly manifests as neurological symptoms, with reports in the literature suggesting Parkinsonian symptoms (typical gait, tremor and muscle rigidity) and neuropsychiatric symptoms (headache, somnolence, confusion) (Fitzgerald *et al.*, 1999; Nagatomo *et al.*, 1999). As mentioned earlier, manganese miners were first described as having a symptom complex attributed to manganese toxicity. Among the symptoms include an initial manic stage, insomnia, depression and delusions. These symptoms may be followed by anorexia, apathy, arthralgias, asthenia and headaches. Finally, later stages may manifest gait and balance abnormalities with a Parkinson's like tremor and rigidity. Radiologically, manganese toxicity can manifest as deposits seen in the basal ganglia primarily on magnetic resonance imaging (MRI), which may correlate with the development of Parkinsonian-type traits (Takagi *et al.*, 2001). A single case report describes a young girl who suffered a seizure disorder that was associated with elevated serum manganese concentration while receiving PN and a symmetric high-intensity signal on T1-weighted images of the basal ganglia (Hsieh *et al.*, 2007). It appears that many of the neurological symptoms will reverse with the withdrawal of manganese from the PN infusion, as may the MRI findings in the basal ganglia (Mirowitz and Westrich, 1992; Stevens and Rashid, 2008). Milatovic *et al.* found that manganese induces oxidative impairment due to mitochrondrial dysfunction in rat astrocytes *in vitro* (Milatovic *et al.*, 2007).

Manganese's role in liver toxicity is not clearly established. There is no strong evidence as yet to support the theory that manganese actually causes cholestasis. A recent study randomized children receiving PN to high or low manganese supplementation. While there were no statistically significant differences in manganese or serum bilirubin levels, subgroup analysis of children receiving at least 75% of their daily fluid intake from HPN demonstrated that those randomized to higher manganese supplementation had a significantly higher serum direct bilirubin and higher peak direct bilirubin compared with the low manganese group (Fok *et al.*, 2001). In liver disease and especially cholestasis, though, manganese excretion is impaired (Messing *et al.*, 1983). Furthermore, since bile flow is decreased during TPN infusion, it is more likely that the elevated manganese concentration in such patients is a sequela of liver disease rather than a direct cause (Reimund *et al.*, 2000). More recent investigations have even questioned the relationship between elevated serum manganese concentration and cholestasis (McMillan *et al.*, 2008).

Finally, manganese deficiency has been reported to result potentially in bone abnormalities. A case report, described as a preliminary communication, described bone calcification irregularities and bone demineralization in a TPN-dependent neonate who was found to have profoundly low serum manganese concentration (Norose *et al.*, 1992).

Hyperoxaluria is another long-known phenomenon associated with the administration of HPN. In general, hyperoxaluria results from one of two possible mechanisms: (i) increased enteral absorption secondary to intestinal disease and increased permeability (perhaps related to colonic absorption); or (ii) synthesis of oxalate from increased levels of a precursor (Swartz *et al.*, 1984). With respect to the latter, if ileal absorption of bile salts conjugated with glycine occurs, colonic bacteria may deconjugate them and liberate the glycine. Conversion of glycine to glyoxalate occurs, which is then absorbed and oxidized to oxalic acid in the liver

(Hockaday *et al.*, 1965). Another potential precursor is ascorbic acid, to be discussed later in this chapter.

Studies have reported urinary oxalate excretion is increased in patients who receive PN (Hoppe *et al.*, 1993; Buchman *et al.*, 1995; Fairholm *et al.*, 2003; Pena de la Vega *et al.*, 2004; Mohamed *et al.*, 2014). Oxalate is usually bound to calcium in the diet and is excreted unabsorbed in the stool. Parenteral administration of ascorbic acid in HPN can lead to hyperoxaluria and renal insufficiency (Swartz *et al.*, 1984; Fairholm *et al.*, 2003; Pena de la Vega *et al.*, 2004). The mechanism by which renal dysfunction may occur in this setting likely relates to calcium oxalate deposition. Furthermore, there may be a role for increased endogenous production of oxalate in patients receiving long-term HPN. Previously, it was believed that hyperoxaluria would not occur in patients with ileal resections and an ileostomy or proximal colostomy. It has since been shown that some short bowel patients with an ileostomy but on long-term HPN developed hyperoxaluria, suggesting the possibility of an increased endogenous oxalate production (Buchman *et al.*, 1995). Ascorbic acid can be aerobically oxidized to oxalate via dehydroascorbate. Ascorbic acid is also believed to degrade to oxalate following exposure to light, which functions as a potent free radical initiator (Smith *et al.*, 1988). Oxalate can further degrade under ultraviolet light exposure to carbon dioxide and formic acid (Gupta *et al.*, 1971). Rockwell *et al.* reported detectable concentrations of oxalate, presumably from endogenous production, in neonatal TPN solutions (Rockwell *et al.*, 1998). In addition, these investigators found that the presence of increased amino acid concentration appeared to confer a protective effect against the conversion of ascorbic acid to oxalate.

The role of ascorbic acid in hyperoxaluria has come under more scrutiny although the FDA raised the recommended level of ascorbic acid in intravenous multivitamin preparations from 100 mg/day to 200 mg/day (FDA, 2000). More recently, the levels of urinary oxalate excretion at both doses were investigated in patients on long-term HPN. A statistically significant increase in urinary oxalate excretion was seen in patients on the 200 mg/day dose, suggesting that a possible increased risk of nephrolithiasis may exist for such patients (Pena de la Vega *et al.*, 2004). In addition, Fairholm *et al.* showed that decreasing the ascorbic acid dose from 500 mg to 100 mg daily substantially decreased urinary oxalate excretion (Fairholm *et al.*, 2003). In all likelihood, very large doses of ascorbic acid are required to cause true hyperoxaluria (Binder, 1974). Finally, treatment with conjugated bile acid supplementation in patients with suspected hyperoxaluria can be effective in the prevention of nephrolithiasis by reducing fat malabsorption, decreasing intraluminal fat concentration and decreasing calcium soap formation, thereby allowing oxalate to precipitate as its insoluble calcium salt rather than be absorbed in the colon (Emmett *et al.*, 2003).

Rare Cardiopulmonary Complications

The cardiopulmonary system certainly can see deleterious effects of HPN. Pulmonary embolus is a rare but potentially devastating complication of HPN; generally speaking, most cases can be attributed to in-dwelling central venous catheter use, which is discussed later in this volume (Chapter 20). Several case reports in the literature have suggested precipitated crystals as another potential source of microvascular pulmonary emboli. In particular, calcium phosphate precipitation has been well studied as an adverse interaction in HPN solutions. Calcium phosphate crystals generally form as dibasic molecules, which are less soluble than monobasic. Among the apparent risk factors for precipitation of calcium phosphate crystals are high molar concentration of calcium and phosphate in the TPN solution, prolonged standing time, increased infusion rate, increased solution pH, increased environmental temperatures, calcium use as a chloride salt and elevated serum magnesium concentrations (Reedy *et al.*, 1999). Clinically, patients with calcium phosphate emboli present with symptoms typical for pulmonary embolus including fever, cough and shortness of breath. High-resolution computed tomography scan usually reveals pulmonary nodules, and one case report cited the potential value of lung biopsy to confirm the diagnosis (McNearney *et al.*, 2003). Discontinuation of the HPN in some of the reported cases appeared to have led to resolution of symptoms.

After several case reports including deaths attributed to precipitates from HPN, the FDA issued a safety alert in 1994 containing guidelines to minimize the risk of calcium phosphate precipitation. Recommendations included the use of in-line filters, avoidance of the use of three-in-one admixtures when possible, and prescribing practices for calcium and phosphate in PN solutions (Lumpkin, 1994). Lipid emulsion three-in-one admixtures can obscure precipitates. If a lipid emulsion is needed, the FDA recommended using a two-in-one with lipid infusion separately, or if three-in-one is medically necessary, adding calcium before the lipid emulsion. The FDA also recommended calculating the solubility of the calcium from the volume at the time calcium is added, not based upon the final volume of the admixture. All home care personnel administering HPN should visually inspect the solution for the presence of precipitates before and during the infusion. If symptoms of acute respiratory distress, pulmonary embolus or interstitial pneumonitis develop, the PN should be stopped and checked for precipitate, and appropriate medical management of the patient's symptoms should be undertaken.

A retrospective analysis of 64 young children who had received PN for a median of 40 months, and had received a routine annual ventilation/perfusion (V/Q) scan, found 39% were abnormal and all were diagnosed with a pulmonary embolism (Pifarre *et al.*, 2009). Risk factors included frequency of lipid emulsion infusion, the presence of bowel inflammation and haematological abnormalities (protein C or S deficiency).

Summary

The literature on the effects of HPN on the kidneys and cardiopulmonary system, as well as on toxicities from heavy metals and other elements, continues to grow. Many mechanisms remain poorly understood, including the decline in both creatinine clearance and renal tubular function. We also continue to learn more about the important role of the trace elements found in HPN. These important components of nutritional support may sometimes, though rarely, carry serious toxicities if their clinical manifestations go unrecognized. Particularly for patients on long-term HPN support, these potential toxicities should always be considered in certain clinical scenarios, as early recognition can clearly be vital to treatment of these adverse events.

References

Baines, A.D. (1965) Cell renewal following dichromate induced renal tubular necrosis. *American Journal of Pathology* 47, 851–876.

Bengoa, J.M., Sitrin, M.D., Wood, R.J. and Rosenberg I.H. (1983) Amino acid-induced hypercalciuria in patients on total parenteral nutrition. *American Journal of Clinical Nutrition* 38, 264–269.

Bertinet, D.B., Tinivella, M., Balzola, F.A., de Francesco, A., Davini, O., Rizzo, L., Massarenti, P., Leonardi, M.A. and Balzol, F. (2000) Brain manganese deposition and blood levels in patients undergoing home parenteral nutrition. *JPEN Journal of Parenteral and Enteral Nutrition* 24, 223–227.

Binder, H.J. (1974) Intestinal oxalate absorption. *Gastroenterology* 67, 441–446.

Bishop, N.J., Robinson, M.J., Lendon, M., Hewitt, C.D., Day, J.P. and O'Hara, M. (1989) Increased concentration of aluminium in the brain of a parenterally fed preterm infant. *Archives of Disease in Childhood* 64, 1316–1317.

Boncompain-Gerard, M., Robert, D., Fouque, D. and Hadj-Aissa, A. (2000) Renal function and urinary excretion of electrolytes in patients receiving cyclic parenteral nutrition. *JPEN Journal of Parenteral and Enteral Nutrition* 24, 234–239.

Buchman, A.L., Moukarzel, A.A. and Ament, M.E. (1992) The role of chromium and cadmium toxicity in TPN-induced nephropathy. *Journal of Clinical Nutrition and Gastroenterology* 7, 39–41.

Buchman, A.L., Moukarzel, A.A., Ament, M.E., Gorbein, J., Goodson, B., Carlson, C. and Hawkins, R.A. (1993) Serious renal impairment is associated with long-term parenteral nutrition. *JPEN Journal of Parenteral and Enteral Nutrition* 17, 438–444.

Buchman, A.L., Moukarzel, A.A. and Ament, M.E. (1995) Excessive urinary oxalate excretion occurs in long-term TPN patients both with and without ileostomies. *Journal of the American College of Nutrition* 14, 24–28.

Buchman, A.L., Neely, M., Grossie, V.B. Jr, Truong, L., Lykissa, E. and Ahn, C. (2001) Organ heavy-metal accumulation during parenteral nutrition is associated with pathologic abnormalities in rats. *Nutrition* 17, 600–606.

Emmett, M., Guirl, M.J., Santa Ana, C.A., Porter, J.L., Neimark, S., Hoffmann, A.F. and Fordtran, J.S. (2003) Conjugated bile acid replacement therapy reduces urinary oxalate excretion in short bowel syndrome. *American Journal of Kidney Disease* 41, 230–237.

Fairholm, L., Saqui, O., Baun, M. and Allard, J. (2003) Influence of multivitamin regimen on urinary oxalate in home parenteral nutrition patients. *Nutrition in Clinical Practice* 18, 366–369.

FDA (US Food and Drug Administration) (1998) Aluminum in large and small volume parenterals used in total parenteral nutrition – FDA. Proposed rule. *Federal Register* 63, 176–185.

FDA (US Food and Drug Administration) (2000) Parenteral multivitamin products; drugs for human use; drug efficacy study implementation; amendment. *Federal Register* 65, 21200–21201.

FDA (US Food and Drug Administration) (2013) Specific labeling requirements for specific drug products. [Aluminum]. *Code of Federal Regulations* Title 21, vol 4. 21CFR201.323.

Fitzgerald, K., Mikalunas, V., Rubin, H., McCarthey, R., Vanagunas, A. and Craig, R.M. (1999) Hypermanganesemia in patients receiving total parenteral nutrition. *JPEN Journal of Parenteral and Enteral Nutrition* 23, 333–336.
Fok, T.F., Chui, K.K., Cheung, R., Ng, P.C., Cheung, K.L. and Hjelm, M. (2001) Manganese intake and cholestatic jaundice in neonates receiving parenteral nutrition: a randomized controlled study. *Acta Paediatrica* 90, 1009–1015.
Gupta, R.P., Rao, G.A. and Gyani, B.P. (1971) Photo-oxidation of oxalic acid. *Indian Journal of Chemistry* 9, 888.
Hambridge, K.M., Sokol, R.J., Fidanza, S.J. and Goodall, M.A. (1989) Plasma manganese concentrations in infants and children receiving parenteral nutrition. *JPEN Journal of Parenteral and Enteral Nutrition* 13, 168–171.
Hockaday, T.D.R., Frederick, E.W., Clayton, J.E. and Smith, L.H. Jr (1965) Studies on primary hyperoxaluria in patients with ileal resection and diarrhea. *Gastroenterology* 56, 960 (abstract).
Hoppe, B., Hesse, A., Neuhaus, T., Fanconi, S., Forster, I., Blau, N. and Leumann, E. (1993) Urinary saturation and nephrocalcinosis in preterm infants: effect of parenteral nutrition. *Archives of Disease in Childhood* 69, 299–303.
Howard, L., Ashley, C., Lyon, D. and Shenkin, A. (2007) Autopsy tissue trace elements in 8 long-term parenteral nutrition patients who received the current US Food and Drug Administration formulation. *JPEN Journal of Parenteral and Enteral Nutrition* 31, 388–396.
Hsieh, C.T., Liang, J.S., Pend, S.S. and Lee, W.T. (2007) Seizure associated with total parenteral nutrition-related hypermanganesemia. *Pediatric Neurology* 36, 181–183.
Jeejeebhoy, K.N., Chu, R.C., Marliss, E.B., Greenberg, G.R. and Bruce-Robertson, A. (1977) Chromium deficiency, glucose intolerance, and neuropathy reversed by chromium supplementation, in a patient receiving long-term total parenteral nutrition. *American Journal of Clinical Nutrition* 30, 531–538.
Lauverjat, M., Hadj Aissa, A., Vanhems, P., Boulereau, P., Fouque, D. and Chambrier, C. (2006) Chronic dehydration may impair renal function in patients with chronic intestinal failure on long-term parenteral nutrition. *Clinical Nutrition* 25, 75–81.
Lumpkin, M.M. (1994) Safety alert: hazards of precipitation associated with parenteral nutrition. *American Journal of Hospital Pharmacy* 51, 1427–1428.
McMillan, N.B., Mulroy, C., MacKay, N.W., McDonald, C.M. and Jackson, W.D. (2008) Correlation of cholestasis with serum copper and whole blood manganese levels in pediatric patients. *Nutrition in Clinical Practice* 23, 161–165.
McNearney, T., Bajaj, C., Boyars, M., Cottingham, J. and Haque, A. (2003) Total parenteral nutrition associated crystalline precipitates resulting in pulmonary artery occlusions and alveolar granulomas. *Digestive Diseases and Sciences* 48, 1352–1354.
Messing, B., Bories, C., Kunstlinger, F. and Bernier, J.J. (1983) Does total parenteral nutrition induce gallbladder sludge formation and lithiasis? *Gastroenterology* 84, 1012–1019.
Milatovic, D., Yin, Z., Gupta, R.C., Sidoryk, M., Albrecht, J., Aschner, J.L. and Aschner, M. (2007) Manganese induces oxidative impairment in cultured rat astrocytes. *Toxicological Sciences* 98, 198–205.
Mirowitz, S.A. and Westrich, T.J. (1992) Basal ganglial signal intensity alterations: reversal after discontinuation of parenteral manganese administration. *Radiology* 185, 535–536.
Mohamed, G.B., Ibrahiem, M.A. and Abdel Hameed, W.M. (2014) Nephrocalcinosis in pre-term neonates: a study of incidence and risk factors. *Saudi Journal of Kidney Diseases and Transplantation* 25, 326–332.
Morris, B.W., MacNeil, S., Hardisty, C.A., Heller, S., Burgin, C. and Gray, T.A. (1999) Chromium homeostasis in patients with type 2 (NIDDM) diabetes. *Journal of Trace Elements in Medicine and Biology* 13, 57–61.

Moukarzel, A.A., Ament, M.E., Buchman, A., Dahlstrom, K.A. and Vargas, J. (1991) Renal function of children receiving long-term parenteral nutrition. *Journal of Pediatrics* 119, 864–868.

Moukarzel, A.A., Song, M.K., Buchman, A.L., Vargas, J., Guss, W., McDiarmid, S., Reyen, L. and Ament, M.E. (1992) Excessive chromium intake in children receiving total parenteral nutrition. *The Lancet* 339, 385–388.

Nagatomo, S., Umehara, F., Hanada, K., Nobuhara, Y., Takenaga, S., Arimura, K. and Osame, M. (1999) Manganese intoxication during total parenteral nutrition: report of two cases and review of the literature. *Journal of Neurological Sciences* 162, 102–105.

Norose, N., Terai, M. and Norose, K. (1992) Manganese deficiency in a child with very short bowel receiving long-term parenteral nutrition. *Journal of Trace Elements and Experimental Medicine* 5, 100–101 (abstract).

Pena de la Vega, L., Lieske, J.C., Milliner, D., Gonyea, J. and Kelly, D.G. (2004) Urinary oxalate excretion increases in home parenteral nutrition patients on a higher intravenous ascorbic acid dose. *JPEN Journal of Parenteral and Enteral Nutrition* 28, 435–438.

Pifarre, P., Roca, I., Irastorza, I., Simo, M., Hill, S., Biassoni, L. and Gordon, I. (2009) Lung ventilation-perfusion scintigraphy in children on long-term parenteral nutrition. *European Journal Nuclear Medicine and Molecular Imaging* 36, 1005–1008.

Ravina, A., Slezak, L., Mirsky, N., Bryden, N.A. and Anderson, R.A. (1999) Reversal of corticosteroid-induced diabetes with supplemental chromium. *Diabetics Medicine* 16, 164–167.

Reedy, J.S., Kuhlman, J.E. and Voytovich, M. (1999) Microvascular pulmonary emboli secondary to precipitated crystals in a patient receiving total parenteral nutrition: a case report and description of the high-resolution CT findings. *Chest* 115, 892–895.

Reimund, J.M., Dietemann, J.L., Warter, H.M., Baumann, R. and Duclos, B. (2000) Factors associated to hypermanganesemia in patients receiving home parenteral nutrition. *Clinical Nutrition* 19, 343–348.

Rockwell, G.F., Campfield, T., Nelson, B.C. and Uden, P.C. (1998) Oxalogenesis in parenteral nutrition solution components. *Nutrition* 14, 836–839.

Scheinkestel, C.D., Adams, F., Mahony, L., Bailey, M., Davies, A.R., Nyulasi, I. and Tuxen, D.V. (2003) Impact of varying parenteral protein loads on amino-acid balance in critically-ill anuric patients on CAVHDF. *Nutrition* 19, 733–740.

Siepler, J.K., Nishikawa, R.A., Diamntidis, T. and Okamoto, R. (2003) Asymptomatic hypermanganesemia in long-term home parenteral nutrition patients. *Nutrition in Clinical Practice* 18, 370–373.

Smith, J.L., Canham, J.E. and Wells, P.A. (1988) Effect of phototherapy light, sodium bisulfite, and pH on vitamin stability in total parenteral nutrition admixtures. *JPEN Journal of Parenteral and Enteral Nutrition* 12, 394–402.

Stevens, L. and Rashid, M. (2008) Manganese toxicity in patients on long term HPN therapy. *JPEN Journal of Parenteral and Enteral Nutrition* 23, 197–198.

Swartz, R.D., Wesley, J.R., Somermeyer, M.G. and Lau, K. (1984) Hyperoxaluria and renal insufficiency due to ascorbic acid administration during total parenteral nutrition. *Annals of Internal Medicine* 100, 530–532.

Takagi, Y., Okada, A., Sando, K., Wasa, M., Yoshida, H. and Hirabuki, N. (2001) On–off study of manganese administration to adult patients undergoing home parenteral nutrition: new indices of in vivo manganese level. *JPEN Journal of Parenteral and Enteral Nutrition* 25, 87–92.

Tandon, S.K., Saxena, D.K., Gaur, J.S. and Chandra, S.V. (1978) Comparative toxicity of trivalent and hexavalent chromium. Alterations in blood and liver. *Environmental Research* 15, 90–98.

Tsapakos, M.J., Hampton, T.H. and Wetterhahn, K.E. (1983) Chromium (VI)-induced DNA lesions and chromium distribution in rat kidney, liver, and lung. *Cancer Research* 43, 5662–5667.
Vargas, J.H., Klein, G.L., Ament, M.E., Ott, S.M., Sherrard, D.J., Horst, R.L., Berquist, W.E., Alfrey, A.C., Slatopolsky, E. and Coburn, J.W. (1988) Metabolic bone disease of total parenteral nutrition: course after changing from casein to amino acids in parenteral solutions with reduced aluminum content. *American Journal of Clinical Nutrition* 48, 1070–1078.
Verhage, A.H., Cheong, W.K. and Jeejeebhoy, K.N. (1996) Neurologic symptoms due to possible chromium deficiency in long-term parenteral nutrition that closely mimic metronidazole-induced syndromes. *JPEN Journal of Parenteral and Enteral Nutrition* 20, 123–127.
Wardle, C.A., Forbes, A., Roberts, N.B., Jawhari, A.V. and Shenkin, A. (1999) Hypermanganesemia in long-term intravenous nutrition and chronic liver disease. *JPEN Journal of Parenteral and Enteral Nutrition* 23, 350–355.
Wongseelashote, O., Daly, M.A. and Frankel, E.H. (2004) High insulin requirement versus high chromium requirement in patients nourished with total parenteral nutrition. *Nutrition* 20, 318–320.

19 Venous Access-related Complications: Infections

Geert Wanten[1*] and Michael Staun[2]

[1]Radboud University Nijmegen Medical Centre, Nijmegen, The Netherlands; [2]Department of Medical Gastroenterology, Rigshospitalet, Copenhagen, Denmark

Key Points

- The nutrition support team is of paramount importance for patient education and for minimizing the rate of infectious complications.
- General barrier precautions are of utmost importance.
- Infections with fungi always require a line shift.
- Repeated line infections may be reduced by antibiotic lock.

Introduction

Since its introduction in the late 1960s, home parenteral nutrition (HPN) has become the mainstay of treatment for patients with severe long-term intestinal failure. But although the clinical relevance of HPN to supply these patients' nutritional needs is beyond doubt, its associated high complication rate remains a worry. Whereas patient survival depends mainly on the underlying disease leading to intestinal failure, the most frequent problem in HPN support is infection related to the presence of a venous access device. HPN delivery requires safe access to a large-bore central vein because of the formulation's high osmolarity. Surgically created arteriovenous fistulae (AVFs) in the arm, similar to those used in haemodialysis, were initially used to administer HPN but became rare with the advent of intravenous catheters in the 1970s. Ever since, central venous access for long-term HPN is almost invariably obtained via a subcutaneously tunnelled catheter or a fully implanted port; whereas, because of their higher infection risk, non-tunnelled catheters are exclusively used for short-term bridging of

E-mail: geert.wanten@radboudumc.nl

parenteral nutrition (PN) during a hospital stay. Tunnelled catheters are usually implanted into the subclavian, internal jugular or femoral vein and have a subcutaneous cuff that inhibits migration of microbes into the catheter tunnel tract. Totally implantable ports are inserted into the same veins as catheters and tunnelled beneath the skin, where the subcutaneous port is accessed with a needle. These ports improve the patient's self-image and lack the requirement for local exit-site care, but in the case of problems they have to be removed surgically.

Catheter-related infections (CRIs) severely impair the patient's quality of life, increase treatment costs and eventually, upon repeated catheter loss, compromise the options to obtain adequate venous access. This chapter focuses on venous access-related infectious complications, their treatment and preventive strategies that promise to limit such complications and improve treatment outcomes. For non-infectious access-related issues we refer the reader to Chapter 20.

Infectious Complications Related to Catheter Insertion and Catheter Type

To decrease infections, tunnelled single-lumen catheters made of polyurethane or silicone should be used whenever possible in the setting of HPN (Tokars *et al.*, 1999; Gillanders *et al.*, 2008; Pittiruti *et al.*, 2009; O'Grady *et al.*, 2011). Tunnelled catheters and fully implanted ports have an equally low risk for extraluminal contamination in the setting of HPN, whereas evidence to support the use of peripherally inserted central catheters (PICC lines) in long-term HPN is lacking (Pittiruti *et al.*, 2009; O'Grady *et al.*, 2011). In order to prevent bacterial contamination, catheter insertion should be carried out using maximal surgical sterile barrier precautions, including wearing masks, caps, sterile gowns and gloves (Raad *et al.*, 1994; O'Grady *et al.*, 2011). Regarding the choice of central vein to insert a tunnelled catheter, data for long-term HPN are lacking (O'Grady *et al.*, 2011). Importantly, the exit site of any catheter should be at a place, mostly the anterior chest, which enables self-management by the patient under visual control. Catheter exchange over a guide wire is contraindicated in the case of an infected catheter or exit site.

Catheter-related Infections: Pathogenesis, Definitions and Symptoms

CRIs might be local, including infections of the catheter exit site, port pocket or subcutaneous catheter tunnel, or systemic, in the form of catheter-related bloodstream infections (CRBSIs) (Pearson, 1996). CRBSIs are defined by a positive culture of the catheter (on removal) or paired blood cultures from a peripheral vein and the catheter (when left in place), with isolation of identical organisms (both species and antibiograms) from cultures of catheter segments and blood drawn from a peripheral vein in a patient with clinical symptoms of sepsis and the absence of another source of infection (Pearson, 1996). A survey of 527 patients in the USA identified CRIs, mainly CRBSIs (80%), exit-site (17%) and tunnel (2%) infections, as the most common problems of HPN support (Buchman *et al.*, 1994). It is assumed that CRIs develop after colonization of the device from the luminal or the outer catheter surface. Infections can be bacterial or fungal in origin, but most problems are caused by skin-derived flora. An Italian survey of 296 HPN patients found that 76% of CRBSIs were caused by Gram-positive *Staphylococcus epidermidis* (51%) or *Staphylococcus aureus* (7%), whereas Gram-negative microbes comprised 16%, fungi 3% and poly-microbial cultures 6% of infections (Santarpia *et al.*, 2010). When investigating differences in bacteriology between colonized catheters and CRBSIs in 354 HPN patients, the authors found that culturing of fungi invariably indicated catheter infection, whereas Gram-positive culture results rather indicated colonization (Lin *et al.*, 2003). These findings corroborate clinical experience that fungal CRBSI requires removal of the catheter, whereas in case of bacterial CRBSI the line can be salvaged in 30–80% of cases (Jeppesen *et al.*, 1998; Clare *et al.*, 2008; O'Grady *et al.*, 2011). The catheter hub is regarded as a common cause of endoluminal CRIs, whereas infections originating from the exit site or tunnel tract are considered extraluminal in nature.

Local signs of CRIs include limited redness of the skin, pain and discharge of pus from the exit site or tunnel, which may also appear elevated due the inflammation. The signs of systemic infection cover a broad range of symptoms; typically patients will complain of fever and chills immediately or hours after the start of PN infusion. Non-specific signs include cardiopulmonary symptoms (shortness of breath, arrhythmias) or gastrointestinal complaints. In any HPN patient, symptoms of infection without another confirmed source should raise the concern for a CRI. That the signs of even CRBSIs may be very subtle was shown in a retrospective study from the UK (Clare *et al.*, 2008). When looking at consecutive HPN patients presenting with proven CRBSI, the authors found that this diagnosis should be suspected in any patient with a newly raised C-reactive protein and/or serum bilirubin, decreased serum albumin and in non-specifically unwell patients, despite the presence of normal white cell counts and apyrexia in one-third of all patients. Of note, CRIs may also cause thromboembolic complications and catheter obstruction (Wechsler *et al.*, 1993).

For clinical purposes strict definitions for colonization and infection, such as presented by Pearson (1996), are important tools. Here, catheter colonization is defined as growth of >15 colony-forming units in semi-quantitative cultures or $>10^3$ colony-forming units in quantitative cultures from a proximal or distal catheter segment, in the absence of clinical symptoms. Local CRIs are defined by similar criteria, with the presence of inflammation (redness, heat, swelling, pain) at the device site. Exit-site infections are defined by inflammation or purulence within 2 cm of the skin at the catheter exit, whereas tunnel infections are characterized by inflammation of tissue overlying the catheter with a distance of >2 cm from the exit site. In patients using implantable ports, pocket infections may occur, with inflammation and necrosis of the skin overlying the reservoir.

Catheter-related Bloodstream Infections: Risk Factors, Diagnosis and Treatment

A prospective study of 827 patients receiving home infusion therapy because of infections (67%), cancer (24%), nutritional and digestive disease (17%), transplants and HIV (18%) diagnosed 69 episodes of CRBSI during nearly 70,000 catheter-days (Tokars *et al.*, 1999). Independent risk factors for infection were, among others: (i) the administration of PN regardless of whether lipids were included; (ii) the use of multi-lumen catheters; and (iii) previous CRBSIs. A large survey (12 centres, 447 HPN patients) by the Home Artificial Nutrition Working Group of the European Society for Enteral and Parenteral Nutrition (ESPEN) a decade ago reported on experience in >100,000 catheter-days and found that 25% of patients developed catheter problems during 6 years, which were caused by infections in 50% and resulted in catheter removal in 50% of these cases (Bozzetti *et al.*, 2002). Implantable ports and daily PN were identified as risk factors, whereas use of catheters for non-nutritional purposes reduced the infection risk (Bozzetti *et al.*, 2002). CRBSI incidence rates in experienced referral centres range from 0.16 to 1.09 per catheter-year and account for about 70% of hospital admissions in HPN patients (Buchman *et al.*, 1994; O'Keefe *et al.*, 1994; Jeppesen *et al.*, 1998; Pironi *et al.*, 2003; Freshwater *et al.*, 2004; Clare *et al.*, 2008). Jeppesen *et al.* (1998) identified the presence of a stoma and high age as risk factors for CRBSI, while others found a reduced infection risk in HPN patients who were under the care of a dedicated nutrition support team (Dimick *et al.*, 2003).

Once a CRBSI is suspected, two sets of blood cultures should be taken, one percutaneously and one from the catheter, to evaluate the possibility of bacteraemia. Paired quantitative blood cultures or paired qualitative blood cultures that are monitored for the differential time to positivity are the preferred means to diagnose a CRBSI (Pittiruti *et al.*, 2009). A probable CRBSI is characterized by a colonized catheter in association with clinical signs suggesting septicaemia, despite the lack of a positive peripheral blood culture. Blood cultures should not be taken on a routine basis in the absence of suspicion for a CRI (O'Grady *et al.*, 2011).

Concerning CRBSI treatment in general, in HPN patients a conservative approach with systemic and local (locks) use of antibiotics is advocated for simple infections due to *S. aureus*, coagulase-negative staphylococci and Gram-negative bacilli, before removing the catheter (Pittiruti *et al.*, 2009; Staun *et al.*, 2009; O'Grady *et al.*, 2011). Catheter removal is inevitable in the case of tunnel infections, port abscesses, in patients with septic shock or in complicated infections, including endocarditis, metastatic infections, septic thrombosis and when paired blood cultures are positive for fungi or virulent bacteria. Successful salvage of infected implanted ports by antibiotic treatment is rare and most of these devices have to be removed (Kuizon *et al.*, 2001). Re-insertion of long-term devices should be postponed until appropriate systemic therapy is administered based on susceptibility of pathogens in cultures and after repeated samples yield negative results, or ideally when negative culture results are obtained 5 to 10 days after completion of antibiotic therapy (Pittiruti *et al.*, 2009).

While thrombolysis with urokinase, streptokinase or tissue plasminogen activator has been successfully used to unblock clogged catheters, these agents are also used in some centres as part of a CRBSI treatment protocol to remove a (possibly infected) thrombus from the catheter tip (Gillanders *et al.*, 2008; Versleijen *et al.*, 2009).

Catheter-related Infections: Prevention

A randomized trial has provided evidence that interactive video-based education of both staff and patients reduces CRIs in HPN patients and improves problem-solving capacities and quality of life (Smith *et al.*, 2003). Such training of all individuals who are involved in HPN care is currently considered a key strategy to decrease CRIs. The same applies for the implementation of an adequate policy of hand-washing by patients and staff, and for the use of chlorhexidine 2% for skin antisepsis of the hands, catheter exit site and of the skin before catheter insertion (Pittiruti *et al.*, 2009; O'Grady *et al.*, 2011). Especially in HPN patients who repeatedly develop CRBSIs, preventive interventions other than changing of the line should be considered, including re-education of the patient or his/her caregiver to self-perform all relevant procedures. Stopcocks, catheter hubs and other sampling ports should always be disinfected, preferably using chlorhexidine 2% in 70% isopropyl alcohol. Intravenous administration sets should be changed every 24 h (for lipid-based PN) or 72 h (for lipid-free PN). There is no definitive proof that the use of needle-free connectors reduces CRBSIs in HPN patients.

Strategies that have been proved not to be effective to prevent CRIs include the use of in-line filters, routine replacement of catheters, antibiotic prophylaxis and the use of heparin (Pittiruti *et al.*, 2009; Staun *et al.*, 2009; O'Grady *et al.*, 2011).

Catheter locking

Other techniques have been tested and implemented to prevent CRBSIs, including the use of several types of catheter lock and flush solutions. Catheter locking is a technique by which an antimicrobial solution is used to fill the catheter lumen and then dwell for a period of time when the catheter is not in use: antibiotics, either alone or in combinations, have been used to this end as well as antiseptic substances such as ethanol, taurolidine and trisodium citrate. These agents are frequently combined with an anticoagulant such as heparin or EDTA.

Antibiotics

Evidence is lacking that prophylactic use of antibiotic locks (or systemic antibiotics for that matter) reduces the incidence of CRBSIs in HPN patients (Pittiruti *et al.*, 2009), while this strategy carries an inherent risk for the development of microbial resistance, especially in patients requiring long-term HPN.

Ethanol

Seventy per cent ethanol has not only been used to dissolve debris and unclog PN catheters, but ethanol locking therapy (ELT) has also been shown to be a promising therapy for the prevention of CRBSIs in small studies in both adult and paediatric HPN patients (Metcalf *et al.*, 2004; Opilla *et al.*, 2007; Maiefski *et al.*, 2009). Benefits over antibiotics include the lack of development of microbial resistance, potent bactericidal and fungicidal properties, and low cost. For instance, Opilla *et al.* (2007) studied nine HPN patients with a crossover design using ELT. Patients developed 81 CRBSIs before ELT and nine CRBSIs thereafter (8.3 versus 2.7 per 1000 catheter-days). In a larger group of 31 HPN patients in the USA who were studied pre- and post-ELT (John *et al.*, 2012), there were 273 admissions due to CRBSIs prior to ELT in comparison to 47 admissions post-ELT, with an adjusted drop in admission rate due to CRBSI from 10.1 to 2.9 per 1000 catheter-days, without any reported side-effects or complications in any patient undergoing ELT.

Taurolidine

Taurolidine, a derivative of the amino acid taurine, prevents microbial adhesion to catheter surfaces and biofilm formation by an irreversible reaction of its metabolites with bacterial cell walls. Taurolidine has a very broad spectrum of activity against bacterial and fungal pathogens and also neutralizes bacterial endo- and exotoxins (Watson *et al.*, 1995; Shah *et al.*, 2002). Experience with taurolidine as a catheter lock from studies in the setting of HPN initially came from work by Jurewitsch and Jeejeebhoy (2005), who used taurolidine in a non-controlled study in seven HPN patients and found a decreased infection rate from 10.8 infections per 1000 catheter-days pre-treatment to 0.8 thereafter. Bisseling *et al.* (2010) conducted the only prospective controlled trial so far by randomizing HPN patients open label after treatment for CRBSI to receive either 2% taurolidine ($n = 16$) or heparin (150 U/ml, $n = 14$). This study was terminated early due to an interim analysis demonstrating that taurolidine locking decreased re-infections by more than 90% when compared with heparin, with a mean infection-free period of 641 catheter-days in the taurolidine group and 176 in the heparin group ($P < 0.0001$). There were no reported adverse effects or catheter occlusions. In addition, these authors also showed that there was no evidence for the development of microbial resistance to taurolidine in cultures from patients who developed CRBSIs while being treated with taurolidine locks (Olthof *et al.*, 2013). Similar findings have been reported in several small retrospective and non-controlled studies. Important issues that remain to be solved in future studies are whether addition of anticoagulants such as citrate to taurolidine affects its efficacy, whether the use of 0.9% sodium chloride (saline) as catheter lock is as effective as taurolidine, or superior to heparin, and whether locks should be withdrawn or flushed into the patient upon the next catheter use.

Overall, at this point, general recommendations for the use of any catheter lock cannot be given due to the fact that: (i) the only studies available are underpowered; (ii) a wide variety of compounds have been used; and (iii) the patient populations that were studied are heterogeneous (O'Grady *et al.*, 2011). Potential problems related to the use of these locks include the development of side-effects, toxicity, allergic reactions and the emergence of microbial resistance.

Arteriovenous fistulae

That an almost forgotten technique, i.e. the use of AVFs constructed in the forearm, is a feasible alternative to catheters in the setting of HPN was reported recently in a Dutch study (Versleijen *et al.*, 2009). In 127 consecutive patients receiving HPN between 2000 and 2006, comprising 344 access-years of tunnelled catheters/ports and 194 access-years of AVFs, the rate of bloodstream infections per year was 0.03 for AVFs and 1.37 for ports and tunnelled catheters, with occlusion rates of 0.60 and 0.35 per year, respectively, showing that although occlusions were somewhat more frequent for AVFs than for tunnelled catheters, the incidence of bloodstream infections was much lower. Of note, these authors consider the use of PICC lines contraindicated in patients in whom creation of an AVF is considered due to the PICC-associated risk for thrombosis.

Summary

This chapter describes the most frequent complications related to venous access, including those related to insertion and placement, catheter-related infections, catheter obstruction and venous thrombosis. Management and preventive measures are also discussed.

References

Bisseling, T.M., Willems, M.C., Versleijen, M.W., Hendriks, J.C., Vissers, R.K. and Wanten, G.J. (2010) Taurolidine lock is highly effective in preventing catheter-related bloodstream infections in patients on home parenteral nutrition: a heparin-controlled prospective trial. *Clinical Nutrition* 29, 464–468.

Bozzetti, F., Mariani, L., Bertinet, D.B., Chiavenna, G., Crose, N., De Cicco, M., Gigli, G., Micklewright, A., Moreno Villares, J.M., Orban, A., Pertkiewicz, M., Pironi, L., Vilas, M.P., Prins, F. and Thul, P. (2002) Central venous catheter complications in 447 patients on home parenteral nutrition: an analysis of over 100,000 catheter days. *Clinical Nutrition* 21, 475–485.

Buchman, A.L., Moukarzel, A., Goodson, B., Herzog, F., Pollack, P., Reyen, L., Alvarez, M., Ament, M.E. and Gornbein, J. (1994) Catheter-related infections associated with home parenteral nutrition and predictive factors for the need for catheter removal in their treatment. *JPEN Journal of Parenteral and Enteral Nutrition* 18, 297–302.

Clare, A., Teubner, A. and Shaffer, J.L. (2008) What information should lead to a suspicion of catheter sepsis in HPN? *Clinical Nutrition* 27, 552–556.

Dimick, J.B., Swoboda, S., Talamini, M.A., Pelz, R.K., Hendrix, C.W. and Lipsett, P.A. (2003) Risk of colonization of central venous catheters: catheters for total parenteral nutrition vs. other catheters. *American Journal of Critical Care* 12, 228–235.

Freshwater, D.A., Saadeddin, A., Deel-Smith, P., Digger, T. and Jones, B.J.M. (2004) Can home parenteral nutrition be provided by non-specialized centres? 2300 weeks experience at a district general hospital in United Kingdom. *Clinical Nutrition* 24, 229–235.
Gillanders, L., Angstmann, K., Ball P., Chapman-Kiddell, C., Hardy, G., Hope, J., Smith, R., Strauss, B. and Russell, D. (2008) AuSPEN clinical practice guideline for home parenteral nutrition patients in Australia and New Zealand. *Nutrition* 24, 998–1012.
Jeppesen, P.B., Staun, M. and Mortensen, P.B. (1998) Adult patients receiving home parenteral nutrition in Denmark from 1991 to 1996: who will benefit from intestinal transplantation? *Scandinavian Journal of Gastroenterology* 33, 839–846.
John, B.K., Khan, M.A. and Speerhas, R. (2012) Ethanol lock therapy in reducing catheter related bloodstream infections in adult home parenteral nutrition patients: results of a retrospective study. *JPEN Journal of Parenteral and Enteral Nutrition* 36, 603–610.
Jurewitsch, B. and Jeejeebhoy, K.N. (2005) Taurolidine lock: the key to prevention of recurrent catheter-related bloodstream infections. *Clinical Nutrition* 24, 462–465.
Kuizon, D., Gordon, S.M. and Dolmatch, B.L. (2001) Single-lumen subcutaneous ports inserted by interventional radiologists in patients undergoing chemotherapy: incidence of infection and outcome of attempted catheter salvage. *Archives of Internal Medicine* 161, 406–410.
Lin, C., Lin, M.T., Hsieh, D.Y., Chao, Y.F., Yeh, S.L., Wu, M.S., Lin, J.T., Lee, P.H., Chang, K.J. and Chen, W.J. (2003) Microbiology difference between colonized catheters and catheter-related bloodstream infections. *Hepatogastroenterology* 50, 1821–1824.
Maiefski, M., Rupp, M.E. and Hermsen, E.D. (2009) Ethanol lock technique: review of the literature. *Infection Control and Hospital Epidemiology* 30, 1096–1108.
Metcalf, S.C., Chambers, S.T. and Pithie, A.D. (2004) Use of ethanol locks to prevent recurrent central line sepsis effective. *Journal of Infectious Diseases* 49, 20–22.
O'Grady, N.P., Alexander, M., Burns, L.A., Dellinger, E.P., Garland, J., Heard, S.O., Lipsett, P.A., Masur, H., Mermel, L.A., Pearson, M.L., Raad, I.I., Randolph, A.G., Rupp, M.E., Saint, S. and Healthcare Infection Control Practices Advisory Committee (2011) Guidelines for the prevention of intravascular catheter-related infections. *American Journal of Infection Control* 39, 1–4.
O'Keefe, S.J., Burnes, J.U. and Thompson, R.L. (1994) Recurrent sepsis in home parenteral nutrition patients: an analysis of risk factors. *JPEN Journal of Parenteral and Enteral Nutrition* 18, 256–263.
Olthof, E.D., Rentenaar, R.J., Rijs, A.J. and Wanten, G.J. (2013) Absence of microbial adaptation to taurolidine in patients on home parenteral nutrition who develop catheter related bloodstream infections and use taurolidine locks. *Clinical Nutrition* 32, 538–542.
Opilla, M.T., Kirby, D.F. and Edmond, M.B. (2007) Use of ethanol lock therapy to reduce the incidence of catheter related blood stream infections in home parenteral nutrition patients. *JPEN Journal of Parenteral and Enteral Nutrition* 31, 302–305.
Pearson, M.L. (1996) Guideline for prevention of intravascular device-related infections. Part I. Intravascular device-related infections: an overview. The Hospital Infection Control Practices Advisory Committee. *American Journal of Infection Control* 24, 262–277.
Pironi, L., Paganelli, F., Labate, A.M., Merli, C., Guidetti, C., Spinucci, G. and Miglioli, M. (2003) Safety and efficacy of home parenteral nutrition for chronic intestinal failure: a 16-year experience at a single centre. *Digestive and Liver Disease* 35, 314–324.
Pittiruti, M., Hamilton, H., Biffi, R., MacFie, J. and Pertkiewicz, M. (2009) ESPEN guidelines on parenteral nutrition: central venous catheters. *Clinical Nutrition* 28, 365–377.
Raad, I.I., Hohn, D.C., Gilbreath, B.J., Suleiman, N., Hill, L.A., Bruso, P.A., Marts, K., Mansfield, P.F. and Bodey, G.P. (1994) Prevention of central venous catheter-related infections by using maximal sterile barrier precautions during insertion. *Infection Control and Hospital Epidemiology* 15, 231–238.

Santarpia, L., Alfonsi, L., Tiseo, D., Creti, R., Baldassarri, L. and Pasanisi, F. (2010) Central venous catheter infections and antibiotic therapy during long-term home parenteral nutrition: an 11-year follow-up study. *JPEN Journal of Parenteral and Enteral Nutrition* 34, 254–262.

Shah, C.B., Mittelman, M.W., Costerton, J.W., Parenteau, S., Pelak, M. and Arsenault, R. (2002) Antimicrobial activity of a novel catheter lock solution. *Antimicrobial Agents and Chemotherapy* 46, 1674–1679.

Smith, C.E., Curtas, S., Kleinbeck, S.V., Werkowitch, M., Mosier, M., Seidner, D.L. and Steiger, E. (2003) Clinical trials of interactive and videotaped educational interventions reduce infection, reactive depression, and rehospitalizations for sepsis in patients on home parenteral nutrition. *JPEN Journal of Parenteral and Enteral Nutrition* 27, 137–145.

Staun, M., Pironi, L., Bozzetti, F., Baxter, J., Forbes A., Joly, F., Jeppesen, P., Moreno, J., Hébuterne, X., Pertkiewicz, M., Mühlebach, S., Shenkin, A. and Van Gossum, A. (2009) ESPEN guidelines on parenteral nutrition: home parenteral nutrition (HPN) in adult patients. *Clinical Nutrition* 28, 467–479.

Tokars, J.I., Cookson, S.T., McArthur, M.A., Boyer, C.L., McGeer, A.J. and Jarvis, W.R. (1999) Prospective evaluation of risk factors for bloodstream infection in patients receiving home infusion therapy. *Annals of Internal Medicine* 131, 340–347.

Versleijen, M.W., Huisman-de Waal, G., Kock, M.C., Elferink, A., van Rossum, L.G., Feuth, T., Willems, M.C. and Wanten, G.J. (2009) Arteriovenous fistulae as an alternative to central venous catheters for delivery of long-term home parenteral nutrition. *Gastroenterology* 136, 1577–1584.

Watson, R.W., Redmond, H.P., McCarthy, J. and Bouchier-Hayes, D. (1995) Taurolidine, an antilipopolysaccharide agent, has immunoregulatory properties that are mediated by the amino acid taurine. *Journal of Leukocyte Biology* 58, 299–306.

Wechsler, R.J., Spirn, P.W., Conant, E.F., Steiner, R.M. and Needleman, L. (1993) Thrombosis and infection caused by thoracic venous catheters: pathogenesis and imaging findings. *American Journal of Roentgenology* 160, 467–471.

20 Non-septic Catheter-related Complications

CRISTINA CUERDA[1]* AND MICHAEL STAUN[2]

[1]*Nutrition Unit, Hospital General Universitario Gregorio Marañón, Madrid, Spain;* [2]*Department of Medical Gastroenterology, Rigshospitalet, Copenhagen, Denmark*

Key Points

- Catheter thrombotic complications may lead to catheter replacement and loss of venous access in patients on home parenteral nutrition (HPN).
- Adequate flushing with saline after parenteral nutrition infusion can prevent catheter occlusion, while there is insufficient evidence to recommend heparin lock or other interventions.
- Venous thrombosis can develop soon after catheter insertion or be delayed in patients with long-term catheterization.
- The decision to start thromboprophylaxis with warfarin or low-molecular-weight heparin in people on HPN should be decided on an individual basis.

Introduction

Home parenteral nutrition (HPN) is administered through central catheters of different type (tunnelled, ports, peripheral inserted central catheters (PICCs)). The use of such devices implies a risk of septic and non-septic complications. Septic complications are the most frequent in patients on HPN. On the other hand, non-septic catheter-related complications may lead to catheter replacement and loss of venous access. Currently, thrombosis in two of the central venous vessels (subclavian, jugular or femoral) is one of the criteria for considering small bowel transplantation (Abu-Elmagd, 2006).

*E-mail: mcuerda.hgugm@salud.madrid.org

This chapter covers the non-septic catheter-related complications, including the catheter occlusions, catheter-related vein thrombosis (CRVT) and other complications that may appear less frequently in patients with long-term catheterization such as catheter breakage and tip migration. The mechanical complications related with the catheter insertion (pneumothorax, artery lesion, malposition) are similar to those patients with short-term catheterization and are not discussed in this chapter (Grant, 2002).

Catheter Occlusions

Catheter tip occlusion during catheter dwell is a common complication, causing difficulty with infusion therapy. The incidence of catheter occlusion in HPN patients is about 0.07 episodes/catheter/year (range 0.059–0.083) (Howard and Ashley, 2003). It is usually unpredictable and may occur at any time, but can be associated with the lifespan of the catheter, the type of catheter used, handling procedures, repeated events of blood flushing back and possibly also the type of intravenous (IV) nutrition used.

The most common cause of catheter occlusion is catheter thrombosis, but it can also be due to HPN formula components, such as lipids and calcium phosphate precipitates. Adequate flushing with saline when the infusion of parenteral nutrition (PN) is completed can prevent catheter occlusion. It is not advised to use the catheter for blood sampling and the use of infusion pumps for HPN may reduce the risk of this complication (Pittiruti *et al.*, 2009). There is no evidence that flushing with heparin or other interventions (pressure caps, heparin-bonded catheters) prevents catheter occlusion, and published studies are merely case reports. Thus there is no evidence that flushing catheters with heparin is more effective than flushing with saline (Mitchell *et al.*, 2009). Future research may identify the ideal flush solution and the best flushing procedures for long-term central venous access devices. According to the guidelines of the European Society for Parenteral and Enteral Nutrition (ESPEN), saline can be used to flush/lock most of the catheters for HPN (evidence grade B) and heparin is recommended in ports, open-ended catheters or when indicated by the manufacturer and in catheters that are not in use (Pittiruti *et al.*, 2009).

If the catheter has been used for a significant period of time it is advised to replace rather than attempting to restore function. Case reports on the use of alcohol, saline, heparin, thrombolytic agents, surgical and radiological procedures have been published. In a double-blind randomized study, Ponec *et al.* (2001) used recombinant tissue plasminogen activator (alteplase) for restoring catheter function with success in 74% of cases compared with 17% in the placebo group. The central venous device had been in use for a median time of 35 days and more studies on long-term patients are warranted. This is supported by the conclusion of a systematic review (van Miert *et al.*, 2012) in which interventions for restoring patency of occluded central lines were evaluated; the authors found that either urokinase or alteplase may be effective in treating catheters occluded by a thrombus.

Catheter-related Vein Thrombosis

Incidence and aetiology

Thrombotic complications of the catheter is a dynamic process with varying severity, from the appearance of the fibrin sheath at the tip of the catheter, to intraluminal blood clot, mural thrombosis and venous thrombosis (Baskin *et al.*, 2009). The fibrin sheath does not usually affect catheter function; it can occur within 24 h after catheter placement and often develops within 2 weeks. Intraluminal clots usually cause catheter occlusion. Mural thrombosis is a blood clot that adheres to the vessel wall and can occlude the tip of the catheter but does not completely occlude the vein. A CRVT occludes the vein and is the most significant thrombotic complication. Its incidence is about 0.027 episodes/catheter/year (range 0.02–0.03) (Howard and Ashley, 2003).

CRVT can be symptomatic or asymptomatic. Symptomatic venous thrombosis may present clinically with pain, tenderness to palpation, oedema, warmth, erythema and the development of regional collateral vessels, usually along with catheter malfunction. The prevalence of asymptomatic vein thrombosis is unknown and probably it is underestimated. In some series it has been reported in up to 66% of adults and 50% of children with a central venous catheter for cancer treatment (Balestreri *et al.*, 1995; Luciani *et al.*, 2001). However, in a recent prospective study including 62 patients on HPN the incidence of venous thrombosis, using serial Doppler ultrasonography measurements, was much lower, 0.05 episodes/catheter/year (Cuerda *et al.*, 2012).

In a large series investigating use of central venous catheters in home infusion care including 50,470 patients, thrombotic catheter dysfunction was higher in PICCs (0.4 per 1000 catheter-days) than in tunnelled (0.06) and chest ports (0.06) ($P<0.01$) (Moureau *et al.*, 2002). In this study 44% of the episodes occurred in the first week after catheter placement.

The pathogenesis of CRVT is multifactorial and includes the following: (i) vessel injury during the procedure of insertion; (ii) venous stasis due to in-dwelling of the device and damage to the endothelium caused by infusion of PN with a high osmolality; and (iii) mechanical rubbing of the catheter against the vessel wall.

Venous thrombosis can develop soon after catheter insertion or be delayed in patients with long-term catheterization. The former cause is probably related to damage to the endothelium of the vein during the insertion and may be decreased by using ultrasound guidance (Pittiruti *et al.*, 2009). Other important factors are: (i) the proper selection of the vein (the right internal jugular vein is the preferred one due to its direct direction to the right atrium versus the left-sided catheters); (ii) the proper selection of the catheter (less thrombogenic material, lowest calibre and single-lumen); and (iii) the correct location of the tip of the catheter (in the lower third of the superior vena cava (SVC), at the atriocaval junction or in the upper portion of the right atrium) (Pittiruti *et al.*, 2009). The risk for thrombosis is also higher in patients with cancer, thrombotic diathesis, multiple catheterizations, catheter infection or treatment with chemotherapy (Kucher, 2011). PICCs

Table 20.1. Risk factors for venous thrombosis.

Catheter
Material (polyvinylchloride and polyethylene are more thrombogenic than silicone and polyurethane)
Number of lumens
Diameter of the catheter
Location of the tip of the catheter
Traumatic insertion (previous catheterizations)
Infection
Patient
Underlying disease (cancer)
Thrombotic diathesis
Previous thrombosis
HPN, chemotherapy, thoracic radiation
Immobilization

should not be inserted in paretic or immobilized arms since the risk of thrombosis is particularly high in these conditions (Pittiruti *et al.*, 2009). Table 20.1 summarizes the main risk factors for venous thrombosis.

Diagnosis

The diagnosis of venous thrombosis may be suspected in patients with certain symptoms (pain, swelling) and signs (oedema, collateral circulation) in the territory drained by the vein in which the catheter is located. Due to its low specificity (14%), the D-dimer test is not a useful method in screening for deep-vein thrombosis (DVT) of upper extremities (Kucher, 2011). The preferred method for screening is Doppler ultrasonography, which may be employed in both symptomatic and asymptomatic thrombosis as it is a non-invasive method with high sensitivity (97%) and specificity (96%) (Di Nisio *et al.*, 2010). The gold standard method for diagnosis is venography, but it is invasive and requires exposure to IV contrast agents and radiation. Computed tomography (CT) angiography or magnetic resonance angiography have recently been introduced, but data on their diagnostic accuracy are limited.

Complications

The main complications of venous thrombosis are infection, pulmonary thromboembolism and post-thrombotic syndrome (Baskin *et al.*, 2009; Kucher, 2011). The infection of the thrombus leads to a septic thrombophlebitis that is a serious complication requiring catheter removal. On the other hand, catheter infection facilitates the development of thrombosis due to adhesion of the components of the thrombus to the biofilm. Pulmonary thromboembolism is symptomatic in

4–14% of patients with venous thrombosis of the upper limbs and is asymptomatic in 15–36%, sometimes delayed months or years after catheter withdrawal. The post-thrombotic syndrome affects only 5% of patients with DVT of the upper limbs.

Prevention

To prevent venous thrombosis it is very important to minimize the damage to the vein wall during catheter insertion. The ESPEN guidelines recommend to use ultrasound-guided catheterization (grade C), to choose a catheter with the smallest calibre compatible with the infusion therapy (grade B) and to place the tip of the catheter at or near to the atriocaval junction (grade B), to decrease the risk of thrombotic complications (Pittiruti *et al.*, 2009). It is also important to prevent catheter infections in patients on HPN.

In the prevention of CRVT, several drugs have been used including heparin (in the catheter lock, inside the HPN bag or administered subcutaneously) and oral anticoagulation agents (vitamin K antagonists).

At least nine meta-analysis and systematic reviews have studied the use of thromboprophylaxis in patients with central vein catheters with different results, probably due to the heterogeneity of the studies as they included a variety of patients (HPN, cancer and other clinical settings), different types of central catheters (short- and long-term) and different preventive treatments (heparin, warfarin) (Randolph *et al.*, 1998; Klerk *et al.*, 2003; Cunningham *et al.*, 2006; Kirkpatrick *et al.*, 2007; Rawson and Newburn-Cook, 2007; Akl *et al.*, 2008, 2011; Chaukiyal *et al.*, 2008; Yacopetti, 2008).

It is also important to consider the benefits and risks of these treatments. Adverse effects of long-term heparin administration are common and include bleeding, thrombocytopenia, metabolic bone disease and loss of hair, as well as concerns about formation of precipitates with lipid components of the feed. Warfarin is associated with increased risk of bleeding (annual risk of 0.4–0.2% for non-intracranial and 0.1–0.9% for intracranial haemorrhage, depending on the INR (international normalized ratio) target range) (Hylek, 2003).

The ESPEN Home Artificial Nutrition group performed a survey reporting the experience of 12 centres, a total of 447 patients with a total of 110,896 HPN-days. The study showed that the use of heparin flushes was associated with more infections, removals and occlusions (Bozzetti *et al.*, 2002).

Based on analysis of the literature, different societies have made recommendations on the prevention of CRVT in people with long-term catheterization. Guidelines of the American Society for Parenteral and Enteral Nutrition (A.S.P.E.N.) recommend a low dose of anticoagulation in patients on long-term HPN (grade B) (A.S.P.E.N. Board of Directors and the Clinical Guidelines Task Force, 2002). ESPEN guidelines recommend prophylaxis with a daily subcutaneous low-molecular-weight heparin (LMWH) only in patients at high risk for thrombosis (cancer, chronic inflammatory disease or those with a family or personal past history of idiopathic venous thrombotic events) (grade C) (Pittiruti *et al.*,

2009). However, the American College of Chest Physicians' guidelines do not support routine prophylaxis with LMWH or vitamin K antagonists in outpatients with cancer and in-dwelling central catheters (grade 2b) (Kahn *et al.*, 2012).

In view of the differing guidelines, prospective studies in selected patients to balance the risk and benefits of thromboprophylaxis are warranted. While awaiting such data, the decision to start thromboprophylaxis should be made on an individual basis.

Treatment

The optimum management of CRVT is controversial as there are few prospective studies to rely on (Staun *et al.*, 20009). This implies that the grade of evidence-based recommendation is low for most of the decisions (grade C) (Kearon *et al.*, 2008).

CRVT is usually treated with anticoagulation, usually LMWH or oral anticoagulants. Initial anticoagulation treatment usually involves LMWH, followed by vitamin K antagonists, except in patients with cancer and patients with poor oral absorption, for whom LMWH is preferred. Compared with warfarin, the LMWHs exhibit a superior safety profile and a more predictable effect without the need for monitoring. The role of the new oral anticoagulants (dabigatran and rivaroxaban) in the treatment of CRVT in patients with intestinal failure may be promising as they need little monitoring (Van Ommen and Tabbers, 2010).

The algorithm of treatment is summarized in Fig. 20.1. The length of time a patient should receive treatment is individual (risk factors, extent and characteristics of the thrombus, catheter removal) but generally is 3–6 months and many centres will continue treatment for as long the patient has a central line (Kucher, 2011).

The decision to remove or leave the catheter *in situ* must be decided on a case-by-case basis (Pittiruti *et al.*, 2009). Moreover, there is a risk of embolization of the thrombus attached to the catheter during the removal. Removal is generally warranted when HPN is no longer necessary, if there is a line infection, if the line is occluded or if there is contraindication to anticoagulation treatment; removal is also necessary if there are persistent symptoms and signs despite anticoagulation (Kucher, 2011).

Thrombolytic agents are not usually employed in upper limb thrombosis, except in cases of massive thrombosis with severe symptoms and signs, if the bleeding risk is low and if the thrombus is recent (less than 10 days old).

In some cases it may be necessary to place an SVC filter if there is contraindication to anticoagulant treatment, if the thrombus progresses despite anticoagulation or if there is a symptomatic pulmonary thromboembolism despite anticoagulation. Catheter mechanical interventions (aspiration, fragmentation, thrombectomy, balloon angioplasty or stenting) or surgical procedures (thrombectomy, venoplasty, venous bypass or descompression at the venous thoracic outlet) will be indicated only in those patients with persistent symptoms and signs and failure of anticoagulation or thrombolysis (Kucher, 2011).

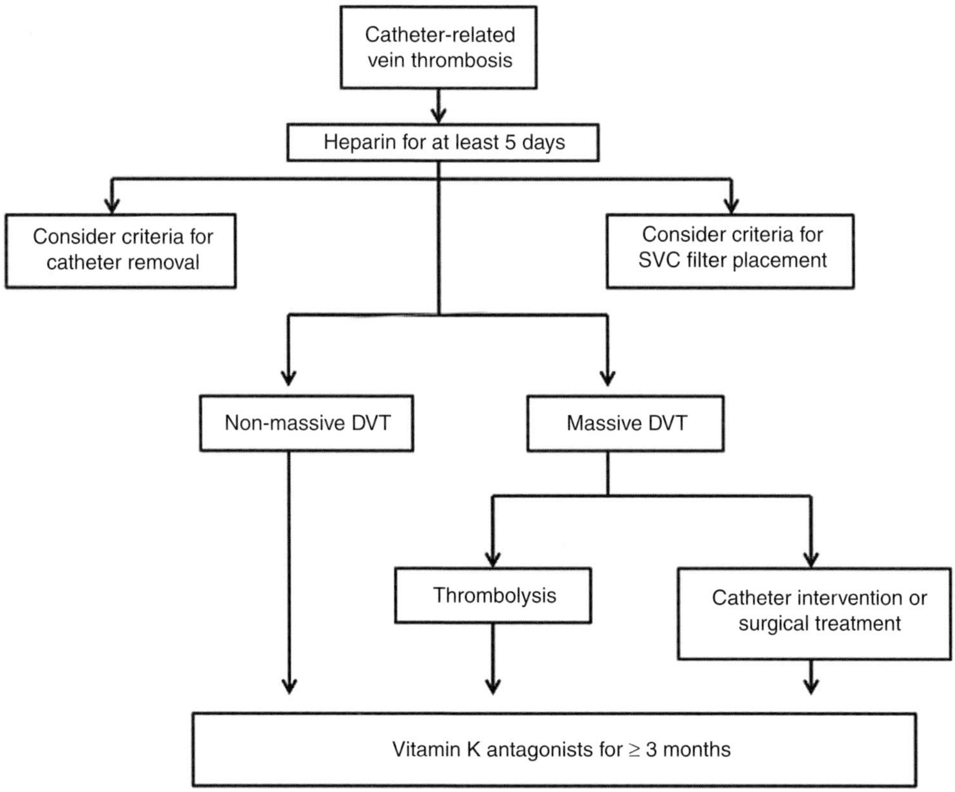

Fig. 20.1. Algorithm for treatment of CRVT.

Other Non-septic Catheter-related Complications

Other mechanical complications that cause dysfunctional catheters in patients on long-term HPN are the following: (i) a kinked catheter; (ii) a tight retaining suture; (iii) inadvertent clamping; and (iv) catheter pinch-off at the junction of the clavicle and the first rib (Grant, 2002).

The kinked catheter usually occurs at or near the exit site. It may be just under the skin, which can only be identified if the catheter is withdrawn a short distance.

If a suture used at the exit site (not recommended) is tied too tight around the catheter it may cause obstruction.

Catheters and infusion tubes frequently have slide or roller occlusion clamps and one of these may have been left closed, or partially closed, after use.

Catheter pinch-off occurs in catheters placed by the percutaneous subclavian vein approach. The result is an intermittent mechanical occlusion of the catheter for both aspiration and infusion of fluids that is relieved by rolling the shoulder or raising the arm of the ipsilateral side. The diagnosis is confirmed by obtaining a chest radiograph in which a narrowing can be observed of the catheter lumen as it passes between the clavicle and the first rib (Arenas-Márquez *et al.*, 2001). If the damage continues, the catheter can break and migrate, causing distal embolization.

In a prospective study of 1457 tunnelled silastic catheters placed by the percutaneous subclavian vein approach, pinch-off was identified in 16 patients (1.1%) by X-ray and in 15 of those patients clinically by positional obstruction. Fractured catheters occurred in three patients who presented with shoulder pain and swelling of the clavicular region (Andris *et al.*, 1994).

Catheter pinch-off can be avoided by inserting the catheter more laterally when using the percutaneous subclavian approach or by using a different access vein. When diagnosed, the catheter should be replaced before catheter fracture and distal migration of the catheter tip occur (Steiger, 2006).

Catheter damage is a common complication due to the use of a hard and long-term clamp, careless removal of the dressing or use of scissors close to the catheter. Although it is usually diagnosed by direct observation, sometimes the leak is very small and can be documented only by injecting saline into the catheter under pressure while the proximal catheter is clamped. In case of damage, the catheter should be clamped near the skin until ready to either repair or replace (Grant, 2002).

Erosion through the skin is a rare event that occurs mostly in emaciated patients with very little subcutaneous fat.

Catheter embolization is rare. The distal tip is usually lodged in the right atrium or right ventricle or embolized into the pulmonary artery and its branches. Embolism can occur during the insertion, as the result of cutting of the catheter during dressing changes or breakage at a weakened or damaged area. The distal tip should be removed because of the risk of arrhythmias and infection. The preferred technique for removal of an embolized catheter is transfemoral IV snaring of the fragment under fluoroscopic guidance by vascular radiology. When the fragment is lodged in the distal pulmonary arterioles, a thoracotomy may be necessary (Grant, 2002).

Loss of Vascular Access

Patients maintained on HPN for many years may encounter repeated line complications with thrombosis and loss of vascular access may eventually be the result. The upper body venous access sites usually will be occluded first. Attempts to recanalize can be done with endovascular intervention. If unsuccessful the femoral veins may be accessed, but it must be kept in mind that the rate of complications with this route generally is significantly higher.

In difficult-access situations, upper extremity venography, ultrasound examination or magnetic resonance venography may be helpful in the assessment of potential alternative venous access routes. Such routes may involve the inferior vena cava, hepatic vein, translumbar vein, azygous vein, other large collateral veins or even direct right atrial catheterization (Sands, 2006). The use of an external arteriovenous graft for IV nutritional support may also be an unconventional option (Versleijen *et al.*, 2009). With the advancement in the results of intestinal transplantation the clinician should consider this option, at the latest when one vascular access route remains open, since this is what the patient will need for the nutritional and intensive care support if a transplant is performed.

Summary

Non-septic catheter-related complications may lead to catheter replacement and loss of venous access in patients on HPN. The most important are catheter occlusions and CRVT. Catheter thrombosis is the most frequent cause of catheter occlusion, although it can be also due to HPN formula components, such as lipids and calcium phosphate precipitates. Adequate flushing with saline after the infusion of PN is completed can prevent catheter occlusion, and there is no evidence that flushing with heparin or other interventions (pressure caps, heparin-bonded catheters) prevent catheter occlusion. Fibrinolytic agents (urokinase, alteplase) are effective in treating catheters occluded by a thrombus.

Venous thrombosis can develop soon after catheter insertion or be delayed in patients with long-term catheterization. The preferred method for screening is Doppler ultrasonography, but the gold standard method for diagnosis is venography or CT. The main complications of venous thrombosis are infection, pulmonary thromboembolism and post-thrombotic syndrome. To prevent venous thrombosis it is very important to minimize the damage to the vein wall during catheter insertion with the use ultrasound guidance, to choose a catheter with the smallest calibre compatible with the infusion therapy and to place the tip of the catheter at or near to the atriocaval junction. The decision to start thromboprophylaxis with warfarin or LMWH in people on HPN should be decided on an individual basis. CRVT is usually treated with anticoagulation, usually LMWH or oral anticoagulants for 3–6 months, and in some cases it can continue for as long as the patient has a central line. The decision to remove or leave the catheter *in situ* must be made from case to case.

References

Abu-Elmagd, K.M. (2006) Intestinal transplantation for short bowel syndrome and gastrointestinal failure: current consensus, rewarding outcomes, and practical guidelines. *Gastroenterology* 130, 132–137.

Akl, E.A., Kamath, G., Yosuico, V., Young Kim, S., Barba, M., Sperati, F., Cook, D.J. and Schünemann, H.J. (2008) Thromboprophylaxis for patients with cancer and central venous catheters: a systematic review and meta-analysis. *Cancer* 112, 2483–2492.

Akl, E., Vasireddi, S., Gunukula, S., Yosuico, V.E., Barba, M., Sperati, F., Cook, D. and Schünemann, H. (2011) Anticoagulation for cancer patients with central venous catheters. *Cochrane Database of Systematic Reviews* issue 2, CD006468, doi: 10.1002/14651858.CD006468.pub3.

Andris, D.A., Krzywda, E.A., Schulte, W., Ausman, R. and Quebbeman, E.J. (1994) Pinch-off syndrome: a rare aetiology for central venous catheter occlusion. *JPEN Journal of Parenteral and Enteral Nutrition* 18, 531–533.

Arenas-Márquez, H., Anaya-Prado, R., Barrera-Zepeda, L.M. and González-Ojeda, A. (2001) Complications of central venous catheters. *Current Opinion in Clinical Nutrition and Metabolic Care* 4, 207–210.

A.S.P.E.N. Board of Directors and the Clinical Guidelines Task Force (2002) Guidelines for the use of parenteral and enteral nutrition in adult and pediatric patients. *JPEN Journal of Parenteral and Enteral Nutrition* 26(1 Suppl.), 1SA–138SA.

Balestreri L., De Cicco, M., Matovic, M., Coran, F. and Morassut, S. (1995) Central venous catheter-related thrombosis in clinically asymptomatic oncologic patients: a phlebographic study. *European Journal of Radiology* 20, 108–111.

Baskin, J.L., Poi, C.H., Reiss, U., Wilimas, J.A., Metzger, M.L., Ribeiro, R.C. and Howard, S.C. (2009) Management of occlusion and thrombosis associated with long-term indwelling central venous catheters. *The Lancet* 374, 159–169.

Bozzetti, F., Mariani, L., Bertinet, D.B., Chiavenna, G., Crose, N., De Cicco, M., Gigli, G., Micklewright, A., Moreno-Villares, J.M., Orban, A., Pertkiewicz, M., Pironi, L., Vilas, M.P., Prins, F. and Thul, P. (2002) Central venous catheter complications in 447 patients on home parenteral nutrition: an analysis of over 100,000 catheter days. *Clinical Nutrition* 21, 475–485.

Chaukiyal, P., Nautiyal, A., Radhakrishnan, S., Singh, S. and Navaneethan, S.D. (2008) Thromboprophylaxis in cancer patients with central venous catheters: a systematic review and meta-analysis. *Journal of Thrombosis and Haemostasis* 99, 38–43.

Cuerda, C., Joly, F., Puiggrós, C., Gil, C., Pironi, L. and HAN-CIF ESPEN Group (2012) Prospective study on the incidence of central vein thrombosis in patients on home parenteral nutrition: preliminary results. *Clinical Nutrition* 7(Suppl. 1), 71–72.

Cunningham, M.S., White, B., Hollywood, D. and O'Donnell, J. (2006) Primary thromboprophylaxis for cancer patients with central venous catheters – a reappraisal of the evidence. *British Journal of Cancer* 94, 189–194.

Di Nisio, M., Van Sluis, G.L., Bossuyt, P.M., Buller, H.R., Porreca, E. and Rutjes, A.W. (2010) Accuracy of diagnostic tests for clinically suspected upper extremity deep vein thrombosis: a systematic review. *Journal of Thrombosis and Haemostasis* 8, 684–692.

Grant, J. (2002) Recognition, prevention, and treatment of home parenteral nutrition central venous access complications. *JPEN Journal of Parenteral and Enteral Nutrition* 26, 21–28.

Howard, L. and Ashley, C. (2003) Management of complications in patients receiving home parenteral nutrition. *Gastroenterology* 124, 1651–1661.

Hylek, E.M. (2003) Complications of oral anticoagulant therapy: bleeding and nonbleeding, rates and risk factors. *Seminars in Vascular Medicine* 3, 271–278.

Kahn, S.R., Lim, W., Dunn, A.S., Cushman, M., Dentali, F., Akl, E.A., Cook, D.J., Balekian, A.A., Klein, R.C., Le, H., Schulman, S. and Murad, M.H.; American College of Chest Physicians (2012) Prevention of VTE in nonsurgical patients: Antithrombotic Therapy and Prevention of Thrombosis, 9th ed: American College of Chest Physicians Evidence-Based Clinical Practice Guidelines. *Chest* 141, e195S–e226S.

Kearon, C., Kahn, S.R., Agnelli, G., Goldhaber, S., Raskob, G.E. and Comerota, A.J.; American College of Chest Physicians (2008) Antithrombotic therapy for venous thromboembolic disease: American College of Chest Physicians Evidence-Based Clinical Practice Guidelines (8th Edition). *Chest* 133, 454–545.

Kirkpatrick, A., Rathbun, S., Whitsett, T. and Raskob, G. (2007) Prevention of central venous catheter-associated thrombosis: a meta-analysis. *American Journal of Medicine* 120, 901–910.

Klerk, C.P.W., Smorenburg, S.M. and Büller, H.R. (2003) Thrombosis prophylaxis in patient populations with a central venous catheter: a systematic review. *Archives of Internal Medicine* 163, 1913–1921.

Kucher, N. (2011) Deep-vein thrombosis of the upper extremities. *New England Journal of Medicine* 364, 861–869.
Luciani, A., Clement, O., Halimi, P., Goudot, D., Portier, F., Bassot, V., Luciani, J.A., Avan, P., Frija, G. and Bonfils, P. (2001) Catheter-related upper extremity deep venous thrombosis in cancer patients: a prospective study based on Doppler US. *Radiology* 220, 655–660.
Mitchell, M.D., Anderson, B.J., Williams, K. and Umscheid, C.A. (2009) Heparin flushing and other interventions to maintain patency of central venous catheters: a systematic review. *Journal of Advanced Nursing* 65, 2007–2021.
Moureau, N., Poole, S., Murdock, M.A., Gray, S.M. and Semba, C.P. (2002) Central venous catheters in home infusion care: outcomes analysis in 50,470 patients. *Journal of Vascular Intervention Radiology* 13, 1009–1016.
Pittiruti, M., Hamilton, H., Biffi, R., MacFie, J. and Pertkiewicz, M. (2009) ESPEN guidelines on parenteral nutrition: central venous catheters (access, care, diagnosis and therapy of complications). *Clinical Nutrition* 28, 365–377.
Ponec, D., Irwin, D., Haire, W.D., Hill, P.A., Li, X., McCluskey, E.R. and COOL Investigators (2001) Recombinant tissue plasminogen activator (alteplase) for restoration of flow in occluded central venous access devices: a double-blind placebo-controlled trial – the Cardiovascular Thrombolytic to Open Occluded Lines (COOL) efficacy trial. *Journal of Vascular Intervention Radiology* 12, 951–955.
Randolph, A.G., Cook, D.J., Gonzales, C.A. and Andrew, M. (1998) Benefit of heparin in central venous and pulmonary artery catheters: a meta-analysis of randomized controlled trials. *Chest* 113, 165–171.
Rawson, K.M and Newburn-Cook, C.V. (2007) The use of low-dose warfarin as prophylaxis for central venous catheter thrombosis in patients with cancer: a meta-analysis. *Oncology Nursing Forum* 34, 1037–1043.
Sands, M.J. (2006) Vascular access in the adult home infusion patient. *JPEN Journal of Parenteral and Enteral Nutrition* 30, 57–64.
Staun, M., Pironi, L., Bozzetti, F., Baxter, J., Forbes, A., Joly, F., Jeppesen, P., Moreno, J., Hébuterne, X., Pertkiewicz, M., Mühlebach, S., Shenkin, A. and Van Gossum, A. (2009) ESPEN guidelines on parenteral nutrition: home parenteral nutrition (HPN) in adult patients. *Clinical Nutrition* 28, 467–479.
Steiger, E. (2006) Dysfunction and thrombotic complications of vascular access devices. *JPEN Journal of Parenteral and Enteral Nutrition* 30, 70–72.
van Miert, C., Hill, R. and Jones, L. (2012) Interventions for restoring patency of occluded central venous catheter lumens. *Cochrane Database of Systematic Reviews* issue 4, CD007119, doi: 10.1002/14651858.CD007119.pub2.
Van Ommen, C.H. and Tabbers, M.H. (2010) Catheter-related thrombosis in children with intestinal failure and long-term parenteral nutrition: how to treat and to prevent? *Thrombosis Research* 126, 465–470.
Versleijen, M.W., Huisman-de Waal, G.J., Kock, M.C., Elferink, A.J., van Rossum, L.G., Feuth, T., Willems, M.C., Jansen, J.B. and Wanten, G.J. (2009) Arteriovenous fistulae as an alternative to central venous catheters for delivery of long-term home parenteral nutrition. *Gastroenterology* 136, 1577–1584.
Yacopetti, N. (2008) Central venous catheter-related thrombosis: a systematic review. *Journal of Infusion Nursing* 31, 241–248.

IV Practical Issues

21 Adult Fluid and Nutritional Requirements for Home Parenteral Nutrition

Beth Rye* and Jeremy Nightingale

St Mark's Hospital, Harrow, UK

Key Points

- When HPN is considered there need to be clear objectives/targets to be achieved and criteria for stopping.
- Patients having HPN usually eat, so absorb a proportion of the macronutrients, vitamins and trace elements consumed.
- The HPN prescription can be predicted by knowledge of the patient's remaining gut anatomy and underlying disease(s). Fistula/stomal losses need to be taken into account.
- The estimated energy given commonly falls between 25 and 35 kcal/kg/day before oral/enteral intake is accounted for.
- If abnormal LFTs occur, consideration should be given to reducing the parenteral lipid.
- PN bags should contain vitamins and trace elements.
- An aim of a PN regimen is to give patients 24-h periods without having PN (usually as 'nights off').

Introduction

Home parenteral nutrition (HPN) is needed for patients with acute or chronic intestinal failure in whom nutritional and/or water and electrolyte balance cannot be corrected by oral or enteral feeding and in whom parenteral nutrition (PN) is feasible at home (Messing *et al.*, 2001). The nutritional and fluid requirements

*E-mail: bethrye@nhs.net

for patients needing HPN are very variable, largely because these patients continue to eat and absorb some nutrition from their gastrointestinal tract. In addition, they may have large fluid losses from one or more stomas or fistulas. It is relatively unusual for patients to depend totally upon PN for their nutritional requirements unless they have bowel obstruction, a gastric/duodenal stoma/fistula or severe dysmotility. HPN when begun needs to have clear objectives (e.g. treat dehydration/undernutrition, reduce diarrhoea, fit for surgery, etc.) and criteria for stopping (e.g. oral intake resumed, surgical resolution, unethical, etc.). The patients are managed by a multidisciplinary nutrition support team consisting at least of a clinician, dietician, specialist nurse and pharmacist (Nightingale, 2010).

Due mainly to the variability in absorption, gastrointestinal losses and patient activity, the initial requirements are a best estimate and with careful monitoring they are adjusted according to the patient's state of hydration and target weight. The final HPN prescription will depend not only upon nutritional/fluid requirements, but upon patient preferences.

This chapter shows how patients are stabilized, established on a regimen and how this is adjusted with time. The aim of HPN is to give the patient as near a normal life as possible with as few hours as possible connected to a feed.

Initial Stabilization in Hospital

Anatomical considerations

If the gut is short (includes an enterocutaneous fistula that drains all gut contents) but has normal function, then the long-term type of nutritional/fluid support can be predicted (Table 21.1) from knowledge of the small intestinal length in circuit and the presence or absence of a colon in continuity. With time (up to 3 years) patients with a colon in continuity are likely to have a degree of anatomical (villus hypertrophy) and functional adaptation (slowing transit and improvement in some biochemical pathways), so that less parenteral support is needed. This is not the case for patients with a jejunostomy, whose nutritional/fluid requirements change little with time (Nightingale *et al.*, 1992).

Table 21.1. Small bowel length and route of long-term nutrition/fluid. (From Gouttebel *et al.*, 1986; Nightingale *et al.*, 1992; Messing *et al.*, 1999.)

	Jejunostomy		Jejunum–colon
Jejunum (cm)	Nutrition	Fluid	Nutrition
0–50	Parenteral	Saline	Parenteral
51–100	Parenteral[a]	Saline	Oral/enteral
101–150	Oral/enteral	OGS	None
151–200	None	OGS	None

OGS, oral (or enteral) glucose/saline solution.
[a]At 85–100 cm may need parenteral saline only.

Establishing a regimen

PN requirements are based upon a careful assessment (Table 21.2) which, if the patient is eating, will involve an estimate of how much total fluid/nutrition is being absorbed and lost in secretions.

While the initial regimen will be relatively standardized for the hospital, the prescription at home will be designed around the patient's wishes/preferences (e.g. nights off feed, duration/timing of feed, frequency of lipid, desired weight, frequency of deliveries, etc.).

Adult Requirements for Water and Electrolytes

Baseline water and electrolyte requirements are calculated (Tables 21.3 and 21.4) and to this is added an estimate of intestinal losses (Table 21.5). The losses will vary as medical and dietary therapy is maximized (e.g. for high-output jejunostomy: restricting oral hypotonic fluid restriction, sipping an oral glucose/saline solution and taking anti-diarrhoeal and anti-secretory drugs).

Standard prescribing ranges that assume normal organ function and no intestinal losses are used to estimate electrolyte requirements (Table 21.4). Depending on the clinical situation and intestinal anatomy, additional sodium,

Table 21.2. Assessment prior to starting PN.

Underlying illness and co-morbidities
Gastrointestinal anatomy (e.g. length of small bowel, fistula(s), etc.)
Fluid status (e.g. gut losses, oral/intravenous intake, urine output, etc.)
Nutritional status (BMI, percentage weight loss, mid-arm muscle circumference)
Current oral/enteral intake
Outcome targets

Table 21.3. Estimation of fluid (water) requirements before gastrointestinal losses are taken into account. (From Tyler, 1989.)

18–60 years old	35 ml/kg body weight
>60 years old	30 ml/kg body weight
Pyrexia	Add 2–2.5 ml/kg body weight for each °C body temperature is above 37°C

Table 21.4. Estimation of electrolyte requirements before gastrointestinal losses are taken into account. (From Micklewright and Todorovic, 1997.)

Sodium	1–1.5 mmol/kg body weight
Potassium	1–1.5 mmol/kg body weight
Magnesium	0.1–0.2 mmol/kg body weight
Calcium	0.1–0.15 mmol/kg body weight
Phosphate	0.5–0.7 mmol/kg body weight or 10 mmol/1000 kcal
Chloride	1–1.5 mmol/kg body weight

potassium and magnesium may be required. Table 21.5 gives some indication of the amount of sodium/potassium lost in different gastrointestinal secretions.

Adult Nutritional Requirements

Energy

Predictive equations can be used to estimate basal metabolic rate (BMR), such as those of Harris and Benedict (1919), Schofield (1985) and currently Henry (2005) (Table 21.6). A physical activity level (Table 21.7) and stress factor if appropriate are added to the BMR to give the total energy requirement. Additional energy (400–1000 kcal) can be added if weight gain is needed.

Care should be taken not to provide excess energy as occurred in the 1970s and 1980s and resulted in hyperglycaemia, liver function test abnormalities and high rates of infection.

The estimated amount of energy commonly falls within the range 20–35 kcal/kg body weight/day (A.S.P.E.N. Board of Directors and the Clinical Guidelines

Table 21.5. Approximate daily volume and composition of intestinal secretions produced in response to food.

	Volume (l)	pH	Na^+ (mmol/l)	K^+ (mmol/l)	Cl^- (mmol/l)	HCO_3^- (mmol/l)	Mg^{2+} (mmol/l)	Ca^{2+} (mmol/l)
Saliva	0.5	7	45	20	44	60	0.7	1.3
Gastric juice	2.0	2	10	10	130	0	0.5	2.0
Pancreatic juice	0.6	8	140	10	30	110	0.2	0.3
Hepatic bile	0.9	7	145	5	100	28	0.6	2.5
Small bowel secretion	1.8[a]	7	138	6	141	<5	<0.1	2.5
Serum		7.4	140	4	100	24	1.0	2.4
Jejunostomy fluid		6.0	100	15	–	–	4.2	16.1

[a]This fluid is released and absorbed on the mucosa and rarely needs to be taken into account in calculating fluid losses; estimates of its electrolyte composition are unreliable.

Table 21.6. Equations for estimating BMR from gender, age and weight (*W*). (From Henry, 2005.)

Gender	Age (years)	BMR (kcal/day)
Male	18–30	16.0 *W*+545
	30–60	14.2 *W*+593
	60–70	13.0 *W*+567
	70+	13.7 *W*+481
Female	18–30	13.1 *W*+558
	30–60	9.74 *W*+694
	60–70	10.2 *W*+572
	70+	10.0 *W*+577

Task Force, 2002; NICE, 2006; Staun *et al.*, 2009), and only rarely more than 40 kcal/kg body weight/day (Koea *et al.*, 1995). Oral and enteral intake is taken into account with an estimate of a malabsorption factor. In patients with a short bowel and jejunostomy at 100 cm from the duodenojejunal flexure, approximately 40% of the oral diet is absorbed and at 50 cm only 20% (Nightingale *et al.*, 1990).

Energy and protein requirements in obesity (body mass index (BMI) > 30 kg/m^2) are adjusted to avoid overfeeding (Table 21.8). Regular anthropometry in this patient group is used to monitor changes in body composition, in particular preventing rapid muscle loss.

Nitrogen

Large nitrogen losses are documented in sepsis, major trauma and burns. An unstressed patient with normal organ function will require 0.14–0.2 g nitrogen/kg body weight/day (Elia, 1990). If a patient has a low muscle mass and requires more nitrogen, 0.3–0.6 g nitrogen/kg body weight/day may be used (Keys *et al.*, 1950).

It has been customary in some countries, including the UK, not to include nitrogen energy (usually 200–300 kcal) in the quoted total energy in a regimen (unlike with enteral nutrition, where the total energy quote includes the nitrogen energy).

Table 21.7. Guidelines for estimating energy and protein requirements in the unstressed/clinically stable patient. (From A.S.P.E.N. Board of Directors and the Clinical Guidelines Task Force, 2002; NICE, 2006.)

Energy	Protein
25–35 kcal/kg body weight/day	0.8–2 g protein/kg body weight/day
Obese patients	*Obese patients*
BMI > 30 kg/m^2 who are not metabolically stressed: calculate energy requirements as normal and subtract 400–1000 kcal/day for a decrease in energy stores	BMI > 30 kg/m^2: use 75% of the value estimated from actual weight BMI > 50 kg/m^2: use 65% of the value estimated from actual weight

Table 21.8. Calculated physical activity level (PAL) of adults; BMR is multiplied by PAL give total energy requirements. (From Department of Health, 1991.)

	Occupational activity					
	Light		Moderate		Moderate/heavy	
Non-occupational activity	Males	Females	Males	Females	Males	Females
Non-active	1.4	1.4	1.6	1.5	1.7	1.5
Moderately active	1.5	1.5	1.7	1.6	1.8	1.6
Very active	1.6	1.6	1.8	1.7	1.9	1.7

Energy sources

Carbohydrate

Carbohydrate and lipid are the main energy sources in PN. Glucose requirements can be set at 3–6 g/kg body weight/day (Staun *et al.*, 2009); being aware that excess glucose provision can cause problems, particularly hyperglycaemia or abnormal liver function tests. Glucose oxidation rate can be calculated (4–7 mg × kg body weight × 60 × 24/1000 × 4) to give an indication of the maximum amount of glucose that can be utilized. However, it is possible to exceed these requirements in malnourished patients requiring weight gain. While the ratio of glucose to lipid may be 50:50 (or 60:40) at first, this is reduced within the first month to be approximately 70–85% from glucose and 15–30% from lipid for long-term HPN (Staun *et al.*, 2009).

Lipid

Most patients are provided with some lipid, in particular in those patients with little enteral intake. Long-term intravenous lipid provision is kept below 1 g/kg body weight/day (500 ml of Intralipid® provides 550 kcal and usually in long-term HPN fewer than three of these are given per week), as above this chronic cholestasis is common (Cavicchi *et al.*, 2000). A 20% soy-based lipid emulsion given weekly is adequate to prevent essential fatty acid deficiency; if a patient is having no lipid and has a dry skin, he/she can apply 10 ml sunflower or safflower oil to the skin daily (Press *et al.*, 1974; Miller *et al.*, 1987).

If a central line catheter tip becomes high (in the superior vena cava or brachiocephalic vein) and replacement is not an immediate option, the feed may be adjusted to have a much lower osmolality (to reduce the risk of venous thrombosis) by relying on a high lipid, low glucose content.

Micronutrients

Vitamins and trace elements are included in the HPN prescriptions (Tables 21.9 and 21.10), especially if the patient has no enteral nutrition or poor gastrointestinal absorption. The commercial preparations used in PN generally provide amounts in excess of basal requirements as they are intended for patients who are nutritionally depleted. Depending on nutritional status and enteral absorption, these preparations can be given daily or on alternate days.

Additional iron, vitamin D and selenium supplementation may be needed in addition to PN if serum levels remain low.

Adjustment of Regimen during Hospital Stay and the Final Prescription for HPN

Often during the hospital stabilization period sepsis is treated and a stoma/fistula output becomes more established, as does the patient's oral intake. Fluid balance usually dominates the clinical picture and a stable regimen with regard to water,

Table 21.9. Daily requirements and sources for parenteral micronutrients. (From American Medical Association, 1979a.)

Trace element	Daily requirement (μmol)	Additrace® (μmol/10 ml)	Decan® (μmol/40 ml)
Zinc	38–100	100	153
Copper	8–24	20	7.5
Selenium	0.4	0.4	0.9
Iron	20	20	18
Manganese	3–15	5	3.6
Chromium	0.2–0.3	0.2	0.3
Molybdenum	0.2	0.2	0.26
Cobalt	–	–	0.025
Iodine	1.0	1.0	0.01
Fluoride	50	50	76

Table 21.10. Daily requirements and sources for parenteral vitamins. (From American Medical Association, 1979b.)

	Daily requirement (μg)	Vitlipid Adult® (μg)	Cernevit® (μg)
Fat-soluble vitamins			
Vitamin A	1000	990	1000
Vitamin E	10	9.1	10.2
Vitamin K	150	150	–
Vitamin D	5	5	5
Water-soluble vitamins			
Vitamin B_1	3.0	3.1	3.5
Vitamin B_2	3.6	4.9	4.1
Vitamin B_6	4.0	4.9	5.5
Niacin	40	40	46
Folic acid	400	400	414
Vitamin B_{12}	5.0	5.0	6.0
Biotin	60	60	69
Vitamin C	100	11	125

sodium and magnesium is gradually established. Fluid balance, weight, clinical symptoms/signs of dehydration (thirst/dry mouth)/overhydration (oedema, raised jugular venous pressure) are assessed daily and blood tests (renal and liver function) done as needed (usually two or more times per week). A urine output greater than 1 l/24 h with random urine sodium level of 20 mmol/l or more is desirable. The energy given depends upon the oral intake, the estimated absorption (which can be better predicted if the bowel length has been measured either at surgery or more commonly radiologically) (Nightingale *et al.*, 1991), blood glucose and weight/muscle mass (which should increase in hospital).

The HPN prescription is formulated towards the end of the patient's hospital admission when he/she is medically stable and consuming a similar amount of food and drink each day. Depending upon his/her nutritional and fluid status, the patient is reviewed in an outpatient clinic 1–8 weeks after discharge and subsequently every 3–6 months.

Monitoring and Adjusting the HPN Prescription in Outpatients

During the multidisciplinary clinic visit a brief clinical examination assessing hydration (postural blood pressure), nutritional status and underlying condition is performed. Weight, mid-arm muscle circumference and triceps skinfold thickness are measured so that BMI and mid-arm muscle mass can be calculated, and a diet history is collected. Blood tests include renal and liver function, minerals (especially magnesium), trace elements and vitamins (mainly fat-soluble ones) (NICE, 2006), and a random urine sample is collected for sodium concentration.

Over time, intestinal adaptation in patients with a retained colon may reduce the parenteral requirement for energy and nitrogen. In addition, it is common for a patient's oral intake to improve at home and this may result less PN being needed.

Special Factors with HPN that May Result in Adjusting the Feeding Regimen

Poor sleep

Patients are often kept awake at night by the pump noise and/or its bright lights and they may get up two or three times during the night to pass urine. These problems can be reduced by having nights free from feed, keeping the feed volume as low as possible to maintain hydration and running the feed through as fast as is safe.

One of the main aims is to give the feed on as few nights as possible. This can usually be done easily in patients with a colon in continuity, but not in patients with a jejunostomy who rapidly become salt and water depleted and need fluid daily.

Some patients prefer to feed during the day and may have a backpack containing a pump and the feeding bag.

Cramps

Many complain of cramps during the feed (Elphick *et al.*, 2009). This may be due to a feed with low sodium concentration that is given quickly or due to sodium depletion. In the long term these can be corrected by increasing the sodium content in the feed, but in the short term immediate relief can be obtained by taking oral table salt. Magnesium depletion may be a contributing factor.

Thirst

While thirst is most commonly due to water and sodium depletion, it can also be due to high concentrations of sodium in the feed. A low random urinary sodium concentration gives an indication of this cause.

Faint/nausea when feed stops

This can be due to reactive hypoglycaemia and may be avoided if the feed is slowed gradually over the last hour of feeding.

Unwell after feeds containing lipid

Many patients complain of malaise, joint pains and/or nausea after a lipid feed; lipid can be given less frequently (e.g. once weekly) or occasionally it is omitted altogether. Sometimes a different lipid preparation helps.

Frequent feeding bag deliveries (feed bag stability)

If a bag has good stability it may be delivered every two or more weeks, if not it may be weekly. Stability is more likely to be a problem if lipid is in the feed or if the feed is of a very large volume (e.g. 4 l or more).

Summary

Most patients should have a good quality of life on HPN with minimal sleep disruption, a stable bag with adequate nutrients, vitamins and trace elements and, if possible, one to four nights off the feed per week. HPN requirements may change over time and careful assessments/monitoring should predict/pick these up. Some patients may achieve the goals set at the start of HPN and so be able to stop HPN. An HPN regimen needs to combine the fluid/nutrition necessary with patients' wishes so that they can have a good quality of life.

References

American Medical Association, Department for Foods and Nutrition (1979a) Guidelines for essential trace element preparations for parenteral use – a statement by an expert panel. *Journal of the American Medical Association* 241, 2051–2054.

American Medical Association, Department for Foods and Nutrition (1979b) Multivitamin preparations for parenteral use – a statement by the Nutrition Advisory Group. *JPEN Journal of Parenteral and Enteral Nutrition* 3, 258–262.

A.S.P.E.N. Board of Directors and the Clinical Guidelines Task Force (2002) Guidelines for the use of parenteral and enteral nutrition in adult and pediatric patients. *JPEN Journal of Parenteral and Enteral Nutrition* 26(Suppl. 1), 1SA–138SA.

Cavicchi, M., Beau, P., Crenn, P., Degott, C. and Messing, B. (2000) Prevalence of liver disease and contributing factors in patients receiving home parenteral nutrition for permanent intestinal failure. *Annals of Internal Medicine* 132, 525–532.

Department of Health (1991) *Dietary Reference Values for Food Energy and Nutrients for the UK.* HMSO, London.

Elia, M. (1990) Artificial nutritional support. *Medicine International* 82, 3392–3396.

Elphick, D.A., Baker, M., Baxter, J.P., Nightingale, J.M., Bowling, T., Page, K.B. and McAlindon, M.E. (2009) Muscle cramps are the commonest side effect of home parenteral nutrition. *Clinical Nutrition* 28, 351–354.

Gouttebel, M.C., Saint-Aubert, B., Astre, C. and Joyeux, H. (1986) Total parenteral nutrition needs in different types of short bowel syndrome. *Digestive Diseases and Sciences* 31, 718–723.

Harris, J.A. and Benedict, F.G. (1919) *A Biometric Study of Basal Metabolism in Man. Carnegie Institute Publication No. 279.* Carnegie Institute, Washington, DC.

Henry, C.J.K. (2005) Basal metabolic rate studies in humans: measurement and development of new equations. *Public Health Nutrition* 8, 1133–1152.

Keys, A., Brozek, J. and Henschel, A. (1950) *The Biology of Human Starvation.* University of Minnesota Press, Minneapolis, Minnesota.

Koea, J.B., Wolfe, R.R. and Shaw, J.H. (1995) Total energy expenditure during total parenteral nutrition: ambulatory patients at home versus patients with sepsis in surgical intensive care. *Surgery* 118, 54–62.

Messing, B., Crenn, P., Beau, P., Boutron-Ruault, M.C., Rambaud, J.C. and Matuchansky, C. (1999) Long-term survival and parenteral nutrition dependence in adult patients with the short bowel syndrome. *Gastroenterology* 117, 1043–1050.

Messing, B., Hebuterne, X. and Nightingale, J. (2001) Home enteral and parenteral nutrition in adults. In: Nightingale, J.M.D. (ed.) *Intestinal Failure.* Greenwich Medical Media Limited, London, pp. 407–430.

Micklewright, A. and Todorovic, V. (1997) *A Pocket Guide to Clinical Nutrition.* British Dietetic Association, London.

Miller, D., Williams, S., Palombo, J., Griffin, R., Bistrian, B. and Blackburn, G. (1987) Cutaneous application of safflower oil in preventing essential fatty acid deficiency in patients on home parenteral nutrition. *American Journal of Clinical Nutrition* 46, 419–423.

NICE (2006) *Nutrition Support for Adults: Oral Nutrition Support, Enteral Tube Feeding and Parenteral Nutrition. NICE Clinical Guideline No. 32.* National Institute for Health and Clinical Excellence, London.

Nightingale, J.M.D. (2010) Nutrition support teams: how they work, are set up and maintained. *Frontline Gastroenterology* 1, 171–177.

Nightingale, J.M.D., Lennard-Jones, J.E., Walker, E.R. and Farthing, M.G. (1990) Jejunal efflux in short bowel syndrome. *The Lancet* 336, 765–768.

Nightingale, J.M.D., Bartram, C.I. and Lennard-Jones, J.E. (1991) Length of residual small bowel after partial resection: correlation between radiographic and surgical measurements. *Gastrointestinal Radiology* 16, 305–306.

Nightingale, J.M.D., Lennard-Jones, J.E., Gertner, D.J., Wood, S.R. and Bartram, C.I. (1992) Colonic preservation reduces the need for parenteral therapy, increases the incidence of renal stones but does not change the high prevalence of gallstones in patients with a short bowel. *Gut* 33, 1493–1497.

Press, M., Hartop, P.J. and Prottey, C. (1974) Correction of essential fatty-acid deficiency in man by cutaneous application of sunflower-seed oil. *The Lancet* ii, 597–599.

Schofield, W.N. (1985) Predicting basal metabolic rate, new standards and review of previous work. *Human Nutrition, Clinical Nutrition* 39C(Suppl. 1), 5–41.

Staun, M., Pironi, L., Bozzetti, F., Baxter, J., Forbes, A., Joly, F., Jeppesen, P., Moreno, J., Hébuterne, X., Pertkiewicz, M., Mühlebach, S., Shenkin, A. and Van Gossum, A. (2009) ESPEN guidelines on parenteral nutrition: home parenteral nutrition (HPN) in adult patients. *Clinical Nutrition* 28, 467–479.

Tyler, D.S. (1989) Fluid and electrolytes. In: Lyerly, H.K. (ed.) *The Handbook of Surgical Intensive Care*, 2nd edn. Year Book Medical Publishers, Inc., Chicago, Illinois, pp. 223–250.

22 Carbohydrates

LUC TAPPY*

Department of Physiology, University of Lausanne and Division of Endocrinology, Diabetes and Metabolism, Lausanne University Hospital, Lausanne, Switzerland

Key Points

- Carbohydrates are present in our everyday diet as starch and disaccharides, and to a small extent as free hexoses. Only glucose can be used as an energy substrate during total parenteral nutrition (TPN) because there is no active disaccharidase enzyme outside the gut in humans.
- It is currently recommended that carbohydrates should account for about 55% of daily energy consumption; sugars (i.e. sucrose, glucose/fructose mixtures) should represent less than 10% of total energy intake according to the Food and Agriculture Organization/World Health Organization.
- Glucose is the only energy substrate that can be used by all cells of the organism; it is the sole substrate used by the brain in normal, non-starved conditions.
- When a carbohydrate-rich meal is ingested, part of the glucose absorbed from the gut can be temporarily stored as hepatic glycogen, to be subsequently released into the blood when glucose absorption declines. The capacity to store hepatic glycogen is, however, limited to about 100 g.
- During sustained administration of high amounts of carbohydrate, whether with TPN or with continuous enteral nutrition, hepatic and muscle glycogen stores become saturated and some glucose is converted into fat by *de novo* lipogenesis. This may cause deposition of intracellular lipids in various organs and tissues; in the liver, it may be a cause of hepatic steatosis.

*E-mail: luc.tappy@unil.ch

Introduction

Carbohydrate intake accounts for 45–55% of total dietary energy intake in most industrialized countries and can be considerably larger in rural areas of Asia and Africa. Digestible carbohydrates can be ingested as starch, which represents the bulk of total carbohydrates in the diet, disaccharides or simple sugars. In North America, high-fructose corn syrup, containing in its most usual form 55% free fructose and 42% free glucose, has become a major source of dietary monosaccharides (White, 2008). Nowadays consumption of mono- and disaccharides represents approximately 20% of our total energy intake (Ervin *et al.*, 2012). Starch and disaccharides require digestion to simple sugars by saliva and pancreatic amylases and by disaccharidases present in the brush border of the small intestine, before being absorbed as simple sugars through carrier-mediated facilitated transport through the enterocytes.

Recommended dietary intake of carbohydrates is 55% of total energy. There is no consensus regarding an upper intake level for mono- and disaccharides, but several organizations recommend that it is limited to 10% of total energy or less (Johnson *et al.*, 2009). Due to the high consumption of sweetened carbonated beverages in industrialized countries and the use of high-fructose corn syrup as a sweetening agent, fructose consumption has increased markedly over the past decades and become a major public health concern because of its potential deleterious metabolic effects (Bray *et al.*, 2004). Besides digestible carbohydrates, foods of plant origin also contain non-digestible complex carbohydrates, i.e. soluble and unsoluble fibres that do not deliver quantitative amounts of energy to the organism but play an important role in maintaining gut microbial flora and gut function (Asp, 1995). In total parenteral nutrition (TPN), starch and disaccharides – which require digestion into simple sugars – cannot be administered and carbohydrates are provided exclusively as simple sugars (essentially glucose, since fructose is no longer used in parenteral nutrition owing to its potential serious adverse effects (Bode *et al.*, 1973)). In home parenteral nutrition (HPN), a variable portion of total energy is provided by oral feeding and includes starch, simple sugars and fibres. This oral feeding is completed with parenteral nutrition to meet the energy requirements. Completion of ingested carbohydrates with intravenous glucose has the consequence that the proportion of simple sugars is increased in HPN.

Role of Glucose in Intermediary Metabolism

Glucose is the carbohydrate of the human body and can be used by virtually all cell types and all organs of the body as a source of energy. In addition, it can be temporarily stored as glycogen in muscle and the liver, or be converted into fatty acids in the liver. It can also be produced from amino acids, glycerol or lactate in the liver and kidneys (Fig. 22.1). Dietary starch and part of the disaccharides are absorbed from the gut as glucose through a secondary, active sodium glucose transport at the apical membrane and a facilitated glucose transport mediated by a glucose transporter GLUT2 at the basolateral side of the enterocytes (Bizeau and Pagliassotti, 2005). Fructose resulting from sucrose digestion or from fructose

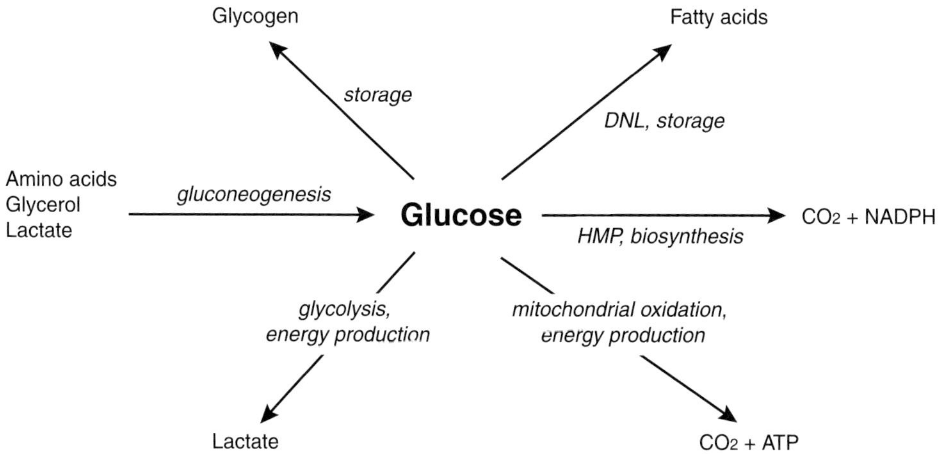

Fig. 22.1. Metabolic pathways for glucose disposal. DNL, *de novo* lipogenesis; HMP, hexose-monophosphate pathway.

intake is absorbed through a facilitated transport mediated by a transporter GLUT5 at the apical side of enterocytes. Its absorption is slower and more easily saturated than that of glucose, and many individuals present significant malabsorption after ingestion of large amounts of fructose. Once absorbed, fructose is taken up rapidly by liver cells, where it is degraded into triose phosphates and/or converted into glucose. As a result of this hepatic metabolism, fructose concentrations in the systemic circulation remain very low and extrahepatic tissues mostly metabolize fructose-derived glucose and lactate (Tappy and Le, 2010) (Fig. 22.1). Most tissues of the human body can switch between glucose and lipid as energy source. The brain, kidney medulla and red blood cells, however, lack the enzymatic machinery required for fat metabolism and rely exclusively on glucose metabolism under normal conditions. Given the central role of the brain in controlling the activities of the various constituents of the body, it is not surprising that strong regulatory mechanisms have evolved to ensure a constant plasma glucose concentration and a constant glucose supply to the brain.

Glucoregulation

In normal individuals, plasma glucose is tightly regulated to remain between 4 and 5.5 mmol/l even when no food intake occurs over several hours. Under such conditions, glucose utilization by the brain and other tissues amounts to about 2 mg/kg body weight/min and is balanced by a production of glucose, essentially from the liver, with a minor contribution from the kidneys (Fig. 22.2a). Glucose production is made possible by the presence of glucose stored as limited amounts of glycogen (about 70–100 g after an overnight fast) in the liver, which can be reconverted into glucose through glycogenolysis and released into the circulation.

In addition, glucose can be synthesized from lactate, glycerol or the carbon skeleton of amino acids through the process of gluconeogenesis. Both glycogenolysis and gluconeogenesis are reciprocally regulated by insulin, on the one hand, and a group of catabolic or stress hormones, including adrenaline, glucagon, cortisol and human growth hormone, on the other. Insulin inhibits both glycogenolysis and gluconeogenesis whereas stress hormones are potent activators of these processes. The balance between insulin secretion (which is low in fasting conditions) and stress hormones allows for the fine tuning of glucose production required to maintain constant fasting plasma glucose concentration (Gerich, 1993; Tappy, 1995) (Fig. 22.2a). Additional intrahepatic mechanisms however, known as 'hepatic autoregulation', contribute to this process (Cherrington, 1999). The efficiency with which these processes allow maintenance of normoglycaemia is illustrated by the metabolic adaptations to physical exercise. During exercise, the energy and glucose consumption of skeletal muscle increases markedly and total glucose utilization increases several-fold. Physical exercise, however, leads to only a small drop in glucose level because it decreases insulin concentration and increases stress hormone release, allowing stimulation of glucose production in proportion with the enhanced muscle glucose utilization (Kjaer, 1998).

In fasting conditions, glucose utilization occurs mainly in the brain, kidney medulla and red blood cells, which are obligatory glucose consumers. In red blood cells, glucose is degraded into pyruvate, which cannot be metabolized further owing to the absence of mitochondria in red blood cells. Pyruvate is then converted into lactate and released as such into the systemic circulation to be reconverted into glucose in the liver. This 'glucose–lactate–glucose' cycling occurs not only in red blood cells, but also in skeletal muscle, inflammatory cells and scar tissues (Cori cycle). Glucose utilization by adipose tissue, resting skeletal muscle, fibroblasts, etc. is low in fasted conditions due to the low insulin concentration, and these tissues rely mostly on fat as an energy substrate. After carbohydrate ingestion or intravenous glucose administration, the rise in glucose level elicits a stimulation of insulin release that acutely increases glucose uptake, oxidation and, if in excess of oxidative capacities, storage as glycogen (Fig. 22.2b). This process occurs in all insulin-sensitive tissues, but is quantitatively most important in skeletal muscle (Gerich, 1993; Tappy, 1995). Of interest, it has now been documented that a portion of the glucose may be oxidized through the action of so-called 'lactate shuttles'. In this process, glucose is converted into lactate by one cell type, to be transferred to another adjacent cell where it is oxidized to CO_2. This has been described in glycolytic–oxidative skeletal muscle fibres and in astrocytes–neurons (Brooks, 2002). Although the functional significance of these shuttles remains incompletely understood, it is likely that lactate may work as a regulatory signal molecule under some circumstances.

Besides oxidation to CO_2 (in all tissues) and glycogen storage (in liver cells and skeletal muscle essentially), small amounts of glucose can be metabolized by the hexose-monophosphate pathway, a process that allows synthesis of NADPH to be used in various biosynthetic processes (lipogenesis) and in the defence against oxidants (glutathione reductase). This pathway also produces ribose-5-phosphate, which is used for the synthesis of nucleic acids. Glucose can also be converted into

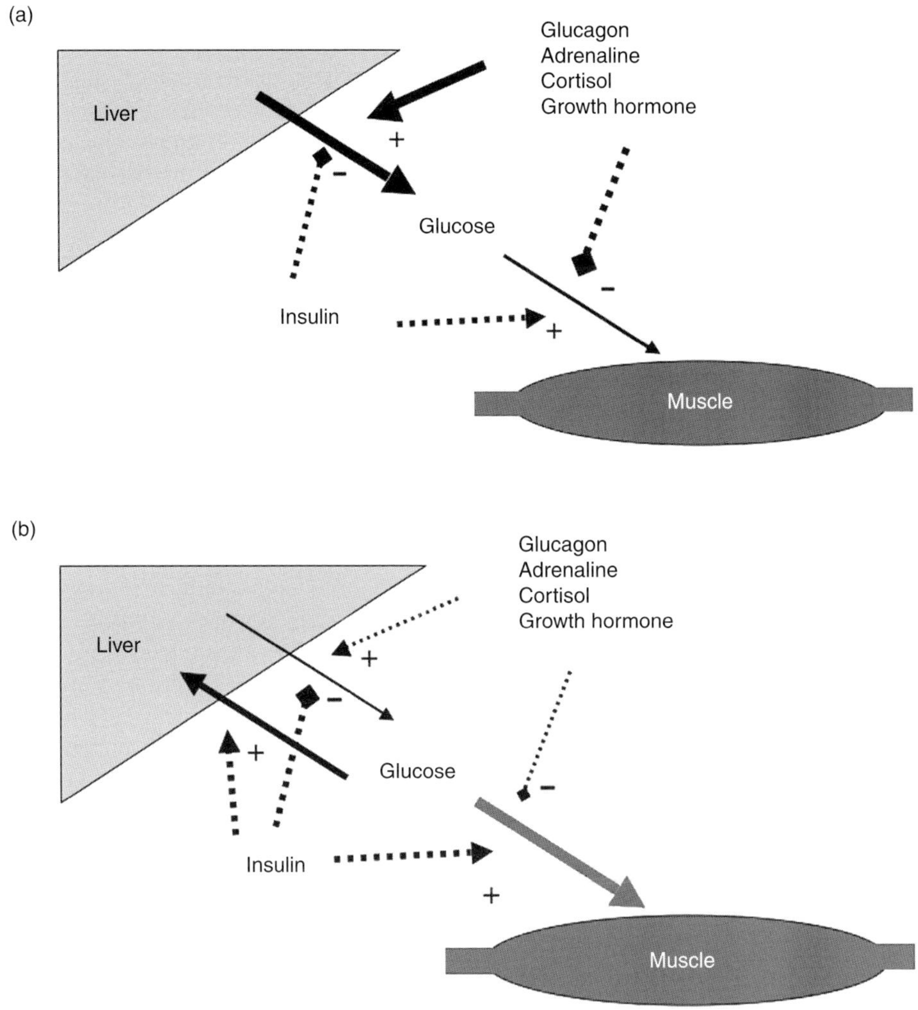

Fig. 22.2. Regulation of glucose metabolism by insulin and stress hormones (glucagon, adrenaline, cortisol and growth hormone) in normal postprandial conditions (a) and in critically ill patients during continuous nutrition (b). –, inhibition; +, activation.

lipids, essentially in liver cells, but also in adipocytes, although this pathway is quantitatively minor in normal conditions (Hellerstein *et al.*, 1996; Minehira *et al.*, 2003).

Energetics of Glucose Oxidation

Complete glucose oxidation to CO_2 releases a total of 32 mol ATP/mol glucose, which will subsequently be used for the energy-requiring processes of the organism (transmembrane ion transports, biosynthetic processes, etc.). However, hydrolysis of a few moles of ATP is also required for glucose absorption to metabolize glucose to fructose-1,6-diphosphate, or to convert glucose into glycogen or lipids. As a result, the net ATP yield of complete glucose oxidation is less than 32 mol ATP/mol glucose and varies according to the metabolic pathways used for glucose metabolism. As a consequence of this extra ATP hydrolysis required for glucose metabolism, resting energy expenditure increases after glucose administration, a process known as glucose-induced thermogenesis. It usually corresponds to energy expenditure equal to 5–10% of the glucose energy administered. Besides the obligatory use of ATP for glucose metabolism, a glucose/insulin-induced stimulation of the sympathetic nervous system also occurs and may contribute to this thermic effect (Tappy and Jéquier, 1993).

Effects of Nutrition on Glucose Metabolism

Healthy individuals can have a wide range of fuel mix in their diet. Several studies have shown that whole-body glucose oxidation adapts rapidly to changes in glucose or carbohydrate intake. Such an adaptation appears essential since the amount of glucose that can be stored as glycogen is very limited (about 100 g in the liver and up to ~1 kg in skeletal muscle under extreme conditions) and conversion of massive amounts of glucose into lipid is an energetically very inefficient process. Thus, when a subject is switched from a low- to a high-carbohydrate diet, net glucose storage (glycogen synthesis) will occur initially. However, over the next few days there is a marked stimulation of glucose oxidation, allowing an even carbohydrate balance to be restored (Elwyn and Bursztein, 1993) (Fig. 22.3a). If carbohydrate intake is in excess of energy requirements, then alternative pathways for glucose disposal have to take place. This occurs through a stimulation of *de novo* lipogenesis (Fig. 22.3b), which takes place under these extremely unusual circumstances in extrahepatic tissues (most likely adipose tissue) (Acheson *et al.*, 1988; Aarsland *et al.*, 1997; Minehira *et al.*, 2003). At the opposite, an acute reduction of carbohydrate intake leads, over a few days, to the reverse adaptation, i.e. a decrease in glucose oxidation. If glucose intake drops below a minimal daily intake (corresponding to the minimal needs of the brain and obligatory glucose-using organs), additional adaptations have to occur. This is what occurs during starvation when no carbohydrate is taken up for several consecutive days (Owen *et al.*, 1990). During the initial days of starvation, hepatic glycogenolysis and gluconeogenesis increase to ensure sufficient amounts of glucose to the brain. After about 36 h, hepatic glycogen stores are depleted and glucose production relies exclusively on gluconeogenesis, essentially from amino acids. The consequence of this is a substantial catabolism of protein (about 2 g protein required for the synthesis of 1 g glucose). In healthy individuals, however, hepatic ketogenesis is stimulated and increases progressively after 3–4 days of starvation while the brain adapts to use ketone bodies as energy fuels. This coordinated liver–brain metabolic adaptation allows the sparing of endogenous proteins and extends survival time.

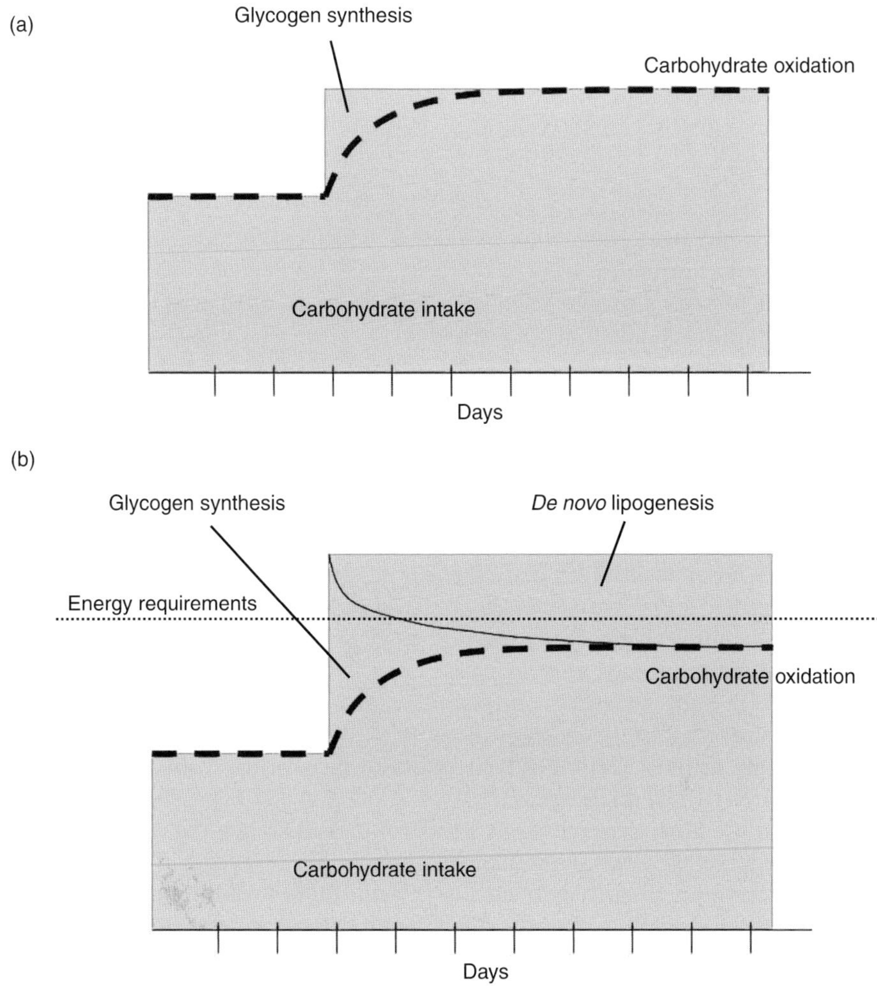

Fig. 22.3. Evolution of carbohydrate oxidation and *de novo* lipogenesis when carbohydrate intake is acutely changed: (a) when carbohydrate intake is modestly increased, carbohydrate oxidation increases to match intake, restoring carbohydrate balance; (b) when carbohydrate intake exceeds energy requirements, *de novo* lipogenesis is stimulated.

Glucose Metabolism in Critically Ill Patients

Patients requiring HPN have a nutrition pattern that differs markedly from normal physiological food intake. First, based on mixed oral/parenteral nutrition, with parenteral carbohydrate being exclusively glucose, they receive a higher proportion of total calories as simple sugars than provided on a normal diet. Second, due to night-time infusion of nutrients, they often have a near-continuous nutrition compared with the essentially episodic food intake of normal individuals. Third, patients submitted to HPN have underlying disorders that may themselves alter energy and substrate metabolism. No study has specifically evaluated glucose utilization in HPN patients, but observations done in critically ill patients with total parenteral or enteral nutrition may still be relevant.

Acute illnesses produce well-characterized alterations of glucose and energy metabolism (Fig. 22.3) (Wolfe *et al.*, 1987; Wilmore and Robinson, 1993), which include:

- an increase in total energy expenditure;
- an increased production of glucose, which can be attributed to increases in stress hormones; and
- a decreased insulin sensitivity, which can be attributed to both stress hormones and inflammatory cytokines.

As a result of these metabolic changes, plasma glucose increases and its rise appears proportional to the severity of the underlying disorders. Furthermore, the subsequent hyperglycaemia appears to have deleterious effects, presumably by production of reactive oxygen species and oxidative damage. In support of this deleterious effect of hyperglycaemia, it has been observed that aggressive treatment of hyperglycaemia in critically ill patients may improve patient outcome and decreases mortality (Van den Berghe *et al.*, 2001). This initial observation, made on cardiac surgery patients, suggested that attaining a tight glycaemic control would improve patient outcome in critically ill patients at large. Subsequent multicentre randomized clinical trials, however, failed to confirm clear beneficial effects of tight glycaemic control and reported an increased incidence of hypoglycaemia. Based on these observations, it is currently recommended to avoid severe hypoglycaemia (>10 mmol/l) in critically ill patients, with insulin therapy if required (Ichai and Preiser, 2010).

It has been observed that critically ill patients retain the capacity to adapt to changes in carbohydrate intake and to maintain an even carbohydrate balance. This has been observed both during TPN and during continuous enteral nutrition (Tappy *et al.*, 1998; Schwarz *et al.*, 2000). However, high carbohydrate intakes were associated with stimulation of hepatic *de novo* lipogenesis. Such stimulation of hepatic *de novo* lipogenesis is also observed in healthy individuals submitted to an isocaloric diet rich in simple sugars but not in complex carbohydrates (Hudgins *et al.*, 1998). It appears therefore that the carbohydrate proportion in the diet and the nature of the carbohydrate play an important role in this process. Furthermore, in critically ill patients, both the mode of carbohydrate administration (i.e. continuous versus episodic) and critical illness per se may be additional factors that stimulate *de novo* lipogenesis (Minehira *et al.*, 2002). In the long term, there is concern that increased *de novo* lipogenesis may either favour the development of non-alcoholic fatty liver disease or lead to hypertriglyceridaemia with possible adverse vascular effects.

Summary

Due to technical constraints, carbohydrate delivery during HPN differs from a normal feeding pattern by: (i) a near-continuous glucose delivery; and (ii) a higher proportion of glucose to total carbohydrate. Risks secondary to this feeding pattern (with possible additional aggravating factors due to the underlying illness) are hyperglycaemia and stimulation of *de novo* lipogenesis, which can be prevented by avoiding excess glucose administration.

References

Aarsland, A., Chinkes, D. and Wolfe, R.R. (1997) Hepatic and whole-body fat synthesis in humans during carbohydrate overfeeding. *American Journal of Clinical Nutrition* 65, 1774–1782.

Acheson, K., Schutz, Y., Bessard, T., Anantharaman, K., Flatt, J. and Jéquier, E. (1988) Glycogen storage capacity and *de novo* lipogenesis during massive carbohydrate overfeeding in man. *American Journal of Clinical Nutrition* 48, 240–247.

Asp, N.G. (1995) Classification and methodology of food carbohydrates as related to nutritional effects. *American Journal of Clinical Nutrition* 61(4 Suppl.), 930–937.

Bizeau, M.E. and Pagliassotti, M.J. (2005) Hepatic adaptations to sucrose and fructose. *Metabolism Clinical and Experimental* 54, 1189–1201.

Bode, J.C., Zelder, O., Rumpelt, H.J. and Wittkamp, U. (1973) Depletion of liver adenosine phosphates and metabolic effects of intravenous infusion of fructose or sorbitol in man and in the rat. *European Journal of Clinical Investigation* 3, 436–441.

Bray, G.A., Nielsen, S.J. and Popkin, B.M. (2004) Consumption of high-fructose corn syrup in beverages may play a role in the epidemic of obesity. *American Journal of Clinical Nutrition* 79, 537–543.

Brooks, G.A. (2002) Lactate shuttles in nature. *Biochemical Society Transactions* 30, 258–264.

Cherrington, A.D. (1999) Control of glucose uptake and release by the liver *in vivo*. *Diabetes* 48, 1198–1214.

Elwyn, D.H. and Bursztein, S. (1993) Carbohydrate metabolism and requirements for nutritional support: part I. *Nutrition* 9, 50–66.

Ervin, R.B., Kit, B.K., Carroll, M.D. and Ogden, C.L. (2012) Consumption of added sugar among US children and adolescents, 2005–2008. *NCHS Data Brief* (87), 1–8.

Gerich, J.E. (1993) Control of glycaemia. *Baillière's Clinical Endocrinology and Metabolism* 7, 551–586.

Hellerstein, M.K., Schwarz, J.M. and Nees, R.A. (1996) Regulation of hepatic *de novo* lipogenesis in humans. *Annual Review of Nutrition* 16, 523–557.

Hudgins, L.C., Seidman, C.E., Diakun, J. and Hirsch, J. (1998) Human fatty acid synthesis is reduced after the substitution of dietary starch for sugar. *American Journal of Clinical Nutrition* 67, 631–639.

Ichai, C. and Preiser, J.C.; Société Française d'Anesthésie-Réanimation; Société de Réanimation de langue Française; Experts group (2010) International recommendations for glucose control in adult non diabetic critically ill patients. *Critical Care* 14, R166.

Johnson, R.K., Appel, L.J., Brands, M., Howard, B.V., Lefevre, M., Lustig, R.H., Sacks, F., Steffen, L.M., Wylie-Rosett, J.; American Heart Association Nutrition Committee of the Council on Nutrition, Physical Activity, and Metabolism and the Council on Epidemiology and Prevention (2009) Dietary sugars intake and cardiovascular health: a scientific statement from the American Heart Association. *Circulation* 120, 1011–1020.

Kjaer, M. (1998) Hepatic glucose production during exercise. *Advances in Experimental Medicine and Biology* 441, 117–127.

Minehira, K., Tappy, L., Chioléro, R., Vladimirova, V., Berger, M.M., Revelly, J.P. and Schwarz, J.M. (2002) Fractional hepatic *de novo* lipogenesis in healthy subjects during near-continuous oral nutrition and bed rest: a comparison with published data in artificially fed, critically ill patients. *Clinical Nutrition* 21, 345–350.

Minehira, K., Bettschart, V., Vidal, H., Vega, N., Di Vetta, V., Rey, V., Schneiter, P. and Tappy, L. (2003) Effect of carbohydrate overfeeding on whole body and adipose tissue metabolism in humans. *Obesity Research* 11, 1096–1103.

Owen, O.E., Tappy, L., Mozzoli, M.A. and Smalley, K.J. (1990) Acute starvation. In: Cohen, R.D., Lewis, B., Alberti, K.G.M.M. and Denman, A.M. (eds) *The Metabolic and Molecular Basis of Acquired Disease*, vol. 1. Baillière Tindall, London, pp. 550–570.

Schwarz, J.M., Chioléro, R., Revelly, J.-P., Cayeux, C., Schneiter, P., Jéquier, E., Chen, T. and Tappy, L. (2000) Effects of enteral carbohydrates on *de novo* lipogenesis in critically ill patients. *American Journal of Clinical Nutrition* 72, 940–945.

Tappy, L. (1995) Regulation of hepatic glucose production in healthy subjects and patients with NIDDM. *Diabetes and Metabolism* 21, 233–240.

Tappy, L. and Jéquier, E. (1993) Fructose and dietary thermogenesis. *American Journal of Clinical Nutrition* 58, 766–770.

Tappy, L. and Le, K.A. (2010) Metabolic effects of fructose and the worldwide increase in obesity. *Physiological Reviews* 9, 23–46.

Tappy, L., Schwarz, J.M., Schneiter, P., Cayeux, C., Revelly, J.P., Fagerquist, C.K., Jéquier, E. and Chioléro, R. (1998) Effects of isoenergetic glucose-based or lipid-based parenteral nutrition on glucose metabolism, *de novo* lipogenesis, and respiratory gas exchanges in critically ill patients. *Critical Care Medicine* 26, 860–867.

Van den Berghe, G., Wouters, P., Weekers, F., Verwaest, C., Bruyninckx, F., Schetz, M., Vlasselaers, D., Ferdinande, P., Lauwers, P. and Bouillon, R. (2001) Intensive insulin therapy in the critically ill patients. *New England Journal of Medicine* 345, 1359–1367.

White, J.S. (2008) Straight talk about high-fructose corn syrup: what it is and what it ain't. *American Journal of Clinical Nutrition* 88, 1716–1721.

Wilmore, D.W. and Robinson, M.K. (1993) Metabolism and nutritional support. In: Fischer, J.E. and Holmes, C.R. (eds) *Surgical Basic Science*. Mosby Year Book, St Louis, Missouri, pp. 125–169.

Wolfe, R.R., Herndon, D.N., Jahoor, F., Miyosi, H. and Wolfe, M. (1987) Effect of severe burn injury on substrate cycling by glucose and fatty acids. *New England Journal of Medicine* 317, 403–408.

23 Use of Lipids in Home Parenteral Nutrition

Benoît Dupont[1], Marie-Astrid Piquet[1], Marietta Musikas[1], Corinne Joubert[1] and Jean-Marie Reimund[2,3*]

[1]Service d'Hépato-Gastro-Entérologie et Nutrition, Centre Hospitalier Universitaire de Caen, Caen, France; [2]Service d'Hépato-Gastroentérologie et d'Assistance Nutritive, Hôpitaux Universitaires de Strasbourg, Hôpital de Hautepierre, Strasbourg, France; [3]INSERM U1113, Laboratoire 'Voies de signalisation du développement et du stress cellulaire dans les cancers digestifs et urologiques', Faculté de Médecine, Université de Strasbourg, Strasbourg, France

Key Points

- There is consensus regarding the advantage of including fat emulsions as a component of nutritional provisions in home parenteral nutrition (HPN) patients.
- The physiochemical stability of lipid emulsions in HPN admixtures represents an important issue, with possible deleterious clinical implications.
- In adult patients, minimal fat supply should be about 1 g/kg body weight/week in order to avoid essential fatty acid deficiency. Supply of fat should not exceed 1 g/kg body weight/day to prevent severe HPN-associated liver disease.
- Adequate vitamin E must be supplied to limit lipid peroxidation in HPN patients.
- Fat emulsions containing long-chain triacylglycerols or a mixture of long-chain triacylglycerols/medium-chain triacylglycerols have successfully been used as an essential component of HPN. The safety of newer lipid emulsions (olive oil and structured lipids) has recently been demonstrated in adults as well as in children.

*E-mail: jm.reimund.gcb@gmail.com

Introduction

Lipid emulsions have been developed for use in parenteral nutrition (PN) for several reasons, one of them being the limited capacity of an organism under PN to oxidize glucose. Lipids provide a concentrated and rapidly usable energy supply. They represent a dense caloric source (9 kcal/g metabolized fatty acids), but also cover the requirements in essential fatty acids (EFAs) (linoleic acid and α-linolenic acid) and fat-soluble vitamins. In addition to their direct nutritional effects, they also modify the phospholipid composition of cell membranes, thereby influencing numerous key regulatory functions such as membrane receptor activities and membrane fluidity, eicosanoid metabolism, cytokine production, cell signalling, apoptosis and gene expression (Wanten and Calder, 2007).

Today, a consensus has been reached concerning the advantage of including fat emulsions as a regular component of nutritional provision in home parenteral nutrition (HPN) patients. Currently available lipid emulsions (Tables 23.1 and 23.2) include: (i) 10%, 20% or 30% emulsions of soybean oil (composed of 100% long-chain triacylglycerols (LCTs) including more than 50% of the polyunsaturated fatty acid (PUFA) linoleic acid (18:2*n*-6)) (Intralipid®, Fresenius Kabi AG, Germany; Ivelip®, Clintec Nutrition Clinique, France/Baxter SA, Belgium; Endolipide®, B. Braun Melsungen AG, Germany) (Fig. 23.1 and Table 23.3); (ii) 10% and 20% medium-chain triacylglycerol (MCT)/LCT (1:1 weight for weight) emulsions (Medialipide® or Lipofundin® MCT, B. Braun Melsungen AG) (Table 23.1); (iii) 20% structured-lipid emulsions (Structolipid®, Fresenius Kabi

Table 23.1. Composition (per 1000 ml) of the fat emulsions mainly used for parenteral lipid provision.

	Intralipid®	Ivelip®	Endolipide®	Medialipide®	Clinoleic®	Structolipid®
Manufacturer	Fresenius Kabi	Clintec/ Baxter	B. Braun	B. Braun	Clintec/ Baxter	Fresenius Kabi
Components						
Soy oil (g)	200/300	200	200	100	40	100
MCT fatty acids[a] (g)	–	–	–	100	–	100
Olive oil (g)	–	–	–	–	160	–
Fish oil (g)	–	–	–	–	–	–
Phospholipids (g)	12	12	12	12	12	12
Glycerol (g)	22.5	25	25	25	22.5	25
Available products						
Glass bottles (ml)	200/500	100/250/ 500/1000	100/250/ 500	100/250/ 500	100/250/ 500	–
Plastic bags (ml)	100/250/ 500/333 (30%)	100/250/ 500	–	100/250/ 500	–	500
Caloric provision (kcal/l)	1100/2000/ 3000	2000	2000	1968	2000	1960

[a]MCT fatty acids used for PN are extracted mainly from coconut or palm oil.

AG) (Table 23.1); and (iv) an olive oil-based lipid emulsion (80% olive oil, i.e. monounsaturated oleic acid/20% soybean oil) (Clinoleic®, Clintec Nutrition Clinique/Baxter SA) (Fig. 23.1, Tables 23.1 and 23.3).

In addition, more specific and/or complex lipid emulsions have been developed that may be used as either: (i) a ready-for-use emulsion (e.g. Smoflipid® (Fresenius Kabi AG), a physical mixture of soybean oil, MCT, olive oil, fish oil and additional α-tocopherol; Lipidem® (B. Braun Melsungen AG), composed of MCTs/LCTs/*n*-3 fatty acids in a 5:4:1 (wt/wt/wt) proportion) (Schlotzer and Kanning, 2004; Ton *et al.*, 2005); or (ii) a fraction of the infused lipids (*n*-3 fatty acids: Omegaven®, Fresenius Kabi AG) (Tables 23.2 and 23.3, Fig. 23.1).

This growing diversity of lipids available for intravenous administration in human nutrition and/or therapeutics opens a large research avenue for clinicians interested in the optimization of fat emulsion use in both short-term PN and patients on HPN (Deckelbaum *et al.*, 2004).

Table 23.2. Composition (per 1000 ml) of the fat emulsions mainly used for parenteral lipid provision (continued).

	Omegaven®	Lipidem®	Smoflipid®
Manufacturer	Fresenius Kabi	B. Braun	Fresenius Kabi
Components			
Soy oil (g)	–	80	60
MCT fatty acids[a] (g)	–	100	60
Olive oil (g)	–	–	50
Fish oil (g)	100	20	30
Phospholipids (g)	12	12	12
Glycerol (g)	25	25	25
Available products			
Glass bottles (ml)	50/100	100/250/500	250/500
Plastic bags (ml)	–	–	–
Caloric provision (kcal/l)	1120	1910	2000

[a]MCT fatty acids used for PN are extracted mainly from coconut or palm oil.

Table 23.3. Major fatty acids composition (%) of oils used to manufacture the classical PN lipid emulsions (minor fatty acids are not indicated).

	Soybean oil	Olive oil	MCT fatty acids[a]	Fish oil
Linoleic acid (18:2*n*-6)	54	10	–	–
α-Linolenic acid (18:3*n*-3)	7	–	–	–
Oleic acid (18:1*n*-9)	23	75	–	–
Capric acid (C10:0)	–	–	40	–
Caprylic acid (C8:0)	–	–	54	–
Eicosapentaenoic acid (20:5*n*-3)	–	–	–	7
Docosahexaenoic acid (22:6*n*-3)	–	–	–	24

[a]MCT fatty acids used for PN are extracted mainly from coconut or palm oil.

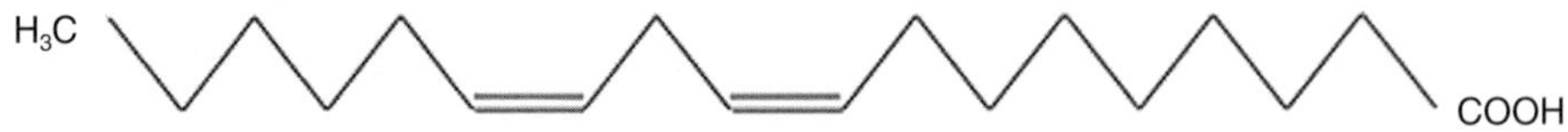

Linoleic acid (18:2*n*-6)

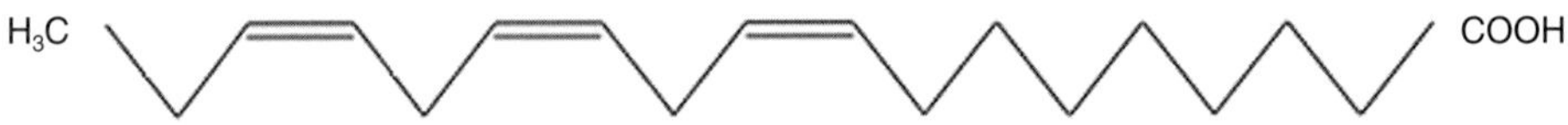

α-Linolenic acid (18:3*n*-3)

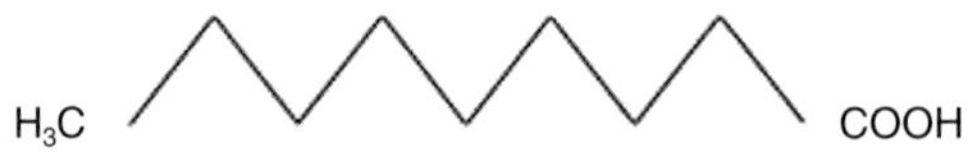

Caprylic (octaenoic) acid (18:0)

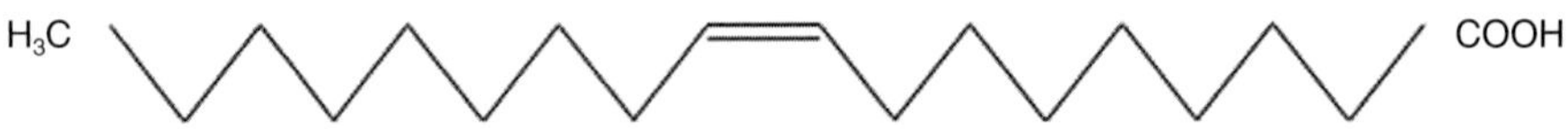

Oleic acid (18:1*n*-9)

Fig. 23.1. Chemical structures of the principal fatty acids composing various lipid emulsions: linoleic acid (LCT from soybean oil), α-linolenic acid (fish oil), caprylic (octaenoic) acid (MCT from coconut or palm oil) and oleic acid (olive oil). For more information on composition of lipid emulsions used in human nutrition see Tables 23.1–23.3.

General Composition and Stability Issues

Formulation components and process parameters of PN admixtures are critical points to consider before their administration. Stability problems may occur during preparation, storage and use of complex PN formulations. They can result from the intrinsic composition of the lipid emulsions used, but more frequently from chemical instabilities arising from incompatibility with other components of the PN admixture. Checking systematically the composition of all PN formulations before using them in human therapeutics is crucial as the administration of an unstable or incompatible admixture may have serious clinical consequences (Lumpkin, 1994).

Structure and composition of lipid emulsions

The aim of the intravenously administered lipids is to mimic the flow of chylomicrons that, when delivered into the blood via the intestinal lymph, provides newly absorbed lipids to normally fed subjects. In PN, lipids necessarily have to be administered in the form of an emulsion, i.e. a dispersion of small oil particles in a vector constituted by a continuous aqueous phase usually containing glycerol. In addition to these two phases, a stabilizing/emulsifying agent is indispensable both for the dispersion of the oil and the stability of the resulting emulsion. The first phase is formed by triacylglycerol-rich particles (TGRPs) modelled on the endogenous natural chylomicron. This phase is stabilized in the liquid hydrophilic phase by a surface layer composed mainly by phospholipids (Ferezou and Bach, 1999). In the case of lipid emulsions for parenteral use in humans, lecithins from an animal source (usually egg-yolk) or a vegetable source (usually soybean) are commonly used (Davis, 1983). They contain up to six phospholipids, and provide both a mechanical/physical barrier and an electrically charged barrier to prevent coalescence of TGRPs. In lipid emulsions, compared with the amount strictly required for stabilization of the triacylglycerol content, the emulsifier is present in relative excess, leading to the formation of liposome-like phospholipid-rich particles. When present in large amounts, these particular emulsion particles can impede lipid and lipoprotein metabolism and modify cell membrane lipid composition (Haumont *et al.*, 1989, 1992; Kalfarentzos *et al.*, 1998). Therefore, because phospholipid excess is particularly noticeable in 10% emulsions, the use of 20% or 30% preparations (providing a more limited phospholipid/triacylglycerol ratio) is recommended (Carpentier and Dupont, 2000).

Stability of intravenous lipid emulsions

A very large number of chemical and physicochemical interactions can potentially occur between lipid emulsions and the other components of the PN admixture. In particular, this can be the case in HPN based on the use of personalized 'all-in-one' (AIO) admixtures varying widely in composition from one patient to another, but also in the same patient from time to time depending on his/her specific nutritional requirements. Therefore, it is of paramount importance that pharmacists and/or manufacturers involved in the preparation of AIO bags systematically ascertain the compatibility of the prescribed nutrients and/or drugs, as well as the final stability of the admixture (Hardy and Puzovic, 2009). In the case of lipid emulsions, several basic factors can interfere with stability such as pH, glucose load, and amino acid or electrolyte concentrations. Instability may result in a cracked, a creamed or an aggregated lipid emulsion depending on the factor(s) interfering with its stability. For example, after autoclaving, sterilized glucose solutions have a pH that can range from 3.5 to 6.5, the pH varying among manufacturers and even within batches from the same manufacturer. This results from glucose decomposition, first to form 5-(hydroxymethyl)-2-furanaldehyde, and then formic and levulinic acids during the heating process. The resulting drop in pH may result in a decrease in charge and repulsive forces to droplet aggregation.

These aggregates have a combined size greater than the majority of droplets and their natural Brownian motion is minimized such that they will rise to the surface of the emulsion to form a 'cream' layer. A similar effect can be observed with cationic electrolytes if the 'critical aggregation concentration/number', as defined by Davis (1983), is inadequate. A high amount of cationic electrolytes, which exhibit an opposite charge to that of the surface charge of lipid droplets, will also reduce the surface potential on the droplets and, as a consequence, the repulsive forces between the droplets, leading to aggregation and coalescence. For all these reasons, the physicochemical stability of lipid emulsions incorporated in HPN admixtures represents an important issue with possible deleterious clinical implications such as impairment in plasma clearance in susceptible individuals, increase in infusion of high amounts of potentially embolic fat droplets, or increase in reactive oxygen species generation leading to tissue damage, in particular PN-associated liver disease (Driscoll, 2005, 2006). This is especially a major concern when PN is used in neonates (Driscoll *et al.*, 2007, 2010; Jalabert *et al.*, 2011).

Metabolism of Intravenous Lipid Emulsions

Infusion of fat emulsion leads to the appearance of exogenous lipids in the blood circulation and produces a transitory increase in triacylglycerol and phospholipid concentrations. The metabolic pathways regulating intravascular metabolism of lipid emulsion TGRPs simultaneously involve several steps: (i) exchange and transfer of lipids and proteins; (ii) enzymatic hydrolysis of triacylglycerols and phospholipids; (iii) uptake of hydrolysis products; and (iv) internalization of particles by different tissues. Schematically, these metabolic pathways are comparable to those of chylomicrons (Olivecrona and Olivecrona, 1998; Ferezou and Bach, 1999). However, by contrast to endogenous chylomicrons, artificial emulsion particles contain no apolipoproteins. As soon as they enter the circulation, TGRPs acquire after a short delay several endogenous apolipoproteins (mainly apo C-I, C-II and C-III, apo E) principally taken from the high-density lipoproteins (HDLs) (Richelle *et al.*, 1986). Apolipoproteins CII are essential as they favour the particle binding to the lipoprotein lipase (LPL) receptor site and activate triacylglycerol hydrolysis, whereas apo CIII tend to inhibit this enzymatic activity (Dupont and Carpentier, 1999; Ferezou and Bach, 1999; Simoens *et al.*, 2008). After this first metabolic step, apo E and apo C-I regulate cellular uptake of remnant particles respectively by facilitating and decreasing particle disposal (Dupont and Carpentier, 1999; Ferezou and Bach, 1999; Simoens *et al.*, 2008). This metabolic process is influenced by the physical properties of the TGRP surface layer, which depends on the composition of both emulsion triacylglycerols and phospholipids and therefore will vary from one emulsion to another (Saito *et al.*, 1997; Arimoto *et al.*, 1998; Martins *et al.*, 1998). The composition of lipid emulsions also influences cellular uptake. For example, use of an MCT/LCT/*n*-3 fatty acid admixture in a 5:4:1 ratio (Lipidem®, B. Braun Melsungen AG) in healthy normolipidaemic subjects resulted in a more rapid and substantial cellular acquisition of C20:5*n*-3 PUFAs (eicosapentaenoic acid, an *n*-3 long-chain PUFA known to protect against excessive inflammatory response) than a 5:5 MCT/LCT emulsion (Medialipide®,

B. Braun Melsungen AG) (Simoens *et al.*, 2008). Finally, plasma apolipoprotein content may be influenced by health status: it is often altered markedly in disease and susceptible to change the effectiveness of the inflammatory and immune responses (Chenaud *et al.*, 2004). As a result, apolipoprotein acquisition of TGRPs provided by lipid emulsions in patients receiving PN varies from one clinical situation to another.

After binding, a substantial proportion of core triacylglycerols are hydrolysed and the resulting free fatty acids are either taken up by the adjacent tissues or released into the systemic circulation. This process, as well as the transfer of another fraction of triacylglycerols from TGRPs to HDLs and low-density lipoproteins (LPLs) in the exchange of cholesteryl ester (a process mediated by the cholesteryl ester transfer protein), reduces strongly the particle size and leads to the formation of remnant particles enriched with cholesteryl ester and depleted of triacylglycerols (Dupont and Carpentier, 1999; Ferezou and Bach, 1999). These are largely taken up by the liver (Cooper, 1997; Havel, 1998; Lambert *et al.*, 2001) and to a lesser extent by several other tissues such as muscle, adipose tissue (Karpe *et al.*, 1997), endothelial cells and possibly intestinal cells (Van Aerde *et al.*, 1997).

As mentioned earlier, differences in the composition of lipid emulsions clearly modulate selected metabolic steps (Hyltander *et al.*, 1995; Dupont and Carpentier, 1999; Carpentier and Dupont, 2000; Qi *et al.*, 2002; Schlotzer and Kanning, 2004; Simoens *et al.*, 2004, 2008; Ton *et al.*, 2005). Nevertheless, whether this may influence the efficacy and safety of lipid emulsions in HPN patients remains largely unexplored.

Lipid Requirements in Adults

The daily lipid requirement in healthy adults on an oral diet has been set at 1–1.5 g/kg body weight/day. This amount covers non-protein, non-carbohydrate energy requirements and prevents essential fatty acid (i.e. linoleic acid (18:2*n*-6) and α-linolenic acid (18:3*n*-3)) deficiency (EFAD). An average daily provision of 3–4.5% of total calories as fat appears to prevent EFAD (Burr *et al.*, 1981). In HPN patients a balance has to be found between requirements and potential toxicity, in particular HPN-associated liver disease (see below). Therefore, although no standard lipid requirements have been defined for these patients, the amount of lipid emulsion administered needs to be lower (in all cases it should not be higher than 1 g/kg body weight/day on long-term PN (schematically, an administration for more than 3 months) in order to prevent hepatic toxicity) (Cavicchi *et al.*, 2000) than in short-term PN (patients on PN for several weeks to less than 3 months), or in enteral nutrition, or in healthy or diseased subjects on an oral diet. Usually it varies between 0.3 and 0.9 g/kg body weight/day (Reimund *et al.*, 1999, 2005; Pironi *et al.*, 2003; Chambrier *et al.*, 2004; Vahedi *et al.*, 2005). In advanced cancer patients on HPN, where the mean length of survival was about 4 months, a lipid/glucose calories ratio of 1:1 was well tolerated for a total overall regimen of 25–30 non-protein kcal/kg body weight/day, each day (Bozzetti *et al.*, 1999, 2002). Whether the increase in lipid provision in these patients (alone or in combination with specific pharmacological interventions) modulates tumour growth compared with patients receiving HPN for non-malignant diseases still has to be investigated in future clinical studies in humans (Bozzetti *et al.*, 1996, 2004).

Intravenous Administration of Lipids in HPN: Efficacy and Safety

HPN efficacy depends on numerous factors related not only to the composition of PN admixtures, but also to the patient, e.g. underlying disease (Howard *et al.*, 1991; Messing *et al.*, 1995; Santarpia *et al.*, 2006), the experience and logistics of the HPN centre (Messing *et al.*, 1995; Smith *et al.*, 2002; Reimund, 2003; Freshwater *et al.*, 2005; Jonkers-Schuitema *et al.*, 2005), etc. Several groups have investigated HPN efficacy in single or multiple centres (Messing *et al.*, 1995, 1998; Reimund *et al.*, 1999; Van Gossum *et al.*, 2001; Ireton-Jones and DeLegge, 2005; Violante *et al.*, 2006). In the particular case of lipid provision, efficacy is tightly related to safety. Too low amounts of lipids may lead to EFAD and its biological and clinical consequences, while too much fat provision may induce side-effects that could limit HPN efficacy and, as a consequence, the patient's quality of life and rehabilitation status.

Essential fatty acid deficiency

EFAD (Hamilton *et al.*, 2006) is a major concern in HPN patients. Normally, there are large stores of EFAs in the body. However, in patients on fat-free total PN or in HPN patients receiving a too low fat/too high glucose admixture for a prolonged time, the induction of hyperinsulinaemia suppresses the mobilization of EFAs from fat stores and induces EFAD which can clinically be characterized by dermatitis (Sinclair, 1956, 1990; Jeppesen *et al.*, 1998), hair loss, increased susceptibility to infection (Cederholm *et al.*, 1994) or impaired wound healing (Hulsey *et al.*, 1977). Haematological abnormalities such as haemolytic anaemia, thrombocytopenia or diminished platelet aggregation, liver fatty infiltration, increase in hepatic enzyme activity, impaired chylomicron synthesis and impaired fat malabsorption have also been described (Jeppesen *et al.*, 1997). It is important to note that biochemical evidence of EFAD appears significantly earlier than clinical symptoms and signs. Usually, it can be diagnosed before clinical manifestations appear by assessing the Holman index or triene/tetraene ratio, i.e. the ratio of eicosatrienoic acid (20:3*n*-9) to arachidonic acid (20:4*n*-6) in patients at risk. Initially, an index >0.4 was considered as indicating EFAD even in patients with no clinical signs (Collins *et al.*, 1971). With improvement of methods of fatty acid analysis, work by Holman *et al.* (1979) suggested values >0.2 as more appropriate. Later, a value >0.025 was proposed to be diagnostic when healthy, free-living reference controls were compared with patients with intestinal fat malabsorption and suspected EFAD (Siguel *et al.*, 1987). Several groups have studied the EFA status in HPN patients (Abushufa *et al.*, 1995; Mascioli *et al.*, 1996; Chambrier *et al.*, 1998; Jeppesen *et al.*, 1998; Reimund *et al.*, 1998). The results can be summarized schematically as follows: (i) EFAD depends on the cut-off value considered.

For example, we found a mean Holman index of 0.031 ± 0.017 in 21 HPN patients, which suggested EFAD in several patients as we defined EFAD at a level >0.025 (Siguel *et al.*, 1987; Reimund *et al.*, 1998). However, regarding Holman's definition (Holman *et al.*, 1979) no patient will be considered to have subclinical EFAD; (ii) an amount of 0.7 (or less but under tight biological control) to a maximum of 1 g lipids/kg body weight/day is sufficient to avoid EFAD in HPN patients according Holman *et al.* (1979); (iii) given these data, one can conclude as Jeppesen *et al.* (1998) do: 'Recommendations regarding lipid dosages in parenteral supplements depend on the degree of correction of plasma fatty acids in the phospholipids one aims at. Lipid dosage adjustments may be performed according to repeated blood tests in individual patients.'

Abnormalities of lipid metabolism

Intravenous fat administration can induce several abnormalities in lipid metabolism such as hypercholesterolaemia and lipoprotein-X formation, hypertriglyceridaemia or, exceptionally, the fat overloading syndrome (Wesson *et al.*, 1984; Dahlstrom *et al.*, 1988; Haber *et al.*, 1988).

Hypercholesterolaemia and lipoprotein-X formation

Hypercholesterolaemia represents the most common alteration in serum lipids in PN patients. The administration of fat emulsions can result in an increase of plasma total cholesterol and phospholipid concentrations and a decrease in HDL-cholesterol while the abnormal lipoprotein-X is formed. Some authors have suggested that hypercholesterolaemia is caused by excessive provision of phospholipids, which mobilizes free cholesterol from extravascular tissue to the vascular compartment (Untracht, 1982). The phospholipid/triacylglycerol ratio is considered to be an important factor affecting these abnormalities: in fact, these changes are more frequent with 10% emulsions, whereas administrations of 20% or 30% emulsions are associated with minor changes only (Rigaud *et al.*, 1984; Haumont *et al.*, 1989; Meguid *et al.*, 1989; Hajri *et al.*, 1990; Garcia-de-Lorenzo *et al.*, 2003). One study, performed in post-operative short-term PN, has also suggested that abnormal lipoprotein-X occurred least with the MCT/LCT 20% fat infusion compared with the 20% LCT emulsion or the 10% MCT/LCT or LCT emulsions (Hailer *et al.*, 1998). However, these effects occur apparently without increasing the atherogenic risk. Usually, unlike associated patient-related factors, hypercholesterolaemia and lipoprotein-X formation may not be deleterious in HPN patients, especially if lipids are not provided in excess (Carpentier (1993) recommends a rate of triacylglycerol administration not exceeding 0.15 g/kg body weight/h in home patients on cyclic nocturnal PN, and other authors recommend rates as low as 0.03–0.05 g/kg body weight/h (Jensen *et al.*, 1990; Miles, 1991)) and patients are assessed regularly for these potential complications.

Hypertriglyceridaemia

Hypertriglyceridaemia (i.e. triglycerides >4.6 mmol/l) appears when the metabolic capacity to clear infused lipids is exceeded. It is important to note that the occurrence of hypertriglyceridaemia depends not only on the amount of infused lipids, but also is greatly influenced by other factors such as accompanying hyperglycaemia, presence of renal insufficiency, concomitant administration of corticosteroids, as well as disease severity. Therefore, correction of hypertriglyceridaemia occurring in a patient on HPN should combine the adjustment of lipid provision and the correction of patient-related factors (Llop *et al.*, 2003). As for hypercholesterolaemia, hypertriglyceridaemia is often simple to avoid or to correct. In addition to correction of the above-mentioned factors, several authors have proposed either a short-term withdrawal of the lipid fraction from the PN admixture (Visschers *et al.*, 2011) or to replace the conventional lipid emulsion by a fish oil intravenous fat emulsion (Gura *et al.*, 2007) for the management of PN-complicating hypertriglyceridaemia. However, these strategies have to be validated in future trials.

Lipid peroxidation in lipid-based HPN

There are two main defence systems in humans against lipid peroxidation: (i) mineral-dependent enzymes (in particular, superoxide dismutase and glutathione peroxidase); and (ii) tocopherols (vitamin E), the most active being α-tocopherol. Vitamin E interacts directly with lipid peroxides to neutralize them in plasma lipoproteins and cell membranes, and therefore vitamin E requirements should be appropriately determined and covered (Biesalski, 2009). Lipid peroxides are labile species that can undergo further decomposition to give products such as malondialdehyde (MDA) and volatile carbohydrates (pentane and ethane), which can be measured in the serum (MDA) and in the breath (pentane). Both breath-pentane output and serum MDA concentration are considered to be sensitive methods to assess *in vivo* lipid peroxidation in humans. In adult HPN patients, high breath pentane (Lemoyne *et al.*, 1988; Van Gossum *et al.*, 1988) and increased MDA concentrations (Pironi *et al.*, 1998; Reimund *et al.*, 2000) have been reported and are associated with decreased vitamin E concentrations (Lemoyne *et al.*, 1988; Van Gossum *et al.*, 1988; Pironi *et al.*, 1998; Reimund *et al.*, 2000) and the PUFA load (Pironi *et al.*, 1998). However, increased lipid peroxidation in adult HPN patients has until now not been associated with a detectable biological or clinical deleterious effect. The question is more critical in paediatric HPN, in particular in neonates or preterm infants, where some reports suggested that depending on the composition of the PN, oxidative stress triggering an inappropriate systemic inflammatory response could occur under certain conditions such as a high exposure to oxygen (Lavoie *et al.*, 2010). Nevertheless, this question remains a matter of debate (Roggero *et al.*, 2010) and no clear correlation with a significant decrease in PN efficacy or an increase in morbidity has been found (Perrone *et al.*, 2007). Despite the potential low impact on HPN outcome, lipid peroxidation has been studied using an olive oil-based lipid emulsion (Clinoleic®, Clintec/Baxter) as it provides less PUFAs and higher vitamin E levels than traditional LCT or MCT/LCT emulsions. In a double-blinded randomized study conducted in paediatric patients over 60 days of PN, the peroxidation index was significantly lower with the olive oil-based infusion (Goulet *et al.*, 1999).

Comparably, in stable adult HPN patients, despite a decrease in MDA concentrations in adults receiving Clinoleic® for a 3-month period at the same amount as their initial lipid emulsion (LCTs or MCTs/LCTs), the difference did not reach statistical significance (Reimund *et al.*, 2005). In summary, adequate vitamin E (in particular α-tocopherol) supply seems to be the best strategy to limit lipid peroxidation in HPN patients. Whether olive oil-based or newer lipid emulsions may induce lower lipid peroxidation remains to be proven definitively.

Intravenous lipids and infectious risk

Compared with patients receiving no artificial nutrition (Snydman *et al.*, 1982; The Veterans Affairs Total Parenteral Nutrition Cooperative Study Group, 1991) or patients on standard polymeric enteral nutrition (Moore *et al.*, 1992; Bozzetti *et al.*, 2001; Marik and Zagola, 2004) or immune-enhancing enteral nutrition (Braga *et al.*, 1998), PN is associated with a higher rate of infectious complications (Gillanders *et al.*, 2012), despite some studies in selected situations of short-term PN not confirming these results (Pacelli *et al.*, 2001). However, whether lipids in PN, especially in HPN, may be a metabolic bystander of this increased risk still remains a matter of debate. Considering available clinical studies in HPN patients, no strong data incriminate lipid emulsions by themselves (independently of their composition) as a culprit. Furthermore, rare data suggest that the type of fat emulsion used (LCTs, MCTs/LCTs, olive oil-based) does not influence the infectious rate in this patient group (Reimund *et al.*, 2005; Vahedi *et al.*, 2005).

HPN-associated liver disease and lipid emulsions

Shortly after the introduction of PN, a spectrum of PN-associated liver dysfunctions and diseases were reported in children and adult patients at a rate ranging from 15% to 85% (Sheldon *et al.*, 1978; Whitington, 1985; Baker and Rosenberg, 1987; Stanko *et al.*, 1987; Sax and Bower, 1988; Clarke *et al.*, 1991). Reported hepatic disturbances during PN include increase in liver-associated enzyme blood activities, steatosis, steatohepatitis, steatonecrosis, intrahepatic cholestasis, fibrosis and cirrhosis. Usually, these changes are not extreme and are reversible after adapting or, if needed, stopping PN. However, some patients (especially those requiring long-term PN, i.e. HPN patients) may develop progressive hepatic failure that can lead to death in a few cases. A multifactorial pathogenesis has been proposed including both patient-related factors and nutritional factors (Quigley *et al.*, 1993; Gabe, 2013). Lipids are considered one of the principal factors responsible for HPN-associated liver disease both in children (Colomb *et al.*, 2000) and adults (Gerard-Boncompain *et al.*, 1992), as they generate pro-inflammatory eicosanoids (prostaglandin E2, prostacyclin I2, leukotrienes B4, C4 and E4) through arachidonic acid (20:4*n*-6) metabolism and contain potentially toxic phytosterols (Clayton *et al.*, 1998; Iyer *et al.*, 1998; Ellegård *et al.*, 2005). However, the responsibility of lipids should also be considered with respect to the amount provided, as Cavicchi *et al.* (2000) from Messing's group clearly found an association between liver disease and a parenteral lipid intake greater than 1 g/kg body weight/day, with a relative risk of developing chronic cholestasis of 2.3 and a relative risk of advanced disease of 5.5. In the case of lower lipid provision in HPN patients, they may not strongly contribute to HPN-associated liver disease. In that case, other factors such as total calories and intravenous carbohydrate calorie load (Reimund *et al.*, 2001; Luman and Shaffer, 2002; Baker and Nightingale, 2004), underlying disease (in particular, ongoing inflammation) (McCowen *et al.*, 2000; Reimund *et al.*, 2001; Forrest *et al.*, 2002; Baker and Nightingale, 2004), intestinal bacterial overgrowth and translocation (Gunsar *et al.*, 2002) and/or frequent sepsis (catheter-related infection) should be considered and, if necessary, corrected (Dickerson and Karwoski, 2002; Howard and Ashley, 2003; Baker and Nightingale, 2004).

Despite the precise mechanism(s) leading to PN (HPN)-complicating liver disease not being fully understood, it has been hypothesized that infusion of too high amounts of lipids generates a lipid overload in liver macrophages resulting in an impaired phospholipid excretion into bile and thereby causing intrahepatic cholestasis (Cavicchi *et al.*, 2000). Lipid infusion has also been considered to inhibit hepatic triglyceride release (Luman and Shaffer, 2002) and, as stated earlier, to induce phytosterol accumulation (Clayton *et al.*, 1998; Kast *et al.*, 2002; Carter *et al.*, 2007).

Are PN-associated abnormalities related to the composition of lipid emulsions? This question is important but currently not completely resolved. Some studies suggested that lipid emulsions composed of 50% MCTs and 50% LCTs or structured lipids may have a lesser impact on liver function (Baldermann *et al.*, 1991; Jaurrieta *et al.*, 1991; Rubin *et al.*, 2000); however, these data have not reached any consensus. Preliminary observations also suggested that olive oil-based PN may reduce the impact of lipid emulsions on liver tests both in short-term (Garcia-de-Lorenzo *et al.*, 2005) and long-term PN (Reimund *et al.*, 2004). Nevertheless, these data have to be confirmed by prospective large-scale studies.

Studies with the fish oil-based emulsion Omegaven® (Fresenius Kabi AG), which does not contain phytosterols (Fallon *et al.*, 2010), have been performed during the past few years, in particular in paediatric PN. In children with short bowel syndrome who developed chronic cholestasis during HPN containing a soybean oil, Gura *et al.* (2008) showed that the introduction of Omegaven® resulted in a shorter time to cholestasis reversal (9 weeks versus 44 weeks in a historical cohort). This was also observed by Puder *et al.* (2009), who reported that 50% of infants receiving Omegaven® demonstrated reversal of cholestasis compared with 6% of a historical group. These results are encouraging but subject to a potential bias as the amounts of lipids infused were usually lower in the fish oil groups, a factor that by itself could explain the reversal of cholestasis (Colomb *et al.*, 2000). Therefore, further work (ideally randomized studies in children and in adults) is necessary to definitively assess the protective role of *n*-3 fatty acid-based lipid emulsions.

Finally, Smoflipid® (Fresenius Kabi AG) – a complex mixture of MCTs, LCTs, olive oil and fish oil (Table 23.2) – has been evaluated in two randomized controlled clinical trials respectively in paediatric ($n=28$) and adult ($n=73$) patients on long-term PN for stable chronic intestinal failure (Goulet *et al.*, 2010; Klek *et al.*, 2013). Smoflipid® decreased the *n*-6/*n*-3 PUFA ratio, increased plasma α-tocopherol concentrations (without any change in lipid peroxidation parameters) and finally improved transaminase activities and bilirubin concentrations in the study performed in adults.

Summary

Fat emulsions containing LCTs or a mixture of MCTs/LCTs have been used successfully as an essential part of HPN. Until recently HPN has usually been organized in referral centres providing high expertise both in PN management itself and in treating the usually severe underlying diseases. HPN most commonly uses AIO bags, the composition of which depends on patients' requirements. These AIO bags are infused over a 10–14 h cyclic nocturnal period in the majority of patients, via a central venous access, using an infusion pump, and ideally in patients where a minimal oral intake remains possible. The number of AIO bags administered per week may vary from one patient to another according to their specific nutritional needs. Therefore, no standard lipid content can be recommended. In most patients, lipids are present in 1:2 or 1:3 AIO bags/week. In adult patients, minimal fat supply may be about 0.7 (or less, but under repeated control in order to detect subclinical EFAD) to 1 g/kg body weight/day, this value being the maximal lipid provision to protect patients from severe HPN-complicating liver disease. Systematic and frequent surveillance of clinical nutritional parameters as well as biological markers (serum cholesterol and triglyceride concentrations, Holman index, liver function tests, etc.) may allow tight adaptation of the optimal amount of lipid emulsions required by each individual patient. The safety of newer lipid emulsions has been reported in children (Goulet *et al.*, 1999) and adults (Reimund *et al.*, 2005; Vahedi *et al.*, 2005) for an olive oil-based lipid emulsion (Clinoleic®, Clintec/Baxter) as well as for structured lipids (Structolipid®, Fresenius Kabi AG). These studies suggest that these emulsions did not increase the risk of complications in patients with chronic intestinal failure on HPN but, at the same time, do not yet report significant advantages despite some indication for lesser lipid peroxidation in one study in paediatric HPN patients with Clinoleic® (Goulet *et al.*, 1999), an immune neutrality in adult HPN patients after 3-month Clinoleic® administration (Reimund *et al.*, 2005) and some minor data suggesting potentially a better hepatic tolerance for both Clinoleic® (Reimund *et al.*, 2004) and Structolipid® (Rubin *et al.*, 2000). In our study, the observed results are confirmed for a period of more than 2 years, as patients enrolled in the study continue to receive Clinoleic® as lipid source (personal observation). These results have to be confirmed in larger studies on long-term administration. Fish oil-based lipid emulsions are also of particular interest. They do not contain phytosterols (Fallon *et al.*, 2010) and have been advocated to prevent or correct HPN-complicating cholestatic disease in paediatric patients (Gura *et al.*, 2008; Puder *et al.*, 2009). However, additional data are needed to confirm this assumption both in children and adults dependent on HPN. Complex lipid emulsions (i.e. Smoflipid®) seem more encouraging as attested by two recently published studies (Goulet *et al.*, 2010; Klek *et al.*, 2013). Nevertheless, more data in more prolonged PN is necessary to appreciate their real interest in HPN.

References

Abushufa, R., Reed, P., Weinkove, C., Wales, S. and Shaffer, J. (1995) Essential fatty acid status in patients on long-term home parenteral nutrition. *JPEN Journal of Parenteral and Enteral Nutrition* 19, 286–290.

Arimoto, I., Saito, H., Kawashima, Y., Miyajima, K. and Handa, T. (1998) Effects of sphingomyelin and cholesterol on lipoprotein lipase-mediated lipolysis in lipid emulsions. *Journal of Lipid Research* 39, 143–151.

Baker, A.L. and Rosenberg, I.H. (1987) Hepatic complications of total parenteral nutrition. *American Journal of Medicine* 82, 489–497.

Baker, N.L. and Nightingale, J.M.D. (2004) Abnormal liver function tests and parenteral nutrition. *Clinical Nutrition* 23, 864–865 (abstract).

Baldermann, H., Wicklmayr, M., Rett, K., Banholzer, P., Dietze, G. and Mehnert, H. (1991) Changes of hepatic morphology during parenteral nutrition with lipid emulsions containing LCT or MCT/LCT quantified by ultrasound. *JPEN Journal of Parenteral and Enteral Nutrition* 15, 601–603.

Biesalski, H.K. (2009) Vitamin E requirements in parenteral nutrition. *Gastroenterology* 137(5 Suppl.), 92–104.

Bozzetti, F., Cozzaglio, L., Gavazzi, C., Bonfanti, G., Lattarulo, M. and Gennari, L. (1996) Total nutritional manipulation in humans: report of a cancer patient. *Clinical Nutrition* 15, 207–209.

Bozzetti, F., Gavazzi, C., Mariani, L. and Crippa, F. (1999) Artificial nutrition in cancer patients: which route, what composition? *World Journal of Surgery* 23, 577–583.

Bozzetti, F., Braga, M., Gianotti, L., Gavazzi, C. and Mariani, L. (2001) Postoperative enteral versus parenteral nutrition in malnourished patients with gastrointestinal cancer: a randomised multicentre trial. *The Lancet* 358, 1487–1492.

Bozzetti, F., Cozzaglio, L., Biganzoli, E., Chiavenna, G., De Cicco, M., Donati, D., Gilli, G., Percolla, S. and Pironi, L. (2002) Quality of life and length of survival in advanced cancer patients on home parenteral nutrition. *Clinical Nutrition* 21, 281–288.

Bozzetti, F., Gavazzi, C., Mariani, L. and Crippa, F. (2004) Glucose-based total parenteral nutrition does not stimulate glucose uptake by human tumours. *Clinical Nutrition* 23, 417–421.

Braga, M., Gianotti, L., Vignali, A., Cestari, A., Bisagni, P. and Di Carlo, V. (1998) Artificial nutrition after major abdominal surgery: impact of route of administration and composition of the diet. *Critical Care Medicine* 26, 24–30.

Burr, L.H., Dunn, G.D. and Brennan, M.F. (1981) Essential fatty acid deficiency during parenteral nutrition. *Annals of Surgery* 193, 304–311.

Carpentier, Y.A. (1993) Lipid emulsions. In: Fürst, P. (ed.) *New Strategies in Clinical Nutrition.* Zuckschwerdt, San Francisco, California, pp. 52–63.

Carpentier, Y.A. and Dupont, I.E. (2000) Advances in intravenous lipid emulsions. *World Journal of Surgery* 24, 1493–1497.

Carter, B.A., Taylor, O.A., Prendergast, D.R., Zimmermann, T.L., Van Furstenberg, R., Moore, D.D. and Karpen, S.J. (2007) Stigmasterol, a soy lipid-derived phytosterol, is an antagonist of bile acid nuclear receptor FXR. *Pediatric Research* 62, 301–306.

Cavicchi, M., Beau, P., Crenn, P., Degott, C. and Messing, B. (2000) Prevalence of liver disease and contributing factors in patients receiving home parenteral nutrition for permanent intestinal failure. *Annals of Internal Medicine* 132, 525–532.

Clarke, P.J., Ball, M.J. and Kettlewell, M.G.W. (1991) Liver function tests in patients receiving parenteral nutrition. *JPEN Journal of Parenteral and Enteral Nutrition* 15, 54–59.

Cederholm, T.E., Berg, A.B., Johansson, E.K., Hellstrom, K.H. and Palmblad, J.E. (1994) Low levels of essential fatty acids are related to impaired delayed skin hypersensitivity in

malnourished chronically elderly people. *European Journal of Clinical Investigation* 24, 615–620.
Chambrier, C., Garcia, I., Gérard-Boncompain, M. and Boulétreau, P. (1998) Fatty acids composition of plasma lipoproteins in patients receiving home parenteral nutrition. *Clinical Nutrition* 17(Suppl. 1), 52–53.
Chambrier, C., Bannier, E., Lauverjat, M., Dray, J., Bryssine, S. and Bouletreau, P. (2004) Replacement of a long-chain triglyceride with medium-chain triglyceride/long-chain triglyceride lipid emulsion in patients receiving long-term parenteral nutrition: effects on essential fatty acid status and plasma vitamin K1 levels. *JPEN Journal of Parenteral and Enteral Nutrition* 28, 7–12.
Chenaud, C., Merlani, P.G., Roux-Lombard, P., Burger, D., Harbarth, S., Luyasu, S., Graf, J.D., Dayer, J.M. and Ricou, B. (2004) Low apolipoprotein A-I level at intensive care unit admission and systemic inflammatory response syndrome exacerbation. *Critical Care Medicine* 32, 632–637.
Clayton, P.T., Whitfield, P. and Iyer, K. (1998) The role of phytosterols in the pathogenesis of liver complications of pediatric parenteral nutrition. *Nutrition* 14, 158–164.
Collins, F.D., Sinclair, A.J., Royle, J.P., Coats, D.A., Maynard, A.T. and Leonard, R.F. (1971) Plasma lipid in human linoleic acid deficiency. *Nutrition and Metabolism* 13, 150–167.
Colomb, V., Jobert-Giraud, A., Lacaille, F., Goulet, O., Fournet, J.C. and Ricour, C. (2000) Role of lipid emulsions in cholestasis associated with long-term parenteral nutrition in children. *JPEN Journal of Parenteral and Enteral Nutrition* 24, 345–350.
Cooper, A.D. (1997) Hepatic uptake of chylomicron remnants. *Journal of Lipid Research* 38, 2173–2192.
Dahlstrom, K.A., Goulet, O.J., Roberts, R.L., Ricour, C. and Ament, M.E. (1988) Lipid tolerance in children receiving long-term parenteral nutrition: a biochemical and immunologic study. *Journal of Pediatrics* 113, 985–990.
Davis, S.S. (1983) The stability of fat emulsions for intravenous administration. In: Johnston, I.D.A. (ed.) *Advances in Clinical Nutrition.* MTP Press, Lancaster, UK, pp. 213–239.
Deckelbaum, R.J., Calder, P.C. and Carpentier, Y.A. (2004) Using different intravenous lipids: underutilized therapeutic approaches? *Current Opinion in Clinical Nutrition and Metabolic Care* 7, 113–115.
Dickerson, R.N. and Karwoski, C.B. (2002) Endotoxin-mediated hepatic lipid accumulation during parenteral nutrition in rats. *Journal of the American College of Nutrition* 21, 351–356.
Driscoll, D.F. (2005) Stability and compatibility assessment techniques for total parenteral nutrition admixtures: setting the bar according to pharmacopeial standards. *Current Opinion in Clinical Nutrition and Metabolic Care* 8, 297–303.
Driscoll, D.F. (2006) Lipid injectable emulsions: pharmacopeial and safety issues. *Pharmaceutical Research* 23, 1959–1969.
Driscoll, D.F., Ling, P.R. and Bistrian, P.R. (2007) Physical stability of 20% injectable lipid emulsions via simulated syringe infusion: effect of glass vs plastic product packaging. *JPEN Journal of Parenteral and Enteral Nutrition* 31, 148–153.
Driscoll, D.F., Silvestri, A.P. and Bistrian, P.R. (2010) Stability of MCT/LCT-based total nutrient admixture for neonatal use over 30 hours at room temperature: applying pharmacopeial standards. *JPEN Journal of Parenteral and Enteral Nutrition* 34, 305–312.
Dupont, I. and Carpentier, Y.A. (1999) Clinical use of lipid emulsions. *Current Opinion in Clinical Nutrition and Metabolic Care* 2, 139–145.
Ellegård, L., Sunesson, Å. and Bosaeus, I. (2005) High serum phytosterol levels in short bowel patients on parenteral nutrition support. *Clinical Nutrition* 24, 415–420.
Fallon, E.M., Le, H.D. and Puder, M. (2010) Prevention of parenteral nutrition-associated liver disease: role of omega-3 fish oil. *Current Opinion in Organ Transplantation* 15, 334–340.

Ferezou, J. and Bach, A. (1999) Structure and metabolic fate of triacylglycerol- and phospholipids-rich particles of commercial parenteral fat emulsions. *Nutrition* 15, 44–50.

Forrest, E.H., Oien, K.A., Dickson, S., Galloway, D. and Mills, P.R. (2002) Improvement in cholestasis associated with total parenteral nutrition after treatment with an antibody against tumour necrosis factor alpha. *Liver* 22, 317–320.

Freshwater, D.A., Saadeddin, A., Deel-Smith, P., Digger, T. and Jones, B.J. (2005) Can home parenteral nutrition be provided by non-specialised centres? 2300 weeks of experience at a district general hospital in the United Kingdom. *Clinical Nutrition* 24, 229–235.

Gabe, S.M. (2013) Lipids and liver dysfunction in patients receiving parenteral nutrition. *Current Opinion in Clinical Nutrition and Metabolic Care* 16, 150–155.

Garcia-de-Lorenzo, A., Lopez-Martinez, J., Planas, M., Chacon, P., Montejo, J.C., Bonet, A., Ortiz-Leyba, C., Sanchez-Segura, J.M., Ordonez, J., Acosta, J., Grau, T. and Jimenez, F.J. (2003) Safety and metabolic tolerance of a concentrated long-chain triglyceride lipid emulsion in critically ill septic and trauma patients. *JPEN Journal of Parenteral and Enteral Nutrition* 27, 208–215.

Garcia-de-Lorenzo, A., Denia, R., Atlan, P., Martinez-Ratero, S., Le Brun, A., Evard, D. and Bereziat, G. (2005) Parenteral nutrition providing a restricted amount of linoleic acid in severely burned patients: a randomised double-blind study of an olive oil-based lipid emulsion *v.* medium/long-chain triacylglycerols. *British Journal of Nutrition* 94, 221–230.

Gerard-Boncompain, M., Claudel, J.P., Gaussorgues, P., Salord, F., Sirodot, M., Chevallier, M. and Robert, D. (1992) Hepatic cytolytic and cholestatic changes related to a change of lipid emulsions in four long-term parenteral nutrition patients with short bowel. *JPEN Journal of Parenteral and Enteral Nutrition* 16, 494–495.

Gillanders, L., Angstmann, K., Ball, P., O'Callaghan, M., Thompson, A., Wong, T. and Thomas, M. (2012) A prospective study of catheter-related complications in HPN patients. *Clinical Nutrition* 31, 30–34.

Goulet, O., de Potter, S., Antébi, H., Driss, F., Colomb, V., Bereziat, G., Alcindor, L.G., Corriol, O., Le Brun, A., Dutot, G., Forget, D., Perennec, V. and Ricour, C. (1999) Long-term efficacy and safety of a new olive oil-base intravenous fat emulsion in pediatric patients: a double-blind randomized study. *American Journal of Clinical Nutrition* 70, 338–345.

Goulet, O., Antébi, H., Wolf, C., Talbotec, C., Alcindor, L.G., Corriol, O., Lamor, M. and Colomb-Jung, V. (2010) A new intravenous fat emulsion containing soybean oil, medium-chain triglycerides, olive oil, and fish oil: a single-center, double-blind randomized study on efficacy and safety in pediatric patients receiving home parenteral nutrition. *JPEN Journal of Parenteral and Enteral Nutrition* 34, 485–495.

Gunsar, C., Melek, M., Karaca, I., Sencan, A., Mir, E., Ortac, R. and Canan, O. (2002) The biochemical and histopathological effects of ursodeoxycholic acid and metronidazole on total parenteral nutrition-associated hepatic dysfunction: an experimental study. *Hepato-gastroenterology* 49, 497–500.

Gura, K., Strijbosch, R., Arnold, S., McPherson, C. and Puder, M. (2007) The role of an intravenous fat emulsion composed of fish-oil in a parenteral nutrition-dependent patient with hypertriglyceridemia. *Nutrition in Clinical Practice* 22, 664–672.

Gura, K.M., Lee, S., Valim, C., Zhou, J., Kim, S., Modi, B.P., Arsenault, D.A., Strijbosch, R.A., Lopes, S., Duggan, C. and Puder, M. (2008) Safety and efficacy of a fish-oil-based fat emulsion in the treatment of parenteral nutrition-associated liver disease. *Pediatrics* 121, 678–686.

Haber, L.M., Hawkins, E.P., Seilheimer, D.K. and Saleem, A. (1988) Fat overload syndrome. An autopsy study with evaluation of the coagulopathy. *American Journal of Clinical Pathology* 89, 223–227.

Hailer, S., Jauch, K.W. and Wolfram, G. (1998) Influence of different fat emulsions with 10 or 20% MCT/LCT or LCT on lipoproteins in plasma of patients after abdominal surgery. *Annals of Nutrition and Metabolism* 42, 170–180.

Hajri, T., Férézou, J. and Lutton, C. (1990) Effects of intravenous infusions of commercial fat emulsions (Intralipid 10 or 20%) on rat plasma lipoproteins: phospholipids in excess are the main precursor of lipoprotein-X-like particles. *Biochimica et Biophysica Acta* 1047, 121–130.

Hamilton, C., Austin, T. and Seidner, D.L. (2006) Essential fatty acid deficiency in human adults during parenteral nutrition. *Nutrition in Clinical Practice* 21, 387–394.

Hardy, G. and Puzovic, M. (2009) Formulation, stability, and administration of parenteral nutrition with new lipid emulsions. *Nutrition in Clinical Practice* 24, 616–625.

Haumont, D., Deckelbaum, R.J., Richelle, M., Dhalan, W., Coussaert, E., Bihain, B.E. and Carpentier, Y.A. (1989) Plasma lipid and plasma lipoprotein concentrations in low birth weight infants given parenteral nutrition with twenty or ten percent lipid emulsion. *Journal of Pediatrics* 115, 787–793.

Haumont, D., Richelle, M., Deckelbaum, R.J., Coussaert, E. and Carpentier, Y.A. (1992) Effect of liposomal content of lipid emulsions on plasma lipids in low birth weight infants receiving parenteral nutrition. *Journal of Pediatrics* 121, 759–763.

Havel, R.J. (1998) Receptor and non-receptor mediated uptake of chylomicron remnants by the liver. *Atherosclerosis* 141(Suppl. 1), 1–7.

Holman, R.T., Smythe, L. and Johnson, F. (1979) Effect of sex and age on fatty acids composition of human serum lipids. *American Journal of Clinical Nutrition* 32, 2390–2399.

Howard, L. and Ashley, C. (2003) Management of patients receiving home parenteral nutrition. *Gastroenterology* 124, 1651–1661.

Howard, L., Heaphey, L., Fleming, C.R., Liniger, L. and Steiger, E. (1991) Four years of North American registry home parenteral nutrition outcome data and their implications for patients management. *JPEN Journal of Parenteral and Enteral Nutrition* 15, 384–393.

Hulsey, T.K., Burnham, S.J., Neblett, W.W., O'Neill, J.A. Jr and Meng, H.C. (1977) Delayed burn wound healing in essential fatty acids deficiency. *Surgery Forum* 28, 31–32.

Hyltander, A., Sandström, R. and Lundholm, K. (1995) Metabolic effects of structured triglycerides in humans. *Nutrition in Clinical Practice* 10, 91–97.

Ireton-Jones, C. and DeLegge, M. (2005) Home parenteral nutrition registry: a five-year retrospective evaluation of outcomes of patients receiving home parenteral nutrition support. *Nutrition* 21, 156–160.

Iyer, K.R., Spitz, L. and Clayton, P. (1998) BAPS prize lecture: New insights into mechanisms of parenteral nutrition-associated cholestasis: role of plant sterols. British Association of Paediatric Surgeons. *Journal of Pediatric Surgery* 33, 1–6.

Jalabert, A., Grand, A., Steghens, J.P., Barbotte, E., Pique, C. and Picaud, J.C. (2011) Lipid peroxidation in all-in-one admixtures for preterm neonates: impact of amounts of lipid, type of lipid emulsion and delivery condition. *Acta Paediatrica* 100, 1200–1205.

Jaurrieta, E., Biondo, S., Rafecas, A., Moreno-Llorente, P., Murgoitio, G., Llop, J., Fabregat, J. and Figueras, J. (1991) A comparative study of hepatic cholestasis after infusion of a long chain triglycerides and a mixture of medium and long chain triglycerides. *Nutrición Hospitalaria* 6, 152–155.

Jensen, G.L., Masciolo, E.A., Seidner, D.L., Istfan, N.W., Domnitch, A.M., Selleck, K., Babayan, V.K., Blackburn, G.L. and Bistrian, B.R. (1990) Parenteral infusion of long- and medium-chain triglycerides and reticuloendothelial system function in man. *JPEN Journal of Parenteral and Enteral Nutrition* 14, 467–471.

Jeppesen, P.B., Christensen, M.S., Høy, C.-E. and Mortensen, P.B. (1997) Essential fatty acid deficiency in patients with severe fat malabsorption. *American Journal of Clinical Nutrition* 65, 837–843.

Jeppesen, P.B., Høy, C.E. and Mortensen, P.B. (1998) Essential fatty acid deficiency in patients receiving home parenteral nutrition. *American Journal of Clinical Nutrition* 68, 126–133.

Jonkers-Schuitema, C.F., Sauerwein, H.P. and Tas, T.H. (2005) Can home parenteral nutrition be provided by non-specialized centres? The Dutch experience. *Clinical Nutrition* 24, 526–527.

Kalfarentzos, F., Kokkinis, K., Leukaditi, K., Maroulis, J., Onoufriou, A. and Alexopoulos, K. (1998) Comparison between two fat emulsions: Intralipid 30% vs Intralipid 10% in critically ill patients. *Clinical Nutrition* 17, 31–34.

Karpe, F., Humphreys, S.M., Samra, J.S., Summers, L.K. and Frayn, K.N. (1997) Clearance of lipoprotein remnant particles in adipose tissue and muscle in humans. *Journal of Lipid Research* 38, 2335–2343.

Kast, H.R., Goodwin, B., Tarr, P.T., Jones, S.A., Anesfeld, A.M., Stoltz, C.M., Tontonov, P., Kliewer, S., Willson, T.M. and Edwards, P.A. (2002) Regulation of multidrug resistance-associated protein 2 (ABCC2) by the nuclear receptors pregnane X receptor, farnesoid X-activated receptor, and constitutive androstane receptor. *Journal of Biological Chemistry* 277, 2908–2915.

Klek, S., Chambrier, C., Singer, P., Rubin, M., Staun, M., Joly, F., Rasmussen, H., Strauss, B.J., Wanten, G., Smith, R., Abraham, A., Szczepanek, K. and Shaffer, J. (2013) Four-week parenteral nutrition using a third generation lipid emulsion (SMOFlipid) – a double-blind, randomised, multicentre study in adults. *Clinical Nutrition* 32, 224–231.

Lambert, M.S., Avella, M.A., Berhane, Y., Sherville, E. and Botham, K.M. (2001) The fatty acid composition of chylomicron remnants influences their binding and internalization by isolated hepatocytes. *European Journal of Biochemistry* 268, 3983–3992.

Lavoie, P.M., Lavoie, J.C., Watson, C., Rouleau, T., Chang, B.A. and Chessex, P. (2010) Inflammatory response in preterm infants is induced early in life by oxygen and modulated by total parenteral nutrition. *Pediatric Research* 68, 248–251.

Lemoyne, M., Van Gossum, A., Kurian, R. and Jeejeebhoy, K.N. (1988) Plasma vitamin E and selenium and breath pentane in home parenteral nutrition patients. *American Journal of Clinical Nutrition* 48, 1310–1315.

Llop, J., Sabin, P., Garau, M. and the Hospital Pharmacy Artificial Nutrition Group of Catalonia (2003) The importance of clinical factors in parenteral nutrition-associated hypertriglyceridemia. *Clinical Nutrition* 22, 577–583.

Luman, W. and Shaffer, J.L. (2002) Prevalence, outcome and associated factors of deranged liver function tests in patients on home parenteral nutrition. *Clinical Nutrition* 21, 337–343.

Lumpkin, M.M. (1994) Safety alert: hazards of precipitation associated with parenteral nutrition. *American Journal of Hospital Pharmacy* 51, 1427–1428.

Marik, P.E. and Zagola, G.P. (2004) Meta-analysis of parenteral nutrition versus enteral nutrition in patients with acute pancreatitis. *British Journal of Medicine* 328, 1407–1412.

Martins, I.J., Vilchèze, C., Mortimer, B.-C., Bittman, R. and Redgrave, T.G. (1998) Sterol side chain length and structure affect the clearance of chylomicron-like lipid emulsions in rats and mice. *Journal of Lipid Research* 39, 302–312.

Mascioli, E.A., Lopes, S.M., Champagne, C. and Driscoll, D.F. (1996) Essential fatty acid deficiency and home parenteral nutrition. *Nutrition* 12, 245–249.

McCowen, K., Burke, P.A. and Bistrian, B.R. (2000) Liver disease and home parenteral nutrition. *Annals of Internal Medicine* 133, 1009–1010.

Meguid, M.M., Kurzer, M., Hayashi, R.J. and Akahoshi, M.P. (1989) Short-term effects of fat emulsion on serum lipids on postoperative patients. *JPEN Journal of Parenteral and Enteral Nutrition* 13, 77–80.

Messing, B., Lemann, M., Landais, P., Gouttebel, M.C., Gerard-Boncompain, M., Saudin, F., Van Gosuum, A., Beau, P., Guedon, C., Barnoud, D., Beliah, M., Joyeux, H., Bouletreau, P., Robert, D., Matuchansky, C., Leverve, X., Lerebours, E., Carpentier, Y. and Rambaud, J.-C. (1995) Prognosis of patients with non-malignant chronic intestinal failure receiving long-term home parenteral nutrition. *Gastroenterology* 108, 1005–1010.

Messing, B., Barnoud, D., Beau, P., Bornet, J.L., Chambrier, C., Di Costanzo, J.D., Gerard-Boncompain, M., Guedon, C., Hebuterne, X., Heresbach, D., de Ledinghen, V., Lescut, D.,

Reimund, J.M., Senesse, P., Beliah, M., Bouletreau, P., Bretagne, J.F., Descos, L., Duclos, B., Kerjean, A., Lerebours, E., Leverve, X., Morichau-Beauchant, M., Paris, J.C., Robert, D., Saint-Aubert, B. and Rampal, P. (1998) A 1993–1995 epidemiological survey of home parenteral nutrition in approved centers for adults in France. *Gastroentérologie Clinique et Biologique* 22, 413–418.

Miles, J.M. (1991) Intravenous fat emulsions in nutritional support. *Current Opinion in Gastroenterology* 7, 306–311.

Moore, F.A., Feliciano, D.V., Andrassy, R.J., McArdle, A.H., Booth, F.V., Morgenstein-Wagner, T.B., Kellum, J.M. Jr, Welling, R.E. and Moore, E.E. (1992) Early enteral feeding, compared with parenteral, reduces postoperative septic complications. The results of a meta-analysis. *Annals of Surgery* 216, 172–183.

Olivecrona, G. and Olivecrona, T. (1998) Clearance of artificial triacylglycerol particles. *Current Opinion in Clinical Nutrition and Metabolic Care* 1, 143–151.

Pacelli, F., Bossola, M., Papa, V., Malerba, M., Modesti, C., Sgadari, A., Bellantone, R., Doglietto, G.B., Modesti, C. and EN-TPN Study Group (2001) Enteral vs parenteral nutrition after major abdominal surgery: an even match. *Archives of Surgery* 136, 933–936.

Perrone, S., Salvi, G., Bellieni, C.V. and Buonocore, G. (2007) Oxidative stress and nutrition in the preterm newborn. *Journal of Pediatric Gastroenterology and Nutrition* 45(Suppl. 3), 178–182.

Pironi, L., Ruggeri, E., Zolezzi, C., Savarino, L., Incasa, E., Belluzzi, A., Munarini, A., Piazzi, S., Tolomelli, M., Pizzoferrato, A. and Miglioli, M. (1998) Lipid peroxidation and antioxidant status in adults receiving lipid-based home parenteral nutrition. *American Journal of Clinical Nutrition* 68, 888–893.

Pironi, L., Paganelli, F. and Labate, A.M.M. (2003) Safety and efficacy of home parenteral nutrition for chronic intestinal failure: a 16-year experience at a single centre. *Digestive and Liver Disease* 35, 314–324.

Puder, M., Valim, C., Meisel, J.A., Le, H.D., de Meijer V.E., Robinson, E.M., Zhou, J., Duggan, C. and Gura, K.M. (2009) Parenteral fish oil improves outcomes in patients with parenteral nutrition-associated liver injury. *Annals of Surgery* 250, 395–402.

Qi, K., Seo, T., Al-Haideri, M., Vogel, T., Carpentier, Y.A. and Deckelbaum, R.J. (2002) Omega-3 triglycerides modify blood clearance and tissue targeting pathways of lipid emulsions. *Biochemistry* 41, 3119–3127.

Quigley, E.M., Marsh, M.N., Shaffer, J.L. and Markin, R.S. (1993) Hepatobiliary complications of total parenteral nutrition. *Gastroenterology* 104, 286–301.

Reimund, J.M. (2003) Home parenteral nutrition: a continuous challenge. *Gastroentérologie Clinique et Biologique* 27, 692–696.

Reimund, J.M., Devin, V., Wagner, A., Koehl, C., Baumann, R. and Duclos, B. (1998) Fatty acid status in home parenteral nutrition patients. *Clinical Nutrition* 17, 60.

Reimund, J.M., Duclos, B., Cuby, C., Malzac, D., Zimmermann, F., Dietemann, J.L., Beretz, L. and Baumann, B. (1999) Home parenteral nutrition: clinical and laboratory analysis of initial experience (1994–1997). Implications for patient management. *Annals of Nutrition and Metabolism* 43, 329–338.

Reimund, J.M., Arondel, Y., Duclos, B. and Baumann, R. (2000) Vitamins and trace elements in home parenteral nutrition patients. *Journal of Nutrition in Health and Aging* 4, 13–18 (erratum in *Journal of Nutrition in Health and Ageing* 2002, 6, 290).

Reimund, J.M., Duclos, B., Arondel, Y. and Baumann, R. (2001) Persistent inflammation and immune activation contribute to cholestasis in patients receiving home parenteral nutrition. *Nutrition* 17, 300–304.

Reimund, J.M., Arondel, Y., Joly, F., Messing, B., Duclos, B. and Baumann, R. (2004) Potential usefulness of olive oil-based lipid emulsions in selected situations of home parenteral nutrition-associated disease. *Clinical Nutrition* 23, 1418–1425.

Reimund, J.M., Rahmi, G., Escalin, G., Finck, G., Baumann, R. and Duclos, B. (2005) Efficacy and safety of an olive oil-based intravenous fat emulsion in adult patients on home parenteral nutrition. *Alimentary Pharmacology & Therapeutics* 21, 445–454.

Richelle, M., Bury, J., Kasry, A., Deckelbaum, R.J. and Carpentier, Y.A. (1986) *In vitro* exchanges of lipids and apoproteins between HDL and exogenous fat. *Clinical Nutrition* 5, 55.

Rigaud, D., Serog, P., Legrand, A., Cerf, M., Apfelbaum, M. and Bonfils, S. (1984) Quantification of lipoprotein X and its relationship to plasma lipid profile during different types of parenteral nutrition. *JPEN Journal of Parenteral and Enteral Nutrition* 8, 529–534.

Roggero, P., Mosca, F., Gianni, M.L., Orsi, A., Amato, O., Migliorisi, E., Longini, M. and Buonocore, G. (2010) F2-isoprostanes and total radical-trapping antioxidant potential in preterm infants receiving parenteral lipid emulsions. *Nutrition* 26, 551–555.

Rubin, M., Moser, A., Vaserberg, N., Greig, F., Levy, Y., Spivak, H., Ziv, Y. and Lelcuk, S. (2000) Structured triacylglycerol emulsion, containing both medium- and long-chain fatty acids, in long-term home parenteral nutrition: a double-blind randomized cross-over study. *Nutrition* 16, 95–100.

Saito, H., Miyako, Y., Handa, T. and Miyajima, K. (1997) Effect of cholesterol on apolipoprotein A-I binding to lipid bilayers and emulsions. *Journal of Lipid Research* 38, 287–294.

Santarpia, L., Alfonsi, L., Pasanisi, F., De Caprio, C., Scalfi, L. and Contaldo, F. (2006) Predictive factors of survival in patients with peritoneal carcinomatosis on home parenteral nutrition. *Nutrition* 22, 355–360.

Sax, H.C. and Bower, R.H. (1988) Hepatic complications of total parenteral nutrition. *JPEN Journal of Parenteral and Enteral Nutrition* 12, 615–618.

Schlotzer, E. and Kanning, U. (2004) Elimination and tolerance of a new parenteral lipid emulsion (SMOF) – a double-blind cross-over study in healthy male volunteers. *Annals of Nutrition and Metabolism* 48, 263–268.

Sheldon, G.F., Peterson, S.R. and Sanders, R. (1978) Hepatic dysfunction during hyperalimentation. *Archives of Surgery* 113, 504–508.

Siguel, E.N, Chee, K.M., Gong, J. and Schaefer, E.J. (1987) Criteria for essential fatty acid deficiency in plasma assessed by capillary column gas–liquid chromatography. *Clinical Chemistry* 33, 1869–1873.

Simoens, Ch., Deckelbaum, R.J. and Carpentier, Y.A. (2004) Metabolism of defined structured triglyceride particles compared to mixtures of medium and long chain triglycerides intravenously infused in dogs. *Clinical Nutrition* 23, 665–672.

Simoens, C.M., Deckelbaum, R.J., Massaud, J.J. and Carpentier, Y.A. (2008) Inclusion of 10% fish oil in mixed medium-chain triacylglycerol–long-chain triacylglycerol emulsions increases plasma triacylglycerol clearance and induces rapid eicosapentaenoic acid (C20:5*n*-3) incorporation into blood cell phospholipids. *American Journal of Clinical Nutrition* 88, 282–288.

Sinclair, H.M. (1956) Deficiency of essential fatty acids and atherosclerosis, etcetera. *The Lancet* 1, 381–383.

Sinclair, H.M. (1990) Essential fatty acids – a historical perspective. *Biochemical Society Transactions* 18, 756–761.

Smith, C.E., Curtas, S., Werkowitch, M., Kleinbeck, S.V. and Howard, L. (2002) Home parenteral nutrition: does affiliation with a national support and educational organization improve patient outcomes? *JPEN Journal of Parenteral and Enteral Nutrition* 26, 159–163.

Snydman, D.R., Murray, S.A., Kornfeld, S.J., Majka, J.A. and Ellis, C.A. (1982) Total parenteral nutrition-related infections. Prospective epidemiological study using semiquantitative methods. *American Journal of Medicine* 73, 695–699.

Stanko, R.T., Nathan, G., Mendelow, H. and Adibi, S.A. (1987) Development of hepatic cholestasis and fibrosis in patients with massive loss of intestine supported by prolonged parenteral nutrition. *Gastroenterology* 92, 197–202.
Ton, M.N., Chang, C., Carpentier, Y.A. and Deckelbaum, R.J. (2005) *In vivo* and *in vitro* properties of an intravenous lipid emulsion containing only medium chain and fish oil triglycerides. *Clinical Nutrition* 24, 492–501.
Untracht, S.H. (1982) Intravascular metabolism of an artificial transporter of triacylglycerols: alterations of serum lipoproteins resulting from total parenteral nutrition with Intralipid. *Biochimica et Biophysica Acta* 711, 176–192.
Vahedi, K., Atlan, P., Joly, F., Le Brun, A., Evard, D., Perennec, V., Roux-Haguenau, D., Bereziat, G. and Messing, B. (2005) A 3-month double-blind randomised study comparing an olive oil- with a soyabean oil-based intravenous lipid emulsion in home parenteral nutrition patients. *British Journal of Nutrition* 94, 909–916.
Van Aerde, J.E., Keelan, M., Clandinin, M.T. and Thomson, A.B. (1997) Lipids in total parenteral nutrition solutions differentially modify lipids in piglet intestinal brush border and microsomal membranes. *JPEN Journal of Parenteral and Enteral Nutrition* 21, 63–71.
Van Gossum, A., Shariff, R., Lemoyne, M., Kurian, R. and Jeejeebhoy, K.N. (1988) Increased lipid peroxidation after lipid infusion as measured by breath pentane output. *American Journal of Clinical Nutrition* 48, 1394–1399.
Van Gossum, A., Vahedi, K., Abdel-Malik, Staun, M., Pertkiewicz, M., Shaffer, J., Hebuterne, X., Beau, P., Guedon, C., Schmit, A., Tjellesen, L., Messing, B., Forbes, A. and ESPEN-HAN Working Group (2001) Clinical, social and rehabilitation status of long-term home parenteral nutrition patients: results of a European multicentre survey. *Clinical Nutrition* 20, 205–210.
The Veterans Affairs Total Parenteral Nutrition Cooperative Study Group (1991) Perioperative total parenteral nutrition in surgical patients. *New England Journal of Medicine* 325, 525–532.
Violante, G, Alfonsi, L., Santarpia, L., Cillis, M.C., Negro, G., De Caprio, C., Russo, N., Contaldo, F. and Pasanisi, F. (2006) Adult home parenteral nutrition: a clinical evaluation after a 3-years experience in a Southern European centre. *European Journal of Clinical Nutrition* 60, 58–61.
Visschers, R.G., Olde Daminck, S.W., Ghelen, J.M., Winkens, B., Soeters, P.B. and van Gemert, W.G. (2011) Treatment of hypertriglyceridemia in patients receiving parenteral nutrition. *JPEN Journal of Parenteral and Enteral Nutrition* 35, 610–615.
Wanten, G.J.A. and Calder, P.C. (2007) Immune modulation by parenteral lipid emulsions. *American Journal of Clinical Nutrition* 85, 1171–1184.
Wesson, D.E., Rich, R.H., Zlotkin, S.H. and Pencharz, P.B. (1984) Fat overload syndrome causing respiratory insufficiency. *Journal of Pediatric Surgery* 19, 777–778.
Whitington, P.F. (1985) Cholestasis associated with total parenteral nutrition in infants. *Hepatology* 5, 693–696.

24 Amino Acids, Protein and the Gut

Peter B. Soeters* and Marcel C.G. van de Poll

The University of Maastricht, Maastricht, The Netherlands

Key Points

- The gut retains ingested protein, leading to a gradual release of constituent amino acids.
- The gut actively mediates the anabolic effects of enteral nutrition.
- The protein-sparing effect of the gut is facilitated by the 'quality' of ingested protein.
- The gut is crucial in intermediary amino acid metabolism, especially in citrulline production.
- Shortage of bowel mass impairs physiological gut functions.
- By administering parenteral nutrition, the protein-sparing function of the gut is bypassed.
- Loss of enterohepatic recycling may underlie taurine deficiency in patients on parenteral nutrition.
- Beneficial effects of glutamine-enriched parenteral and enteral nutrition have been described, but more supportive evidence is required to prove efficacy conclusively.

Introduction

All living organisms from monocellular organisms to the human species need amino acids. Amino acids characteristically consist of a carbon chain with a carboxyl group and an amino group. Most amino acids are neutral and have an aliphatic or an aromatic carbon chain. Some are, however, di-acidic (glutamic acid, aspartic acid) and some dibasic (lysine, arginine, histidine). Twenty different

*E-mail: pb.soeters@maastrichtuniversity.nl

amino acids are found in human protein (Table 24.1). Of these, eight amino acids are essential (indispensable) because the human body does not have the ability to synthesize them in significant amounts and therefore has to rely on food ingestion for their supply. The other 12 amino acids can be synthesized from the eight essential amino acids, but the capacity to do this may be limited under specific conditions. Optimal diets therefore should contain, in addition to the essential amino acids, also non-essential amino acids (see further in this chapter). There is a growing amount of literature supporting the possibility that in disease conditions the demand for some non-essential amino acids may exceed their endogenous synthesis capacity, so that the normal amino acid composition of the diet may need to be modified to meet requirements (Luiking *et al.*, 2004; Melis *et al.*, 2004). In case of severe liver failure the capacity of the liver to degrade certain essential or non-essential amino acids may become limited, which has led to the suggestion that the diet should contain diminished amounts of some amino acids that rely for their breakdown on the liver (Cabre and Gassull, 2005). Patients on home parenteral nutrition (HPN) often have a short bowel and diminished intestinal mass, which diminishes the capacity to efficiently digest and absorb a bolus meal; in turn, this dictates recommendations on meal size and frequency. This will be discussed in a later part of this chapter.

In plant proteins, amino acids consist in the D- and the L-form. In animals only the L-form is used to synthesize protein. Amino acids with the D-form in the diet therefore are not used, or are less efficiently used, for this purpose. Only D-methionine and D-phenylalanine can be efficiently used for human protein synthesis, because they can be transformed into the L-form via transamination reactions. Some amino acids are produced in the body that are not found in protein but that serve other purposes. Examples are the intermediates of the urea cycle (e.g. citrulline, ornithine).

Proline is not found in muscle protein but is abundantly present in collagen. Similarly, glycine and alanine are present in collagen in far higher concentrations than in most dietary proteins. Taurine is present in the cell in high concentrations and acts as an osmolyte modulating cellular hydration state and a bile acid conjugant; it is not a true amino acid rather an imino acid because it does not contain a carboxyl but a sulfonic group.

Amino Acid Content and Concentrations

The major part of amino acids is present in proteins like muscle protein or collagen, for which they function as building stones. Several types of protein can be distinguished (Table 24.2). Structural proteins are quantitatively the most important group (90% of total body protein, 10–20% of body cell mass) (Guyton and Hall, 1996), whereas plasma and tissue proteins like albumin, immunoglobulins, haemoglobin and fibrinogen comprise less than 10% of the total protein content of the body (Anderson and Anderson, 2002). A third group consists of highly active proteins like enzymes, hormones, cytokines, genes, membrane carrier proteins, signalling proteins and others; they comprise less than 1% of total body protein but are important modulators of metabolism. Free amino acids comprise

Table 24.1. Specific functions of amino acids and their intermediate products.

Amino acid	Products	Function	Claimed supplementation efficacy
Alanine	Pyruvate	Gluconeogenesis in liver Nitrogen and carbon transport Precursor in ureagenesis Highly concentrated in collagen	Part of dipeptide with glutamine with beneficial effects in stressed conditions
Arginine	Nitric oxide (NO) Urea Creatine Agmatine	Vasodilatation Immunomodulation Neurotransmission Cell signalling Ornithine precursor Ammonia detoxification Intermediate in energy metabolism in muscle	Positive effects for use in immunonutrition on morbidity suggested in surgical and trauma patients; further research warranted Positive effects in pulmonary hypertension, cardiac ischaemia, impotence Positive effects suggested in muscle synthesis
Citrulline	Arginine	Intermediate in NO synthesis	Increased NO synthesis with clinical benefit has been claimed but only animal experimental data are at hand
Ornithine	Polyamines	Cell differentiation Proline precursor	May improve healing burn wounds (ornithine α-ketoglutarate)
Proline	Hydroxyproline	Hepatocyte DNA, protein synthesis Collagen synthesis	Possibly collagen synthesis (?)
Asparagine		Aspartic acid precursor	Asparaginase-induced asparagine depletion is therapeutic in leukaemia
Aspartic acid	Oxaloacetate, fumarate, malate	Gluconeogenesis Pyrimidine synthesis Important anaplerotic substrate, produced in transamination reactions with many amino acids	
Methionine	Creatine	Methyl donor Cysteine precursor (see arginine)	
Cysteine (cystine)	Glutathione Taurine	Antioxidant Bile acid conjugation Neuronal cell development Regulation of membrane potential Calcium transport	Improves antioxidant status in undernutrition, inflammatory disease Reduces contrast-induced nephropathy in renal failure Mucolysis, symptom reduction in COPD

Table 24.1. *Continued.*

Amino acid	Products	Function	Claimed supplementation efficacy
Glutamic acid	Glutamine α-oxoglutarate Glutathione Aminobutyric acid	Ammonia disposal Gluconeogenesis Antioxidant Inhibition of CNS Excitation of CNS (NMDA receptor)	
Glutamine	Ammonia Glutamic acid α-oxoglutarate Non-essential amino acids	Interorgan nitrogen transport Renal HCO_3^- production Crucial anaplerotic substrate in TCA cycle Crucial substrate for NADPH production	May reduce infectious morbidity in trauma patients, burn patients and surgical patients
Glycine	Glutathione Creatine Serine	Inhibition of CNS (glycine receptor) Excitation of CNS (NMDA receptor) Antioxidant (see arginine) Donates nitrogen and carbon to form purines	Adjuvant to antipsychotics, probably reduces negative symptoms of schizophrenia Part of dipeptide with glutamine with beneficial effects in inflammatory states
Serine	D-Serine	Excitation of CNS (NMDA receptor) Glycine precursor Cysteine precursor	Adjuvant to antipsychotics, probably reduces negative symptoms of schizophrenia
Threonine	Glycine Serine	Brain development	
Histidine	Histamine	Immunomodulation Gastric acid secretion	
Lysine	Carnitine Glutamate	Mitochondrial oxidation of long-chain fatty acids	Reduction of chronic stress-induced anxiety
Branched-chain amino acids			
Isoleucine		Delivers amino group for glutamine synthesis	Diminishes ammonia production during upper gastrointestinal haemorrhage
Leucine	α-Ketoisocaproic acid	Regulator of protein synthesis Delivers amino group for glutamine synthesis	Improves protein malnutrition and restores amino acid and neurotransmitter balance in hepatic failure and hepatic encephalopathy
Valine	α-Keto-β-methylvaleric acid α-Ketoisovaleric acid	Delivers amino group for glutamine synthesis	

Continued

Table 24.1. *Continued.*

Amino acid	Products	Function	Claimed supplementation efficacy
Aromatic amino acids			
Phenylalanine		Tyrosine precursor	
Tyrosine	L-DOPA Dopamine Noradrenaline, adrenaline Triiodothyronine, thyroxine	Dopamine synthesis Movement, affect, pleasure, motivation Activation of sympathetic nervous system (fight-or-flight response) Regulation of basal metabolic rate	Possible slight improvement of cognitive functions after physical or mental exhaustion Metabolites are powerful pharmacotherapeutic drugs
Tryptophan	Kynureninic acid Quinolinic acid Serotonin Melatonin	CNS inhibition CNS excitation Mood regulation Sleep regulation Intestinal motility Regulation of circadian rhythms	No known benefits of the amino acid itself
Asp, Phe, Tyr, Val, Ile, Met, His, Pro, Arg	Intermediates in TCA cycle	Anaplerotic substrates Supply substrate for gluconeogenesis	Part of regular diet

TCA, tricarboxylic acid; CNS, central nervous system; NMDA, *N*-methyl-D-aspartic acid; COPD, chronic obstructive pulmonary disease.

only a fraction of the total body pool of amino acids, because more than 95% is present in protein. The free plasma pool of amino acids, in turn, is only a small part of all free amino acids. This pool is very similar in concentration to the extracellular extravascular pool of free amino acids. As this compartment is larger than the plasma compartment, its free amino acid quantities will therefore be proportionally larger than the plasma pool (Fig. 24.1). In turn, the intracellular pool is larger than the free extracellular pool (plasma and extravascular) because most intracellular amino acid concentrations are much higher than extracellular concentrations (Guyton and Hall, 1996). The high intracellular concentrations are caused by the fact that most amino acids are actively transported into the cell, leading to a steep uphill gradient between the intra- and extracellular compartments. A similar mechanism underlies the high intracellular concentration of glutathione. These gradients are maintained by sodium-linked transport and must therefore be accompanied by increased Na^+-, K^+-ATPase activity to maintain membrane potential. This is especially true for amino acids like glutamine, alanine and serine. Na^+-, K^+-ATPase activity increases during metabolic stress (Hsieh *et al.*, 2003) but may fail to maintain membrane potential (Shires *et al.*, 1983) due to leakiness of the membrane. This explains that when sodium transport fails in states of severe disease with altered membrane potential, both

Table 24.2. Examples of different proteins in the body.

Type	Examples
Structural proteins	Actin
	Myosin
	Collagen
Extracellular proteins	Albumin
	Haemoglobin
	Fibrinogen
	Cytokines
	Immunoglobulins
	Acute-phase proteins
Intracellular/cell-bound proteins	Enzymes
	Membrane transporters
	Transcription factors
	Heat shock proteins

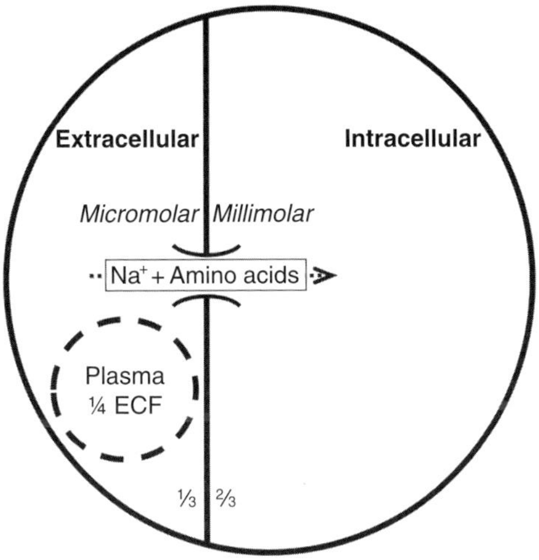

Fig. 24.1. Schematic representation of the distribution and transport of amino acids throughout the intracellular and extracellular compartments. ECF, extracellular fluid.

intracellular and extracellular amino acid concentrations change without necessarily reflecting a state of depletion.

From the foregoing it also follows that the free plasma pool forms only a minute part of the total amino acid content of the body. The amount of free amino acids in the body is primarily dependent on their rate of appearance, which in turn is the sum of protein degradation, synthesis and exogenous intake. Other factors, however, such as the activity of transporters, permeability or leakiness of the plasma membrane and degree of induction of rate-limiting degradative enzymes also influence the concentration within, and concentration gradients between, compartments. Amino acid concentrations in plasma and other compartments should therefore be interpreted with caution. However, in general amino acid levels decrease in inflammatory states, which may be due to the changes in membrane function described earlier. Additionally, increases in extravascular extracellular volume, caused by inflammation (see earlier), lead to dilution of electrolytes, amino acids, albumin and other solutes. An additional cause may consist of a decrease in protein content of the organism, resulting from net protein catabolism, induced by chronic inflammation. This is supported by the fact that these low levels are present despite the release of amino acids (specifically glutamine, alanine, glycine and proline) from peripheral tissues being increased in critical illness (Bruins *et al.*, 2003).

Amino Acid Functions

The availability of a complete and balanced precursor pattern of amino acids is crucial for protein synthesis. If one essential amino acid is lacking, peptide chain elongation will stop. In practice this situation is rare, but it occurs after upper gastrointestinal bleeding. After gastrointestinal haemorrhage substantial amounts of haemoglobin protein are presented to the digestive tract. Haemoglobin however lacks isoleucine, one of the essential branched-chain amino acids. This situation leads to diminished protein synthesis and increased ammonia and urea synthesis (Deutz *et al.*, 1991), which may explain the dismal effects on encephalopathy in patients with liver insufficiency and upper gastrointestinal bleeding (Olde Damink *et al.*, 1999). In the absence of this rare condition and in the absence of exogenous amino acid supply, protein synthesis will not stop however because there is a continuous supply of amino acids from the breakdown of protein. The kinetics of this protein turnover will be discussed in a later part of this chapter.

Specific amino acids may function as precursors of non-protein products playing other roles in human metabolism (Table 24.1). Claims have been made that in specific conditions these amino acids may become limiting for the synthesis of these non-protein products or for the execution of a specific function. This claim is strongest for glutamine, which is produced in high quantities in burns, trauma and infection and which may become limiting when the disease process is prolonged and severe (Melis *et al.*, 2004). Supplementation may be beneficial in these conditions, provided there is a normally functioning liver. In the older literature extremely high plasma glutamine levels (and most other amino acids), suggested to be toxic, have been found in patients with acute fulminant liver failure. In more recent literature glutamine levels have also been found to be elevated in a minority of critically ill patients in an intensive care unit (Rodas *et al.*, 2012). In this last category glutamine supplementation may have deleterious effects. On the basis of clinical studies and the described metabolism, supplementation with glutamine may be beneficial in critically ill patients with long-standing inflammatory disease, but with good liver and kidney function. In addition, amounts of glutamine supplemented should not exceed the amounts produced by the body itself in critical illness.

Claims of benefit have also been made for arginine but this claim is not convincingly supported by clinical data (Luiking *et al.*, 2004). It has been demonstrated that arginine is produced in increased amounts in diseased states due to increased supply by net protein degradation. New formation of arginine by the intestine and kidney contributes not more than 15% of the total production rate (Luiking *et al.*, 2009). It is therefore unlikely that endogenous arginine synthesis is insufficient with regard to the production of nitric oxide, polyamines, etc. If there is a beneficial effect of arginine supplementation this may therefore result from a potential pharmacological action rather than from supplementation of a deficit.

There is still some interest in the effects of sulphur-containing amino acids (e.g. *N*-acetylcysteine) as they play important roles in the maintenance of redox state during oxidative stress. Efficacy of their supplementation has not been convincingly proved, possibly with the exception of iodine contrast-induced nephrotoxicity (Birck *et al.*, 2003) and acetaminophen poisoning (Brok *et al.*, 2002).

Degradation of Amino Acids

In animal and human metabolism there is continuous and simultaneous synthesis and degradation of protein. Both in health and disease exogenous administration of amino acids (as protein and together with other nutrients) is required to achieve an optimal balance. In the healthy organism the full amount of amino acids derived from protein degradation cannot be fully reutilized for protein synthesis because of the specific non-protein functions that are served by amino acids, some of which lead to products that cannot be re-synthesized into the original amino acid. This especially applies to essential amino acids (for instance, branched-chain amino acids). Consequently, even in non-stressed starvation states there is a modest loss of nitrogen, and hence of amino acids and protein, because the kidney continues to excrete nitrogen, largely as ammonia. The amount of nitrogen (in grams) multiplied by a factor of 25 furnishes an estimation of the muscle protein lost in grams. Urinary ammonia is derived from the renal conversion of glutamine to ammonia and glucose. The glucose produced is released in the renal vein whereas at least half of the ammonia is released in the urine. This obligatory loss of protein, even in healthy states, implies that protein losses need to be replenished to cover the deficit. Although losses will be minimized when only protein is administered, ultimately a balanced diet is necessary to maintain body composition. The healthy adult organism is in protein/nitrogen balance when eating well. This implies that the amount of urea and other nitrogenous compounds lost in urine, stools, sweat, hair, nails, etc. equals the amount of food protein absorbed by the intestinal tract. In disease the net loss of protein nitrogen per day is far greater than in health and continues even when adequate food is ingested (see below). Increased amino acid utilization in disease occurs in several ways, which depend on the metabolic condition of the organism. The amino acid may wholly or completely be used for the production of the specific product, described in Table 24.1, but as the products of amino acid degradation provide substrates for further metabolism, net loss is limited. The products of amino acid degradation consist of nitrogenous compounds and compounds derived from the carbon skeleton. The nitrogenous substances can be used for the synthesis of, for example, pyrimidines, purines or non-essential amino acids, whereas the carbon skeletons can be used for the synthesis of several components of biomass (nucleic acids, non-essential amino acids and many other molecules in lower amounts).

In this last process the amino acid carbon skeleton is to a large degree first utilized in the liver and kidney for formation of glucose, which subsequently can act as a building block for cells and matrix. It should be emphasized that in stress starvation and in starvation without stress, very little glucose is fully oxidized as a consequence of insulin resistance. In view of the fact that in (stress) starvation 90% of new glucose formation is derived from amino acid carbon skeletons, preferential use of glucose for synthetic function rather than oxidation limits protein losses (Soeters and Soeters, 2012). Both nitrogenous and carbonic products can be partly utilized for the re-synthesis of their precursor in metabolic cycles such as the Cori cycle or the nitric oxide cycle.

When there is liberal and superfluous supply of nutrients, some amino acids deliver carbon that can only be transformed into fat (from acetyl-coA or oxaloacetyl-coA). However, glucogenic amino acids can also be utilized for fatty acid synthesis. It is of interest that the site of irreversible degradation of amino acids is specific for each amino acid. The group of branched-chain amino acids is largely degraded in peripheral tissues (muscle, adipose tissue), whereas the aromatic amino acids (phenylalanine, tyrosine, tryptophan) are largely irreversibly degraded in the liver. The branched-chain amino acids can be irreversibly degraded in muscle but also in adipose tissue and the resulting carbon skeleton can be wholly (leucine) or partly (isoleucine) reutilized for triglyceride synthesis in adipose tissue itself. In the breakdown of leucine, β-hydroxy-β-methylglutaryl-CoA is produced which is a precursor of cholesterol.

Protein Metabolism in Starvation and Stress

The differences between starvation and stress metabolism of amino acids are well known. Whereas the body is able to limit protein losses during starvation, this is less true during stressed states (trauma, infectious states). In pure starvation all pathways are geared to the preservation of protein stores, specifically muscle protein. Both peripheral protein stores (muscle, bone, skin) and central stores like the splanchnic tissues and the immune system lose protein mass (Romijn, 2000). Kinetically, a decrease in protein turnover is found in all organs with protein synthesis slightly more depressed than protein degradation. In this muscle protein-sparing process, the ability of tissues like the central nervous system to burn ketones (which can cross the blood–brain barrier; fatty acids cannot) as fuel is a crucial mechanism. This allows the organism to decrease the production of new glucose (gluconeogenesis) which would otherwise require carbon skeletons of amino acids. In this manner, healthy individuals can decrease their urea production to about 1–2 g of urea nitrogen per day whereas most of the urinary nitrogen (5–7 g total) consists of ammonia nitrogen, excreted in the urine. On the basis of these findings it has been reasoned (Owen *et al.*, 1969) that in long-term starvation the liver produces almost no glucose from amino acid skeletons; most of the glucose produced arises in the kidney because this yields ammonia, and produces bicarbonate, necessary to maintain acid–base balance and to buffer an acid urine resulting from the net production of organic acids in starvation.

In stressed situations protein turnover of central organs like the liver, the spleen and the other components of the immune system is upregulated, and net protein synthesis is actually increased in well-resuscitated intensive care patients, in well-nourished patients undergoing surgery and in experimental animals challenged with endotoxin (Bruins *et al.*, 2003). Liver protein mass increases, immune cell proliferation is enhanced and more protein and cells are deposited in the wound. In muscle, protein turnover is also increased in previously well-nourished and resuscitated individuals, but protein degradation is clearly increased above protein synthesis, leading to net muscle protein loss. This protein lost from muscle furnishes the amino acids necessary to build protein accrued in the central tissues. In this process the peripheral tissues, in collaboration with the liver, produce substantial amounts of glutamine, alanine, glycine and proline, more than can be explained on the basis of the breakdown of muscle protein. The role of the intestine in the re-routing of amino acids will be discussed further below.

Intermediary Amino Acid Metabolism in the Intestine

Glutamine metabolism in the intestine

Glutamine is an important substrate for the intestine and plays a central role in intermediary amino acid metabolism in the gut. It furnishes building blocks by virtue of its role as an anaplerotic substrate for the tricarboxylic acid (TCA) cycle after its conversion to glutamate by glutaminase and further deamination of glutamate to α-ketoglutarate. Further, it serves as a precursor of protein, glutathione, polyamines and nucleotide synthesis and as a nitrogen carrier. The degradation of glutamine in the gut wall yields as main nitrogenous substance ammonia. The anaplerotic role of glutamine is particularly important in stressed states where intermediates of the TCA cycle are removed from the cycle to serve other processes such as the synthesis of nucleotides, phospholipids, sterols and cellular proteins. Simultaneously glutamine-derived α-ketoglutarate mediates NADPH production within the TCA cycle, which is important in the regulation of the intracellular redox potential (Soeters and Grecu, 2012). Enterocytes incubated *in vitro* in a glutamine-containing medium produce glutamic acid, alanine and ammonia in a time- and concentration-dependent manner (Matsutaka *et al.*, 1973). Windmueller and Spaeth (1974, 1975, 1980) assessed in a large series of semi-*in vivo* experiments the fate of glutamine-derived nitrogen and the contribution of glutamine to the provision of energy in the intestine. Glutamine was taken up from the intestine in a concentration-dependent manner and was metabolized to other amino acids and ammonia. The nitrogen of glutamine was found to be metabolized as follows: 36% in alanine, 7% in proline, 10% in citrulline, 11% in ornithine and 36% in ammonia. Energy coverage was found to be derived as follows: 35% from glutamine carbon, 26% from 3-hydroxybutyrate, 24% from acetoacetate, 7% from glucose, and the remainder from lactates and unesterified fatty acids. Despite these important findings it took another decade before their clinical relevance was appreciated by clinicians, and before research was initiated to explore the potential benefits of glutamine supplementation through *in vivo* experiments (Yoshida *et al.*, 1992) or in clinical settings (Scheltinga *et al.*, 1991; Ziegler *et al.*, 1992).

Glutamine metabolism in the intestine after trauma and in models of sepsis

Souba's group (Souba, 1983, 1993; Souba and Wilmore, 1983; Souba *et al.*, 1985a,b, 1987, 1990; Sarac *et al.*, 1994) has greatly stimulated research in this area and found in experimental animals that endotoxin greatly stimulated the uptake of glutamine by the intestine and the liver. We found in similar experiments in pigs that after both surgical trauma and endotoxin challenge, net release of glutamine by the hindquarter increased whereas the net uptake by the intestine decreased (Deutz *et al.*, 1992a; Bruins *et al.*, 2000). Uptake by the liver and the spleen increased. In these two organs the metabolism of glutamine changed from a modest net release in the control non-stressed situation to net uptake after trauma or endotoxin challenge (Deutz *et al.*, 1992a). This increased net flux of glutamine and is supported by the finding that after trauma and sepsis the A–V difference across the hindquarter or forearm increases (Clowes *et al.*, 1980; Carli *et al.*, 1990; Fong *et al.*, 1990; Mjaaland *et al.*, 1993; Brown *et al.*, 1994). This must imply that the glutamine released by the hindquarter is taken up by central organs like liver and spleen, as found in our experiments (Deutz *et al.*, 1992a).

Rather unexpectedly, whole-body tracer data do not indicate a substantial increase in the turnover of glutamine after trauma or during sepsis (Gore and Jahoor, 1994; Jackson *et al.*, 1999; van Acker *et al.*, 2000). This probably implies that the increased net flux of glutamine from peripheral tissues to central tissues is not generated by increased production in muscle and increased uptake in central tissues, but rather by decreased uptake in muscle and decreased production in central organs. We found in contradistinction with the findings of Souba and Wilmore (1983) and Souba *et al.* (1985a,b, 1987) that peripheral, predominantly muscle tissue produces glutamine that is subsequently taken up by the splanchnic tissues but not by the gut. Our data show that in this process the intestine itself is a rather passive organ that takes up less glutamine in the fasted, traumatized or inflammatory state, whereas the liver and the spleen take up more glutamine even in the presence of lower plasma levels (Deutz *et al.*, 1992a; Bruins *et al.*, 2000). These observations are supported by recent *in vivo* human data showing a diminished splanchnic extraction of glutamine and reduced conversion to citrulline in critically ill patients (Kao *et al.*, 2013). In the semi-*in vivo* setting plasma glutamine level has been suggested to be an important factor determining uptake of glutamine by the intestine (Windmueller and Spaeth, 1974, 1975, 1980).

A–V differences across the jejunum and ileum in humans during abdominal operations were found to correlate with plasma glutamine levels (van der Hulst *et al.*, 1997). The fractional extraction of glutamine was by far the highest (30%) in the jejunum. This was paralleled by the A–V differences of the main products of glutamine degradation: ammonia, citrulline, proline, ornithine and alanine (van der Hulst *et al.*, 1997). The release of these degradation products of glutamine was much larger in the jejunum than in the ileum. A–V differences across the colon showed some uptake of glutamine and a modest release of glutamic acid and ammonia in the venous effluent of the colon in a non concentration-dependent manner. It is possible that ammonia release in the colon is effectuated by a modest degradation of glutamine in the colonocyte and by bacterial degradation of urea and probably amino acids. These findings indicate that uptake of glutamine by the small intestine is concentration dependent (van der Hulst *et al.*, 1997) although it is uncertain what will happen at higher glutamine levels. Furthermore, the negative effects of starvation on intestinal integrity have been demonstrated to be counteracted by infusion of glutamine (van der Hulst *et al.*, 1993). This raises the question as to which factors determine glutamine levels.

In the past, we have claimed that the depleted state causes plasma glutamine levels to drop. Most clinical patients who have lost weight and are considered to be depleted also exhibit symptoms of chronic inflammation. It is therefore often difficult to separate the influences of chronic inflammation and depletion. To separate the influence of these two factors we reviewed our data, and found that patients exhibiting signs of inflammatory activity had low plasma glutamine levels and increased permeability of the bowel. In this subgroup of patients glutamine supplementation appears to reduce intestinal permeability (Hulsewe *et al.*, 2004).

Glutamine uptake in solid tumours of the colon

Studies in cancer cell lines have shown that some cell types take up large quantities of glutamine (Bode *et al.*, 2002) by a process referred to as 'glutaminolysis'. These studies suggest that cancer cells preferentially utilize glutamine-derived α-oxoglutarate instead of pyruvate as an anaplerotic substrate for the TCA cycle (Hensley *et al.*, 2013). It has been suggested that some cancer types may therefore act as a 'sink' for glutamine. In the same experiment in surgical patients in which we studied A–V concentration differences in different parts of the intestine, we also assessed A–V differences across parts of the colon containing malignant tumours. In accordance with observations by Holm's group (Holm *et al.*, 1995), we found that there was no preferential uptake of glutamine by these tumours (van der Hulst *et al.*, 1997). For coverage of their energy requirements colonic cancers appeared to rely on glycolysis, because there was a substantially increased uptake of glucose and stoichiometric release of lactate compared with healthy parts of the colon. In view of many new findings and changed insight in the role of the Warburg phenomenon, it is now becoming clear that any rapidly growing tissue utilizes preferentially glucose, glutamine, glycine, proline and, to a quantitatively lesser degree, other amino acids as building blocks for proliferation and uses fatty acids as fuel to generate energy (Soeters and Soeters, 2012).

The role of the intestine in the routing of nitrogen and carbon

Disease and trauma need to be overcome by the body by an adequate host response, which requires substrate. In these stress conditions the organism is generally starving. The substrate therefore has to be delivered predominantly by peripheral tissues, released in the circulation and taken up by the central and crucial organs like the liver, immune system and wound, in which this host response occurs. The transport needs to be non-toxic and the waste products arising from these substrates need to be presented to the organs involved in their clearance. The two main categories of substrate necessary to sustain host response consist of appropriate fuel and amino acids, necessary for the synthesis of proteins that play important roles in host response. Glutamine carbon is an important building block for white cells in the liver, spleen and remainder of the immune system, as well for wound healing (Newsholme, 1988). In fact, it is necessary for any tissue in which cell proliferation and matrix deposition are required. Glutamine is released by peripheral (muscle) tissues and is derived from three sources: (i) the free intracellular pool; (ii) protein breakdown; and (iii) new formation. The free tissue pool can furnish this glutamine only to a very limited degree, because it is small compared with the flux taken up in the splanchnic area. Also, the amount of glutamine derived from protein degradation is modest because glutamine constitutes only 5% of human muscle protein and the α-amino nitrogen exported from muscle accounts for 30% of glutamine. A substantial part of glutamine release therefore is derived from new formation of glutamine in peripheral, predominantly muscle tissues, where ammonia is taken up from the blood and is bound to glutamic acid. Glutamic acid, in turn, arises from a transamination reaction of branched-chain amino acids with α-ketoglutarate, largely resulting from the degradation of glucose. Another source consists of glutamic acid synthesis in the liver from amino acids taken up by the liver from the systemic circulation and derived from the breakdown of peripheral (muscle) protein.

In conclusion, the catabolic process in muscle furnishes amino acids that function as building blocks for protein synthesis in the liver, wound and immune system, and glutamine that, together with glucose, glycine and to a lesser degree other amino acids, serve to synthesize non-protein cell elements like DNA/RNA in the liver, spleen, wound and immune system. Glutamine is ideally suited for this purpose, because its concentration and flux can differ without toxic side-effects. The carbon skeleton of glutamine can easily be converted (via the TCA cycle) to many elements of biomass and the sites where it is degraded are ideally located, so that the ammonia resulting from the first step in its breakdown in the intestine is presented to the liver, producing urea or glutamine, and to the kidney, excreting at least half of the ammonia produced in the urine. Only a modest amount of ammonia is released in the renal vein and reaches the systemic circulation.

The role of the intestine in the routing of amino acid-derived carbon skeletons

The role of the intestine in the routing of amino acid-derived carbon is not completely elucidated. Part of the glutamine skeleton is oxidized; part is degraded to yield alanine and citrulline. Ubiquitously, ^{14}C-labelled glutamine carbon was shown to be metabolized by the intestine to carbon dioxide (55%), lactate (8–15%), citrate (2%), other organic acids (1%), citrulline (5%), proline (4%), alanine (4%) and glucose (4%) in an *ex vivo* experimental setup (Windmueller, 1982). However, the incubation medium did not contain fatty acids, promoting the oxidation of other substrates including glutamine. It is likely that this does not happen in the *in vivo* situation where fatty acids are available. The formation of alanine in muscle can be considered part of the Cori cycle, in that it is released into the circulation and subsequently serves as precursor for gluconeogenesis in the liver or kidney. Peripheral tissues take up the glucose thus produced, where it acts as an anaplerotic substrate for the TCA cycle or where it serves glycolysis. Pyruvate resulting from glycolysis in turn can be transaminated with branched-chain amino acids to yield alanine, which is released in the circulation and, in turn, can participate in renewed Cori cycling. Badly perfused tissues with low mitochondrial metabolism and deficient fatty acid utilization during sepsis or severe illness may require increased glycolytic flux (generally leading to significantly elevated plasma lactate levels >2.5 mmol/l), which provides energy in compromised tissues, but these situations are relatively rare and are associated with a high mortality risk. In well-perfused organs glycolytic flux, present in traumatized or septic states, does not serve to generate energy but promotes Cori cycling which, similar to the cycling of the TCA cycle, allows branching off of substrate for the synthesis of biomass and to preserve redox potential (Soeters and Soeters, 2012). Plasma lactate levels are elevated but do not rise above 2.5 mmol/l.

The role of the intestine in the production of specific amino acids

Citrulline and arginine

The intestine is the only site that releases substantial amounts of citrulline. Classically it is assumed that citrulline released from the intestine is generated by the consecutive actions of the enzymes glutaminase, ornithine-oxoacid aminotransferase and ornithine transcarbamylase, which degrade glutamine to produce citrulline via glutamate and ornithine. Recent data have suggested that glutamine may be more important as a nitrogen donor than as a carbon donor for citrulline biosynthesis (Marini *et al.*, 2010). This however seems species dependent, since experimental results from murine studies were not supported by subsequent human data (Kao *et al.*, 2013). The production of citrulline is crucial as an intermediate in the urea cycle, but also has been claimed to be crucial because it can be released into the circulation and taken up by the kidney where arginine can be produced via argininosuccinate synthetase and argininosuccinate lyase. Arginine plays an important role in protein synthesis and nitric oxide production and its deficiency has been implicated in numerous diseases (Wu and Morris, 1998). The relevance of intestinal citrulline production for arginine synthesis is underlined by the fact that the length of the remaining small bowel in short bowel syndrome (SBS) has been demonstrated to correlate with citrulline levels (Crenn *et al.*, 2000). In case reports, hyperammonaemic encephalopathy has been described in the presence of a healthy liver but a short bowel (Yokoyama *et al.*, 1996) and has been ascribed to limited supply of urea cycle intermediates. Similarly, focal tubulo-interstitial nephritis has been suggested to result from short bowel and low citrulline and consequently arginine levels (Hebiguchi *et al.*, 2002). This suggestion was supported by the observation that supplementation with arginine reversed the renal pathology.

We found in surgical patients a consistently negative arterial–portal concentration difference for arginine (van der Hulst *et al.*, 1997). This arginine is newly formed in the intestine by argininosuccinate synthetase and argininosuccinate lyase, which are modestly expressed in the adult gut and did not arise from net negative protein balance or from residual absorption from the gut lumen, because no net production by the gut was found for other (conditionally) essential amino acids. The liver takes up arginine and therefore in the fasted state intestinal arginine production does not lead to net splanchnic release and does not contribute to the systemic free arginine pool. It must be noted, however, that the hepatic fractional extraction of arginine is only 25%. This indicates that increasing arginine flux in the portal vein may lead to splanchnic arginine production and explains why systemic arginine levels can be stimulated by enteral arginine supplementation.

Cynober (1994) has suggested that at times of high arginine intake, arginine is taken up from the gut and released into the portal vein. On the other hand, when omnivorous mammals are kept on a low-arginine diet, the intestinal enzymatic machinery adapts and converts most of the enterally administered arginine to citrulline (Cynober *et al.*, 1995). It has been suggested that this change represents an adaptation aimed at prohibiting hepatic nitrogen loss, since it has been suggested that the liver does not take up citrulline in contrast to arginine (Windmueller and Spaeth, 1981). However, the view that the liver cannot take up citrulline is not consistently supported by *in vivo* data in laboratory animals (Remesy *et al.*, 1978; Deutz *et al.*, 1992b) and humans (van de Poll *et al.*, 2007). In fact, citrulline extraction is in the same range as hepatic arginine extraction.

Whether arginine production in the kidney is really crucial at times of dietary shortage is questionable because in such situations whole-body protein catabolism will furnish quantities of arginine that are several-fold larger than renal production (Castillo *et al.*, 1993).

Taurine and glycine

We found unexpectedly high concentration differences across the jejunum and especially the ileum of glycine and taurine in surgical patients who had been starved for at least 12 h and were undergoing surgery (van der Hulst *et al.*, 1997). The release of taurine into the venous effluent of the ileum reached levels of a similar order of magnitude as the uptake of glutamine and the release of alanine. An obvious explanation is that in the process of re-absorption of conjugated bile acids in the small bowel these conjugates are de-conjugated and released into the portal vein as bile acids and free glycine and taurine. This demonstrates that enterohepatic cycling of bile salts is not restricted to the bile acid part but also applies to these amino acids. The consequences of bile acid malabsorption and the coinciding loss of glycine and especially taurine have not received much attention in the literature, but at least one case report suggests that these findings may be clinically relevant.

It has been shown that children receiving parenteral nutrition without supplemental taurine developed low taurine plasma levels and neuronal (especially retinal) dysfunction, which could be counteracted by addition of taurine to the feed (Geggel *et al.*, 1985). The indispensability of taurine in this condition has been ascribed to low expression of taurine biosynthetic enzymes, which account for only a very low renewal of the total body pool of taurine. Taurine may therefore only be dispensable when it can rely on adequate and almost complete conservation of the taurine pool via enterohepatic cycling of taurine (van der Hulst *et al.*, 1997). Most children and adults on long-term parenteral nutrition suffer from intestinal malabsorption, which may induce substantial losses of bile acids, glycine and taurine in their stools. As far as we know, no data are available on this subject.

Intermediary Protein Metabolism in the Intestine

The biological value of protein

It is well known that after a meal a healthy organism retains protein, which implies that at the whole body level more protein is synthesized than is degraded. This retention is balanced after 24 h by net protein loss during the fasting state during the night. It has been suggested (Waterlow, 1995) and evidence has been provided that the splanchnic area and specifically the intestine itself (Volpi *et al.*, 1996; Mariotti *et al.*, 2000; Dangin *et al.*, 2001; Soeters *et al.*, 2001; van der Schoor *et al.*, 2002) accumulates protein after a meal and releases amino acids from this protein in the post-absorptive period. The distinction between intestinal and hepatic utilization of meal-derived protein is difficult for methodological reasons. In addition, the assessment of protein kinetics by the gut is hampered by the fact that amino acids can be metabolized that are derived from both the intestinal lumen and the arterial inflow of amino acids. Also the intestine stores, synthesizes and releases protein both in the gut lumen and in the gut wall. All these factors complicate the precise assessment of what happens with meal-derived protein.

The quality of a protein is generally believed to be dependent on two factors: (i) the digestibility/absorption; and (ii) the composition of the protein. In recent years it has become apparent that a third factor also decisively contributes to protein quality. The old view considered the rapid appearance of amino acids into the portal vein after a bolus meal as evidence for the quality of the protein. At that time it was not appreciated well that this rapid appearance coincided with increased ureagenesis and gluconeogenesis. A more modern view is that the appearance of amino acids after a bolus meal should be slow and prolonged to make amino acids available to the organism over a protracted period of time and at a slow rate (van der Hulst *et al.*, 1993, 1997; van Acker *et al.*, 2000; Bode *et al.*, 2002; Hulsewe *et al.*, 2004; Kao *et al.*, 2013). This increases the efficiency of utilization of these amino acids for protein synthesis and decreases their net breakdown. The mechanism operative in this protein-sparing effect consists of the fact that amino acids derived from the digestion of a bolus meal are to some degree retained in the intestinal region (Windmueller, 1982; Newsholme, 1988; Holm *et al.*, 1995; Marini *et al.*, 2010) and do not immediately appear in the portal vein. There must be a pool of amino acids in the intestine that can enlarge in size after the meal, and that in the post-absorptive state decreases in size and slowly releases amino acids into the portal and subsequently into the systemic circulation

(Mjaaland *et al.*, 1993). The nature of this pool most likely consists of rapidly synthesized or more slowly degraded protein. Support for this mechanism consists of the fact that bolus meals with a composition suitable for protein synthesis decrease and prolong the appearance of amino acids into the portal vein. If a protein is supplied in the bolus meal lacking one essential amino acid and thus disfavouring protein synthesis, amino acids appear more rapidly into the portal vein and induce more ureagenesis (Brown *et al.*, 1994). This also happens when the bolus meal consists only of protein and does not contain calories like carbohydrates or fat (Brown *et al.*, 1994). When a tapered release of amino acids derived from degradation of the protein in the meal and the resulting low production of urea is considered as evidence for the biological value of the protein in question, casein protein has clearly better quality than soy protein (Wu and Morris, 1998) and whey protein (Hebiguchi *et al.*, 2002).

The regulation of protein accretion in the gut

Many authors have confirmed the presence of a positive protein balance after a meal (Melville *et al.*, 1989; Millward *et al.*, 1991; Pacy *et al.*, 1994; Quevedo *et al.*, 1994). In most reports whole-body level protein degradation was diminished whereas protein synthesis decreased or did not exhibit changes (Melville *et al.*, 1989; Pacy *et al.*, 1994; Quevedo *et al.*, 1994; Cayol *et al.*, 1995). After a meal containing either casein or soy as a protein we found that feeding self-evidently increased the net appearance of amino acids in the portal vein. Both proteins increased protein degradation to a similar degree but protein synthesis increased to a greater degree after casein than after soy (Wu and Morris, 1998). This difference was not significant, but the difference between appearance (protein degradation) and disappearance (protein synthesis) of phenylalanine was lower in the casein group than in the soy group. This implies that less of the meal-derived protein appears in the portal vein and that therefore more of the casein protein is temporarily retained in the intestine. Simultaneously urea production was greatly enhanced in the first few hours after initiating tube feeding in these pigs in the soy group, whereas this was not the case in the casein group. When more protein is administered, more of the protein-derived amino acids will be oxidized (van der Schoor *et al.*, 2001). Other groups reported similar findings (Mahe *et al.*, 1996; Volpi *et al.*, 1996; Gaudichon *et al.*, 1999; van Goudoever *et al.*, 2000; van der Schoor *et al.*, 2002).

Beaufrere's group (Boirie *et al.*, 1997; Arnal *et al.*, 2000) employed a dual tracer technique with one leucine tracer given with the meal intravenously and a different tracer intragastrically, and found that more whey protein than casein protein appeared in the first few hours after the meal in the portal vein, that amino acid concentrations were higher in the whey group and that protein synthesis rate was higher. After 2 h, however, protein synthesis dropped in the whey group, whereas in the casein group synthesis remained higher than in the whey group and protein degradation remained suppressed longer in the casein group. All these findings are consistent with the interpretation that despite the fact that the meals are identical, isocaloric and isonitrogenous, different proteins are utilized differently. The rapid appearance and high oxidation of whey proteins has led to the designation 'fast dietary protein', but implies that it has a short-lasting anabolic effect; whereas a 'slow dietary protein' like casein is oxidized to a lesser extent and has a longer-lasting anabolic effect, which makes it a protein with a higher biological value when administered without other nutrients. However, whey is the better protein when given in small boluses (Dangin *et al.*, 2001), divided over time or when other nutrients are added (Deutz *et al.*, 1995).

The nature of the labile protein pool in the intestine

The question may be raised what the nature is of the protein temporarily retained in the gut after a meal. The first possibility includes differences in the rate of digestion and absorption (Dangin *et al.*, 2001). This may apply for casein, which is known to coagulate in the stomach and consequently to be digested at a much slower rate than most other proteins.

The explanation for these findings appears to be complex. After a bolus meal a concerted action of amino acids, glucose, insulin and cholecystokinin stimulates the secretion and synthesis of pancreatic and intestinal digestive enzymes (O'Keefe *et al.*, 1994; Bragado *et al.*, 2000). Part of these enzymes is already present in the pancreas as zymogen stores and waiting to be released during the meal. Control of this process occurs at the post-translational level (Bragado *et al.*, 2000). This process adds protein contained in enzymes to the total protein and amino acid pool in the intestine, which makes the interpretation of tracer studies during enteral feeding difficult. However it does not explain the retention of meal-derived amino acids, because the enzymes released were already present and were not synthesized from amino acids from the meal. These considerations do not fully apply to the synthesis and secretion of enzymes by the intestinal mucosa, because at this location amino acids utilized for enzyme protein synthesis may be derived from both the intestinal lumen and the systemic circulation (Nakshabendi *et al.*, 1995; Bouteloup-Demange *et al.*, 1998). For this to be the case, it must be possible that goblet cells and enterocytes take up amino acids from the intestinal lumen and from the basolateral membrane. Similar considerations apply to the synthesis of mucin in the intestine, pancreas and in bile. The question is whether mucin is directly synthesized from gut-derived substrate or from substrate derived from the systemic circulation.

A second potential store of amino-nitrogen consists of di-, tri-, polypeptides or proteins produced after partial digestion and absorbed from the intestinal lumen, yielding amino acids in the mucosa in varying quantities and potentially partially released into the portal vein. Claims have been made that part of protein-derived amino-nitrogen is released in this manner, but very little quantitative data are available, if at all.

A third and very likely factor contributing to retention of meal-derived protein inside the intestine is proliferation of bacteria and bacterial protein during and after the meal, which subsequently is digested and absorbed by the enterocytes.

These three potential forms of acutely produced protein may form part of the labile protein pool that accumulates during and after the meal, and in the post-absorptive phase is degraded, furnishing amino acids to the organism. The result is that after 24 h a zero protein balance is reached.

The presence of a labile protein pool in the intestine is known to be present in nature. An extreme example is the python that feeds once every 2 months. After the feed there is enormous hypertrophy of the intestine, but also the meal itself is known to be digested and absorbed very slowly. It has the beneficial effect that it tapers the release of meal-derived amino acids to the liver which would otherwise rapidly degrade these amino acids, produce large quantities of urea, burn the resulting carbon skeletons or store them as glycogen or fat. This is beneficial at times when food is scarce and when the organism has to rely on the unforeseen moment that food is available. The ability of the human organism to retain protein in this labile protein pool is very modest, however, compared with other species like reptiles (Holmberg *et al.*, 2002).

The data reviewed also indicate that for the labile protein pool to expand maximally, a protein with a high biological value should be consumed, combined with calories and other essential nutrients to promote maximal protein synthesis. We reported similar findings with regard to casein and soy protein. Soy appeared much faster in the portal vein and stimulated urea production to a much greater extent than casein. These findings have defined casein as a slow protein and whey and soy protein as fast proteins, and support the claim that casein is a better protein in healthy organisms consuming boluses of protein. When whey is delivered in small boluses or when all other nutrients are added to the meal, whey is the better protein.

Consequences for Patients on HPN

The most important indications for long-term parenteral nutrition are SBS and other forms of intestinal failure. These patients often suffer from massive fluid loss and nutrient malabsorption, but also lack the active role the intestine plays in amino acid and protein metabolism.

Intermediary metabolism

Loss of intestinal mass may lead to disturbances in intermediary metabolism, exemplified by the diminished glutamine to citrulline conversion and consequent low plasma citrulline levels. Such changes may induce very specific demands with respect to amino acid composition of the feed and feeding frequency to avoid specific deficiencies and to maintain nitrogen balance. Solid data (especially clinical data) regarding the need for specific amino acid supplementation in patients with SBS are scarce, however.

Glutamine

Much research, considering specific problems in amino acid metabolism in patients with SBS on HPN, focuses on glutamine (partly reviewed above). The beneficence and the possible working mechanisms of glutamine remain subject to debate (Ockenga *et al.*, 2005). The strongest claims for the beneficence of glutamine supplementation are derived from clinical studies concerning the simultaneous administration of glutamine and growth hormone. This combination is suggested to augment intestinal adaptation and to promote weaning from parenteral nutrition (Byrne *et al.*, 2005). These results however are not consistently reproduced in similar studies (Scolapio, 2004), which probably implies that the potential effect of glutamine (plus growth hormone), if it exists at all, is only small. A drawback of growth hormone is that it needs to be administered continuously to keep its beneficial effects. At present treatment with glucagon-like peptide-1 appears to be more promising, but this hormone is also very expensive because continuous administration is most likely required to maintain benefit.

Citrulline

Loss of bowel length and mass impairs the conversion of glutamine to citrulline, which is accompanied by reduced citrulline levels. It has been suggested that these levels actually represent a citrulline deficiency and citrulline supplementation restores citrulline and arginine levels in rats with a short bowel (Osowska *et al.*, 2004). Simultaneously nitrogen balance improves in animals treated with citrulline. Hitherto no clinical data regarding its effectiveness are at hand.

Taurine and cysteine

Patients (especially children) on total parenteral nutrition are at risk of developing taurine deficiency (Lourenco and Camilo, 2002). Taurine normally is a non-essential amino acid, but it relies on enterohepatic cycling to maintain its total body pool (van der Hulst *et al.*, 1997). Taurine deficiency in children on artificial nutrition is generally ascribed to the incomplete development of enzymes involved in taurine synthesis, but the role of (absent) enterohepatic cycling has received no attention. Taurine is a standard component of virtually all parenteral and enteral feeding solutions.

Cysteine can function as a precursor for taurine and it has been shown that cysteine supplementation can restore taurine levels in children on HPN (Helms *et al.*, 1999). In addition, cysteine may have beneficial effects on intestinal mucosa through its antioxidative capacity (Ardite *et al.*, 2000). Clinical data on the potential role of cysteine in parenteral nutrition are lacking, however.

Protein accretion and feeding frequency

During total parenteral nutrition the protein-sparing effects of the intestine, which facilitates gradual release of nutrients after bolus feeding, is obviously absent. In these patients a continuous parenteral or enteral infusion of nutrients is needed to ensure gradual nutrient supply to the body and to maintain body cell mass. Evidently such a continuous infusion limits the mobility of the patient. To improve mobility, in most patients nocturnal enteral (or parenteral nutrition) is instituted through fine-bore feeding tubes. These patients also may benefit from more frequent but smaller enteral meals during the evening and the night.

Feed composition

In cases of severe chronic protein-losing enteropathy, it might become necessary to compensate nitrogen losses by liberal administration of protein/amino acids. This does not guarantee correction of the net loss, but may augment protein synthesis, which may help to (modestly) limit net loss. In severe cases even surgery should be considered. Such conditions, however, can regularly be avoided and in fact electrolyte losses and disorders generally predominate over nitrogen losses in patients with SBS. There are a number of disease-specific parenteral and enteral feeding solutions with varying amounts of, for example, sulfur amino acids, arginine and branched-chain amino acids. In most cases, however, lack of clinical data leaves room for discussion about their clinical efficacy. Large randomized clinical trials are needed to establish the potential advantage of such disease-specific feeds. Similarly, the quality of products for standard HPN of different manufacturers has not been compared with each other in clinical trials, but similarity in protein source and amino acid composition suggests that these differences, if any, are small.

Summary

Amino acids are the building blocks of protein and are involved in numerous specific functions. Adequate amino acid intake is necessary to maintain body cell mass and to support these specific functions. The gut actively regulates the rate at which ingested proteins are degraded and released to the circulation and thereby mediates the anabolic effects of ingested proteins and the duration of the postprandial anabolic phase.

The gut is also a metabolically active organ; it produces citrulline and maintains the body pool of taurine. These specific gut functions may be impaired in patients on parenteral nutrition and/or patients with intestinal failure. In these patients, a gradual long-lasting infusion of amino acids is preferable to bolus administration for improvement of the nitrogen homeostasis.

The composition of parenteral or enteral feeding solutions (e.g. high glutamine or citrulline levels) has been suggested to influence nitrogen balance or specific amino acid functions, but the efficacy of such adjusted compositions is still the subject of debate and ongoing studies.

References

Anderson, N.L. and Anderson, N.G. (2002) The human plasma proteome: history, character, and diagnostic prospects. *Molecular and Cellular Proteomics* 1, 845–867.

Ardite, E., Sans, M., Panes, J., Romero, F.J., Pique, J.M. and Fernandez-Checa, J.C. (2000) Replenishment of glutathione levels improves mucosal function in experimental acute colitis. *Laboratory Investigation* 80, 735–744.

Arnal, M.A., Mosoni, L., Boirie, Y., Gachon, P., Genest, M., Bayle, G., Grizard, J., Antoine, J.M., Beaufrere, B. and Mirand, P.P. (2000) Protein turnover modifications induced by the

protein feeding pattern still persist after the end of the diets. *American Journal of Physiology. Endocrinology and Metabolism* 278, E902–E909.
Birck, R., Krzossok, S., Markowetz, F., Schnulle, P., van der Woude, F.J. and Braun, C. (2003) Acetylcysteine for prevention of contrast nephropathy: meta-analysis. *The Lancet* 362, 598–603.
Bode, B.P., Fuchs, B.C., Hurley, B.P., Conroy, J.L., Suetterlin, J.E., Tanabe, K.K., Rhoads, D.B., Abcouwer, S.F. and Souba, W.W. (2002) Molecular and functional analysis of glutamine uptake in human hepatoma and liver-derived cells. *American Journal of Physiology. Gastrointestinal and Liver Physiology* 283, G1062–G1073.
Boirie, Y., Dangin, M., Gachon, P., Vasson, M.P., Maubois, J.L. and Beaufrere, B. (1997) Slow and fast dietary proteins differently modulate postprandial protein accretion. *Proceedings of the National Academy of Sciences USA* 94, 14930–14935.
Bouteloup-Demange, C., Boirie, Y., Dechelotte, P., Gachon, P. and Beaufrere, B. (1998) Gut mucosal protein synthesis in fed and fasted humans. *American Journal of Physiology* 274, E541–E546.
Bragado, M.J., Tashiro, M. and Williams, J.A. (2000) Regulation of the initiation of pancreatic digestive enzyme protein synthesis by cholecystokinin in rat pancreas *in vivo*. *Gastroenterology* 119, 1731–1739.
Brok, J., Buckley, N. and Gluud, C. (2002) Interventions for paracetamol (acetaminophen) overdoses. *Cochrane Database of Systematic Reviews* (2), CD003328.
Brown, J.A., Gore, D.C. and Jahoor, F. (1994) Catabolic hormones alone fail to reproduce the stress-induced efflux of amino acids. *Archives of Surgery* 129, 819–824.
Bruins, M.J., Soeters, P.B. and Deutz, N.E. (2000) Endotoxemia affects organ protein metabolism differently during prolonged feeding in pigs. *Journal of Nutrition* 130, 3003–3013.
Bruins, M.J., Deutz, N.E. and Soeters, P.B. (2003) Aspects of organ protein, amino acid and glucose metabolism in a porcine model of hypermetabolic sepsis. *Clinical Science* 104, 127–141.
Byrne, T.A., Wilmore, D.W., Iyer, K., Dibaise, J., Clancy, K., Robinson, M.K., Chang, P., Gertner, J.M. and Lautz, D. (2005) Growth hormone, glutamine, and an optimal diet reduces parenteral nutrition in patients with short bowel syndrome: a prospective, randomized, placebo-controlled, double-blind clinical trial. *Annals of Surgery* 242, 655–661.
Cabre, E. and Gassull, M.A. (2005) Nutrition in liver disease. *Current Opinion in Clinical Nutrition and Metabolic Care* 8, 545–551.
Carli, F., Webster, J., Ramachandra, V., Pearson, M., Read, M., Ford, G.C., McArthur, S., Preedy, V.R. and Halliday, D. (1990) Aspects of protein metabolism after elective surgery in patients receiving constant nutritional support. *Clinical Science* 78, 621–628.
Castillo, L., Chapman, T.E., Sanchez, M., Yu, Y.M., Burke, J.F., Ajami, A.M., Vogt, J. and Young, V.R. (1993) Plasma arginine and citrulline kinetics in adults given adequate and arginine-free diets. *Proceedings of the National Academy of Sciences USA* 90, 7749–7753.
Cayol, M., Tauveron, I., Rambourdin, F., Prugnaud, J., Gachon, P., Thieblot, P., Grizard, J. and Obled, C. (1995) Whole-body protein turnover and hepatic protein synthesis are increased by vaccination in man. *Clinical Science* 89, 389–396.
Clowes G.H. Jr, Randall, H.T. and Cha, C.J. (1980) Amino acid and energy metabolism in septic and traumatized patients. *JPEN Journal of Parenteral and Enteral Nutrition* 4, 195–205.
Crenn, P., Coudray-Lucas, C., Thuillier, F., Cynober, L. and Messing, B. (2000) Postabsorptive plasma citrulline concentration is a marker of absorptive enterocyte mass and intestinal failure in humans. *Gastroenterology* 119, 1496–1505.
Cynober, L. (1994) Can arginine and ornithine support gut functions? *Gut* 35(1 Suppl.), S42–S45.
Cynober, L., Le Boucher, J. and Vasson, M.P. (1995) Arginine metabolism in mammals. *Journal of Nutritional Biochemistry* 6, 402–413.

Dangin, M., Boirie, Y., Garcia-Rodenas, C., Gachon, P., Fauquant, J., Callier, P., Ballevre, O. and Beaufrere, B. (2001) The digestion rate of protein is an independent regulating factor of postprandial protein retention. *American Journal of Physiology. Endocrinology and Metabolism* 280, E340–E348.

Deutz, N.E., Reijven, P.L., Bost, M.C., van Berlo, C.L. and Soeters, P.B. (1991) Modification of the effects of blood on amino acid metabolism by intravenous isoleucine. *Gastroenterology* 101, 1613–1620.

Deutz, N.E., Reijven, P.L., Athanasas, G. and Soeters, P.B. (1992a) Post-operative changes in hepatic, intestinal, splenic and muscle fluxes of amino acids and ammonia in pigs. *Clinical Science* 83, 607–614.

Deutz, N.E., Dejong, C.H., Athanasas, G. and Soeters, P.B. (1992b) Partial enterectomy in the rat does not diminish muscle glutamine production. *Metabolism* 41, 1343–1350.

Deutz, N.E.P., Ten Have, G.A.M., Soeters, P.B. and Moughan, P.J. (1995) Increased intestinal amino-acid retention from the addition of carbohydrates to a meal. *Clinical Nutrition* 14, 354–364.

Fong, Y.M., Tracey, K.J., Hesse, D.G., Albert, J.D., Barie, P.S. and Lowry, S.F. (1990) Influence of enterectomy on peripheral tissue glutamine efflux in critically ill patients. *Surgery* 107, 321–326.

Gaudichon, C., Mahe, S., Benamouzig, R., Luengo, C., Fouillet, H., Dare, S. and Van Oycke, M. (1999) Net postprandial utilization of [^{15}N]-labelled milk protein nitrogen is influenced by diet composition in humans. *Journal of Nutrition* 129, 890–895.

Geggel, H.S., Ament, M.E., Heckenlively, J.R., Martin, D.A. and Kopple, J.D. (1985) Nutritional requirement for taurine in patients receiving long-term parenteral nutrition. *New England Journal of Medicine* 312, 142–146.

Gore, D.C. and Jahoor, F. (1994) Glutamine kinetics in burn patients. Comparison with hormonally induced stress in volunteers. *Archives of Surgery* 129, 1318–1323.

Guyton, A.C. and Hall, J.E. (1996) *Textbook of Medical Physiology*. W.B. Saunders, Philadelphia, Pennsylvania.

Hebiguchi, T., Kato, T., Yoshino, H., Mizuno, M., Wakui, H., Komatsuda, A. and Imai, H. (2002) Renal focal tubulointerstitial fibrosis with short bowel syndrome: report of a case. *Surgery Today* 32, 646–650.

Helms, R.A., Storm, M.C., Christensen, M.L., Hak, E.B. and Chesney, R.W. (1999) Cysteine supplementation results in normalization of plasma taurine concentrations in children receiving home parenteral nutrition. *Journal of Pediatrics* 134, 358–361.

Hensley, C.T., Wasti, A.T. and DeBerardinis, R.J. (2013) Glutamine and cancer: cell biology, physiology, and clinical opportunities. *Journal of Clinical Investigation* 123, 3678–3684.

Holm, E., Hagmuller, E., Staedt, U., Schlickeiser, G., Gunther, H.J., Leweling, H., Tokus, M. and Kollmar, H.B. (1995) Substrate balances across colonic carcinomas in humans. *Cancer Research* 55, 1373–1378.

Holmberg, A., Kaim, J., Persson, A., Jensen, J., Wang, T. and Holmgren, S. (2002) Effects of digestive status on the reptilian gut. *Comparative Biochemistry and Physiology. Part A, Molecular & Integrative Physiology* 133, 499–518.

Hsieh, C.C., Hwang, T.L., Chen, H.M., Chen, M.F., Sun, Y.F. and Lau, Y.T. (2003) Sepsis correlated with increased erythrocyte Na^+ content and Na^+/K^+ pump activity. *Journal of Biomedical Science* 10, 389–395.

Hulsewe, K.W., van der Hulst, R.W., van Acker, B.A., von Meyenfeldt, M.F. and Soeters, P.B. (2004) Inflammation rather than nutritional depletion determines glutamine concentrations and intestinal permeability. *Clinical Nutrition* 23, 1209–1216.

Jackson, N.C., Carroll, P.V., Russell-Jones, D.L., Sonksen, P.H., Treacher, D.F. and Umpleby, A.M. (1999) The metabolic consequences of critical illness: acute effects on glutamine and protein metabolism. *American Journal of Physiology* 276, E163–E170.

Kao, C., Hsu, J., Bandi, V. and Jahoor, F. (2013) Alterations in glutamine metabolism and its conversion to citrulline in sepsis. *American Journal of Physiology. Endocrinology and Metabolism* 304, E1359–1364.

Lourenco, R. and Camilo, M.E. (2002) Taurine: a conditionally essential amino acid in humans? An overview in health and disease. *Nutrición Hospitalaria* 17, 262–270.

Luiking, Y.C., Poeze, M., Dejong, C.H., Ramsay, G. and Deutz, N.E. (2004) Sepsis: an arginine deficiency state? *Critical Care Medicine* 32, 2135–2145.

Luiking, Y.C., Poeze, M., Ramsay, G. and Deutz, N.E. (2009) Reduced citrulline production in sepsis is related to diminished *de novo* arginine and nitric oxide production. *American Journal of Clinical Nutrition* 89, 142–152.

Mahe, S., Roos, N., Benamouzig, R., Davin, L., Luengo, C., Gagnon, L., Gausserges, N., Rautureau, J. and Tome, D. (1996) Gastrojejunal kinetics and the digestion of [^{15}N] β-lactoglobulin and casein in humans: the influence of the nature and quantity of the protein. *American Journal of Clinical Nutrition* 63, 546–552.

Marini, J.C., Didelija, I.C., Castillo, L. and Lee, B. (2010) Glutamine: precursor or nitrogen donor for citrulline synthesis? *American Journal of Physiology. Endocrinology and Metabolism* 299, E69–E79.

Mariotti, F., Huneau, J.F., Mahe, S. and Tome, D. (2000) Protein metabolism and the gut. *Current Opinion in Clinical Nutrition and Metabolic Care* 3, 45–50.

Matsutaka, H., Aikawa, T., Yamamoto, H. and Ishikawa, E. (1973) Gluconeogenesis and amino acid metabolism. 3. Uptake of glutamine and output of alanine and ammonia by non-hepatic splanchnic organs of fasted rats and their metabolic significance. *Journal of Biochemistry* 74, 1019–1029.

Melis, G.C., ter Wengel, N., Boelens, P.G. and van Leeuwen, P.A. (2004) Glutamine: recent developments in research on the clinical significance of glutamine. *Current Opinion in Clinical Nutrition and Metabolic Care* 7, 59–70.

Melville, S., McNurlan, M.A., McHardy, K.C., Broom, J., Milne, E., Calder, A.G. and Garlick, P.J. (1989) The role of degradation in the acute control of protein balance in adult man: failure of feeding to stimulate protein synthesis as assessed by L-[1-^{13}C] leucin infusion. *Metabolism* 38, 248–255.

Millward, D.J., Price, G.M., Pacy, P.J. and Halliday, D. (1991) Whole-body protein and amino acid turnover in man: what can we measure with confidence? *Proceedings of the Nutrition Society* 50, 197–216.

Mjaaland, M., Unneberg, K., Larsson, J., Nilsson, L. and Revhaug, A. (1993) Growth hormone after abdominal surgery attenuated forearm glutamine, alanine, 3-methyl-histidine, and total amino acid efflux in patients receiving total parenteral nutrition. *Annals of Surgery* 217, 413–422.

Nakshabendi, I.M., Obeidat, W., Russell, R.I., Downie, S., Smith, K. and Rennie, M.J. (1995) Gut mucosal protein synthesis measured using intravenous and intragastric delivery of stable tracer amino acids. *American Journal of Physiology* 269, E996–E999.

Newsholme, E.A. (1988) A role for muscle in the immune system and its importance in surgery, trauma, sepsis and burns. *Nutrition* 4, 261–268.

Ockenga, J., Borchert, K., Stuber, E., Lochs, H., Manns, M.P. and Bischoff, S.C. (2005) Glutamine-enriched total parenteral nutrition in patients with inflammatory bowel disease. *European Journal of Clinical Nutrition* 59, 1302–1309.

Olde Damink, S.W., Dejong, C.H., Deutz, N.E., van Berlo, C.L. and Soeters, P.B. (1999) Upper gastrointestinal bleeding: an ammoniagenic and catabolic event due to the total absence of isoleucine in the haemoglobin molecule. *Medical Hypotheses* 52, 515–519.

O'Keefe, S.J., Bennet, W.M., Zinsmeister, A.R. and Haymond, M.W. (1994) Pancreatic enzyme synthesis and turnover in human subjects. *American Journal of Physiology* 266, G816–G821.

Osowska, S., Moinard, C., Neveux, N., Loi, C. and Cynober, L. (2004) Citrulline increases arginine pools and restores nitrogen balance after massive intestinal resection. *Gut* 53, 1781–1786.

Owen, O.E., Felig, P., Morgan, A.P., Wahren, J. and Cahill, G.F. Jr (1969) Liver and kidney metabolism during prolonged starvation. *Journal of Clinical Investigation* 48, 574–583.

Pacy, P.J., Price, G.M., Halliday, D., Quevedo, M.R. and Millward, D.J. (1994) Nitrogen homeostasis in man: the diurnal responses of protein synthesis and degradation and amino acid oxidation to diets with increasing protein intakes. *Clinical Science* 86, 103–116.

Quevedo, M.R., Price, G.M., Halliday, D., Pacy, P.J. and Millward, D.J. (1994) Nitrogen homoeostasis in man: diurnal changes in nitrogen excretion, leucine oxidation and whole body leucine kinetics during a reduction from a high to a moderate protein intake. *Clinical Science* 86, 185–193.

Remesy, C., Demigne, C. and Aufrere, J. (1978) Inter-organ relationships between glucose, lactate and amino acids in rats fed on high-carbohydrate or high-protein diets. *The Biochemical Journal* 170, 321–329.

Rodas, P.C., Rooyackers, O., Hebert, C., Norberg, A. and Wernerman, J. (2012) Glutamine and glutathione at ICU admission in relation to outcome. *Clinical Science* 122, 591–597.

Romijn, J.A. (2000) Substrate metabolism in the metabolic response to injury. *Proceedings of the Nutrition Society* 59, 447–449.

Sarac, T.P., Souba, W.W., Miller, J.H., Ryan, C.K., Koch, M., Bessey, P.Q. and Sax, H.C. (1994) Starvation induces differential small bowel luminal amino acid transport. *Surgery* 116, 679–685.

Scheltinga, M.R., Young, L.S., Benfell, K., Bye, R.L., Ziegler, T.R., Santos, A.A. and Antin, J.H. (1991) Glutamine-enriched intravenous feedings attenuate extracellular fluid expansion after a standard stress. *Annals of Surgery* 214, 385–393.

Scolapio, J.S. (2004) Current update of short-bowel syndrome. *Current Opinion in Gastroenterology* 20, 143–145.

Shires, G.T., Peitzman, A.B., Illner, H. and Shires, G.T. (1983) Changes in red blood cell transmembrane potential, electrolytes, and energy content in septic shock. *Journal of Trauma* 23, 769–774.

Soeters, M.R. and Soeters, P.B. (2012) The evolutionary benefit of insulin resistance. *Clinical Nutrition* 31, 1002–1007.

Soeters, P.B. and Grecu, I. (2012) Have we enough glutamine and how does it work? A clinician's view. *Annals of Nutrition and Metabolism* 60, 17–26.

Soeters, P.B., de Jong, C.H. and Deutz, N.E. (2001) The protein sparing function of the gut and the quality of food protein. *Clinical Nutrition* 20, 97–99.

Souba, W.W. (1983) Glucocorticiods alter amino acid metabolism in visceral organs. *Surgical Forum* (Abstract), 79.

Souba, W.W. (1993) Total parenteral nutrition with glutamine in bone marrow transplantation and other clinical applications (editorial; comment). *JPEN Journal of Parenteral and Enteral Nutrition* 17, 403.

Souba, W.W. and Wilmore, D.W. (1983) Postoperative alteration of arteriovenous exchange of amino acids across the gastrointestinal tract. *Surgery* 94, 342–350.

Souba, W.W., Smith, R.J. and Wilmore, D.W. (1985a) Effects of glucocorticoids on glutamine metabolism in visceral organs. *Metabolism* 34, 450–456.

Souba, W.W., Smith, R.J. and Wilmore, D.W. (1985b) Glutamine metabolism by the intestinal tract. *JPEN Journal of Parenteral and Enteral Nutrition* 9, 608–617.

Souba, W.W., Roughneen, P.T., Goldwater, D.L., Williams, J.C. and Rowlands, B.J. (1987) Postoperative alterations in interorgan glutamine exchange in enterectomized dogs. *Journal of Surgical Research* 42, 117–125.

Souba, W.W., Klimberg, V.S., Plumley, D.A., Salloum, R.M., Flynn, T.C., Bland, K.I. and Copeland, E.M. III. (1990) The role of glutamine in maintaining a healthy gut and supporting the metabolic response to injury and infection. *Journal of Surgical Research* 48, 383–391.

van Acker, B.A., Hulsewe, K.W., Wagenmakers, A.J., Soeters, P.B. and von Meyenfeldt, M.F. (2000) Glutamine appearance rate in plasma is not increased after gastrointestinal surgery in humans. *Journal of Nutrition* 130, 1566–1571.

van de Poll, M.C.G., Ligthart-Melis, G.C., Boelens, P.G., Deutz, N.E.P., van Leeuwen, P.A.M. and Dejong, C.H.C. (2007) Intestinal and hepatic metabolism of glutamine and citrulline in humans. *Journal of Physiology* 581, 819–827.

van der Hulst, R.R., van Kreel, B.K., von Meyenfeldt, M.F., Brummer, R.J., Arends, J.W., Deutz, N.E. and Soeters, P.B. (1993) Glutamine and the preservation of gut integrity. *The Lancet* 341, 1363–1365.

van der Hulst, R.R., von Meyenfeldt, M.F., Deutz, N.E. and Soeters, P.B. (1997) Glutamine extraction by the gut is reduced in depleted (corrected) patients with gastrointestinal cancer. *Annals of Surgery* 225, 112–121.

van der Schoor, S.R., van Goudoever, J.B., Stoll, B., Henry, J.F., Rosenberger, J.R., Burrin, D.G. and Reeds, P.J. (2001) The pattern of intestinal substrate oxidation is altered by protein restriction in pigs. *Gastroenterology* 121, 1167–1175.

van der Schoor, S.R., Reeds, P.J., Stoll, B., Henry, J.F., Rosenberger, J.R., Burrin, D.G. and Van Goudoever, J.B. (2002) The high metabolic cost of a functional gut. *Gastroenterology* 123, 1931–1940.

van Goudoever, J.B., Stoll, B., Henry, J.F., Burrin, D.G. and Reeds, P.J. (2000) Adaptive regulation of intestinal lysine metabolism. *Proceedings of the National Academy of Sciences USA* 97, 11620–11625.

Volpi, E., Lucidi, P., Cruciani, G., Monacchia, F., Reboldi, G., Brunetti, P., Bolli, G.B. and De Feo, P. (1996) Contribution of amino acids and insulin to protein anabolism during meal absorption. *Diabetes* 45, 1245–1252.

Waterlow, J.C. (1995) Whole-body protein turnover in humans – past, present, and future. *Annual Review of Nutrition* 15, 57–92.

Windmueller, H.G. (1982) Glutamine utilization by the small intestine. *Advances in Enzymology and Related Areas of Molecular Biology* 53, 201–237.

Windmueller, H.G. and Spaeth, A.E. (1974) Uptake and metabolism of plasma glutamine by the small intestine. *Journal of Biological Chemistry* 249, 5070–5079.

Windmueller, H.G. and Spaeth, A.E. (1975) Intestinal metabolism of glutamine and glutamate from the lumen as compared to glutamine from blood. *Archives of Biochemistry and Biophysics* 171, 662–672.

Windmueller, H.G. and Spaeth, A.E. (1980) Respiratory fuels and nitrogen metabolism *in vivo* in small intestine of fed rats. Quantitative importance of glutamine, glutamate, and aspartate. *Journal of Biological Chemistry* 255, 107–112.

Windmueller, H.G. and Spaeth, A.E. (1981) Source and fate of circulating citrulline. *American Journal of Physiology* 241, E473–E480.

Wu, G. and Morris, S.M. Jr (1998) Arginine metabolism: nitric oxide and beyond. *The Biochemical Journal* 336, 1–17.

Yokoyama, K., Ogura, Y., Kawabata, M., Hinoshita, F., Suzuki, Y., Hara, S., Yamada, A., Mimura, A., Nakayama, M., Kawaguchi, Y. and Sakai, O. (1996) Hyperammonemia in a patient with short bowel syndrome and chronic renal failure. *Nephron* 72, 693–695.

Yoshida, S., Leskiw, M.J., Schluter, M.D., Bush, K.T., Nagele, R.G., Lanza-Jacoby, S. and Stein, T.P. (1992) Effect of total parenteral nutrition, systemic sepsis, and glutamine on gut mucosa in rats. *American Journal of Physiology* 263, E368–E373.

Ziegler, T.R., Young, L.S., Benfell, K., Scheltinga, M., Hortos, K., Bye, R., Morrow, F.D., Jacobs, D.O., Smith, R.J. and Antin, J.H. (1992) Clinical and metabolic efficacy of glutamine-supplemented parenteral nutrition after bone marrow transplantation. A randomized, double-blind, controlled study. *Annals of Internal Medicine* 116, 821–828.

25 Micronutrients in Home Parenteral Nutrition

Alan Shenkin*

Faculty of Medicine, University of Liverpool, Liverpool, UK

Key Point

- In patients on home parenteral nutrition, provision of micronutrients is essential for preventing deficiencies and to optimize nutritional therapy.

Introduction

Most patients who require home parenteral nutrition (HPN) will already have been in hospital for a substantial period and will have been stabilized on a regimen providing amounts of energy and amino acids that meet their requirements. They will no longer be undergoing net catabolism as a result of previous surgery or other therapy and it is unlikely that there is an additional requirement for rapid anabolism. Hence, nutritional requirements for all nutrients, including the micronutrients of vitamins and trace elements, will be similar to those of free-living individuals who are consuming a normal oral diet – variations in requirement will result largely from variations in physical activity. For a minority of patients there may still be issues with regard to regaining tissue mass and function (especially of skeletal muscle) so that requirements will be higher, and for others there may be ongoing substantial losses especially of trace elements, for example through a high-output ileostomy.

This chapter covers typical micronutrient requirements during HPN in adult patients together with some discussion of the requirements of infants and children, how provision of micronutrients may be optimized and some of the risks of excess provision, and suggests a protocol for monitoring safety and adequacy of supply.

*E-mail: shenkin@liv.ac.uk

Micronutrient Requirements in HPN

All patients requiring HPN are either completely dependent for the provision of their trace element and vitamin requirements on their parenteral nutrition (PN) regimen or they may have uncertain or variable intake and absorption from any oral diet they consume. Therefore they need an intravenous supply of all essential vitamins and trace elements to meet their daily requirements. The micronutrient preparations for use in PN have generally been developed to provide more than basal amounts of all micronutrients, to allow particularly for surgical patients who are catabolic, have increased losses or who have commenced PN already in a depleted state. The amount present in each daily dose is therefore more than the amount expected to be absorbed from the Reference Nutrient Intake (the standards used in the UK; Panel of Dietary Reference Values, Department of Health, 1991) or from the US Dietary Reference Intakes (Food and Nutrition Board, Institute of Medicine, 2000, 2002) and, since these additives are given intravenously, they should more than meet the requirement for most individuals. Because of major differences in recommendations in the USA and Europe, the American Society for Parenteral and Enteral Nutrition (A.S.P.E.N.) established a taskforce to consider trace element and vitamin requirements during PN (including HPN) and a comprehensive report has been published (Vanek *et al.*, 2012). It is interesting to note the differences between the recommended oral and intravenous intakes, which reflect the efficiency of intestinal absorption of the different micronutrients from an oral diet (Tables 25.1–25.3). Similar tables for trace element and vitamin

Table 25.1. Trace elements in adult HPN.

	RNI	RDA	Additrace®[a]	Decan®[b]	A.S.P.E.N.
Zinc (μmol) (mg)	145 (9.5)	170 (11)	100 (6.5)	153 (10)	46–77 (3–5)
Copper (μmol) (mg)	19 (1.2)	14 (0.9)	20 (1.3)	7.5 (0.5)	5–8 (0.3–0.5)
Selenium (μmol) (μg)	0.75–0.95 (60–75)	0.7 (55)	0.4 (32)	0.9 (72)	0.75–1.25 (60–100)
Iron (μmol) (mg)	170 (9.5)	140 (8)	360 (20)	320 (18)	NR
Manganese (μmol) (mg)	26 (1.4)	42 (2.3)	5 (0.28)	3.6 (0.2)	1.0 (0.055)
Chromium (μmol) (mg)	0.5 (26)	0.6 (30)	0.2 (10)	0.3 (15)	0.2–0.3 (10–15)
Molybdenum (μmol) (μg)	0.5–4.0 (50–400)	0.5 (50)	0.2 (19)	0.26 (25)	NR
Cobalt (nmol) (μg)	NR	NR	NR	25 (1.5)	NR
Iodine (μmol) (μg)	1.0 (127)	1.2 (150)	1.0 (127)	0.01 (1.27)	NR
Fluoride (μmol) (mg)	200 (3.8)	158 (3)	50 (1)	79 (1.5)	NR

[a]This product is being replaced in some countries with a new product, Addeven®, with lower zinc (77 μmol), copper (6.3 μmol) and manganese (1 μmol) and higher selenium (1 μmol).
[b]This product is being replaced in some countries with a new product, Nutryelt® (Aguettant, France), with lower copper (4.7 μmol), manganese (1 μmol) and fluorine (50 μmol), and higher selenium (0.9 μmol) and iodine (1 μmol).
RNI, Reference Nutrient Intake (UK); RDA, Recommended Dietary Allowance (USA); NR, no recommendation; Additrace®, Fresenius Kabi, Sweden; Decan®, Baxter, France; A.S.P.E.N., from Vanek *et al.* (2012).

Table 25.2. Fat-soluble vitamins in adult HPN.

	RNI	DRI	Vitalipid®	Cemevit®	A.S.P.E.N.
Vitamin A (μg)	700	1000	1000	1000	990
Vitamin E (μg)	5	10	9.1	10.2	10
Vitamin D (μg)	–	5	5	5	5
Vitamin K (μg)	70	80	150	0	150

RNI, Reference Nutrient Intake (UK); DRI, Dietary Reference Intake (USA); Vitalipid®, Fresenius Kabi, Sweden; Cemevit®, Baxter, UK; A.S.P.E.N., from Vanek *et al.* (2012).

Table 25.3. Water-soluble vitamins in adult HPN.

	RNI	DRI	Soluvit N®	Cemevit®	A.S.P.E.N.
Vitamin B_1 (mg)	0.9	15	3.1	3.5	6.0
Vitamin B_2 (mg)	1.3	1.7	4.9	4.1	3.6
Vitamin B_6 (mg)	1.4	2.0	4.0	4.5	6.0
Niacin (mg)	16	19	40	46	40
Folate (μg)	200	200	400	414	600
Vitamin B_{12} (μg)	1.5	2.0	5.0	6.0	5.0
Biotin (μg)	100	150	60	69	60
Vitamin C (mg)	40	60	100	125	200

RNI, Reference Nutrient Intake (UK); DRI, Dietary Reference Intake (USA); Soluvit N®, Fresenius Kabi, Sweden; Cernevit®, Baxter, UK; A.S.P.E.N., from Vanek *et al.* (2012).

requirements in total parenteral nutrition (TPN) have been developed for infants and children (Tables 25.4 and 25.5) (Greene *et al.*, 1988).

Three factors might still put patients at risk of micronutrient deficiency:

1. A small number of patients may be deliberately deprived of certain micronutrient supplements if they develop particular complications. For example, development of cholestasis and hyperbilirubinaemia may lead to concern that copper and manganese may be retained and become toxic due to reduced excretion in the bile. In one case, this led to copper being withdrawn 8 months after commencing TPN and 15 months later the patient developed severe pancytopenia, reversed by copper provision (Fuhrman *et al.*, 2000).

2. More commonly, patients may be given their micronutrient supplements on only a limited number of days per week, for example three to five times. This may be because they require PN only on these days to meet the shortfall in oral intake, or there may be practical reasons due to difficulty in addition of supplements to bags at home. If patients require PN for only a limited number of days per week to maintain body weight and tissue function, it can be assumed that there is sufficient small intestinal function to permit some absorption of macronutrients. It may therefore also be assumed that sufficient micronutrients will have been absorbed from the oral diet that has been consumed. However, this may not be the case since it will depend on the composition of the food and whether there is a suitable balance of all trace elements and vitamins.

Moreover, for those where there are practical difficulties in supply or addition of micronutrients each day, individuals may receive bags with energy/amino

Table 25.4. Trace element requirements during PN in infants and children. (From Greene *et al.*, 1988.)[a]

	Infants >3 months and children (per kg body weight/day)	
	μmol	μg
Iron	1.8	100
Zinc	1.5	100
Copper	0.3	20
Selenium	0.025	2
Manganese	0.02	1
Molybdenum	0.003	0.25
Chromium	0.005	0.2
Iodine	0.008	1
Fluoride	1	20

[a]These amounts are also recommended by A.S.P.E.N. (from Vanek *et al.*, 2012) with the proviso that for neonates, no added chromium should be given, if possible.

Table 25.5. Daily vitamin requirements during PN in infants and children. (From Greene *et al.*, 1988.)[a]

	Infants >3 months and children (per kg body weight/day)
Vitamin A (μg)	700
Vitamin D (μg)	10
Vitamin E (mg)	7
Vitamin K (μg)	200
Vitamin B_1 (mg)	1.2
Vitamin B_2 (mg)	1.4
Vitamin B_5 (mg)	5
Vitamin B_6 (mg)	1.0
Vitamin B_{12} (μg)	1.0
Vitamin C (mg)	80
Folic acid (μg)	140
Biotin (μg)	20
Niacin (mg)	17

[a]These amounts are also recommended by A.S.P.E.N. (from Vanek *et al.*, 2012).

acids/minerals but without certain trace elements or vitamins. For example, fat emulsions may be provided only once or twice per week and hence provision of fat-soluble vitamins may be limited. Although preparations exist that provide fat-soluble vitamins in a water-soluble base, some of these are incomplete. Moreover, some preparations lack certain water-soluble vitamins and use may lead to deficiency, for example of biotin (Carlson *et al.*, 1995).

Patients who receive a reduced supply of micronutrients are at risk of micronutrient depletion and ultimately clinical deficiency, but overall there is only a little evidence of this, probably because of the excess of most micronutrients available from the days when micronutrients are provided.

3. There remains a significant risk of instability of certain micronutrients within the PN mixture. This is probably of most concern for ascorbic acid, which is readily oxidized if oxygen-permeable EVA (ethylene vinyl acetate) bags are used. Oxidation is much more rapid if copper is also present in the PN mixture, which would generally be the case (Allwood and Kearney, 1998). Those patients whose bags are prepared with all additives present before delivery to the home are therefore likely to receive an inadequate amount of vitamin C. Degradation of ascorbate is much reduced if multilayered bags, impermeable to oxygen, are used. Similarly, there is concern about the stability of thiamine and riboflavin to ultraviolet light (Gibbons *et al.*, 2001). Thiamine is also sensitive to degradation by bisulfite, which is present in some amino acid preparations as a preservative (Smith *et al.*, 1988). Vitamin A is also sensitive to ultraviolet radiation, but this is unlikely to be a problem with normal room lighting.

Certain of the trace elements may also undergo chemical change and hence become less bioavailable; for example, zinc may complex with some amino acids, copper may react with hydrogen sulfide that is generated by sterilization of cysteine (Bates *et al.*, 1984) or selenite may be reduced to the non-available elemental selenium (Ganther and Kraus, 1989). The extent to which this is a real risk leading to impaired clinical status has not yet been established, but on theoretical grounds it would seem safer, and more effective, to make all additions of micronutrients immediately before infusion.

Adequacy of Provision of Trace Elements and Vitamins

In the early days of HPN, patients often received incomplete or unbalanced preparations of trace elements and vitamins, leading to a variety of well-documented deficiency states in both adults (Jeejeebhoy *et al.*, 1977; Takagi *et al.*, 1977; Johnson *et al.*, 1981) and children (Dunlap *et al.*, 1974; Weber *et al.*, 1981; Vinton *et al.*, 1987). With the development of modern, more complete parenteral micronutrient preparations, recent studies of trace element and vitamin status have largely confirmed that provided patients receive a regular supply of these supplements, biochemical measurements in plasma will be within or close to 'normal' limits (Davis *et al.*, 1987; Malone *et al.*, 1989). Some studies have shown that biochemical status may not be optimal (Forbes and Forbes, 1997; Reimund *et al.*, 2000a, 2002), especially if micronutrients are pre-added to bags and stored in this way for up to 30 days (Baines *et al.*, 2001). However, provided the regimen is reviewed to ensure regular provision of all essential vitamins and trace elements, it should now be a rare event indeed for a patient to develop clinical signs of deficiency. Nonetheless, for certain micronutrients there continues to be concern about the adequacy of input.

Iron

Iron-deficiency anaemia is still a frequent problem in HPN, one study finding that approximately 30% of patients developed this complication (Forbes and Forbes, 1997). This occurs mainly because preparations of trace elements for TPN contain low amounts of iron, or sometimes no iron, due to concerns about incompatibilities in the PN mixture. Anaemia can be readily treated by provision of small daily doses of iron or by whole-body iron dextran infusions (Khaodhiar *et al.*, 2002). In a study on eight HPN patients on whom autopsy samples were available, tissue iron concentrations were found to be similar to control values, whereas zinc, copper and manganese were more variable (Howard *et al.*, 2007). This suggests that the availability of sensitive functional tests for iron status permits fairly accurate provision of adequate amounts, in contrast to those elements where such functional indices are less available.

Selenium

The Reference Nutrient Intake (UK) or Recommended Dietary Intake (USA) for selenium is about 0.7–1.0 μmol/day (55–75 μg/day) in the oral diet (Panel of Dietary Reference Values, Department of Health, 1991; Food and Nutrition Board, Institute of Medicine, 2000). Since selenium is absorbed efficiently from the small intestine, this is the amount that should be provided intravenously. In a unique study of autopsy material from patients who died while receiving HPN, a supply of 1.1 μmol/day (600 μg/week) was found to maintain an adequate intracellular selenium concentration in most tissues examined (Howard *et al.*, 2005).

One extensively used preparation provides only 0.4 μmol/day and studies have shown that although this may be adequate to maintain selenium status in many patients, it will not be sufficient to correct depleted selenium status, nor maintain the status in those with greater needs (Malone *et al.*, 1989). The best estimate of selenium requirements during intravenous nutrition is within the range of 0.75–1.25 μmol/day (60–100 μg/day), which will meet the basal requirement plus an amount to compensate for ongoing depletion or increased oxidative stress (Shenkin, 2009).

This issue is compounded by ongoing concern about the adequacy of selenium intake in the oral diet, with most countries in Europe having low dietary selenium (Rayman, 2002). So even if patients are consuming a reasonable oral intake, it is unlikely that this will compensate for a low intravenous intake. Patients receiving a low daily intravenous intake may therefore require additional supplements of selenium, possibly in the form of a separate additive of sodium selenite.

Vitamin K

A long-standing recommendation from the Nutritional Advisory Group of the American Medical Association was that patients should not receive daily vitamin K supplements if they were on anticoagulant therapy (Nutrition Advisory Group, 1979). Certain fat-soluble vitamin preparations for PN therefore do not contain vitamin K (Table 25.2). Patients may receive some intake of vitamin K from soybean oil emulsions (Lennon *et al.*, 1993), but this may not be sufficient, and if not given further vitamin K, patients receiving PN have prolonged prothrombin times (Dalton *et al.*, 1984). The Food and Drug Administration therefore now recommends inclusion of vitamin K in the PN regimen at a level of 150 μg/day (Helphingstine and Bistrian, 2003). This may lead to an increased requirement for warfarin for patients requiring anticoagulation, but provided clinicians are aware of this likely requirement, the potential benefits of ensuring all patients maintain vitamin K status should be worthwhile. If patients are receiving a preparation that does not include vitamin K, then a separate injection of vitamin K should be given once per week.

Provision of Micronutrients to Achieve Optimal Tissue Function

Prevention of clinical deficiency is no longer regarded as sufficient evidence of adequacy of provision (Shenkin, 2004). This is especially true for patients receiving HPN, since this may continue for many years, and the main objectives are to ensure the best possible quality of life and freedom from disease over the period of HPN and beyond that period, if patients adapt to an enteral or oral diet. Micronutrients have a key role in the function of many organs and tissues, including brain, muscle, bone and the immune system. It is widely believed that marginal or subclinical deficiency carries some disadvantage, either at the metabolic level or in terms of non-specific symptoms such as tiredness. However, demonstrating benefit from preventing or correcting such subclinical deficiency has proved elusive. Despite some early suggestions of benefit on immune function (Chandra, 1992), these studies have now been discredited (White, 2004) and recent studies have failed to demonstrate any reduction in infections in elderly individuals taking a well-balanced micronutrient supplement (Avenell *et al.*, 2005; El Kadiki and Sutton, 2005). And with a small number of notable exceptions (Clark *et al.*, 1996; Hercberg *et al.*, 2004), long-term trials of antioxidant vitamins and trace elements have failed to demonstrate a reduction in coronary artery disease, cancer incidence or mortality (Shenkin, 2006; Bjelakovic *et al.*, 2012). Some evidence exists for improved outcome in critically ill patients by use of antioxidant micronutrients (Heyland *et al.*, 2005), although this is inconsistent. There have been no long-term studies of micronutrient supply and clinical outcome in patients receiving HPN.

It is now recognized that some changes in tissue function occur as a result of changes in oxidant/antioxidant balance and that micronutrients play multiple roles in achieving adequate antioxidant status (Evans and Halliwell, 2001). There is special concern in relation to oxidative damage to polyunsaturated fatty acids in lipoproteins, which is a key stage in the development of coronary artery disease. Oxidized fatty acids within cell membranes will also alter the function of membranes and non-specifically impair cell function (Evans and Halliwell, 2001). Moreover, damage to nucleic acids will lead to a reduction in the DNA repair mechanisms or to mutagenesis, which in turn may lead to neoplastic disease. These changes are probably of only minimal concern when considering short-term PN in the acutely ill patient, but they take on more significance when optimizing long-term nutritional care.

In our own studies, we have found that total antioxidant status is frequently poor prior to surgery and is not corrected by up to 19 days of PN with standard supplements in the post-operative period (Baines and Shenkin, 2002). During HPN, regular provision of standard supplements maintained plasma concentrations of most micronutrients and plasma antioxidant capacity in most patients, but less consistently if the bag had been stored after addition of the micronutrients (Baines *et al.*, 2001).

Only a few studies have been reported on antioxidant status in PN. Pironi *et al.* (1998) found an increase in serum malondialdehyde (MDA) in HPN patients, indicating increased lipid peroxidation, which correlated with the daily polyunsaturated fatty acid load in the lipid emulsion, and also correlated negatively with the plasma tocopherol concentration. Reimund *et al.* (2000a) also found increased MDA, which was correlated with the reduced plasma vitamin E concentration. Red blood cell (RBC) glutathione peroxidase and plasma selenium were also reduced. MDA may therefore be a sensitive indicator of inadequate/adequate antioxidant status in HPN. In a short-term post-operative TPN study, Linseisen *et al.* (2000) showed that supplementation with a medium-chain triacylglycerol (MCT)/long-chain triacylglycerol (LCT)/*n*-3 fatty acid emulsion enriched with α-tocopherol was not associated with evidence of lipid peroxidation, although rather surprisingly this was also the case for an LCT emulsion that was not supplemented with vitamin E. Schepens *et al.* (2006) found that although there was some evidence of increased oxidative stress in their HPN patients receiving standard additives, there was no evidence of increased oxidative damage.

Taken overall, these studies suggest that increased amounts of tocopherol may be required during HPN depending on the fat emulsion used, and that care is also required to ensure adequate selenium provision. This should, however, also be balanced by the evidence that high-dose tocopherol supplements (>150 μg/day) may be associated with increased all-cause mortality (Miller *et al.*, 2005). Moreover, there is no evidence that the biochemical changes of increased oxidation that have been observed in some, but not all studies have translated into an increased risk of disease or complications. Hence much more work with accurate clinical outcomes is required to optimize long-term parenteral intake of the various micronutrients.

Risks of Excess Provision

For most micronutrients, the safety margin between adequacy of provision and toxicity is large and there is little danger of seriously excessive provision. Moreover, commercial preparations have now been in use in individual patients for many years and few toxic effects have been observed. Nonetheless, the following continue to be of some concern.

Chromium

Most patients receiving long-term PN have elevated plasma levels of chromium (Malone *et al.*, 1989; Moukarzel *et al.*, 1992) and increased tissue content of chromium (Howard *et al.*, 2007). This results from the deliberate provision of chromium to ensure prevention of chromium deficiency states, together with the variable contamination of chromium in PN solutions, especially amino acid preparations. It is not clear whether this high level of chromium is directly harmful, although in neonates on long-term PN, serum chromium was inversely correlated with glomerular filtration rate and the renal function was not improved after stopping chromium supplementation in the PN (Moukarzel *et al.*, 1992). There is no evidence of harm in adults; this is supported by studies on patients with implanted hip prostheses who had very high serum and urine chromium over a 10-year period but showed no change in renal function (Marker *et al.*, 2008).

Manganese

Manganese toxicity is of greater concern, since a number of patients have now been identified with high blood manganese concentrations and associated clinical toxicity. High serum or whole-blood manganese may result from excess provision or from reduced excretion in bile as a result of cholestatic disease (Hambidge *et al.*, 1989). Cholestasis is likely to be less important than excess provision (Wardle *et al.*, 1999), although patients with chronic inflammation are more likely to develop hypermanganesaemia with abnormal biochemical liver function tests (Reimund *et al.*, 2000b).

The main complication of hypermanganesaemia is deposition of manganese in the basal ganglia (Mirowitz and Westrich, 1992), which may be associated with symptoms of Parkinsonism (Ejima *et al.*, 1992; Reynolds *et al.*, 1998). Although withdrawal of manganese provision may reverse deposition in the basal ganglia, as detected by magnetic resonance imaging (Ono *et al.*, 1995), reversal of symptoms is not consistent. Manganese toxicity may also predispose to cholestasis in children (Fell *et al.*, 1996), but other studies have suggested that factors other than manganese are more important in the aetiology of cholestasis in parenterally fed children (Beath *et al.*, 1996).

It seems clear that care must be taken with manganese provision. Over recent years, with better methods of assessing manganese status, recommendations for intravenous provision have fallen progressively from about 40 μmol/day (Wretlind, 1972) to 3–5 μmol/day (Shenkin, 2001) to 1 μmol/day (Takagi *et al.*, 2002; Vanek *et al.*, 2012) or less (Hardy, 2009). Patients receiving long-term PN should have manganese status checked, if possible, on a regular basis, by measurement of whole-blood manganese concentration. Development of unexplained neurological changes or cholestatic disease is an indication for careful assessment of manganese status and provision.

Vitamin D

There is continued uncertainty about how to optimize vitamin D status during HPN. One of the most difficult complications of HPN is a painful metabolic bone disease, with variable histological features and reduced bone mineral density (Jeejeebhoy, 1998). Different studies have suggested overprovision of vitamin D

(Verhage *et al.*, 1995), suppression of normal parathyroid responses (Lipkin, 1998), a role for excess aluminium provision (Klein *et al.*, 1992) or indeed an effect of many other dietary components (New, 2003). Overall, it seems likely that many patients will have inadequate vitamin D status (Vanek *et al.*, 2012), which may have long-term effects on bone strength and muscle and immune function. It would appear to be good practice to maintain vitamin D concentrations at about the level that prevents vitamin D insufficiency and maintains a normal plasma parathyroid hormone concentration. Oral supplements of vitamin D (as much as 500 μg/day) may be adequate if there is some absorptive capacity.

A Protocol for Monitoring Micronutrients during HPN

Based on the discussion above, the following protocol can be proposed for patients on HPN (National Collaborating Centre for Acute Care, 2006):

- Assess the weekly intake of micronutrients from all sources – intravenous, plus oral or enteral – making an approximate allowance for the length of small intestine and the likely efficiency of absorption.
- Ensure that the estimated total intake exceeds the recommended intakes from an adequate oral diet.
- On starting HPN, and every 3–6 months, check the following: plasma concentration of zinc, copper and selenium (with C-reactive protein and albumin to assist interpretation); plasma 25-hydroxyvitamin D and parathyroid hormone; plasma vitamin B_{12} and folate, and RBC folate; RBC manganese; RBC glutathione peroxidase; haemoglobin, haematocrit and mean corpuscular volume; urea and electrolytes; and biochemical liver function tests. The frequency of these checks will vary if there is a change in the patient's condition or if there is a need to change the regimen.
- Certain other measurements of antioxidant status could also be considered that are mainly used for research purposes, for example total antioxidant capacity (Serafini and Del Rio, 2004), and/or are markers of oxidative damage such as MDA or F_2 isoprostanes (Roth *et al.*, 2004).
- Plasma homocysteine may be helpful in optimizing folate status (Young and Woodside, 2000).

Summary

In patients receiving long-term intravenous nutrition, the main objectives of provision of micronutrients are prevention of deficiency and optimization of function. In children, there must also be an allowance for growth. These can largely be achieved by meticulous attention to intake relative to requirements of all the micronutrients, together with a careful protocol for laboratory testing. The use of markers of oxidant stress and of oxidative damage, together with physiological markers of tissue function or markers of immune function may be helpful, and these should be included in future studies. Attention must also be paid to ensure that micronutrients are given safely, that incompatibility or degradation does not take place within the intravenous nutrition bag or mixture, and that patients are not exposed to excess levels of provision. More studies of different levels of provision and long-term outcome are required.

References

Allwood, M.C. and Kearney, M.C. (1998) Compatibility and stability of additives in parenteral nutrition admixtures. *Nutrition* 14, 697–706.

Avenell, A., Campbell, M.K., Cook, J.A., Hannaford, P.C., Kilonzo, M.M., McNeill, G., Milne, A.C., Ramsay, C.R., Seymour, D.G., Stephen, A.I. and Vale, L.D. (2005) Effect of multivitamin and multimineral supplements on morbidity from infections in older people (MAVIS trial): pragmatic, randomised, double blind, placebo controlled trial. *British Medical Journal* 331, 324–329.

Baines, M. and Shenkin, A. (2002) Lack of effectiveness of short-term intravenous micronutrient nutrition in restoring plasma antioxidant status after surgery. *Clinical Nutrition* 21, 145–150.

Baines, M., Barber, D., Davidson, A., Gabe, S.M., Shaffer, J.L. and Shenkin, A. (2001) Effect of differing antioxidant intakes upon plasma antioxidant concentrations of patients on home IVN. *Clinical Nutrition* 20, 46–47.

Bates, C.G., Greiner, G. and Gegenheimer, A. (1984) Precipitate in admixtures of new amino acid injection. *American Journal of Hospital Pharmacy* 41, 1312–1316.

Beath, S.V., Gopalan, S. and Booth, I.W. (1996) Manganese toxicity and parenteral nutrition. *The Lancet* 347, 1773–1774.

Bjelakovic, G., Nikolova, D., Gluud, L.L., Simonetti, R.G. and Gluud, C. (2012) Antioxidant supplements for prevention of mortality in healthy participants and patients with various diseases. *Cochrane Database of Systematic Reviews* issue 3, CD007176.

Carlson, G.L., Williams, N. and Barber, D. (1995) Biotin deficiency complicating long-term total parenteral nutrition in an adult patient. *Clinical Nutrition* 14, 186–190.

Chandra, R.K. (1992) Effect of vitamin and trace-element supplementation on immune responses and infection in elderly subjects. *The Lancet* 340, 1124–1127.

Clark, L.C., Combs, G.F. Jr, Turnbull, B.W., Slate, E.H., Chalker, D.K., Chow, J., Davis, L.S., Glover, R.A., Graham, G.F., Gross, E.G., Krongrad, A., Lesher, J.L. Jr, Park, H.K., Sanders, B.B. Jr, Smith, C.L. and Taylor, J.R. (1996) Effects of selenium supplementation for cancer prevention in patients with carcinoma of the skin. A randomized controlled trial. Nutritional Prevention of Cancer Study Group. *Journal of the American Medical Association* 276, 1957–1963.

Dalton, M.J., Schepers, G., Gee, J.P., Alberts, C.C., Eckhauser, F.E. and Kirking, D.M. (1984) Consultative total parenteral nutrition teams: the effect on the incidence of total parenteral nutrition-related complications. *JPEN Journal of Parenteral and Enteral Nutrition* 8, 146–152.

Davis, A.T., Franz, F.P., Courtnay, D.A., Ullrey, D.E., Scholten, D.J. and Dean, R.E. (1987) Plasma vitamin and mineral status in home parenteral nutrition patients. *JPEN Journal of Parenteral and Enteral Nutrition* 11, 480–485.

Dunlap, W.M., James, G.W. III and Hume, D.M. (1974) Anemia and neutropenia caused by copper deficiency. *Annals of Internal Medicine* 80, 470–476.

Ejima, A., Imamura, T., Nakamura, S., Saito, H., Matsumoto, K. and Momono, S. (1992) Manganese intoxication during total parenteral nutrition. *The Lancet* 339, 426.

El Kadiki, A. and Sutton, A.J. (2005) Role of multivitamins and mineral supplements in preventing infections in elderly people: systematic review and meta-analysis of randomised controlled trials. *British Medical Journal* 330, 871–874.

Evans, P. and Halliwell, B. (2001) Micronutrients: oxidant/antioxidant status. *British Journal of Nutrition* 85, 67–74.

Fell, J.M., Reynolds, A.P., Meadows, N., Khan, K., Long, S.G., Quaghebeur, G., Taylor, W.J. and Milla, P.J. (1996) Manganese toxicity in children receiving long-term parenteral nutrition. *The Lancet* 347, 1218–1221.

Food and Nutrition Board, Institute of Medicine (2000) *Dietary Reference Intakes for Vitamin C, Vitamin E, Selenium, and Carotenoids.* National Academy Press, Washington, DC.

Food and Nutrition Board, Institute of Medicine (2002) *Dietary Reference Intakes for Vitamin A, Vitamin K, Arsenic, Boron, Chromium, Copper, Iodine, Iron, Manganese, Molybdenum, Nickel, Silicon, Vanadium, and Zinc.* National Academy Press, Washington, DC.

Forbes, G.M. and Forbes, A. (1997) Micronutrient status in patients receiving home parenteral nutrition. *Nutrition* 13, 941–944.

Fuhrman, M.P., Herrmann, V., Masidonski, P. and Eby, C. (2000) Pancytopenia after removal of copper from total parenteral nutrition. *JPEN Journal of Parenteral and Enteral Nutrition* 24, 361–366.

Ganther, H.E. and Kraus, R.J. (1989) Chemical stability of selenious acid in total parenteral nutrition solutions containing ascorbic acid. *JPEN Journal of Parenteral and Enteral Nutrition* 13, 185–188.

Gibbons, E., Allwood, M.C., Neal, T. and Hardy, G. (2001) Degradation of dehydroascorbic acid in parenteral nutrition mixtures. *Journal of Pharmaceutical and Biomedical Analysis* 25, 605–611.

Greene, H.L., Hambidge, K.M., Schanler, R. and Tsang, R.C. (1988) Guidelines for the use of vitamins, trace elements, calcium, magnesium, and phosphorus in infants and children receiving total parenteral nutrition: report of the Subcommittee on Pediatric Parenteral Nutrient Requirements from the Committee on Clinical Practice Issues of the American Society for Clinical Nutrition. *American Journal of Clinical Nutrition* 48, 1324–1342.

Hambidge, K.M., Sokol, R.J., Fidanza, S.J. and Goodall, M.A. (1989) Plasma manganese concentrations in infants and children receiving parenteral nutrition. *JPEN Journal of Parenteral and Enteral Nutrition* 13, 168–171.

Hardy, G. (2009) Manganese in parenteral nutrition: who, when, and why should we supplement? *Gastroenterology* 137(5 Suppl.), 29–35.

Helphingstine, C.J. and Bistrian, B.R. (2003) New Food and Drug Administration requirements for inclusion of vitamin K in adult parenteral multivitamins. *JPEN Journal of Parenteral and Enteral Nutrition* 27, 220–224.

Hercberg, S., Galan, P., Preziosi, P., Bertrais, S., Mennen, L., Malvy, D., Roussel, A.M., Favier, A. and Briancon, S. (2004) The SU.VI.MAX Study: a randomized, placebo-controlled trial of the health effects of antioxidant vitamins and minerals. *Archives of Internal Medicine* 164, 2335–2342.

Heyland, D.K., Dhaliwal, R., Suchner, U. and Berger, M.M. (2005) Antioxidant nutrients: a systematic review of trace elements and vitamins in the critically ill patient. *Intensive Care Medicine* 31, 327–337.

Howard, L., Ashley, C., Lyon, D. and Shenkin, A. (2005) Autopsy tissue selenium levels in eight home parenteral nutrition (HPN) patients. *JPEN Journal of Parenteral and Enteral Nutrition* 29, 38.

Howard, L., Ashley, C., Lyon, D. and Shenkin, A. (2007) Autopsy tissue trace elements in 8 long-term parenteral nutrition patients who received the current US Food and Drug Administration formulation. *JPEN Journal of Parenteral and Enteral Nutrition* 31, 388–396.

Jeejeebhoy, K.N. (1998) Metabolic bone disease and total parenteral nutrition: a progress report. *American Journal of Clinical Nutrition* 67, 186–187.

Jeejeebhoy, K.N., Chu, R.C., Marliss, E.B., Greenberg, G.R. and Bruce-Robertson, A. (1977) Chromium deficiency, glucose intolerance, and neuropathy reversed by chromium supplementation, in a patient receiving long-term total parenteral nutrition. *American Journal of Clinical Nutrition* 30, 531–538.

Johnson, R.A., Baker, S.S., Fallon, J.T., Maynard, E.P. III, Ruskin, J.N., Wen, Z., Ge, K. and Cohen, H.J. (1981) An occidental case of cardiomyopathy and selenium deficiency. *New England Journal of Medicine* 304, 1210–1212.

Khaodhiar, L., Keane-Ellison, M., Tawa, N.E., Thibault, A., Burke, P.A. and Bistrian, B.R. (2002) Iron deficiency anemia in patients receiving home total parenteral nutrition. *JPEN Journal of Parenteral and Enteral Nutrition* 26, 114–119.

Klein, G.L., Alfrey, A.C., Shike, M. and Sherrard, D.J. (1992) Aluminum and TPN-related bone disease. *American Journal of Clinical Nutrition* 55, 483–485.

Lennon, C., Davidson, K.W., Sadowski, J.A. and Mason, J.B. (1993) The vitamin K content of intravenous lipid emulsions. *JPEN Journal of Parenteral and Enteral Nutrition* 17, 142–144.

Linseisen, J., Hoffmann, J., Lienhard, S., Jauch, K.W. and Wolfram, G. (2000) Antioxidant status of surgical patients receiving TPN with an omega-3-fatty acid-containing lipid emulsion supplemented with α-tocopherol. *Clinical Nutrition* 19, 177–184.

Lipkin, E.W. (1998) A longitudinal study of calcium regulation in a nonhuman primate model of parenteral nutrition. *American Journal of Clinical Nutrition* 67, 246–254.

Malone, M., Shenkin, A., Fell, G.S. and Irving, M.H. (1989) Evaluation of a trace element preparation in patients receiving home intravenous nutrition. *Clinical Nutrition* 8, 307–312.

Marker, M., Grübl, A., Riedl, O., Heinze, G., Pohanka, E. and Kotz, R. (2008) Metal-on-metal hip implants: do they impair renal function in the long-term? A 10-year follow-up study. *Archives of Orthopaedic and Trauma Surgery* 128, 915–919.

Miller, E.R. III, Pastor-Barriuso, R., Dalal, D., Riemersma, R.A., Appel, L.J. and Guallar, E. (2005) Meta-analysis: high-dosage vitamin E supplementation may increase all-cause mortality. *Annals of Internal Medicine* 142, 37–46.

Mirowitz, S.A. and Westrich, T.J. (1992) Basal ganglial signal intensity alterations: reversal after discontinuation of parenteral manganese administration. *Radiology* 185, 535–536.

Moukarzel, A.A., Song, M.K., Buchman, A.L., Vargas, J., Guss, W., McDiarmid, S., Reyen, L. and Ament, M.E. (1992) Excessive chromium intake in children receiving total parenteral nutrition. *The Lancet* 339, 385–388.

National Collaborating Centre for Acute Care (2006) *Nutrition Support in Adults. Oral Nutrition Support, Enteral Tube Feeding and Parenteral Nutrition.* National Collaborating Centre for Acute Care, London.

New, S.A. (2003) Intake of fruit and vegetables: implications for bone health. *Proceedings of the Nutrition Society* 62, 889–899.

Nutrition Advisory Group (1979) Multivitamin preparations for parenteral use. A statement by the Nutrition Advisory Group. American Medical Association Department of Foods and Nutrition, 1975. *JPEN Journal of Parenteral and Enteral Nutrition* 3, 258–262.

Ono, J., Harada, K., Kodaka, R., Sakurai, K., Tajiri, H., Takagi, Y., Nagai, T., Harada, T., Nihei, A. and Okada, A. (1995) Manganese deposition in the brain during long-term total parenteral nutrition. *JPEN Journal of Parenteral and Enteral Nutrition* 19, 310–312.

Panel of Dietary Reference Values, Department of Health (1991) *Dietary Reference Values for Food Energy and Nutrients for the United Kingdom.* HMSO, London.

Pironi, L., Ruggeri, E., Zolezzi, C., Savarino, L., Incasa, E., Belluzzi, A., Munarini, A., Piazzi, S., Tolomelli, M., Pizzoferrato, A. and Miglioli, M. (1998) Lipid peroxidation and antioxidant status in adults receiving lipid-based home parenteral nutrition. *American Journal of Clinical Nutrition* 68, 888–893.

Rayman, M.P. (2002) The argument for increasing selenium intake. *Proceedings of the Nutrition Society* 61, 203–215.
Reimund, J.M., Arondel, Y., Duclos, B. and Baumann, R. (2000a) Vitamins and trace elements in home parenteral nutrition patients. *Journal of Nutrition Health and Aging* 4, 13–18.
Reimund, J.M., Dietemann, J.L., Warter, J.M., Baumann, R. and Duclos, B. (2000b) Factors associated to hypermanganesemia in patients receiving home parenteral nutrition. *Clinical Nutrition* 19, 343–348.
Reimund, J.M., Arondel, Y., Duclos, B. and Baumann, R. (2002) Vitamins and trace elements in home parenteral nutrition patients – erratum. *Journal of Nutrition Health and Aging* 6, 290.
Reynolds, N., Blumsohn, A., Baxter, J.P., Houston, G. and Pennington, C.R. (1998) Manganese requirement and toxicity in patients on home parenteral nutrition. *Clinical Nutrition* 17, 227–230.
Roth, E., Manhart, N. and Wessner, B. (2004) Assessing the antioxidative status in critically ill patients. *Current Opinions in Clinical Nutrition and Metabolic Care* 7, 161–168.
Schepens, M.A., Roelofs, H.M., Peters, W.H. and Wanten, G.J. (2006) No evidence for oxidative stress in patients on home parenteral nutrition. *Clinical Nutrition* 25, 939–948.
Serafini, M. and Del Rio, D. (2004) Understanding the association between dietary antioxidants, redox status and disease: is the total antioxidant capacity the right tool? *Redox Report* 9, 145–152.
Shenkin, A. (2001) Adult micronutrient requirements. In: Payne-James, J., Grimble, G. and Silk, D. (eds) *Artificial Nutrition Support in Clinical Practice*, 2nd edn. Greenwich Medical Media, London, pp. 193–212.
Shenkin, A. (2004) Trace elements and vitamins in parenteral and enteral nutrition. In: Sobotka, L. (ed.) *Basics in Clinical Nutrition*, 3rd edn. Galen, Prague, pp. 169–175.
Shenkin, A. (2006) The key role of micronutrients. *Clinical Nutrition* 25, 1–13.
Shenkin, A. (2009) Selenium in intravenous nutrition. *Gastroenterology* 137, 61–69.
Smith, J.L., Canham, J.E., Kirkland, W.D. and Wells, P.A. (1988) Effect of Intralipid, amino acids, container, temperature, and duration of storage on vitamin stability in total parenteral nutrition admixtures. *JPEN Journal of Parenteral and Enteral Nutrition* 12, 478–483.
Takagi, Y., Okada, A., Itakura, T., Satani, M., Manabe, H. and Kasahara, N. (1977) Zinc deficiency during intravenous hyperalimentation. A clinical analysis of eleven cases. *Medical Journal of Osaka University* 28, 67–76.
Takagi, Y., Okada, A., Sando, K., Wasa, M., Yoshida, H. and Hirabuki, N. (2002) Evaluation of indexes of *in vivo* manganese status and the optimal intravenous dose for adult patients undergoing home parenteral nutrition. *American Journal of Clinical Nutrition* 75, 112–118.
Vanek, V.W., Borum, P., Buchman, A., Fessler, T.A., Howard, L., Jeejeebhoy, K., Kochevar, M., Shenkin, A. and Valentine, C.J. (2012) A.S.P.E.N. position paper: recommendations for changes in commercially available parenteral multivitamin and multi-trace element products. *Nutrition in Clinical Practice* 27, 440–491.
Verhage, A.H., Cheong, W.K., Allard, J.P. and Jeejeebhoy, K.N. (1995) Harry M. Vars Research Award. Increase in lumbar spine bone mineral content in patients on long-term parenteral nutrition without vitamin D supplementation. *JPEN Journal of Parenteral and Enteral Nutrition* 19, 431–436.
Vinton, N.E., Dahlstrom, K.A., Strobel, C.T. and Ament, M.E. (1987) Macrocytosis and pseudoalbinism: manifestations of selenium deficiency. *Journal of Pediatrics* 111, 711–717.
Wardle, C.A., Forbes, A., Roberts, N.B., Jawhari, A.V. and Shenkin, A. (1999) Hypermanganesemia in long-term intravenous nutrition and chronic liver disease. *JPEN Journal of Parenteral and Enteral Nutrition* 23, 350–355.
Weber, T.R., Sears, N., Davies, B. and Grosfeld, J.L. (1981) Clinical spectrum of zinc deficiency in pediatric patients receiving total parenteral nutrition (TPN). *Journal of Pediatric Surgery* 16, 236–240.

White, C. (2004) Three journals raise doubts on validity of Canadian studies. *British Medical Journal* 328, 67.

Wretlind, A. (1972) Complete intravenous nutrition. Theoretical and experimental background. *Nutrition and Metabolism* 14(Suppl.), 57.

Young, I.S. and Woodside, J.V. (2000) Folate and homocysteine. *Current Opinion in Clinical Nutrition and Metabolic Care* 3, 427–432.

26 Choice of Venous Access in Home Parenteral Nutrition

Mauro Pittiruti[1]* and Paolo Cotogni[2]

[1]Department of Surgery, Catholic University Hospital, Rome, Italy;
[2]Department of Medicine, University of Turin, Turin, Italy

Key Points

- Choice of venous access for home parenteral nutrition (HPN) must reflect nutritional requirements, expected duration of therapy and the patient's choice.
- Short-term devices are not recommended for patients on home treatment.
- Peripherally inserted central catheters are an option also for patients sent home with parenteral nutrition, but self-care is difficult due to the placement of the device.
- The choice between the tunnelled catheter and the port, the most commonly used devices for patients on HPN, depends on the skills of the staff and the patient's preference.

Introduction

The proper choice of a venous access for parenteral nutrition (PN) depends largely on nutrient requirements, expected duration of PN and the setting in which PN will be delivered (August *et al.*, 2009; Pittiruti *et al.*, 2009a; Royal College of Nursing, 2010; Infusion Nurses Society, 2011; O'Grady *et al.*, 2011; Steiger, 2012).

Venous access devices (VADs) can be classified as central (when the tip of the catheter lies between the lower third of the superior vena cava and the upper region of the right atrium) or peripheral (in all other instances; although, for the purpose of infusion of hyperosmolar solutions and PN, the position of the tip in the inferior vena cava – typically after cannulation of the femoral vein – is also sometimes regarded as 'central'). Concerning their performance in terms of

*E-mail: mauro.pittiruti@rm.unicatt.it

duration, they can be classified as short-term, medium-term or long-term (Gallieni *et al.*, 2008).

Much evidence from the medical literature and from clinical practice suggests that home parenteral nutrition (HPN) should preferably be delivered through a central route, with a medium-term or long-term VAD (Pittiruti *et al.*, 2009a).

Short-term VADs

Short-term VADs may be peripheral or central. Short-term peripheral VADs are usually 35–52 mm long Teflon cannulas. They are the most commonly used VADs in hospital practice and are inserted into superficial veins of the upper arm of adult patients or into any superficial vein of children and neonates. They are not appropriate for HPN because: (i) they are associated with a high risk of dislocation and infiltration; and (ii) they require strict surveillance and frequent repositioning (Pittiruti *et al.*, 2009a).

A short-term central VAD is usually a non-tunnelled, 20–30 cm long, polyurethane catheter inserted into a central vein (subclavian vein, internal jugular vein, innominate vein or axillary vein), whose tip is located in the proximity of the cavoatrial junction. These VADs are intended for continuous use and normally should be inserted only in hospitalized patients and used for a limited time (days to weeks) (Ryder, 2006). They are not considered appropriate for HPN owing to their limited performance in terms of duration and their high risk of lumen occlusion, dislocation, venous thrombosis and infection (Gallieni *et al.*, 2008; Gillanders *et al.*, 2008; Pittiruti *et al.*, 2009a).

Medium-term VADs

Medium-term VADs are non-tunnelled devices specifically designed for discontinuous use; they include midline catheters, peripherally inserted central catheters (PICCs) and non-tunnelled centrally inserted silicone catheters (Hohn catheters).

Midline catheters

Midline catheters are 20–25 cm long, polyurethane or silicone non-tunnelled catheters, with a diameter between 3 and 5 Fr. Midline catheters are inserted either into superficial veins of the antecubital area (antecubital or cephalic vein), using a 'blind' percutaneous technique, or into the deep veins of the arm (basilic, brachial or axillary vein), with ultrasound guidance (Pittiruti *et al.*, 2009b). By definition, their tip is not 'central', i.e. is not located in the superior vena cava but in the axillary vein or in the subclavian vein. The guidelines of the US Centers for Disease Control and Prevention (O'Grady *et al.*, 2011) recommend that midline catheters should be taken into consideration as a potential option every time that peripheral intravenous therapy is expected for more than 6 days (Grade B). However, their role in PN is controversial. Most patients who are candidates for PN usually require a central route of delivery. In some situations, however, PN may be safely delivered by a medium-term peripheral access (i.e. a midline catheter).

In conclusion, the use of ultrasound-inserted midline catheters for HPN is a controversial but a possible option in selected patients, as long as the nutritional treatment is not required for too long periods of time and the osmolarity of the solution is kept within safe limits.

PICCs

PICCs are non-tunnelled, central catheters inserted through a peripheral vein of the arm (basilic, brachial, or – less frequently – cephalic); they are 50–60 cm long and are usually made of silicone or second- or third-generation polyurethane (Pittiruti *et al.*, 2009b). They differ from Hohn catheters, which are non-tunnelled, 20 cm long, centrally inserted silicone catheters (Raad *et al.*, 1993). Both PICCs and Hohn catheters can be used for prolonged continuous or intermittent infusion therapies, both in hospitalized patients and in patients treated as outpatients (day-hospital or ambulatory), in a hospice or at home for prolonged HPN (Ryder, 2006).

PICCs are usually placed at the bedside by physicians or more frequently by nurses; nowadays, they should preferably be inserted into a deep vein of the upper mid-arm by ultrasound guidance (Lamperti *et al.*, 2012). One-, two- or three-lumen PICCs are currently available. The use of most types of PICCs is approved by the US Food and Drug Administration for up to 12 months; although many PICCs – if properly inserted and properly managed – may stay in place and in use for a year or two. They are considered ideal for short- and medium-term HPN, but – since the exit site on the arm effectively renders one hand inoperative – self-care may be difficult, so that the patient may require the assistance of a caregiver (Gillanders *et al.*, 2008). The expected duration of use of a PICC depends on several factors: (i) the ratio between the catheter diameter and vein diameter; (ii) the technique of insertion; (iii) the position of the tip; (iv) the location of the exit site; (v) the technique of securing the catheter to the skin; (vi) the patient's compliance; and (vii) last but not least, the competence of the nurse or caregiver in the maintenance policies.

Recently, tunnelled PICCs have entered clinical practice. Tunnelling may be an effective tool to achieve an adequate exit site at the upper mid-arm even when the vein has been cannulated very close to the axilla. Also, tunnelling is also an effective way to protect the catheter from extraluminal contamination, thus reducing the risk of catheter-related infection (Maki *et al.*, 2006). It is uncertain whether they should be regarded as 'medium-term' or 'long term' VADs: the clinical experience with tunnelled PICCs is still quite limited and their expected time of use for parenteral nutrition is unknown.

Hohn catheters

Hohn catheters are also commonly classified as medium-term VAD. Considering the high risk of dislocation, their use for home care is nowadays largely replaced by the use of PICCs, which appear to be safer and more cost-effective. A recent prospective study conducted on cancer patients on HPN, for more than 51,000 catheter-days, showed that Hohn catheters were associated with significantly more frequent catheter-related complications (infection, venous thrombosis, dislocation, etc.) compared with PICCs (Cotogni *et al.*, 2013).

Long-term VADs

Long-term VADs include tunnelled-cuffed central catheters (such as Hickman, Broviac, Pro-Line, cuffed Groshong) and totally implanted venous ports. They are specifically designed for prolonged infusion of nutrition and/or chemotherapy (for a period longer than 3–4 months).

Tunnelled-cuffed catheters

Tunnelled-cuffed catheters are made of silicone (Hickman, Broviac, Groshong) or polyurethane (Pro-Line); the tunnel protects the VAD from extraluminal contamination, while the Dacron cuff increases its stability (Pratt *et al.*, 2007). Tunnelled catheters have been shown to be associated with lower catheter-related infection than non-tunnelled catheters (Maki *et al.*, 2006). The cuff stimulates an inflammatory response within the subcutaneous tunnel, leading to tissue fibrosis and consequent catheter stabilization that is usually optimal 3 or 4 weeks after insertion.

Cuffed silicon catheters with a distal valve (Groshong) have the theoretical advantage of not requiring heparin flushes but are far more expensive. In a controlled study, they were not superior to the traditional, open-ended devices in terms of performance and early and late complications (Biffi *et al.*, 2001). On the other hand, many recent guidelines do not recommend the use of heparin, even with open-ended catheters (Pratt *et al.*, 2007), especially when infusing PN, since heparin may favour lipid precipitation. Therefore, there is little evidence to support the use of valved catheters for HPN. Tunnelled-cuffed catheters made of power-injectable polyurethane (such as Pro-Line) may have the advantage of being more resistant and less prone to fracture; also, they can be used for injection of contrast medium during radiological investigations.

In recent times, cuffed-tunnelled PICCs have entered into clinical use: their performance in terms of duration and prevention of complications (infection, dislodgement) is still unknown.

Totally implanted ports

Totally implanted ports consist of a reservoir (usually made of titanium and/or plastic) connected to a central catheter (usually made of silicone), which may be valved or not. Ports have a lower risk of infection compared with both tunnelled and non-tunnelled external VADs (Maki *et al.*, 2006), but a higher risk of occlusion when used for infusion of lipid emulsions (Cotogni *et al.*, 2013). Most ports have only one lumen. Double-lumen ports are used for specific purposes, as in patients who require simultaneous infusion of potentially non-compatible drugs (e.g. fluorouracil) with 'all-in-one' PN bags (mainly with lipids or phosphates). Ports allow bathing and swimming, which are more difficult to manage with external VADs, and they may appeal to patients concerned about the alteration of their body image. On the other hand, ports are more expensive to insert and remove, and they leave larger scars. Their use implies the periodic percutaneous placement of a specialized, non-coring needle (Huber needle) into the reservoir.

Thus, the choice between tunnelled catheters and ports depends on several factors, mainly related to the patient's choice and compliance, the skill of the nursing staff and the frequency of VAD use. According to many guidelines (Gallieni *et al.*, 2008; Pittiruti *et al.*, 2009a; O'Grady *et al.*, 2011), ports should be preferred in patients who require long-term intermittent use of the VAD (e.g. chemotherapy treatment scheduled on a weekly or monthly basis), whereas tunnelled-cuffed catheters should be used in patients requiring frequent or continuous access (e.g. for HPN based on a frequency of five or more accesses per week). However, the evidence for this recommendation is weak (Grade C of the European Society for Parenteral and Enteral Nutrition (ESPEN) guidelines) (Pittiruti *et al.*, 2009a).

Tunnelled-cuffed central catheters versus PICCs

Some controversy still exists about the choice between tunnelled-cuffed central catheters versus PICCs for medium-term HPN. The ESPEN guidelines suggest that tunnelled-cuffed catheters should be preferred when HPN is planned for more than 3 months (Pittiruti *et al.*, 2009a), while the Australasian Society for Parenteral and Enteral Nutrition (AuSPEN) guidelines consider that PICCs may be acceptable for HPN expected for a long period of time, up to 12–18 months (Gillanders *et al.*, 2008). The clinical experience with PICCs is increasing in Europe, and PICCs are now inserted and managed according to strict protocols of care that minimize complications (maximal barrier precautions at insertion, ultrasound guidance, accurate verification of the catheter tip, stabilization with sutureless devices, skin antisepsis with 2% chlorhexidine); this is apparently associated with fewer and fewer complications (Pittiruti *et al.*, 2012). Also, PICCs are far more cost-effective than tunnelled-cuffed catheters, particularly should a catheter-related complication occur when the patient is at home; management of PICC-related complications do not usually require hospitalization and even repositioning of the device can be safely performed at home or in hospice. Very recently, two prospective studies have demonstrated the advantages of PICCs for HPN in terms of catheter-related complications (Botella-Carretero *et al.*, 2013; Cotogni *et al.*, 2013). Both studies have shown that PICCs are associated with a significantly reduced risk of catheter-related bacteraemia compared with tunnelled-cuffed catheters. Also, in both studies there was no significant advantage of tunnelled-cuffed catheters over PICCs in terms of duration.

Summary

Medium-term (mainly PICCs) and long-term VADs are both adequate for HPN. The use of short-term central venous catheters for non-hospitalized patients should be strongly discouraged, considering their high susceptibility to infection and the risk of obstruction or dislocation of the device, as well as of catheter-related venous thrombosis (Pittiruti *et al.*, 2009a).

According to international guidelines, choosing the most appropriate type of VAD for PN is the result of a cooperative process among the patient, nurses and the different physicians involved in the patient's care, as well as the other members of nutrition support team (dietician and pharmacist). The choice of VAD must take into account the duration of therapy, physical assessment, patient's health history, support system and resources, patient–caregiver ability to care for the VAD, device availability and – last but not least – the patient's preference. The patient should receive clear, complete and comprehensive verbal and written information explaining the risks, benefits and care of the VAD.

At present, patients and their caregivers still play a small role in the choice of VAD at the beginning of treatment, despite the emerging evidence showing that their early involvement is associated with greater patient and caregiver satisfaction, shorter length of hospital stay, fewer emergency room visits and decreased treatment costs (Barton *et al.*, 1998).

In conclusion, before the insertion of the VAD, we suggest the use of 'proactive vascular planning' (Kokotis, 2005) based on interventions for reducing the risk of catheter-related complications and increasing patient safety and cost-effectiveness.

References

August, D.L., Huhmann, M.B. and the American Society for Parenteral and Enteral Nutrition Board of Directors (2009) A.S.P.E.N. clinical guidelines: nutrition support therapy during adult anticancer treatment and hematopoietic cell transplantation. *JPEN Journal of Parenteral and Enteral Nutrition* 33, 472–500.

Barton, A.J., Danek, G., Johns, P. and Coons, M. (1998) Improving patient outcomes through CQI: vascular access planning. *Journal of Nursing Care Quality* 13, 77–85.

Biffi, R., De Braud, F., Orsi, F., Pozzi, S., Arnaldi, P., Goldhirsch, A., Rotmensz, N., Robertson, C., Bellomi, M. and Andreoni, B. (2001) A randomized, prospective trial of central venous ports connected to standard open-ended or Groshong catheters in adult oncology patients. *Cancer* 92, 1204–1212.

Botella-Carretero, J.I., Carrero, C., Guerra, E., Valbuena, B., Arrieta, F., Calanas, A., Zamarron, I., Balsa, J.A. and Vazquez, C. (2013) Role of peripherally inserted central catheters in home parenteral nutrition: a 5-year prospective study. *JPEN Journal of Parenteral and Enteral Nutrition* 37, 544–549.

Cotogni, P., Pittiruti, M., Barbero, C., Monge, T., Palmo, A. and Boggio Bertinet, D. (2013) Catheter-related complications in cancer patients on home parenteral nutrition: a prospective study of over 51,000 catheter days. *JPEN Journal of Parenteral and Enteral Nutrition* 37, 375–383.

Gallieni, M., Pittiruti, M. and Biffi, R. (2008) Vascular access in oncology patients. *CA – A Cancer Journal for Clinicians* 58, 323–346.

Gillanders, L., Angstmann, K., Ball, P., Chapman-Kiddell, C., Hardy, G., Hope, J., Smith, R., Strauss, B. and Russell, D. (2008) AuSPEN clinical practice guideline for home parenteral nutrition patients in Australia and New Zealand. *Nutrition* 24, 998–1012.

Infusion Nurses Society (2011) Infusion Nursing Standards of Practice. *Journal of Infusion Nursing* 34(Suppl. 1S), S1–S109.

Kokotis, K. (2005) Cost containment and infusion services. *Journal of Infusion Nursing* 28(3), 22–32.

Lamperti, M., Bodenham, A.R., Pittiruti, M., Blaivas, M., Augoustides, J.G., Elbarbary, M., Pirotte, T., Karakitsos, D., LeDonne, J., Doniger, S., Scoppettuolo, G., Feller-Kopman, D., Schummer, W., Biffi, R., Desruennes, E., Melniker, L.A. and Verghese, S.T. (2012) International evidence-based recommendations on ultrasound-guided vascular access. *Intensive Care Medicine* 38, 1105–1117.

Maki, D.G., Kluger, D.M. and Crnich, C.J. (2006) The risk of bloodstream infection in adults with different intravascular devices: a systematic review of 200 published prospective studies. *Mayo Clinic Proceedings* 81, 1159–1171.

O'Grady, N.P., Alexander, M., Burns, L.A., Dellinger, E.P., Garland, J., Heard, S.O., Lipsett, P.A., Masur, H., Mermel, L.A., Pearson, M.L., Raad, I., Randolph, A.G., Rupp, M.E. and Saint, S. (2011) Healthcare Infection Control Practices Advisory Committee. Guidelines for the prevention of intravascular catheter-related infections. *American Journal of Infection Control* 39, 1–34.

Pittiruti, M., Hamilton, H., Biffi, R., MacFie, J. and Pertkiewicz, M. (2009a) ESPEN guidelines on parenteral nutrition: central venous catheters (access, care, diagnosis and therapy of complications). *Clinical Nutrition* 28, 365–377.

Pittiruti, M., Scoppettuolo, G., Emoli, A., Dolcetti, L., Migliorini, I., LaGreca, A. and Malerba, M. (2009b) Parenteral nutrition through ultrasound-placed PICCs and midline catheters is associated with a low rate of complications: an observational study. *Nutritional Therapy & Metabolism* 27, 142–148.

Pittiruti, M., Brutti, A., Celentano, D., Pomponi, M., Biasucci, D.G., Annetta, M.G. and Scoppettuolo, G. (2012) Clinical experience with power-injectable PICCs in intensive care patients. *Critical Care* 16, R21.

Pratt, R.J., Pellowe, C.M., Wilson, J.A., Loveday, H.P., Harper, P.J., Jones, S.R., McDougall, C. and Wilcox, M.H. (2007) EPIC2: national evidence-based guidelines for preventing healthcare-associated infections in NHS hospitals in England. *Journal of Hospital Infection* 65(Suppl. 1), S1–S64.

Raad, I., Davis, S., Becker, M., Hohn, D., Houston, D., Umphrey, J. and Bodey, G.P. (1993) Low infection rate and long durability of nontunneled silastic catheters. A safe and cost-effective alternative for long-term venous access. *Archives of Internal Medicine* 153, 1791–1796.

Royal College of Nursing (2010) Standards for Infusion Therapy. Available at: http://ivtherapyathome.heartofengland.nhs.uk/wp-content/uploads/2013/05/RCN-Guidlines-for-IV-therapy.pdf (accessed 15 February 2013).

Ryder, M. (2006) Evidence-based practice in the management of vascular access devices for home parenteral nutrition therapy. *JPEN Journal of Parenteral and Enteral Nutrition* 30, 82–93.

Steiger, E. (2012) Obtaining and maintaining vascular access in the home parenteral nutrition patient. *JPEN Journal of Parenteral and Enteral Nutrition* 26(5), 17–20.

27 Venous Access Care in Home Parenteral Nutrition

Giancarlo Scoppettuolo[1*] and Mauro Pittiruti[2]

[1]*Department of Infectious Diseases, Catholic University Hospital, Rome, Italy;* [2]*Department of Surgery, Catholic University Hospital, Rome, Italy*

Key Points

- Obtain venous access by selecting the most suitable access device and inserting it safely.
- Maintain the device effectively by ensuring patency and reducing the risk of sepsis, catheter-related thrombosis and catheter fracture.

Introduction

Home parenteral nutrition (HPN) is the ideal treatment for patients with chronic intestinal failure who cannot meet their nutritional requirements through oral or enteral feeding and who do not require hospitalization (Staun *et al.*, 2009). However, HPN can only be safely delivered if a medium-term or long-term vascular access device (VAD) is appropriately inserted and appropriately maintained in use (Gillanders *et al.*, 2008; Pittiruti *et al.*, 2009; Staun *et al.*, 2009).

Indeed, most HPN-related complications are basically VAD-related complications, such as infection – particularly catheter-related bloodstream infection (CRBSI) – venous thrombosis or lumen occlusion (Dibb *et al.*, 2013). A recent prospective study on HPN patients (Gillanders *et al.*, 2012) showed an overall incidence of 3.6 complications per 1000 catheter-days (11.6 when the VAD was not used exclusively for parenteral nutrition (PN) but also for other treatments), with a higher occurrence in paediatric patients (8.4) versus adults (2.5). The authors found an incidence of 2.5 CRBSI per 1000 catheter-days (6.9 in children and 0.8 in adults); the average cost of each septic episode was €6480.

In another 11-year study in 296 patients on HPN (Santarpia *et al.*, 2010), the incidence of infection was 2.0 per 1000 catheter-days and the mean time between

*E-mail: g.scoppettuolo@gmail.com

starting HPN and the first episode of infection was highly variable (237.4 ± 229.6 days, range 39–1560). The microorganisms causing the infection were *Staphylococcus epidermidis* (51%), *Staphylococcus aureus* (7%), other Gram-positive (18%) and Gram-negative (16%) bacteria and yeasts (3%).

Other studies report even higher rates of infection. In a recent study, the occurrence of infection (both local and bacteraemic) during the first 6 months of HPN was 11.5 per 1000 catheter-days (Zhao *et al.*, 2013). Further studies have found a different risk of infection related to the type of VAD; a very recent prospective study on 289 VADs (51,308 catheter-days) used for HPN in cancer patients (Cotogni *et al.*, 2013) detected a mean incidence of 0.35 bacteraemic infections per 1000 catheter-days, which was particularly low in ports (0.19/1000 days) and in peripherally inserted central catheters (PICCs) (0/1000 days). Interestingly, this same study detected a significant inverse correlation between the risk of infection and use of evidence-based technologies such as ultrasound-guided venepuncture and stabilization of the VAD with suture-less devices.

Finally, a recent systematic review of 39 studies published between 1984 and 2012, analysing a total of 1796 cuffed-tunnelled catheters, 1061 ports and 143 PICCs used for HPN (Dreesen *et al.*, 2013), showed that the overall incidence of CRBSI was 0.38–4.58 per 1000 catheter-days (median 1.31), although somewhat lower (0.19–2.41 per 1000 catheter-days, median 0.82) in those studies considering HPN mostly for benign disease compared with studies on cancer patients (1.9–6.8 per 1000 catheter-days, median 1.31). Several factors were significantly associated with a high risk of CRBSI: some of them being related to the VAD (number of lumens, tunnelled versus non-tunnelled, calibre, etc.), some to the patient (neoplastic versus benign diseases), some to the treatment (modality of HPN, etc.) and some to venous access care (training of the caregiver, competence of the nurses, etc.).

All these studies show that the VAD has a crucial role in determining the incidence of complications during HPN: appropriate care of the catheter exit site and of the infusion line is of paramount importance for reducing the catheter-related complications and especially catheter-related infections. Any strategy aimed to reduce the risk of infection will actually increase the safety and the cost-effectiveness of HPN.

Routes of Infection

VAD-related infections are secondary to the colonization of the catheter, which may occur via two different routes: (i) the extraluminal route; and (ii) the intraluminal route (Crnich and Maki, 2002).

Colonization by the extraluminal route occurs when microorganisms migrate from the skin of the patient or from the hands of the health provider to the external surface of the catheter, first colonizing the extravascular and then the intravascular tract of the catheter. Among the effective strategies that may reduce colonization of the VAD via the extraluminal route are: (i) an adequate policy of hand washing; (ii) appropriate skin antisepsis during and after VAD insertion;

(iii) adequate protection of the exit site with transparent membranes; (iv) tunnelling of the VAD; and (v) an appropriate policy of dressing of the exit site.

Colonization by the intraluminal route occurs when microorganisms enter the infusion line through the hubs, connectors, stopcocks and all the add-on devices of the intravenous line. Effective strategies for reducing this type of colonization are: (i) an adequate policy of hand washing before taking care of the line; (ii) scrubbing the hubs and the needle-free connectors (NFCs) before any access to the line; and (iii) an adequate policy of periodic replacement of the infusion lines.

Targeting Zero

Although many of these strategies have been known for many years, the incidence of CRBSI has not decreased significantly for decades and it has sometimes been fatalistically accepted as inevitably connected to the use of a central VAD. Recently, a new 'philosophy' has been introduced into clinical practice: the idea that catheter-related infections should not be regarded as unpreventable or only partially preventable events, but as operator-dependent complications that can be minimized and even abolished by a proper aptitude of the health operators. This new approach, termed 'Targeting Zero', has been developed by APIC, the US Association for Professionals in Infection Control and Epidemiology, and was adopted by the most recent edition of the Centers for Disease Control and Prevention (CDC) guidelines in 2011 (O'Grady *et al.*, 2011). As a matter of fact, in recent years many clinical studies have shown that 'zero CRBSI' is a target which can really be achieved. The most known study in this regard was conducted in 108 intensive care units (the so-called Michigan Keystone Project) a few years ago (Pronovost *et al.*, 2006). The key strategy for achieving zero CRBSI was the 'bundle', i.e. the simultaneous, consistent and systematic implementation of a small number of evidence-based recommendations that act synergistically to reduce the risk of a specific undesired event. The effectiveness of this bundle is based on its consistent adoption by all health operators in all patients. The approach developed in the Michigan study consisted of five strategies: (i) hand washing; (ii) maximal barrier precautions at VAD insertion; (iii) rational choice of the insertion site; (iv) skin antisepsis with 2% chlorhexidine; and (v) immediate removal of the VAD when no longer needed. In the following years, many other 'bundles' for achieving zero CRBSI have been developed, such as the bundle of GAVeCeLT, the Italian Association for Long Term Venous Access, reported in Table 27.1 (Scoppettuolo *et al.*, 2011).

In a very recently published paper, AHRQ – the US Agency for Healthcare Research and Quality – recommends the adoption of bundles for prevention of CRBSI, classifying this intervention as 'strongly encouraged' for clinical practice (Shekelle *et al.*, 2013).

Infection Prevention

Most guidelines agree that an effective prevention of CRBSI should include both 'behavioural' strategies and 'technological' strategies that should be adopted before, during and after VAD insertion (Pratt *et al.*, 2007; Marshall *et al.*, 2008; Pittiruti *et al.*, 2009; O'Grady *et al.*, 2011).

- *Before insertion*: choice of the most appropriate VAD, taking into consideration the planning of the therapy, the needs of the patient, the experience of the staff who will care for the VAD, etc.
- *At insertion*: adoption of appropriate asepsis, maximal barrier precautions, skin antisepsis with 2% chlorhexidine, ultrasound-guided venepuncture, careful choice of the insertion site and the exit site, etc.
- *After insertion*: appropriatc carc of the exit site and appropriate management of the infusion line (Ryder, 2006).

The following lists the cornerstones of CRBSI prevention that can be considered valid for any kind of VAD (short-, medium- or long-term), in any setting (hospital, hospice, home care) (see Table 27.2 for a comparison of the most important guidelines between recommendations).

Table 27.1. GAVeCeLT bundle for prevention of infections associated with PICCs and CVCs.

Hand hygiene and maximal sterile barrier precautions during VAD insertion
Proper choice of insertion site (preferred sites, in decreasing order: mid-arm, infraclavicular, supraclavicular, neck, groin)
Ultrasound-guided insertion for both CVCs and PICCs
Use of 2% chlorhexidine for skin antisepsis before insertion and for continuous or discontinuous antisepsis of the exit site
Use of suture-less devices for securing the catheter, whenever possible
Use of transparent dressings, whenever possible
Prompt removal of unnecessary lines

CVC, central venous catheter.

Table 27.2. Strength of recommendation of the main strategies for CRBSI prevention: comparison between the most recent guidelines.

	EPIC2 2007	SHEA/IDSA 2008	ESPEN 2009	CDC 2011
Education	D	A-II	A	I-A
Maximal sterile barrier precautions	C	A-I	B	I-B
Hand hygiene	A	B-II	A	I-B
Ultrasound-guided insertion	–	–	A	I-B
Skin antisepsis with chlorhexidine	A	A-I	A	I-A
Chlorhexidine-impregnated sponges	–	B-I	B	I-B
Suture-less devices	–	–	C	II
Catheter site dressing regimens	D	A-I	C	I-A
Scrub the hub with appropriate antiseptic	D	B-II	C	I-A
Replacement of administration sets	D	A-II	C	I-A

SHEA/IDSA, Society for Healthcare Epidemiology of America/Infectious Diseases Society of America.

Behavioural strategies

- *Education* of all health operators involved in the choice, insertion and care of the VAD (Pratt *et al.*, 2007; Marshall *et al.*, 2008; Pittiruti *et al.*, 2009; O'Grady *et al.*, 2011), including training of the patient and the caregivers, who play a crucial role in HPN (Kumpf and Tillman, 2012). A most important educational tool is the implementation of a specific 'checklist' for each manoeuvre (Marshall *et al.*, 2008). Other useful tools include practical handbooks and brochures, DVDs, web-based tutorials, etc. (Gifford *et al.*, 2010). Studies have shown (MacRitchie, 1978; Moukarzel *et al.*, 1994; Smiths *et al.*, 2002; Fitzgerald *et al.*, 2011) that proper education and information has a significant beneficial effect not only on the risk of complications but also on the psychological aptitude of the patient, making him/her feel more 'in control' of his/her condition.
- *Hand washing.* An appropriate policy of hand washing is the most effective and inexpensive strategy for CRBSI prevention. Health operator, patient and caregiver should be instructed to wash their hands with an alcohol-based gel before and after any contact with the VAD or with the infusion line. It is well known that health professionals unfortunately do not consistently adopt such a cost-effective strategy (Pratt *et al.*, 2007; Marshall *et al.*, 2008; Pittiruti *et al.*, 2009; World Health Organization, 2009; O'Grady *et al.*, 2011).
- *Maximal barrier precautions at insertion.* Use of non-sterile beret, non-sterile mask, sterile gloves, sterile gown and wide sterile field covering most of the patient ('full body' drape) (Pratt *et al.*, 2007; Marshall *et al.*, 2008; Pittiruti *et al.*, 2009; O'Grady *et al.*, 2011; Lamperti *et al.*, 2012).

Technological strategies

- *Ultrasound guidance at insertion.* Ultrasound-guided choice of the most appropriate vein and ultrasound-guided venepuncture have been proved to reduce not only the risk of mechanical complications, the time needed and the cost of the manoeuvre, but also the risk of infection (Pratt *et al.*, 2007; Pittiruti *et al.*, 2009; O'Grady *et al.*, 2011; Lamperti *et al.*, 2012; Moreau *et al.*, 2013).
- *Skin antisepsis with 2% chlorhexidine.* When used at concentration >1%, chlorhexidine is one of the most effective tools for reducing hospital-acquired infections and in particular catheter-related infections. Since 2007 it has been proved that 2% chlorhexidine is superior to povidone iodine for prevention of CRBSI (Pratt *et al.*, 2007; Marshall *et al.*, 2008; Pittiruti *et al.*, 2009; O'Grady *et al.*, 2011). The best formula for skin antisepsis before insertion or for disinfecting the skin around the exit site of the catheter is 2% chlorhexidine gluconate in 70% isopropyl alcohol.
- *Protection of the exit site with an appropriate dressing.* Transparent dressings are preferred because they stabilize the catheter and allow simultaneously good visibility and complete protection of the exit site (Pratt *et al.*, 2007). The exit site of cuffed-tunnelled catheters should also be protected with a transparent dressing, at least for the first months (O'Grady *et al.*, 2011).

- *Accurate disinfection of the hub before any access to the infusion line.* The hub should be vigorously scrubbed for 10–15 s with chlorhexidine or alcohol or povidone iodine, to reduce the risk of intraluminal colonization (Kaler and Chinn, 2007).
- *Protection of the line with appropriate NFCs.* NFCs were introduced into clinical practice more than a decade ago and play an important role in decreasing the risk of accidental contamination by the healthcare provider. Many different NFCs are available and although choice of the most appropriate NFC is a controversial issue, most guidelines suggest the use of a transparent NFC with neutral displacement, easy to swab, with minimal dead space (O'Grady *et al.*, 2011; Hadaway, 2012). The NFC should be scrubbed before each access, as with any hub, and should be replaced each time that the infusion line is replaced (every 24–72 h).
- *Periodic replacement of the infusion line* and of all the add-on devices every 24 h (if used for infusion of lipids or blood products) or every 48–72 h (if used for 'clear' infusions); recent evidence suggests that in the latter case the infusion lines may be replaced every 96 h (Pratt *et al.*, 2007; Marshall *et al.*, 2008; Pittiruti *et al.*, 2009; O'Grady *et al.*, 2011).
- *Periodic replacement of the Huber needle* inserted in the totally implantable VAD, at least every 7 days (O'Grady *et al.*, 2011).
- *Antimicrobial lock in selected patients.* According to the latest edition of the CDC guidelines, long-term VADs with a history of relapsing CRBSI should be locked with an antimicrobial solution when not in use (O'Grady *et al.*, 2011). Which antimicrobial lock to use is still a controversial issue, since very few data are available. Recent studies or case reports have shown the effectiveness of vancomycin/heparin (Safdar and Maki, 2006), vancomycin/ciprofloxacin/heparin (Henrickson *et al.*, 2000), 70% ethanol (Opilla *et al.*, 2007; John *et al.*, 2012) and 1.35% taurolidine/4% citrate (Touré *et al.*, 2012). Particularly, taurolidine seems promising for long-term users of VAD and more studies are awaited.

Prevention of Lumen Occlusion

Recent studies have shown that effective prevention of lumen occlusion should be based not on the heparinization of the catheter when not in use (the so-called 'heparin lock'), but on a well-defined policy of flush with saline, before and after each infusion. With the only exception of VADs used for haemodialysis and pheresis, there is no convincing evidence that heparin has any role in preventing the occlusion of central or peripheral venous catheters (Pratt *et al.*, 2007). On the other hand, an evidence-based protocol for prevention of lumen occlusion should include the following strategies (Pratt *et al.*, 2007; Pittiruti *et al.*, 2009):

- Flush the VAD with 10 ml saline (in the adult patient) before and after each infusion, using the so-called 'push–pause' technique; 20 ml saline should be used in adults after blood sampling or after infusion of lipids, blood products or contrast medium. A smaller amount of saline should be used in children and neonates, depending on the age of the patient and on the dead space of the VAD.

- Do not use heparin lock routinely and in particular do not use heparin when the line is used for lipid infusion (as this increases the risk of lipid precipitates).
- Use preferably a pump when infusing PN.
- Do not mix drugs and do not infuse drugs in the same line as PN.
- Use preferably a neutral-displacement NFC, to avoid 'backflow' at disconnection.
- Remove the Huber needle with a 'positive pressure' technique.
- Choose VAD of appropriate calibre and preferably made of power-injectable polyurethane (since this is associated with higher flow rates, easier flushing and easier unblocking of the catheter).

Prevention of Catheter-related Venous Thrombosis

Prevention of venous thrombosis is based mostly upon an accurate technique of VAD selection and insertion, which should include: (i) choice of a catheter with a calibre not larger than ⅓ of the inner diameter of the vein; (ii) appropriate choice of the insertion site and the exit site; (iii) ultrasound-guided venepuncture; (iv) proper verification that the tip of the central VAD is located in the proximity of the cavoatrial junction; and (v) adequate stabilization of external VADs with sutureless devices and transparent adhesive dressing.

The role of pharmacological prophylaxis with low-molecular-weight heparin has been strongly criticized in the most recent guidelines and its cost-effectiveness is quite controversial. Most likely, it should be reserved only for patients with previous episodes of catheter-related thrombosis and/or known genetic abnormalities associated with a high risk of venous thrombosis (Biffi *et al.*, 2007; Pittiruti *et al.*, 2009; Debourdeau *et al.*, 2012). Patients who are at particular risk of thrombosis can be offered prophylactic treatment with warfarin (Klerk *et al.*, 2003).

Prevention of Mechanical Complications

Common mechanical complications include: (i) rupture of the external or internal tract of the VAD; (ii) tip migration; (iii) partial or total dislocation of external VADs; and (iv) mechanical problems of the reservoir of totally implanted VADs.

Prevention is based upon:

- proper choice of the VAD (preferred choice of power-injectable polyurethane catheter for external VADs, since silicone is more prone to rupture);
- an accurate, state-of-the-art technique of insertion (proper choice of the insertion site and the exit site, ultrasound-guided venepuncture, real-time verification of the proper position of the tip, proper positioning of the cuff at least 2 cm inside the tunnel, proper planning of the pocket of the reservoir,

adequate stabilization of external VADs with suture-less devices and transparent adhesive membranes); and

- careful management during venous access care (surveillance of the VAD, weekly replacement of the suture-less device and transparent dressing, avoidance of scissors and blades while removing the dressing, use of contrast medium injection only if the VAD is certified to be power-injectable).

Summary

Healthcare professionals taking care of patients on HPN must translate evidence for best practice of catheter care into procedures to reduce the risk of catheter-related complications.

References

Biffi, R., Pittiruti, M. and Campisi, C. (2007) Catheter-related central venous thrombosis: the development of an Italian nationwide consensus paper. *Nutritional Therapy & Metabolism* 25, 173–182.

Cotogni, P., Pittiruti, M., Barbero, C., Monge, T., Palmo, A. and Boggio Bertinet, D. (2013) Catheter-related complications in cancer patients on home parenteral nutrition: a prospective study of over 51,000 catheter days. *JPEN Journal of Parenteral and Enteral Nutrition* 37, 375–383.

Crnich, C.Y. and Maki, D.G. (2002) The promise of novel technology for the prevention of intravascular device-related bloodstream infections. Pathogenesis and short-term device. *Clinical Infectious Disease* 34, 1232–1242.

Debourdeau, P., Farge, D., Beckers, M., Baglin, C., Bauersachs, R.M., Brenner, B., Brilhante, D., Falanga, A., Gerotzafias, G.T., Haim, N., Kakkar, A.K., Khorana, A.A., Lecumberri, R., Mandala, M., Marty, M., Monreal, M., Mousa, S.A., Noble, S., Pabinger, I., Prandoni, P., Prins, M.H., Qari, M.H., Streiff, M.B., Syrigos, K., Büller, H.R. and Bounameaux, H. (2013) International clinical practice guidelines for the treatment and prophylaxis of thrombosis associated with central venous catheters in patients with cancer. *Journal of Thrombosis and Haemostasis* 11, 71–80.

Dibb, M., Teubner, A., Theis, V., Shaffer, J. and Lai, S. (2013) The management of long-term parenteral nutrition. *Alimentary Pharmacology & Therapeutics* 37, 587–603.

Dreesen, M., Foulon, V., Spriet, I., Goossens, G.A., Hiele, M., De Pourcq, L. and Willems, L. (2013) Epidemiology of catheter related infections in adult patients receiving home parenteral nutrition: a systematic review. *Clinical Nutrition* 32, 16–26.

Fitzgerald, S.A., Macan Yadrich, D., Wercowitch, M., Piamjariyaku, U. and Smith, C.E. (2011) Creating patient and education web sites. Design and content of the home parenteral nutrition family caregivers web sites. *Computer, Informatics, Nursing* 29, 637–645.

Gifford, H., DeLegge, M. and Epperson, L.A. (2010) Education methods and techniques for training home parenteral nutrition patients. *Nutrition in Clinical Practice* 25, 443–450.

Gillanders, L., Angstmann, K., Ball, P., Chapman-Kiddell, C., Hardy, G., Hope, J., Smithe, R., Strauss, B. and Russel, D. (2008) Australasian Society of Parenteral and Enteral Nutrition. AuSPEN clinical practice guidelines for home parenteral nutrition patients in Australia and New Zealand. *Nutrition* 24, 988–1002.

Gillanders, L., Angstmann, K., Ball, P., O'Callaghan, M., Thomson, A., Wong, T. and Thomas, M. (2012) A prospective study on catheter-related complications in HPN patients. *Clinical Nutrition* 31, 30–34.
Hadaway, L. (2012) Needleless connectors for IV catheters. *American Journal of Nursing* 112(11), 32–44.
Henrickson, K.J., Axtell, R.A., Hoover, S.M., Kuhn, S.M., Pritchett, J., Kehl, S.C. and Klein, J.P. (2000) Prevention of central venous catheter-related infections and thrombotic events in immunocompromised children by the use of vancomycin/ciprofloxacin/heparin flush solution: a randomized, multicenter, double-blind trial. *Journal of Clinical Oncology* 18, 1269–1278.
John, B.K., Khan, M.A., Speerhas, R., Rhoda, K., Hamilton, C., Dechicco, R., Lopez, R., Steiger, E. and Kirby, D.F. (2012) Ethanol lock therapy in reducing catheter-related bloodstream infections in adult home parenteral nutrition patients: results of a retrospective study. *JPEN Journal of Parenteral and Enteral Nutrition* 36, 603–610.
Kaler, W. and Chinn, R. (2007) Successful disinfection of needleless access port: a matter of time and friction. *Journal of the Association for Vascular Access* 12, 140–142.
Klerk, C.P.W., Smorenburg, S.M. and Buller, H.R. (2003) Thrombosis prophylaxis in patient populations with a central venous catheter. *Archives of Internal Medicine* 163, 1913–1921.
Kumpf, V.J. and Tillman, E.M. (2012) Home parenteral nutrition: safe transition from hospital to home. *Nutrition in Clinical Practice* 27, 749–757.
Lamperti, M., Bodenham, A.R., Pittiruti, M., Blaivas, M., Augoustides, J.G., Elbarbary, M., Pirotte, T., Karakitsos, D., Ledonne, J., Doniger, S., Scoppettuolo, G., Feller-Kopman, D., Schummer, W., Biffi, R., Desruennes, E., Melniker, L.A. and Verghese, S.T. (2012) International evidence-based recommendations on ultrasound-guided vascular access. *Intensive Care Medicine* 38, 1105–1117.
MacRitchie, K.J. (1978) Life without eating or drinking: total parenteral nutrition outside hospital. *Canadian Psychiatric Association Journal* 23, 379–399.
Marshall, J., Mermel, L.A., Classen, D., Arias, K.M., Podgorny, K., Anderson, D.J., Burstin, H., Calfee, D.P., Coffin, S.E., Dubberke, E.R., Fraser, V., Gerding, D.N., Griffin, F.A., Gross, P., Kaye, K.S., Klompas, M., Lo, E., Nicolle, L., Pegues, D.A., Perl, T.M., Saint, S., Salgado, C.D., Weinstein, R.A., Wise, R. and Yokoe, D.S. (2008) Strategies to prevent central line-associated bloodstream infections in acute care hospital. *Infection Control and Hospital Epidemiology* 29(Suppl. 1), S22–S30.
Moreau, N., Lamperti, M., Kelly, L.J., Dawson, R., Elbarbary, M., van Boxtel, A.J. and Pittiruti, M. (2013) Evidence-based consensus on the insertion of central venous access devices: definition of minimal requirements for training. *British Journal of Anaesthesia* 110, 347–356.
Moukarzel, A.A., Haddad, I., Ament, M.E., Buchman, A.L., Reyen, L., Maggioni, A., Baron, H.I. and Vargas, J. (1994) 230 patient years of experience with long-term parenteral nutrition in childhood: natural history and life of central venous catheters. *Journal of Pediatric Surgery* 29, 1323–1327.
O'Grady, N.P., Alexander, M., Burns, L.A., Dellinger, E.P., Garland, J., Heard, S.O., Lipsette, P.A., Masur, H., Mermel, L.A., Pearson, M.L., Raad, I.I., Randolph, A.G., Rupp, M.E. and Saint, S., Healthcare Infection Control Practices Advisory Committee (2011) Guidelines for the prevention of intravascular catheter-related infections. *Clinical Infectious Disease* 52(9), e162–e193.
Opilla, M., Kirby, D.F. and Edmond, M.B. (2007) Use of ethanol lock therapy to reduce the incidence of catheter-related bloodstream infections in home parenteral nutrition patients. *JPEN Journal of Parenteral and Enteral Nutrition* 31, 302–305.
Pittiruti, M., Hamilton, H., Biffi, R., MacFie, J. and Pertkiewicz, M. (2009) ESPEN Guidelines on parenteral nutrition. *Clinical Nutrition* 28, 365–377.

Pratt, R.J., Pellowe, C.M., Wilson, J.A., Loveday, H.P., Harper, P.J., Jones, S.R., McDougall, C. and Wilcox, M.H. (2007) EPIC2: national evidence-based guidelines for preventing healthcare-associated infections in NHS hospitals in England. *Journal of Hospital Infection* 65(Suppl. 1), S1–S64.

Pronovost, P., Needham, D., Berenholtz, S., Sinopoli, D., Chu, H., Cosgrove, S, Sexton, B., Hyzy, R., Welsh, R., Roth, G., Bander, J., Kepros, J. and Goeschel, C. (2006) An intervention to decrease catheter-related bloodstream infections in the ICU. *New England Journal of Medicine* 355, 2725–2732.

Ryder, M. (2006) Evidence-based practice in tha management of vascular access devices for home parenteral nutrition therapy. *JPEN Journal of Parenteral and Enteral Nutrition* 30(1 Suppl.), S82–S93.

Safdar, N. and Maki, D.G. (2006) Use of vancomycin-containing lock or flush solutions for prevention of bloodstream infection associated with central venous access devices: a meta-analysis of prospective, randomized trials. *Clinical Infectious Disease* 43, 474–484.

Santarpia, L., Alfonsi, L., Tiseo, D., Creti, R., Baldassarri, L., Pasanisi, F. and Contaldo, F. (2010) Central venous catheter infections and antibiotic therapy during long-term home parenteral nutrition: an 11-year follow-up study. *JPEN Journal of Parenteral and Enteral Nutrition* 34, 254–261.

Scoppettuolo, G., Dolcetti, L., Taraschi, C. *et al.* (2011) Targeting zero CLABSI in patients with PICC lines: a case–control study. Presented at the *Association for Vascular Access Annual Scientific Meeting*, San José, California, 3–6 October 2011 (poster #37).

Shekelle, P.G., Pronovost, P.J., Wachter, R.M., McDonald, K.M., Schoelles, K., Dy, S.M., Shojania, K., Reston, J.T., Adams, A.S., Angood, P.B., Bates, D.W., Bickmann, L., Carayon, P., Donaldson, L., Duan, N., Farley, D.O., Greenhalgh, T., Haughorn, J.L., Lake, E., Lilford, R., Lohr, K.N., Meyers, G.S., Miller, M.R., Neuhauser, D.V., Ryan, G., Saint, S., Shortell, S.M., Stevens, D.P. and Walshe, K. (2013) The top patient safety strategies that can be encouraged for adoption now. *Annals of Internal Medicine* 158, 365–368.

Smith, C.S., Curtas, S., Wercowitch, M., Kleinbeck, S.V. and Howard, L. (2002) Home parenteral nutrition: does affiliation with a national support and educational organization improve patient outcome? *JPEN Journal of Parenteral and Enteral Nutrition* 26, 159–163.

Staun, M., Pironi, L., Bozzetti F., Baxter, J., Forbes, A., Joly, F., Jeppesen, P., Moreno, J., Hébuterne, X., Pertkiewicz, M., Mühlebach, S., Shenkin, A. and Van Gossum, A. (2009) ESPEN Guidelines on parenteral nutrition: home parenteral nutrition (HPN) in adult patients. *Clinical Nutrition* 28, 467–469.

Touré, A., Lauverjat, M., Peraldi, C., Boncompain-Gerard, M., Gelas, P., Barnoud, D. and Chambrier, C. (2012) Taurolidine lock solution in the secondary prevention of central venous catheter-associated bloodstream infections in home parenteral nutrition patients. *Clinical Nutrition* 31, 567–570.

World Health Organization (2009) *WHO Guidelines on Hand Hygiene in Health Care*. WHO, Geneva, Switzerland.

Zhao, V.M., Griffith, D.P., Blumberg, H.M., Dave, N.J., Battey, C.H., McNally, T.A., Easley, K.A., Galloway, J.R. and Ziegler, T.R. (2013) Characterization of post-hospital infections in adults requiring home parenteral nutrition. *Nutrition* 29, 52–59.

28 Teaching the Home Parenteral Nutrition Patient

Kurt Boeykens*

AZ Nikolaas, Sint-Niklaas, Belgium

Key Points

- Carefully select patients who may benefit from home parenteral nutrition (HPN).
- A (home) nutritional support team can play an important role in the preparation, training and follow-up of the patient on HPN.
- Training should start pre-discharge.
- If accurately managed, HPN can be safely provided.
- A well-organized, individualized and multifaceted approach can prevent complications and improve quality of life.

Introduction

Parenteral nutrition (PN) can be managed in the home care setting for a short- or long-term (sometimes lifelong) period. This management differs from that of hospitalized patients because there is a shift in primary responsibility from healthcare professionals to patients and caregivers. The general goals in the education process are to: (i) improve or maintain quality of life (QoL); (ii) promote independence with the infusion; (iii) (self-) monitor the HPN; and (iv) prevent complications (Gifford *et al.*, 2010). A multidisciplinary team can play an important role in the individualized decision-making process and guide all the necessary measures or steps that have to be taken.

*E-mail: kurt.boeykens@aznikolaas.be

The Role of a Multidisciplinary Team

Patients receiving PN in the hospital setting are often monitored by a (home) nutrition support team ((H)NST). It is generally accepted that optimal nutritional care is provided by a multidisciplinary expert team in which each member has a specific role in the nutrition care process (nutritional assessment, nutrition care plan, monitoring, discharge planning and outpatient care). For HPN there are no published trials that compare the outcome of patients cared for by different types of professional groups and/or institutions (Gillanders *et al.*, 2008). Some data even indicate that smaller centres can produce similar results to large centres for line sepsis (Bozzetti *et al.*, 2002). On the other hand, retrospective studies have shown improved benefit of HPN therapy when patients are referred early to expert centres where multidisciplinary teams exist (Ireton-Jones and De Legge, 2005; Gillanders *et al.*, 2008). The key team members are generally a clinical nutrition nurse specialist, a (clinical) pharmacist, a nutrition support physician and a dietician. Also other health professionals (psychologists, social workers, psychiatrists, case managers, physiotherapists and occupational therapists) can be involved. HPN indeed requires coordination of care between several healthcare disciplines within and outside the hospital (Kumpf and Tillman, 2012).

Patient Selection

The indication to start HPN in patients with benign long-term intestinal failure, who cannot meet their nutritional requirements by enteral intake, is rather obvious when they can be treated outside the acute care setting. For intestinal failure due to malignant disease there is more debate and the practice in Europe differs among countries. In 1997 a European survey reported that some countries such as Denmark and the UK rarely give HPN to cancer patients (Van Gossum *et al.*, 1999). In the case of malignancies with bowel obstruction HPN should not be given to patients with a short life expectancy, a low performance status, metastasis to vital organs and a high level of palliative care (Staun *et al.*, 2009). An HPN questionnaire by the European Society for Parenteral and Enteral Nutrition (ESPEN) Home Artificial Nutrition (HAN) working group revealed that centres in Europe exclude patients from their HPN programme because of several criteria including intellect (33%), physical disability (24%), social situation (25%), underlying disease (18%) and age (16%) (Micklewright *et al.*, 2002; Judson *et al.*, 2006).

QoL is an important outcome parameter in all patients. A good overall QoL can be achieved (Huisman-de Waal *et al.*, 2007) but is especially important in patients with cancer. That is why HPN should be started only after a thorough discussion with the patient and/or family about the pros and cons. Once started, the same discussion has to take place in case of withholding the HPN and in accordance with the guidelines. The problem is often how to determine the impact of QoL from symptoms related to the underlying disease versus the impact of HPN. An important aspect of QoL is trying to maintain as much as possible the patient's freedom in terms of not being 'online' all the time. Administering the PN overnight is usually done but when it disturbs the patient's sleep too much, infusing at daytime should be considered. Sometimes it will not be necessary to give a total parenteral nutrition (TPN) bag every day (Kirby *et al.*, 2012).

Transition to HPN and Home Assessment

The transition of the patient from the hospital to the home not only involves consideration of the proper indication, the disease state or the QoL. HPN should also be safely administered and adequately monitored. Ideally, a nurse should first visit the patient's home to have a clear view on the discharge facilities. Items that should be assessed are listed in Table 28.1 (Hamilton, 1999; Ireton-Jones *et al.*, 2003; Kovacevich *et al.*, 2005).

Education of Patients/Caregivers

In 2012 a systematic review of global practices on HPN care was published. This review included recommendations derived from different national or international guidelines. In most guidelines, education, monitoring, preventing complications and the involvement of a multidisciplinary support team are discussed as specific topics (Dreesen *et al.*, 2012). Patient and/or caregiver education is indeed important and should start before discharge. It will make the transition less stressful. Education and training should be performed in a quiet environment. Patients can be overwhelmed by the complexity of the teaching programme, so this needs to be tailored to each individual depending on the established learning goals and necessary learning skills needed for the appropriate management of HPN. The

Table 28.1. Assessment criteria for HPN.

Appropriate indication for HPN
Appropriate venous access site for mid-term or long-term use
Nutritional assessment: fluid, calorie, electrolyte and micronutrient requirements
Stable HPN regimen before discharge
Medical and physical suitability/stability
Functional ability and rehabilitative potential
Psychological and emotional suitability
Social and financial status
Lifestyle/activities of daily living
Home care environment evaluation
General cleanliness (e.g. is there a clean area for aseptic/sterile procedures?)
Presence of animals?
Basic home safety (telephone access, clean storage for supplies, dedicated refrigerator, toilet/bathroom, sanitary water supply, etc.)
Competency and independence of the patient/caregivers
Reimbursement sources for payment of products, services, equipment or supplies
Consistent delivery of products, equipment or supplies
Around-the-clock (on-call) availability of an experienced home care provider
Post-discharge monitoring possibilities

teaching programme for an independent patient may take from several days to weeks. A possible way of organizing education is that in the first period, patients will have to learn all necessary skills and afterwards will have to demonstrate that they can manage their HPN unsupervised by the trainers who are of course available in back up for advice or assistance. Important aspects of the educational programme are summarized in Table 28.2 (Andris and Krzywda, 2008). Of course, it is not always necessary to discuss all items in every patient. This depends on patient skills, the duration of the HPN and the underlying condition.

Multiple education interventions are available including methods such as one-on-one counselling, written or printed materials, group meetings, demonstrations, videotapes, CDs/DVDs and Internet education (Gifford *et al.*, 2010). A

Table 28.2. Home TPN education checklist and/or learning goals.

- Indication for HPN
- HPN telephone numbers and resources
- Storage, handling of admixtures, medications and supplies
- Adding medications or multivitamins to the TPN bag
- Compounding
- Preparing the TPN bag and IV tubing
  - Spiking of the TPN bag
  - Priming the IV tubing
  - Loading/inserting the IV tubing into the pump
- Infusion pump
  - Programming and commencing
  - Troubleshooting/pump alarms/pump failure/emergency backup
  - Discontinuing TPN
- Aseptic/sterile techniques or procedures according to institutional protocol guidelines
  - Hand washing
  - Flushing the catheter
  - Catheter care and dressings
  - Connecting IV line to the catheter
  - Blood draws
- Preventing, recognizing and managing HPN-related complications
  - TPN bag: fluid leaks, changes in colour or presence of particles/precipitates
  - Catheter: blood in catheter, blockage (clot), tear, suspected infection (exit-site/systemic), dislodgement, breakage, venous thrombosis
  - Metabolic complications and symptoms: hyper/hypoglycaemia, dehydration, electrolyte disturbances
  - Trace element/vitamin deficiencies/toxicities
  - PN-associated liver disease (long-term HPN)
- Most common mistakes
- TPN self-monitoring
  - Intake and output record (hydration status)
  - Weight gain or loss
  - Temperature
  - Glycaemic control
  - Shortness of breath
  - Signs of electrolyte or nutrient imbalances

(patient-specific) manual with information and instructions for HPN should be used for the patient and/or caregiver (see Table 28.3).

The combination of different teaching strategies seems to be the best option but no time limits for training are set because patients learn at different rates. It is important that the consequences of non-compliance are stressed, and the fact that they can be life threatening. Proper education is essential for HPN patients in gaining independence, preventing complications or re-hospitalizations and achieving an acceptable QoL. HPN education does not end with the initial demonstration of skills included in the checklist. After discharge, regular home visits by a nurse and/or telephone calls are a possibility to further assess the competency of the patient or caregiver. In the case of problems and questions a hotline should be available.

Preventing Complications and Monitoring

Preventing complications, mainly catheter-related complications, are of major importance because these catheters are literately lifelines for patients. A catheter-related bloodstream infection (CRBSI) is the most common complication; it can result in catheter removal in up to 50% of patients and is the greatest cause of morbidity and mortality in HPN patients (Bozzetti *et al.*, 2002). Another consequence is readmission to the hospital, which will have a negative impact on QoL and will account for extra high costs to healthcare. Besides infectious complications, other complications that should be discussed include mechanical complications, metabolic disturbances, PN-associated liver disease and metabolic bone disease.

Patients who receive detailed written and oral instructions on aseptic catheter care and recognizing complications seem to benefit in terms of preventing central venous catheter-related sepsis. As shown by Santarpia *et al.* (2002) in a retrospective study, the group that received standard information had more infections than the well-educated group.

Patients on HPN must be seen and assessed on a regular basis by the multidisciplinary team. Of course, timing will depend on the status of the patient. All patients should have a baseline nutritional assessment (Gillanders *et al.*, 2008). Evidence to guide monitoring of patients on long-term HPN is scarce. European guidelines (Staun *et al.*, 2009; Wanten *et al.*, 2011) advocate periodical monitoring.

Table 28.3. Possible content of an HPN patient/caregiver manual.

Names and telephone numbers of healthcare professionals/resources available for providing expert advice and problem solving
General information about TPN/HPN
Prescription for the nutrition solution, duration of therapy and additives
Instructions for bag preparation, adding additives, mixing and pump use
Procedures for catheter care
List of the required equipment for administering HPN
Home nutrition support (self-) monitoring records
Potential solutions (problem solving) in the event of complications

Summary

HPN is a complex therapy that requires coordination of many healthcare providers. The expertise of a multidisciplinary support team is recommended to provide proper and patient-tailored education or therapy. Self-management and preventing complications are important goals to improve QoL and to avoid unnecessary costs to healthcare.

References

Andris, D. and Krzywda, E.A. (2008) *The A.S.P.E.N. Nutritional Support Patient Education Manual.* American Society for Parenteral and Enteral Nutrition, Silver Spring, Maryland.

Bozzetti, F., Mariani, L., Boggio Bertinet, D., Chiavenna, G., Crose, N., De Cicco, M., Gigli, G., Micklewright, A., Moreno Villares, J.M., Orban, A., Pertkiewicz, M., Pironi, L., Planas Vilas, M., Prins, F. and Thul, P. (2002) Central venous catheter complications in 447 patients on home parenteral nutrition: an analysis of over 100,000 catheter days. *Clinical Nutrition* 21, 475–485.

Dreesen, M., Foulon, V., Vanhaecht, K., De Pourcq, L., Hiele, M. and Willems, L. (2012) Guidelines recommendations on care of adult patients receiving home parenteral nutrition (HPN): a systematic review of global practices. *Clinical Nutrition* 31, 602–608.

Gifford, H., DeLegge, M. and Epperson, L.A. (2010) Education methods and techniques for training home parenteral nutrition patients. *Nutrition in Clinical Practice* 25, 443–450.

Gillanders, L., Angstmann, K., Ball, P., Chapman-Kiddell, C., Hardy, G., Hope, J., Smith, R., Strauss, B., Russell, D. and Australian Society of Parenteral and Enteral Nutrition (2008) AuSPEN clinical practice guideline for home parenteral nutrition patients in Australia and New Zealand. *Nutrition* 24, 998–1012.

Hamilton, H. (1999) *Total Parenteral Nutrition: A Practical Guide for Nurses*, 1st edn. Churchill Livingstone, London.

Huisman-de Waal, G., Schoonhoven, L., Jansen, J., Wanten, G. and van Achterberg, T. (2007) The impact of home parenteral nutrition on daily life – a review. *Clinical Nutrition* 26, 275–288.

Ireton-Jones, C. and De Legge, M. (2005) Home parenteral nutrition registry: a five-year retrospective evaluation of outcomes of patients receiving home parenteral nutrition support. *Nutrition* 21, 156–160.

Ireton-Jones, C., De Legge, M., Epperson, L.A. and Alexander, J. (2003) Management of the home parenteral nutrition patient. *Nutrition in Clinical Practice* 18, 310–317.

Judson, K., Field, J. and Wengler, A. (2006) Teaching patients home parenteral nutrition. In: Bozzetti, F., Staun, M. and Van Gossum, A. (eds) *Home Parenteral Nutrition*, 1st edn. CAB International, Wallingford, UK, pp. 285–291.

Kirby, F., Mandy, L.C., Rex, A.S. and Emery, D.M. (2012) Home parenteral nutrition tutorial. *JPEN Journal of Parenteral and Enteral Nutrition* 36, 632–644.

Kovacevich, D.S., Frederick, A., Kelly, D., Nishikawa, R. and Young, L. (2005) Standards for specialized nutrition support: home care patients. *Nutrition in Clinical Practice* 20, 579–590.

Kumpf, V. and Tillman, E. (2012) Home parenteral nutrition: safe transition from hospital to home. *Nutrition in Clinical Practice* 27, 749–757.

Micklewright, A., Wengler, A., Prins, F., Bozetti, F., Hebuterne, X., Moreno Villares, J.M., Pertkiewicz, M., Pironi, L., Staun, M., Thul, P., Van Gossum, A. and the ESPEN-HAN Working Group (2002) Home parenteral nutrition (HPN) teaching practice in Europe. *Clinical Nutrition* 21, 42.

Santarpia, L., Pasanisi, F., Alfonsi, L., Violante, G., Tiseo, D., De Simone, G. and Contaldo, F. (2002) Prevention and treatment of implanted central venous catheter (CVC)-related sepsis: a report after six years of home parenteral nutrition (HPN). *Clinical Nutrition* 21, 207–211.

Staun, M., Pironi, L., Bozzetti, F., Baxter, J., Forbes, A., Joly, F., Jeppesen, P., Moreno, J., Hebuterne, X., Pertkiewicz, M., Mühlebach, S., Shenkin, A. and Van Gossum, A. (2009) ESPEN guidelines on parenteral nutrition: home parenteral nutrition (HPN) in adult patients. *Clinical Nutrition* 28, 467–479.

Van Gossum, A., Bakker, H., Bozzetti, F., Staun, M., Leon-Sanz, M., Hebuterne, X., Pertkiewicz, M. and Shaffer, J. (1999) Home parenteral nutrition in adults: a European multicentre survey in 1997: ESPEN-Home Artificial Nutrition Working Group. *Clinical Nutrition* 18, 135–140.

Wanten, G., Calder, P.C. and Forbes, A. (2011) Managing adult patients who need home parenteral nutrition. *British Medical Journal* 342, d1447.

29 Preparation and Provision of Home Parenteral Nutrition Solutions

Pilar Gomis*

The Pharmacy Service, Hospital 12 de Octubre, Madrid, Spain

Key Points

- The guarantee of adequate technique is based on the strict following of the parenteral nutrition (PN) preparation protocol, the validation of the preparation process and the training of personnel.
- In order to increase stability of the PN solution and decrease lipid peroxidation, the use of photo-protection and multilayer bags is recommended, as well as organic phosphates and lipid emulsions with low content of polyunsaturated fatty acids.
- For the sake of safety, 1.2 µm filters should be used.
- It is important for patients and caregivers to be aware of the correct storage conditions for PN bags.
- Some pharmaceutical companies have 'ready-to-use' bags with predefined compositions, the stability of which is guaranteed for longer periods of time.

Introduction

In contrast to most hospitalized patients who require parenteral nutrition (PN) for a few days, home parenteral nutrition (HPN) is provided for long periods of time and the caloric intake needs to be adjusted to avoid weight loss or overfeeding complications. Some patients need extra fluid or electrolyte supplementation that can be incorporated into the bag or administered separately. Many of these patients are also receiving drugs intravenously that can sometimes be added to the PN bag to facilitate their administration.

*E-mail: pgomis.hdoc@salud.madrid.org

Although initially, in most of the HPN programmes in Europe, preparation was performed almost completely by hospital pharmacies, nowadays some pharmaceutical companies have 'ready-to-use' bags with predefined composition, the stability of which is guaranteed for longer periods of time, or individualized PN bags are prepared for delivery to patients. It is recommended that a multidisciplinary team, of which the pharmacist must be a part, performs the management of HPN patients (Bischoff *et al.*, 2009).

Preparation

Essential prerequisites include secure venous access and the availability of medical, nursing, dietetic and pharmacy staff skilled in the management of HPN. Most pharmacies in large hospitals have specific units for PN bag preparation where a strict aseptic technique is followed under the supervision of a pharmacist. The guarantee of aseptic technique is based on: (i) strictly following the PN preparation protocol; (ii) the use of laminar flow cabins in a specific clean area; (iii) the quality of solutions; (iv) the validation of the preparation process; (v) microbiological controls; and (vi) the training of personnel.

The main problems we encounter in PN preparation are emulsion stability and calcium phosphate precipitation. Some authors have recommended the separate administration of lipids, arguing that we do not know if the emulsion is stable and that we cannot see calcium phosphate precipitations if they occur – because of the opacity of lipids. But, as we shall see later, calcium phosphate precipitation can be avoided by using organic phosphates, and most PN emulsions are stable if we follow preparation protocols. For the sake of safety, 1.2 μm filters should be used.

In addition, when lipids are administered separately, two different lines are needed – or two-lumen lines can be used – because if we administer PN and lipids in the same line, simultaneously, we may also have stability problems; and if one is administered before the other, there could be side-effects or it could be inconvenient for the patient because he/she cannot afford to be disconnected for any length of time. 'All-in-one' PN solutions have other important advantages in HPN: (i) they need less line manipulation; (ii) they are less costly; (iii) they need only an administration pump; and (iv) microorganisms reproduce with more difficulty than in lipids alone.

The major problems of PN stability or compatibility are the following.

Emulsion stability

Emulsion stability depends mainly on pH, temperature, amino acid concentration, electrolyte concentration – particularly divalent cations – and type of lipids used. It is also fundamental to follow the right sequence of addition. Adding amino acids first is recommended, because they stabilize the emulsion and counteract the deleterious effects of highly concentrated glucose and electrolytes. With higher amino acid concentration the emulsion is more stable.

It has been also shown that very low lipid concentration can decrease stability of PN solutions. Some studies have found that olive oil-based lipid emulsions and medium-chain triacylglycerol (MCT)/long-chain triacylglycerol (LCT) emulsions are more stable than LCT emulsions (Driscoll *et al.*, 2001). The new lipid emulsions containing *n*-3 polyunsaturated fatty acids (PUFAs) also seem to be quite stable in PN (Driscoll *et al.*, 2009). In HPN, the use of more stable fat emulsions would be recommended, because these PN solutions need a more extended shelf-life. Filter use is also recommended to increase safety.

Calcium phosphate precipitation

High concentrations of calcium and phosphate can cause calcium phosphate precipitation. This depends on the concentration of calcium and phosphate ions, pH, amino acid concentration, type of calcium and phosphate salts, ambient temperature, infusion speed and storage time. There are reference curves which indicate calcium and inorganic phosphate compatibility (Poole *et al.*, 1983; Dunham *et al.*, 1991); when inorganic phosphates are used, we have to be very cautious not to exceed calcium and phosphate concentration limits. Amino acids have a protective effect, forming complexes with calcium or phosphate, diminishing precipitation risk. Addition order is also very important. Calcium or phosphate can be added at the beginning and the other components should be added at the end, when the final volume is reached. It is important that if, for example, the phosphate is added at the beginning, the calcium is not added until the volume at which they are compatible is reached. Sometimes, particularly in paediatrics, calcium and inorganic phosphate limits are below patient requirements. Nevertheless, organic phosphates are also stable within PN admixtures (Ronchera *et al.*, 1995) and their limits are higher than the concentrations usually used (Hanning *et al.*, 1989; Raupp *et al.*, 1991; Prinzivalli and Ceccerelli, 1999; Chaieb *et al.*, 2008; Ribeiro *et al.*, 2009). The use of filters is recommended: 0.22 μm filters in no-fat PN and 1.22-μm filters in all-in-one PN.

Vitamin degradation

Long-term PN patients generally need daily administration of vitamins to prevent deficiencies (Mikalunas *et al.*, 2001). Many years ago, some studies showed that vitamins could degrade in PN solutions and that trace elements could interact with vitamins, thus diminishing their stability. Because of that, their addition was recommended just before PN administration and every other day with trace elements.

The most unstable vitamins in PN are thiamine, retinol, riboflavin and ascorbic acid. Thiamine instability is due to its reduction by metabisulfites, which was important when amino acid solutions used to contain sulfites, but nowadays most of them are sulfite free. Retinol and riboflavin degradation are mainly due to photo-degradation, but all-in-one PN and protection from light diminish this degradation. Ascorbic acid is oxidized in the presence of oxygen and copper catalyses this oxidation. This degradation decreases in all-in-one bags and with high cysteine concentration.

In PN hospital preparation there are two main reasons why vitamin C is in contact with oxygen, increasing its oxidation: (i) at the preparation site when the bag is filled by gravity or pumps; and (ii) bag permeability. The first can be avoided or diminished by using nitrogen for filling bags or by decreasing both oxygen contact during the filling and residual oxygen inside the bag as much as possible. The second is responsible for vitamin C degradation over time and can be inhibited by using multilayer bags (Gomis *et al.*, 1996; Dupertuis *et al.*, 2002, 2005; Vazquez *et al.*, 2009). These bags prevent passage of oxygen and also provide some photoprotection. Nowadays, using multilayer and photo-protection bags we can introduce vitamins and trace elements in PN bags with 5-day stability.

Peroxidation

Lipid peroxidation in all-in-one bags seems to be directly related to the PUFA content and inversely related to the α-tocopherol/PUFA ratio of the emulsion (Pironi *et al.*, 2003). The main factors that influence oxidation in PN solutions are: (i) light; (ii) contact with oxygen during the preparation or oxygen permeability of the bag; (iii) trace elements like iron or copper; and (iv) temperature (Steger and Muhlebach, 2000).

In HPN patients there is an increased oxidative stress and inadequate antioxidant status (Massarenti *et al.*, 2004). In order to avoid peroxide formation, refrigeration of PN solutions throughout storage is recommended, as well as avoidance of high temperatures during administration, protection of PN bags from light and avoiding contact with oxygen. Multilayer bags significantly reduce hydroperoxide generation (Balet *et al.*, 2004). If one-layer, ethyl vinyl acetate (EVA) bags are used, it is better to utilize low-PUFA lipid emulsions because hydroperoxide content depends on this (Balet *et al.*, 2004).

Drug stability

Drugs can only be added to PN solutions or be infused via a Y-site when studies regarding their drug compatibility and emulsion stability have been performed. Some medications, like insulin, ranitidine or octreotide, are stable in all-in-one PN bags and can be added at the preparation site, avoiding patient or caregiver work and line manipulation.

Preparation Sheets and Labelling

HPN orders, in general, do not change frequently; the PN formulations usually change their composition when patients have had medical revisions or complications. Occasionally they can continue for years without any change in PN formulation. It is very important to avoid re-transcription errors. Sometimes it may be necessary to separate home PN- from hospitalized PN-order transcriptions to avoid daily or weekly copying of PN composition. It would be good practice with these patients not to change the preparation sheet unless a new prescription order is sent. It is also very important to have open communication with prescribing physicians to avoid prescription or legibility problems. An error in HPN composition can have more serious consequences than with a hospitalized patient, because it can be difficult to detect and the problem can exist for a longer period of time. For instance, forgetting to add vitamins or trace elements is not a problem for 1 or 2 days, but can be damaging for long periods of time. Computer programs can help when preparation sheets are generated. Labelling is also important, and patients or caregivers should check the labels every time they receive their bags and contact the pharmacist if something does not match.

The Location of Solution Preparation and Provision

HPN patients, in contrast to hospitalized patients for whom PN can be prepared on almost a daily basis, cannot collect bags every day; therefore, a long PN shelf-life is essential.

In this respect there are many differences between countries – and even between hospitals within the same country. Sometimes preparations have much to do with delivery availability. There are three main scenarios, the advantages and disadvantages of which are summarized in Table 29.1.

Preparation in hospital

The advantage of this kind of preparation is that patients receive all their needs or almost all their needs in one bag. Patient manipulation is minimal. Vitamins and trace elements are included, and also some stable drugs. Although there can be

Table 29.1. Advantages and disadvantages of different types of site preparations.

	Hospital-made PN	Ready-to-use PN (multi-chamber bags)	Individualized company preparation
Shelf-life	5 days (mean)	>1 year	5–6 days
Composition	Individualized	Standard	Individualized
Vitamins and trace elements	Included	Not included	Included
Drugs	Included if stable	Not included	Included if stable
Delivery to patients	Pick up in the hospital/ delivery to patient's residence[a]	Pick up in the hospital/ delivery to patient's residence[a]	Delivery to patient's residence
Schedule	Once or twice per week	Depends on patient's storage capacity	Daily
Price	++	+++	+++++

[a]If home care services are available.

many different individual situations, in most cases patients or their relatives have to pick up the PN bags at a pharmacy once or twice per week.

Ready-to-use PN bags

These are multi-chamber bags made by pharmaceutical companies with predefined compositions. Almost every day, more different newly registered compositions appear. Companies ensure both emulsion stability and the absence of compatibility problems for long periods of time while the chambers are not joined, and for 5–8 days after joining. They also guarantee the stability if some electrolytes are introduced. The solutions do not contain vitamins or trace elements, which should be added before administration. When the composition does not match patients' exact requirements, patients – or their carers – must also add electrolytes and/or administer fluid bags, drugs, etc.

Individualized company preparations

Some companies prepare individualized PN bags for HPN prescribed in hospitals. Usually, PN orders are sent from pharmacy services by computer and bags are sent to the patient's residence. Vitamins, trace elements and some drugs can be included. The only disadvantage is price. In some countries there are home care companies that provide not only PN solutions and PN-related supplies, but also health services that can include caregiver training on PN and pumps prior to discharge, assessment of the home environment, 24 h telephone line for problem resolution and home nursing visits (Norman and Crill, 2011).

Delivery

There are different forms of bag delivery, depending on hospitals and availability in each country. In some countries, there are companies that have home care services with or without PN compounding. They deliver PN bags, disposable items such as infusion sets and even pumps, refrigerators, etc. Some of them also offer nursing support at home. In some places this is carried out by primary care. In other cases, patients or caregivers pick up the bags at the hospital and they should be taught that if delivery distance is long, or ambient temperature is high, they need to refrigerate the bags – using ice if necessary – but avoiding the possibility of freezing.

Administration of HPN

It is recommended that 1.2 μm filters be used because they avoid not only precipitates but also the coalescence of oil droplets and other particles from the preparation process (rubber, glass, etc.). These particles can be deposited in the lungs

(Walpot *et al.*, 1989). Although there are no studies concerning deleterious particle effects in the long-term PN patient, HPN patients will receive a large amount of intravenous fluids over the course of their life. The fewer particles they receive, the fewer side-effects they could have. There are filters incorporated in the administration set that provide the advantage of diminishing home line manipulation. It is important that patients or caregivers, besides being familiar with line care, know about integrity of the PN solution and the necessity of storing it under refrigeration. They also need to know that the product should be administered below 25°C and not to remove the photo-protection from the bag. When infusion is not cyclic, patients have to be aware not to be outside on a day when temperatures are >28°C (Lee *et al.*, 2003).

Role of the Pharmacist in HPN

It is important for pharmacists be part of HPN teams, contributing their knowledge (Mühlebach *et al.*, 2009) of:

- products and equipment used for PN;
- potential interactions or incompatibilities between PN components or other medications administered;
- stability of PN regimens and their correct handling (storage, light protection, administration);
- selection and composition of PN regimens; and
- education and training.

The pharmacist's role depends on the development of HPN. If, as would be desirable, HPN monitoring is concentrated in experienced hospitals, pharmacists should continue to be part of HPN teams, helping design PN compositions in accordance with stability issues and patient necessities. If all patients or caregivers pick bags up in the pharmacy, the pharmacist could educate them concerning issues related to PN bag storage and administration. If, on the other hand, HPN can be ordered by any hospital, pharmacists could also have an important role in hospitals where there is no nutritional support unit or team, helping physicians in charge of patients to prescribe PN.

The pharmacist's contribution depends in part on his/her medical specialization and knowledge of the subject. In some hospitals, the PN guidelines and the follow-up are done by Pharmaceutical Services, although normally the doctor prescribes the diet and the pharmacist checks it before preparing it or sending it to an external provider for preparation. For example, the guidelines for trace elements and vitamins are of special importance with HPN patients. The quantity of manganese must be carefully checked, given that many commercially available trace elements contain quantities substantially greater than those recommended and accumulations of this trace element in basal ganglia have been chronicled. In patients with renal or hepatic failure, it is important to provide appropriate amounts of some micronutrients in order to avoid accumulation. Aluminium is a contaminant found in many of the products used in the preparation of PN solutions. It is important to minimize the content as much as possible.

In addition to the preparation of PN, the HPN patient may need Pharmaceutical Services to prepare other types of intravenous medications for them such as antibiotics (in the case of catheter infection), iron (given that it cannot always be added to the PN formulation) or solutions such as 70% alcohol to seal the catheter, among others. Cancer patients also need medications for pain control or chemotherapy for the control of the disease that are generally prepared by Pharmaceutical Services. The pharmacist also plays an important role by providing information to the doctor and/or the patient regarding the compatibility and stability of both the PN and the other medications that these patients receive.

Summary

HPN preparation can be performed by hospitals or by the pharmaceutical industry using either long shelf-life, multi-chamber bags or individualized ones. In order to increase stability of the PN solution and decrease lipid peroxidation, the use of photo-protection and multilayer bags is recommended, as well as organic phosphates and low-PUFA lipid emulsions. The use of filters of 1.2 μm diameter can increase safety. Preparation site and distribution depend on the hospital and the types available within the country.

When home care services are available, bags are delivered to the patient's residence, frequently with materials. Sometimes nursing care is also provided. Depending on the country, these services can be provided by the pharmaceutical industry or by primary care. If these services are not available, patients/care providers must collect the bags once or twice per week. It is important for them to be aware of the correct storage conditions for PN bags.

References

Balet, A., Cardona, D., Jane, S., Molins-Pujol, A.M., Sanchez-Quesada, J.L., Gich, I. and Mangues, M.A. (2004) Effects of multilayered bags vs. ethylvinyl-acetate bags on oxidation of parenteral nutrition. *JPEN Journal of Parenteral and Enteral Nutrition* 28, 85–91.

Bischoff, S.C., Kester, L., Meier, R., Radziwill, R., Schwab, D., Thul, P. and the working group for developing the guidelines for parenteral nutrition of The German Association for Nutritional Medicine (2009) Organisation, regulations, preparation and logistics of parenteral nutrition in hospitals and homes; the role of the nutrition support team – Guidelines on Parenteral Nutrition, Chapter 8. *GMS German Medical Science* 7, Document 20.

Chaieb, D.S., Chaumeil, J.C., Jebnoun, S., Khrouf, N., Hedhili, A. and Sfar, S. (2008) Effect of the intravenous lipid emulsions on the availability of calcium when using organic phosphate in TPN admixtures. *Pharmaceutical Research* 25, 2545–2554.

Driscoll, D.F., Giampietro, K., Wichelhaus, D.P., Nehne, J., Niemann, W. and Bistrian, B.R. (2001) Physicochemical stability assessments of lipid emulsions of varying oil composition. *Clinical Nutrition* 20, 151–157.

Driscoll, D.F., Ling, P. and Bistrian, B.R. (2009) Pharmacopeial compliance of fish oil-containing parenteral lipid emulsion mixtures: globule size distribution (GSD) and fatty acid analyses. *International Journal of Pharmaceutics* 379, 125–130.

Dunham, B., Marcuard, S., Khazanie, P.G., Meade, G., Craft, T. and Nichols, K. (1991) The solubility of calcium and phosphorus in neonatal total parenteral nutrition solutions. *JPEN Journal of Parenteral and Enteral Nutrition* 15, 608–611.
Dupertuis, Y.M., Morch, A., Fathi, M., Sierro, C., Genton, L., Kyle, U.G. and Pichard, C. (2002) Physical characteristics of total parenteral nutrition bags significantly affect the stability of vitamins C and B_1: a controlled prospective study. *JPEN Journal of Parenteral and Enteral Nutrition* 26, 310–316.
Dupertuis, Y.M., Ramseyer, S., Fathi, M. and Pichard, C. (2005) Assessment of ascorbic acid stability in different multilayered parenteral nutrition bags: critical influence of the bag wall material. *JPEN Journal of Parenteral and Enteral Nutrition* 29, 125–130.
Gomis, P., Míguelez, S., Navarro, J.A., Estenoz, J., Alegre, E., Moreno, J.M., Zannuy, M.A. and León-Sanz, M. (1996) Estabilidad de vitaminas en nutrición parenteral: comparación de bolsas multicapa frente a unicapa. *Nutrición Hospitalaria* 11, 259–264.
Hanning, R.M., Mitchell, M.K. and Atkinton, S.A. (1989) *In vitro* solubility of calcium glycerophosphate versus conventional mineral salts in pediatric parenteral nutrition solutions. *Journal of Pediatric Gastroenterology and Nutrition* 9, 67–72.
Lee, M.D., Yoon, J.E. and Kim, S.I. (2003) Stability of total nutrient admixtures in reference to ambient temperatures. *Nutrition* 19, 886–890.
Massarenti, P., Biasi, F., De Francesco, A., Pauletto, D., Rocca, G., Silli, B., Vizio, B., Serviddio, G., Leonarduzzi, G., Poli, G. and Palmo, A. (2004) 4-Hydroxynonenal is markedly higher in patients on a standard long-term home parenteral nutrition. *Free Radical Research* 38, 73–80.
Mikalunas, V., Fitzgerald, K., Rubin, H., McCarthy, R. and Craig, R.M. (2001) Abnormal vitamin levels in patients receiving home total parenteral nutrition. *Journal of Clinical Gastroenterology* 33, 393–396.
Mühlebach, S., Franken, C., Stanga, Z. and working group for developing the guidelines for parenteral nutrition of The German Association for Nutritional Medicine (2009) Practical handling of AIO admixtures – Guidelines on Parenteral Nutrition, Chapter 10. *GMS German Medical Science* 7, Document 18.
Norman, J.L. and Crill, C.M. (2011) Optimizing the transition to home parenteral nutrition in pediatric patients. *Nutrition in Clinical Practice* 26, 273–285.
Pironi, L., Guidetti, M., Zolezzi, C., Fasano, M.C., Paganelli, F., Merli, C., Bersani, G., Pizzzoferrato, A. and Miglioni, M. (2003) Peroxidation potential of lipid emulsions after compounding in all-in-one solutions. *Nutrition* 19, 784–788.
Poole, R.L., Rupp, C.A. and Kerner, J.A. (1983) Calcium and phosphorus in neonatal parenteral nutrition solutions. *JPEN Journal of Parenteral and Enteral Nutrition* 7, 358–360.
Prinzivalli, M. and Ceccerelli, S. (1999) Sodium D-fructose-1, 6-diphosphate vs. sodium monohydrogen phosphate in total parenteral nutrition: a comparative *in vitro* assessment of calcium/phosphate compatibility. *JPEN Journal of Parenteral and Enteral Nutrition* 23, 326–332.
Raupp, P., Kries, R.V., Pfahl, H.G. and Manz, F. (1991) Glycero vs. glucose-phosphate in parenteral nutrition of premature infants: evaluation of calcium/phosphorus compatibility. *JPEN Journal of Parenteral and Enteral Nutrition* 15, 469–473.
Ribeiro, D.O., Lobo, B.W., Volpato, N.M., da Veiga, V.F., Cabral, L.M. and de Sousa, V.P. (2009) Influence of the calcium concentration in the presence of organic phosphorus on the physicochemical compatibility and stability of all-in-one admixtures for neonatal use. *Nutrition Journal* 8, 51.
Ronchera, C.L., Jiménez, N.V. and Peidro, J. (1995) Stability of parenteral nutrition admixtures containing organic phosphates. *Clinical Nutrition* 14, 373–380.

Steger, P.J. and Muhlebach, S.F. (2000) Lipid peroxidation of intravenous lipid emulsions and all-in-one admixtures in total parenteral nutrition bags: the influence of trace elements. *JPEN Journal of Parenteral and Enteral Nutrition* 24, 37–41.
Vazquez, R., Hoang, M.L. and Martin, J., Yahia, Y.A., Graffard, H., Guyon, F. and Do, B. (2009) Simultaneous quantification of water-soluble and fat-soluble vitamins in parenteral nutrition admixtures by HPLC–UV–MS/MS. *European Journal of Hospital Pharmacy Science* 15, 28–35.
Walpot, H., Franckle, R.P., Buchard, W.G., Agternkamp, C. and Mueller, F.G. (1989) Particulate contamination of intravenous solution and drug additives during long term intensive care. *Anasthesist* 38, 544–548.

30 Administration of Home Parenteral Nutrition

Asuncion Ballarin[1*], Viviane Lievin[2] and André Van Gossum[3]

[1]Hôpital Erasme, Brussels, Belgium; [2]Department of Hospital Pharmacy, Hôpital Erasme, Brussels, Belgium; [3]Clinic of Intestinal Diseases and Clinical Nutrition, Hôpital Erasme, Free University of Brussels, Brussels, Belgium

Key Points

- In the majority of patients on home parenteral nutrition (HPN), infusions are administered on a cyclical nocturnal basis.
- The duration of administration must take into consideration the infusion volume, the tolerance of the patient and the vascular patency.
- Although it has been generally recommended, the benefit of using a heparin lock has not been proved.
- The use of infusion pumps is increasing and may improve quality of life for patients on HPN.

Introduction

The administration of parenteral nutrition (PN) at home should meet some specific goals: safety, tolerance and patient autonomy. Taking into account these parameters, the main objective is primarily to combine an optimal nutritional support with the best quality of life for patients on home parenteral nutrition (HPN).

Administration of HPN must consider various issues:

1. Patient's characteristics: age, indication for HPN and underlying disease, co-morbidity, degree of rehabilitation and professional activity, and willingness.
2. The type of perfusion: volume, composition, compounding.
3. The type of venous access as well as the patient's vascular patency.

*E-mail: asuncion.ballarin@erasme.ulb.ac.be

Patient's Characteristics

In the majority of HPN patients, PN is administered on a cyclical nocturnal basis (Van Gossum *et al.*, 2001). This regimen has the advantage of providing autonomy during the daytime for 6–12 h and of encouraging oral food intake. Nevertheless, the cyclical nocturnal regimen may induce some discomfort such as sleep disturbance due to frequent urine excretion (Scolapio *et al.*, 2002; Persoon *et al.*, 2005). Moreover, the sleep period can also be disturbed by the control pump's alarm. A small percentage of patients prefer a cyclical diurnal regimen and, more rarely, a continuous daily administration. The latter is more frequently observed in patients with advanced cancer for whom autonomy is already very limited.

The duration of administration must take into consideration the volume of infusion and the patient's tolerance. The rate of administration should be progressively adapted over time and according to the patient's feeling/well-being. Some factors may limit the rate of administration: the need for a large volume, the existence/presence of some degree of cardiac failure, the vascular patency. Indeed, in patients with previous venous thrombosis and/or a superior vena cava syndrome, the rate of administration must be very cautious.

The timing of HPN administration is also dependent on who is doing the intravenous line connection and disconnection. It is much more flexible for a patient who performs the manipulation himself than for a patient requiring the assistance of a relative or a community nurse. The handling of HPN is performed by the patient himself, a relative who has been educated in the technique or community nurses. In many countries, the role of commercial providers for HPN is becoming more and more important (Tappenden, 2012). A close collaboration between the hospital nutrition team, the patient and the home care services is mandatory for assuring the best quality of care (Wanten *et al.*, 2011; Guenter *et al.*, 2012). Another factor that may interfere with the period of HPN infusion is the volume of intestinal fluid output. Indeed, patients having a high-output jejunostomy may experience fatigue, malaise and thirst only a few hours after stopping the infusion, concomitant with hypovolaemia.

The use of portable infusion pumps may improve independence of patients and quality of life; this technique was developed mainly for adolescents who required large infusion volume (Boutin and Hagan, 1992).

Type of Perfusion

Usually HPN is administered as an 'all-in-one' bag. This is more comfortable and requires only one giving/infusion set. Moreover, the risk of bacterial contamination is minimal. Individually prepared bags have to be stored in a refrigerator. It is advisable to remove the bag from the fridge some hours before starting the infusion. The commercially available bags can be stored at room temperature and are reconstituted immediately before their administration. For patients receiving commercially prepared bags in the long term, there is a need to add vitamins and trace elements before administration. This has to be done in sterile conditions.

In addition to sterile handling of giving sets, needles and bags, HPN administration requires a suitable environment. It is highly recommended to visit the home facilities where the manipulations are performed in order to assure a sufficient level of hygiene. A Canadian survey showed that community agency, socio-economic or educational status was not significant in determining line sepsis (Chang *et al.*, 2005). Patients who had intravenous administration of medication or blood samples that were drawn through the catheter, a higher number of dependants or a trained family member involved in HPN were in the high-risk category for line sepsis, in addition to patients who were part-time students or receiving social assistance.

Type and Handling of Venous Access

The administration of HPN must also consider the venous access and the type of device that is used. In the majority of patients, HPN is administered through a central venous catheter (CVC). The selection of the venous access is based on the vascular anatomy, the expected duration of HPN, the patient's activity and willingness, and the ability of the patient himself or his caregiver in handling the access. Further considerations include body image and costs.

It has been shown that the use of peripherally inserted central catheters (PICCs) has a statistically increased risk of catheter infection (DeLegge *et al.*, 2005). PICC lines are not currently recommended for long-term HPN, although evidence to support this statement is scarce. However, Botella-Carretero *et al.* recently reported a series of 48 patients receiving HPN through PICCs. They observed the same ratio of catheter-related complications as for other CVC lines, especially for oncology patients with HPN lasting less than 6 months (Botella-Carretero *et al.*, 2013).

In short bowel, fistula and some other gastrointestinal diseases, salt, water and magnesium balance may continue to be negative despite oral supplements, even in patients with adequate nutritional status (Martinez-Riquelme *et al.*, 2005). It has been recently shown that subcutaneous self-administered fluid infusion (0.5–1.0 l of 0.9% saline + 0.5 l of 5% dextrose with 2 to 4 mmol $MgSO_4$) at home could be an easily managed, safe and effective method for restoring and maintaining water, salt and magnesium balance. That could be of special interest in the frail or elderly in whom HPN may be difficult.

There are no guidelines for changing needles when ports are used. Manufacturers recommend changing the needle daily. This is uncomfortable for the patient and extremely expensive. In clinical practice most of the needles are changed once weekly. An analysis of over 100,000 catheter-days showed that 36% of the needles were changed every day (Bozzetti *et al.*, 2002). A daily puncture of the port was associated with more complications and removals of the device than when punctures were less frequent. An inviolate skin barrier over the port loses its significance if patients are infused every day. The risk of infection increases by daily needle perforation of the skin over the port. Some patients prefer to leave the needle in the site in the interval between HPN administrations to avoid the discomfort of repeated piercing. The safety of this practice should be confirmed by performing a prospective randomized trial.

Some teams systematically use a multi-purpose, closed, needle-free connector for blood sampling, intermittent injections or continuous infusion of PN. This closed system is likely to increase the safety of patients and to eliminate the use of an obturator.

Use of a heparin lock has been recommended for a long time in patients receiving HPN to prevent catheter thrombosis (Lyons *et al.*, 1981). When a heparin lock is employed, a large range of doses are used (from 50 to 500 units in 5 ml of 0.9% saline). Although there was no randomized trial for supporting this concept, the use of low-dose (50 units in 5 ml of 0.9% saline) heparin block has been recommended. The analysis of 110,869 days with CVC in patients on HPN by the European Society for Parenteral and Enteral Nutrition (ESPEN) Home Artificial Nutrition (HAN) Group showed significant disadvantages of using a heparin flush (Bozzetti *et al.*, 2002). There have been significantly more infections, removals and occlusions when heparin flush was used. Heparin has severe adverse effects, such as thrombocytopenia, bone disease and loss of hair. There is no randomized prospective study that shows the potential benefit of heparin flush to prevent catheter thrombosis in long-term HPN patients. Many teams have selected to flush the catheter using a few millilitres of 0.9% saline.

For preventing catheter-related sepsis, the use of ethanol lock (John *et al.*, 2012; Pieroni *et al.*, 2013) or taurolidine lock (Bisseling *et al.*, 2010; Touré *et al.*, 2012) has shown very promising results. Prospective randomized trials are ongoing. This is detailed in Chapter 19.

Thromboprophylaxis using either low-molecular-weight heparin or vitamin K antagonists is still debatable despite some positive results (Vegting *et al.*, 2012).

Infusion/giving sets for HPN are discarded after each use. Administration sets for separate fat emulsions should be discarded after each unit of fat is infused if it is not consecutively (Driscoll *et al.*, 1996). Containers and administration sets free of the plasticizer di-2-ethylhexylphthalate (DEHP) should be used to prevent DEHP contamination of infusions, especially those containing fat emulsions. Since DEHP is highly lipophilic, fat emulsions are capable of extracting DEHP from the polyvinylchloride administration sets. This is important in long-term patients. There may be adverse effects from DEHP related to its potential for neurotoxicity, carcinogenicity and hepatotoxicity in animals. Most of the infusion containers used in Europe are made from ethylvinyl acetate; the use of DEHP should be totally discontinued.

In the clinical setting, intravenous infusion pumps are an integral component of PN administration. Use of an electronic infusion pump to safely administer infusions in hospital is recommended. This is different in long-term PN in home patients: the infusion time in HPN is regularly between 10 and 14 h, and it is usually adjusted by the patient and not the physician. There is no difference when infusion time is not exactly as suggested by the physician. The best time is that preferred by the patient, if there is no hyperglycaemia or hyperlipidaemia. If patients have experience with and without infusion pumps, they may refuse pumps giving the reasons that there are frequent alarms and sleeping is interrupted. If there is no regulation by law, infusion pumps are not necessary in patients on total PN at home. The use of pumps is very variable from one to another country throughout Europe (Van Gossum *et al.*, 2001). In HPN patients who are not using pumps, the use of flow control devices (Dialaflow®) is recommended.

In conclusion, administration of HPN should follow some general guidelines but may be individually adapted to each patient.

Summary

In the majority of the patients, PN is administered on a cyclical nocturnal basis. This regimen may induce some discomfort such as sleep disturbance. The rate of administration must take into account the volume of infusion, the patient's tolerance and the vascular patency.

Usually, HPN is administered as an all-in-one bag. The selection of venous access is based on several parameters. There are no guidelines for changing needles when ports are used. Although it is largely used, the benefit of a heparin lock has not been proved. The use of pumps is variable from one country to another. Administration of HPN must follow some general guidelines, but may be individually adapted to each patient in order to improve the quality of life.

References

Bisseling, T.M., Willems, M.C., Versleijen, M.W., Hendriks, J.C., Vissers, R.K. and Wanten, G.J. (2010) Taurolidine lock is highly effective in preventing catheter-related bloodstream infections in patients on home parenteral nutrition: a heparin-controlled prospective trial. *Clinical Nutrition* 29, 464–468.

Botella-Carretero, J.L., Carrero, C., Guerra, E., Valbuena, B., Arrieta, F., Calañas, A., Zamarrón, I., Balsa, J.A. and Vázquez, C. (2013) Role of peripherally central catheters in home parenteral nutrition: a 5-year prospective study. *JPEN Journal of Parenteral and Enteral Nutrition* 37, 544–549.

Boutin, J. and Hagan, E. (1992) Patients' preference regarding portable pumps. *Journal of Intravenous Nursing* 15, 230–232.

Bozzetti, F., Mariani, L., Bertinet, D.B., Chiavenna, G., Crose, N., De Cicco, M., Gigli, G., Micklewright, A., Moreno Villares, J.M., Orban, A., Pertkiewicz, M., Pironi, L., Vilas, M.P., Prins, F. and Thul, P. (2002) Central venous catheter complications in 447 patients on home parenteral nutrition: an analysis of over 100,000 catheter days. *Clinical Nutrition* 21, 475–485.

Chang, A., Enns, R., Saqui, O., Chatur, N., Whittaker, S. and Allard, J.P. (2005) Line sepsis in home parenteral nutrition patients: are there socioeconomic risks factors? A Canadian study. *JPEN Journal of Parenteral and Enteral Nutrition* 29, 408–412.

DeLegge, M., Borak, G. and Moore, N. (2005) Central venous access in the home parenteral nutrition population – you PICC. *JPEN Journal of Parenteral and Enteral Nutrition* 29, 425–428.

Driscoll, D., Bacon, M. and Bistrian, B. (1996) Effects of in-line filtration on lipid particle size distribution in total nutrient admixtures. *JPEN Journal of Parenteral and Enteral Nutrition* 20, 296–301.

Guenter, P., Robinson, L., DiMaria-Ghalili, R.A., Lyman, B., Steiger, E. and Winkler, M.F. (2012) Development of Sustain™: A.S.P.E.N.'s National Patient Registry for Nutrition Care. *JPEN Journal of Parenteral and Enteral Nutrition* 36, 399–406.

John, B.K., Khan, M.A., Speerhas, R., Rhoda, K., Hamilton, C., Dechicco, R., Lopez, R., Steiger, E. and Kirby, D.F. (2012) Ethanol lock therapy in reducing catheter-related bloodstream infections in adult home parenteral nutrition patients: results of a retrospective study. *JPEN Journal of Parenteral and Enteral Nutrition* 36, 603–610.

Lyons, J., Falkenbach, L. and Cerra, F. (1981) Home parenteral nutrition with full-time home care nurses. *JPEN Journal of Parenteral and Enteral Nutrition* 5, 528–530.

Martinez-Riquelme, A., Rawlings, J., Morley, S., Kendall, J., Hosking, D. and Allison, S. (2005) Self-administered subcutaneous fluid infusion at home in the management of fluid depletion and hypomagnesemia in gastrointestinal diseases. *Clinical Nutrition* 24, 158–163.

Persoon, A., Huisman-deWaal, G., Naber, T., Schoonhoven, L., Tas, T., Saverwein, H. and van Achterberg, T. (2005) Impact of long-term HPN on daily life in adults. *Clinical Nutrition* 24, 304–313.

Pieroni, K.P., Nespor, C., Ng, M., Garcia, M., Hurwitz, M., Berquist, W.E. and Kerner, J.A. Jr (2013) Evaluation of ethanol lock therapy in pediatric patients on long-term parenteral nutrition. *Nutritional in Clinical Practice* 28, 226–231.

Scolapio, J., Savoy, A., Kaplan, J., Burger, C. and Lin, S. (2002) Sleep patterns of cyclic parenteral nutrition, a pilot study: are these sleepless nights? *JPEN Journal of Parenteral and Enteral Nutrition* 26, 214–217.

Tappenden, K.A. (2012) A challenge to providers of clinical nutrition therapy. *JPEN Journal of Parenteral and Enteral Nutrition* 36, 377.

Touré, A., Lauverjat, M., Peraldi, C., Boncompain-Gerard, M., Gelas, P., Barnoud, D. and Chambrier, C. (2012) Taurolidine lock solution in the secondary prevention of central venous catheter-associated bloodstream infection in home parenteral nutrition patients. *Clinical Nutrition* 31, 567–570.

Van Gossum, A., Vahedi, K., Abdel-Malik, M., Staun, M., Pertkiewicz, M., Shaffer, J., Hebuterne, X., Beau, P., Guedon, C., Schmit, A., Tjellesen, L., Messing, B. and Forbes, A.; ESPEN-HAN Working Group (2001) Clinical, social and rehabilitation status of long-term parenteral nutrition: results of a European multicentre survey. *Clinical Nutrition* 20, 205–210.

Vegting, I.L., Tabbers, M.M., Benninga, M.A., Wilde, J.C., Serlie, M.J., Tas, T.A., Jonkers, C.F. and van Ommen, C.H. (2012) Prophylactic anticoagulation decreases catheter-related thrombosis and occlusion in children with home parenteral nutrition. *JPEN Journal of Parenteral Enteral Nutrition* 36, 456–462.

Wanten, G., Calder, P.C. and Forbes, A. (2011) Managing adult patient who need home parenteral nutrition. *British Medical Journal* 342, d1447.

31 Monitoring Patients on Home Parenteral Nutrition

MICHAEL STAUN[1]* AND LORIS PIRONI[2]

[1]*Department of Medical Gastroenterology, Rigshospitalet, Denmark;*
[2]*Center for Chronic Intestinal Failure, Department of Medical and Surgical Science, University of Bologna, Bologna, Italy*

Key Points

- Monitoring of patients on home parenteral nutrition (HPN) usually takes place at the discharging hospital with access to the specialized team. Monitoring can also be carried out by a home care agency involving the local or discharging hospital and the general practitioner.
- Intervals between monitoring visits for the stable patient are 2–4 months. Consider that unstable patients may need more attention.
- Parameters monitored at each visit should include biochemical variables and anthropometry; every 6 months or annually, trace element and vitamin status and bone mineral density should be measured.
- To ensure the quality of treatment, assign the responsibility for monitoring to a specific healthcare professional associated with the specialized team in hospital.
- Prospective studies on the impact of different monitoring regimens on outcome, including the quality of life of HPN patients, are warranted.

Introduction

When patients are sent home with parenteral nutrition (HPN), a plan for monitoring the effect of the treatment must be established. The purpose of monitoring is to ensure that treatment goals are achieved and that patients obtain the best possible quality of life (QoL). Although well trained, patients must be able to recognize and cope with complications, including infections and mechanical problems with the catheter, venous thrombosis as well as metabolic disturbances. Supplying

*E-mail: staun@rh.dk

parenteral nutrition is technically demanding, involves considerable costs and may in some cases cause serious complications. A successful clinical outcome requires clinical supervision at regular intervals and careful attendance of the patients. Monitoring serves a number of purposes and this includes evaluating the patient's well-being, nutritional and more technical issues, as well as QoL.

Guidelines for Monitoring

The guidelines on HPN published recently by the European Society of Parenteral and Enteral Nutrition (ESPEN) (Staun *et al.*, 2009) outline monitoring schedules, recommending measurement of biochemistry and anthropometry at 3-month intervals and suggesting measurement of trace elements and vitamins every 6 months and bone density measurements at annual intervals. The American Society for Parenteral and Enteral Nutrition (A.S.P.E.N.) recommends slightly different monitoring intervals for certain parameters such as trace elements and liver function tests (Klein, 1997; Payne-James, 1997; A.S.P.E.N. Board of Directors, 1999). In the A.S.P.E.N. document a need for an annual assessment of QoL is stated, but this is not included in the ESPEN guidelines.

Monitoring should ideally be carried out by a nutrition team taking into consideration the clinical situation of the patient, his or her individual wishes and the resources of the attending institution. No quality assurance studies on the monitoring process of HPN patients are available, so the current monitoring practice of HPN patients is based mainly on experience. The organization usually involves the multidisciplinary nutrition team and management is in some cases underpinned by local guidelines provided by the national society of clinical nutrition (Van Gossum *et al.*, 1999).

Parameters Monitored at Visits

When evaluating how patients manage at home and which parameters to monitor, there are no comparative studies telling the significance in relation to outcome or QoL. However, we know from a European survey conducted in 2002 (Wengler *et al.*, 2006) how the monitoring of HPN patients is performed. Also, a study from 2010 (Hallum *et al.*, 2010) outlines the monitoring practice for HPN in Scotland.

In the European study, 42 HPN centres were asked questions on: (i) the use of written guidelines; (ii) the structure of the department, including the presence of an HPN team responsible for monitoring this specific group of patients after discharge from the hospital; (iii) home visits; (iv) where monitoring took place; (v) the personnel involved; (vi) to whom the responsibility for the monitoring process was assigned; (vii) intervals between monitoring visits; (viii) the clinical parameters evaluated at monitoring visits; and (ix) how handling of complications and monitoring were managed. The HPN experience of the centres was in the range 2–30 years and ranged in size from 0 to 125 HPN patients, representing a total number of 934 of whom 54% had received HPN for more than 2 years. The primary disease was non-malignant in 90% while 10% had been diagnosed with active cancer.

Based on the results of this questionnaire-based study, the following scheme (Table 31.1) for monitoring practice can be outlined. This would provide information of the clinical status and response to the nutrition therapy. The intervals between visits and activities carried out must, of course, be individualized since the need of the patient will vary significantly. In particular, shortly after discharge patients may need more advice and attention from those responsible for the treatment.

In the first month after starting HPN, the patient will need special attention and review of his/her psychosocial status. The patient may develop depression after being in hospital for a long time and then being at home coping with this new situation with relatives, everyday life activities and, for some patients, a job. Assessment of QoL of the HPN patient can be measured routinely by using the SF-36® or equivalent to evaluate the impact of the infusion therapy on daily activities. A valuable tool could be specific questionnaires designed for this patient population in order to study QoL with HPN, but no such studies have been reported.

Body weight should be monitored once per week. The patients can do it themselves at home and if body weight does not increase as expected, the team should consider other causes like metabolic disturbances, sepsis or the impact of an underlying disease. If by contrast the weight increases very quickly, the team must consider if the patient is over-hydrated and appropriate measures should be taken. In the case of severe metabolic disturbance, patients must be admitted and some centres will routinely assess the HPN treatment during short admissions or by monitoring electrolyte and water balance in a home care setting. For patients with significant malabsorption or short bowel syndrome, measurement of intestinal function may guide the clinician with regard to the needs of parenteral supply (Jeppesen and Mortensen, 2002). The impact of such measures for HPN patients on outcome and QoL has not been reported.

The European study (Wengler *et al.*, 2006) showed that all HPN centres measured body weight or anthropometry at every visit and 48% of centres assessed blood pressure and pulse at every visit. Nearly all centres in the study evaluated the state of hydration and 74% of the centres asked patients about oral intake. The mood of the HPN patient was considered in 86% of the centres at every monitoring visit. So these appear to be key parameters that the majority agrees should be evaluated as a routine. Questionnaires specifically addressing this population of patients have been developed (see Chapter 34 in this volume).

The following biochemical parameters should be evaluated at every monitoring visit: haematology, biochemical tests for liver function, serum creatinine and electrolytes, serum calcium, serum magnesium and serum phosphate. Intervals between measurements depend on the clinical situation, but for the stable patient 2–3 months usually are sufficient. This is also reflected in the European study (Wengler *et al.*, 2006) since all centres reported that these biochemical parameters were monitored at each visit. Biochemical abnormalities are not uncommon in this patient population; a broad range of changes have been reported regarding haematology and electrolytes as well as trace element deficiencies (Burnes *et al.*, 1992).

Table 31.1. Scheme for monitoring practice of long-term HPN (serum, plasma or whole-blood concentration unless mentioned otherwise; U, 24 h urine or urine concentration).

	Before starting	Monthly (up to first 6 months)	Quarterly or at 4-month intervals	Annually
Body weight	X	X	X	
Body temperature	X	X	X	
Blood pressure	X	X	X	
Heart rate	X	X	X	
Hydration status	X	X	X	
Fluid balance	X	X	X	
Oral intake	X	X	X	
Mood	X		X	
QoL	X		X	
CVC examination	X		X	
Haemogram	X	X	X	
Ferritin	X	X	X	
Iron	X	X	X	
Total protein	X	X	X	
Albumin	X	X	X	
Pre-albumin	X	X	X	
Glucose	X	X	X	
Triglycerides	X	X	X	
Cholesterol	X	X	X	
Electrolytes (Na, Cl, K, Mg, Ca, P)	X	X	X	
Electrolytes – U (Na, Cl, K, Mg, Ca, P)	X	X	X	
Bicarbonate	X	X	X	
Creatinine	X	X	X	
Urea	X	X	X	
Urinalysis	X	X	X	
Bilirubin total and direct	X	X	X	
AST/ALT	X	X	X	
Alkaline phosphatase	X	X	X	
γ-Glutamyl transferase	X	X	X	
Prothrombin time (INR)	X	X	X	
Lipase	X	X	X	
Abdominal ultrasound	X			X
Parathyroid hormone	X			X
Osteocalcin	X			X
Collagen cross-laps	X			X
BMD (DEXA)	X			X
25-Hydroxyvitamin D	X			X
Vitamin A	X			X
Vitamin E	X			X
Vitamin B12	X			X
Folate	X			X
Vitamin C	X			X
Zinc	X			X
Copper	X			X
Manganese	X			X
Selenium	X			X

CVC, central venous catheter; AST, aspartate aminotransferase; ALT, alanine aminotransferase; INR, international normalized ratio.

In general, elevated levels of serum triglycerides are not a problem if manufacturer's guidelines regarding dosing of parenteral lipid are taken into consideration. Many centres will routinely measure levels of triglycerides and in the European study about 50% of centres performed such measurements. In that study, 14% of centres measured the levels of vitamins A, E, D, B_{12} and folic acid, but not at every visit, rather in the case of problems (Wengler *et al.*, 2006).

Considering that secondary osteoporosis is frequently observed (Pironi *et al.*, 2002; Haderslev *et al.*, 2004), measurement of bone mineral density (BMD) using dual-energy X-ray absorptiometry (DEXA) scans is recommended at annual intervals for the majority of patients, while a small group presenting with very low BMD entering treatment protocols may require DEXA scans at 6-month intervals. Regarding monitoring practice, 64% of European centres measured BMD in all patients once or twice per annum, the rest less often (Wengler *et al.*, 2006).

The patient/caregiver must be able to: (i) recognize vascular access device complications and carry out routines (Figs 31.1 and 31.2); (ii) recognize signs and symptoms of fluid imbalance; (iii) perform testing of the urine for glucose; and (iv) recognize signs and symptoms of hyperglycaemia or hypoglycaemia (A.S.P.E.N. Board of Directors, 1999).

Patients sent home with HPN due to an active malignant disease might have problems (pain relief, psychosocial problems) (see Chapter 13 of this volume) that differ significantly from those generally seen in benign disorders. Thus when monitoring, it is important that the nutrition support team works closely together with the palliative unit or the oncologists, in order to solve specific issues.

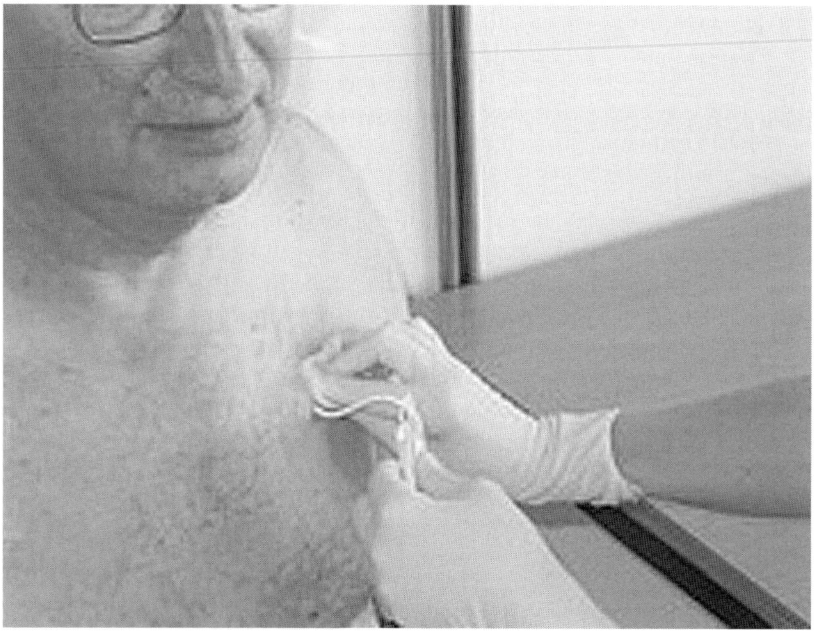

Fig. 31.1. Some patients use a transparent dressing to cover the exit site.

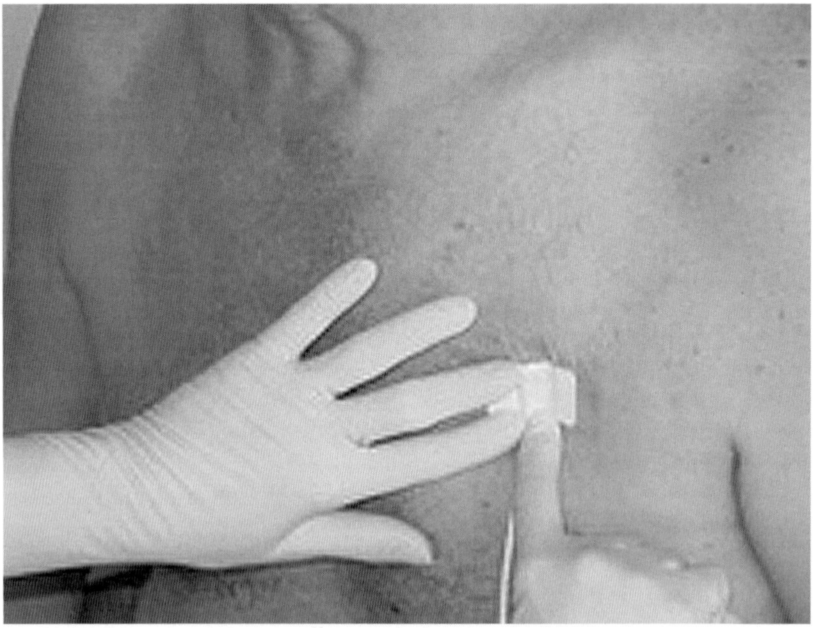

Fig. 31.2. The dressing is changed in the HPN outpatient clinic or in the home of the patient.

The study by Hallum *et al.* (2010) was not able to show any difference in complication rate between patients reviewed as recommended and those monitored less often. Overall, their study revealed that less than one-third of patients met recommended monitoring intervals.

Location and Personnel Involved in Monitoring the HPN Patient

The monitoring usually takes place at the discharging hospital with access to the specialized team. The members of the team could be a physician, nutrition nurse, dietician, pharmacist, psychologist and a social worker. The main responsibility for monitoring the patient should be assigned to one specific person (contact person), for example the physician or the nutrition nurse.

Monitoring can also be carried out by a home care agency involving the hospital or the general practitioner. It is important to keep close contact with the patient when starting treatment until the patient/caregiver is confident with the situation. The patient should have at least one nursing visit at home to assess and monitor the initiation of parenteral nutrition in the home. In Europe, stable patients on HPN were monitored at the discharging hospital (73%), at a local hospital (12%), by the general practitioner (11%) or by a home care agency (4%) (Wengler *et al.*, 2006).

Almost all European centres (90%) reported that the main responsibility for monitoring the patient was assigned to one specific person (Wengler *et al.*, 2006) and this is in line with the framework of the guidelines presented by the A.S.P.E.N.

Board of Directors (1999). Home visits after discharge for monitoring purposes were carried out by 31 of the centres involving a specialized HPN team, general practitioner, and community nurse or home care agency.

Intervals between Monitoring Visits

The interval between monitoring visits varies according to the needs of the patient. When starting HPN treatment, visits should be two weeks after discharge, very much depending on how stable the patient's condition is. When the parenteral nutrition is stable and the patient is confident with the treatment, intervals between monitoring visits are 1–3 months. The unstable patient needs more attention.

In the case of problems/complications, the patient will get in touch with the HPN team, outpatient clinic, local hospital, community nurse, general practitioner or home care agency.

Intervals between monitoring visits for the stable HPN patient in Europe were in the range 1–6 months and 52% of responders evaluated the patient at intervals of 2–3 months (Wengler *et al.*, 2006).

It should be checked regularly if parenteral therapy is still required, if the patient can be weaned off or if nutritional support by the enteral route can be increased.

Summary

Monitoring of patients on HPN is essential for evaluation of treatment effect and management of the complications associated with this treatment. Monitoring is most often carried out at the discharging hospital with access to the specialized nutrition team. Monitoring can also be performed by a home care agency involving the hospital or the general practitioner. Intervals between visits vary, being on average 3 months. The unstable patient may need more attention.

Assignment of responsibility for monitoring is probably very important for the quality of the process. A previous questionnaire-based study indicated that in general responsibility is assigned to a specific person most often associated with the specialized team in hospital.

Biochemistry and anthropometry should be measured at all visits; trace elements, vitamins and bone mineral density only occasionally, annual intervals are recommended.

Official guidelines for monitoring are not available and prospective studies on the impact of different monitoring regimens on outcome, including the QoL of HPN patients, are warranted.

References

A.S.P.E.N. Board of Directors (1999) Standards for home nutrition support. *Nutrition in Clinical Practice* 14, 151–162.

Burnes, J.U., O'Keefe, S.J., Fleming, C.R., Devine, R.M., Berkner, S. and Herrick, L. (1992) Home parenteral nutrition. A 3-year analysis of clinical and laboratory monitoring. *JPEN Journal of Parenteral and Enteral Nutrition* 16, 327–332.

Haderslev, K.V., Tjellesen, L., Haderslev, P.H. and Staun, M. (2004) Assessment of the longitudinal changes in bone mineral density in patients receiving home parenteral nutrition. *JPEN Journal of Parenteral and Enteral Nutrition* 28, 289–294.

Hallum, N.S., Baxter, J.P., O'Reilly, D. and Mckee, R.F. (2010) Home parenteral nutrition in Scotland: frequency of monitoring, adequacy of review and consequences for complication rate. *Clinical Nutrition* 26, 1139–1145

Jeppesen, P.B. and Mortensen, P.B. (2002) Intestinal failure defined by measurements of intestinal energy and wet weight absorption. *Gut* 46, 701–706.

Klein, S. (1997) Nutrition support in clinical practice: review of published data and recommendations for future research directions. *JPEN Journal of Parenteral and Enteral Nutrition* 21, 133–156.

Payne-James, J. (1997) Cost-effectiveness of nutrition support teams. Are they necessary? *Nutrition* 13, 928–930.

Pironi, L., Labate, A.M., Pertkiewicz, M., Przedlacki, J., Tjellesen, L., Staun, M., De Francesco, A., Gallenca, P., Guglielmi, F.W., Van Gossum, A., Orlandoni, P., Contaldo, F., Villares, J.M. and ESPEN-Home Artificial Nutrition Working Group (2002) Prevalence of bone disease in patients on home parenteral nutrition. *Clinical Nutrition* 21, 289–296.

Staun, M., Pironi, L., Bozzetti, F., Baxter, J., Forbes, A., Joly, F., Jeppesen, P., Moreno, J., Hébuterne, X., Pertkiewicz, M., Mühlebach, S., Shenkin, A. and Van Gossum, A. (2009) ESPEN guidelines on parenteral nutrition: home parenteral nutrition (HPN) in adult patients. *Clinical Nutrition* 28, 467–479.

Van Gossum, A., Bakker, H., Bozzetti, F., Staun, M., Leon-Sanz, M., Hebuterne, X., Pertkiewicz, M., Shaffer, J. and Thul, P. (1999) Home parenteral nutrition in adults: a European multicentre survey in 1997. ESPEN-Home Artificial Nutrition Working Group. *Clinical Nutrition* 18, 135–140.

Wengler, A., Micklewright, A., Hebuterne, X., Bozzetti, F., Pertkiewicz, M., Moreno, J., Pironi, L., Thul, P., Van Gossum, A., Staun, M. and the ESPEN HAN Working Group (2006) Monitoring of patients on home parenteral nutrition (HPN) in Europe. A questionnaire based study on monitoring practice in 42 centres. *Clinical Nutrition* 25, 693–700.

32 Dietary Care in Home Parenteral Nutrition and Intestinal Failure

Cora F. Jonkers-Schuitema*

Home TPN and Intestinal Failure Team, Academic Medical Center, Amsterdam, The Netherlands

Key Points

The main clinical responsibilities of a dietician working within a multidisciplinary team in the field of home parenteral nutrition (HPN) are:

- assessment and monitoring of nutritional status;
- assessment and monitoring of enteral intake;
- designing appropriate parenteral nutrition regimens;
- monitoring HPN regimens and ensuring that nutritional deficiencies do not occur;
- providing advice and evidence-based nutrition education material for patients/carers;
- participating in audit and research as part of the clinical governance strategy; and
- being a point of contact for patients, providing some psychological support.

Introduction

Since the mid-1980s dietetics has developed significantly in the field of medical nutrition support. There has been a transition from physically preparing diets and modular tube feeds to an evidence-based, educational role. Dietetic practice is nowadays 'the singular ability to translate complex clinical nutritional concepts into simple everyday language coupled with acceptable strategies for implementing nutritional change' (Howard *et al.*, 1999). A home total parenteral nutrition (TPN) support team should include a dietician due to these translation techniques/

*E-mail: c.f.jonkers@amc.uva.nl

challenges; an effective communication with clinicians, nurses, pharmacists, patients and carers is imperative. When providing home TPN, a trained dietician can act as case manager for these patients by working together with the multidisciplinary team.

The main responsibilities of a dietician working within the multidisciplinary team in the field of HPN are: (i) assessing nutritional status; (ii) assessing, advising on and evaluating dietary intake; (iii) designing and monitoring appropriate TPN regimens; (iv) evaluating the transition from TPN to oral and/or enteral nutrition; (v) advising on and providing evidence-based nutritional education material for patients and caretakers; (vi) participating in research; and (vii) being a point of contact for the patient, providing (psychological) support.

Assessment of Nutritional Status

Assessment of nutritional status should include anthropometric and biochemical indices, and take into account intestinal absorption and total intake from the enteral and parenteral route. The goal of parenteral nutrition is to replenish and maintain nutritional and functional status, therefore optimizing body image and ultimately quality of life. The ease of this will depend on the clinical condition of the patient. In palliative care, HPN should provide the best balance between quality and length of life.

Anthropometric assessment

Body weight is the most widely recognized objective tool used in nutritional assessment, as it is simple to measure and equipment is readily available. Caution is required in patients with precarious fluid balance like in high-output stomas, fistulas, kidney failure, oedema and/or severely malnourished patients undergoing initial re-feeding, as rapid fluctuations in weight are likely to reflect changes in hydration, rather than lean body mass.

Weight can be compared with the height of the patient by calculating body mass index (BMI; BMI = weight/height^2), where a BMI between 18.5 and 25 kg/m^2 in adults is considered desirable. A BMI of <18.5 kg/m^2 (for patients over 65 years of age, <20 kg/m^2) is used to define undernutrition (Roche, 1981).

In paediatric patients malnutrition is defined by growth charts. If the weight-for-height is two standard deviations or more below the mean of the reference population (<–2 SD), the child is classified as malnourished. Also children who drop –1 SD in weight-for-height are malnourished (World Health Organization, 2006, 2007).

It is generally accepted that unintentional loss of body weight in adults over 5% in one month or 10% in the preceding 6 months is considered significant, in terms of clinical outcome (Dewys *et al.*, 1980), and that 20% recent weight loss is evidence of protein–energy malnutrition (Kinney, 1988). Patients attending HPN clinics should routinely have weight and BMI measured at every visit and the outcome should be used to evaluate the TPN prescription.

Weight, BMI and recent weight loss give limited information on body composition. Patients with normal weight or obesity can be defined as malnourished if their lean tissue mass is low compared with their fat mass. Especially older persons with a low activity pattern should be evaluated for this sarcopenic obesity (Zamboni *et al.*, 2008).

Body composition status determining fat reserves and fat-free mass can be estimated from bedside techniques such as triceps skinfold thickness (measured using skinfold callipers) and mid-arm muscle circumference (MAMC) (Blackburn *et al.*, 1977). Initial measurements of upper-arm anthropometry can be compared with standardized tables (Jelliffe, 1966; Frisancho, 1981), but consideration must be given to the demographics of the original populations recruited, the sample size and whether these reference tables apply to a HPN population of today. It is vital that the same, experienced individual performs all the measurements as these are limited by intra/inter-observer variability (Hall *et al.*, 1980).

Other techniques such as bioelectrical impedance analysis or spectrometry (BIA or BIS) could be used to evaluate the individual patient, but the outcome is not validated in routine clinical practice in patients with extremely low BMI ($<16\,kg/m^2$) and/or deranged fluid balance (Earthman *et al.*, 2007).

To evaluate nutritional status, handgrip strength can be used as a single parameter to evaluate the outcome of nutrition over time. Patients should be encouraged in the home situation to exercise in order to have the best outcome of the (infused) nutrients (Norman *et al.*, 2010).

Biochemical assessment

Biochemical data evaluating the effect of the parenteral formula should be performed according to the clinical presentation of the patient. Stable outpatients should be routinely checked every 3 months, in unstable situations this could be intensified to daily or weekly until the patient is stable again. Table 32.1 shows biochemical parameters and monitoring advice. The dietician should be able to interpret the outcome of the biochemical data and know the dietary interventions related to the prescribed TPN, oral and/or enteral formula in the case of findings outside the normal range.

Failure to improve nutritional status may be due to sepsis or acute disease state, rather than the inadequate provision of nutrition. Markers of the inflammatory response, such as C-reactive protein, albumin, white blood cell count and platelets, are useful in indicating sepsis or acute disease.

Albumin level is considered to reflect disease severity rather than nutritional status, as levels of inflammatory markers can fall following surgery and can be normal in cases of severe malnutrition, such as anorexia nervosa. Albumin is an important marker to evaluate calcium levels of the patient. Calcium is bound to albumin and a low albumin status will derange the outcome of calcium. In case of a low albumin status it is preferred to measure ionized calcium or use the formula:

Table 32.1. Biochemical parameters: monitoring advice.

Parameter	Evaluation in clinical setting	Evaluation in outpatient setting
Electrolytes Sodium Potassium Magnesium Phosphate Calcium (albumin)	Daily to weekly	Stable patients: every 3 months Unstable patients: weekly
Kidney function Urea Creatinine	Twice weekly	Stable patients: every 3 months Unstable patients: weekly
Liver function Total bilirubin Aspartate transaminase (ASAT) Alanine transaminase (ALAT) γ-Glutamyltransferase (γ-GT) Alkaline phosphatase	Twice weekly	Stable patients: every 3 months Unstable patients: weekly
25-Hydroxyvitamin D, parathyroid hormone	Once at start of TPN, every 3 months	Every 3 months
Vitamin B_{12}, folate, thiamine, vitamin A	Once at start of TPN, every 3 months	Once at start of TPN, every 3 months
Iron status (haemoglobin, iron saturation, iron, ferritin)	Weekly	Once at start of TPN, every 3 months

$$\text{Corrected calcium} = [0.02 \times (\text{standard albumin} - \text{serum albumin})] + \text{serum } Ca^{2+}.$$

HPN is associated with hepatobiliary complications, from mild elevation of liver function tests to hepatic steatosis and intrahepatic cholestasis. Hepatobiliary complications are found less frequently when patients receive oral feeding because utilization of the gastrointestinal tract stimulates biliary secretion (Guglielmi *et al.*, 2001). An inverse relationship between raised alkaline phosphatase and remaining length of small bowel, especially in patients with <100 cm of small bowel, is reported (Lumen and Shaffer, 2002). The dietician should advise the best oral intake, unless it is contraindicated, e.g. in cases of bowel perforation with intra-abdominal collections or high-output fistulas. For more on HPN-related liver complications, see Chapter 16 in this volume.

Besides the oral and/or enteral intake, the dietary advice could also focus upon the content of the TPN. Hypercaloric TPN (>40 kcal/kg body weight/day) as well as the use of lipid emulsions could cause cholestasis. Normocaloric TPN and restriction of the lipids in the formula up to 1 g/kg body weight/day could prevent the patient developing severe hepatic complications due to TPN. In infants lipid emulsions can be used to a maximum of 3 g/kg body weight/day; the caloric intake depends on age and growth.

The use of *n*-3 fatty acid (fish oil) emulsions is increasing and could influence the hepatic disturbance. These lipid emulsions should not fully replace the usual lipid emulsion when the hepatic complications are cured. The use of single fish oil emulsions should only be pharmaceutical, not continuous (Cober *et al.*, 2012).

Assessment and Monitoring of Enteral Intake

The contribution of oral intake to meeting total nutritional requirements should be assessed, considering both intake and nutrient losses such as malabsorption. Determination of habitual dietary intake is fraught with difficulty and requires a detailed dietary assessment. Oral nutritional intake can be estimated from a food diary of actual intake, or from a dietary history based on recall. The dietary assessment should consider food items, dietary supplements, frequency of consumption, day-to-day variability, cooking methods and portion sizes.

Dietary intake is associated with many cultural, behavioural, social and psychological factors, as well as being a means of providing the body with macro- and micronutrients. Patients may have experienced many different forms of oral/enteral tube feeding with limited success and this can have an impact on whether the enteral and/or oral route should be used again.

The use of intravenous nutrients could influence the intake of oral and/or enteral nutrition. This can be a reason for a diminished oral intake. Using cyclic TPN (e.g. during the night) could stimulate the oral intake if necessary (Stratton and Elia, 1999).

Estimation of Nutrient Intake

The absorption of enterally provided nutrition is influenced by the length of the remaining small bowel, functional capacity, intestinal adaptation, the capacity of digestive organs like bile, the pancreas and liver, pharmacological therapy and the composition of the dietary intake (DiBaise *et al.*, 2006; Thompson *et al.*, 2012; Matarese, 2013).

Balance studies are used to assess intestinal absorption, where all oral input is controlled (food, fluid and medication) and output is measured over a defined time period. Balance studies can be performed in fresh stools to evaluate the absorption of fat (fat malabsorption test) or of all nutrients (like in bomb calorimetry) (Wierdsma *et al.*, 2011).

These techniques are often impractical to perform on all patients in the clinical setting and as no routine bedside technique is available, the degree of malabsorption is often estimated. Percentage absorption of the total energy intake ingested may vary between 20 and 80% but when interpreting the research studies, consideration must be given to the diversity of the population (in terms of anatomy and time since last surgical resection). The easiest way to evaluate the impact of the oral and/or enteral nutrition is to follow the weight of the patient. If weight is gaining fast following the intravenous provision of nutrients, the absorption of food is good. Tapering of the TPN in volume or frequency is required if the target weight is reached (Matarese, 2013).

Short Bowel With or Without Colon in Continuity and the Use of Nutrients

The colon can partially adapt the function of the small bowel (jejunum, ileum). If the colon is *in situ*, adaptation can be progressive up to 3 years (Messing *et al.*, 1999). If adaptation is completed the total absorption will mostly remain less than 100%. Patients should be hyperphagial and be advised to consume hypercaloric food, 4–6 meals daily.

The use of macronutrients and fluids should be advised according to the remaining function of the bowel (Matarese, 2013); whether there is an intact ileocoecal valve, colon or just the stoma bag at the end of the small bowel. Table 32.2 lists the main differences in oral nutrient intake depending on the presence of colon in continuity. Based on theory, a low-fat, high-carbohydrate diet could be used for patients with a preserved colon. In practice, this is difficult since such a diet is not palatable being with a higher volume and this may reduce the total energy intake. For patients with a colon in function, malabsorbed carbohydrates lead to increased production of gases. Usually the patients themselves find a balance in order to maximize the intake and absorption. Intensive dietary care can help patients find the best diet to balance between good nutritional intake, manageable output and good quality of life (see Table 32.3).

Table 32.2. Diet for short bowel syndrome. (From Prado *et al.*, 2012.)

	Colon in continuity	No colon in continuity
Fluids	ORS and hypotonic	Isotonic, ORS
Carbohydrate	50–60% of energy intake from complex carbohydrates Limit simple sugars	40–50% of energy intake complex carbohydrates Limit simple sugars
Fat	Low fat (20–30% of energy intake) Adequate intake of essential fatty acids In weight loss, MCTs	30–40% of energy intake Adequate intake of essential fatty acids
Protein	1.2–1.5 g/kg body weight/day High biological value	1.2–1.5 g/kg body weight/day High biological value
Fibre	Added soluble 5–10 g	Added soluble 5–10 g Normal to low
Oxalate	Restricted	Not restricted

ORS, oral rehydration solution; MCT, medium-chain triglycerides.

Table 32.3. Nutritional goals in paediatric patients. (From Koletzko *et al.*, 2006.)

Age	Energy (kcal/kg body weight/day)	Protein (g/kg body weight/day)
Preterm	110–120	1.5–4
0–1 years	90–100	1.5–3
1–7 years	75–90	1.5–2.5
7–12 years	60–75	1.5–2.5
12–18 years	30–60	1.5

Fluids

Isotonic fluids are the easiest to absorb in the bowel, with or without a colon. Plain water should be avoided in large quantities (maximum of 1–2 glasses of 150 ml/day) and the best choices are bouillon, lemonade with added salt, tea with a dash of sugar, iso-osmotic sports drinks (with added salt 1 g/l), vegetable juices with added salt and oral rehydration solutions (ORS). Sports drinks have low salt content and can be used if salt is added up to 90 mmol/l (1 g/l); this will optimize water and sodium absorption in the proximal jejunum and prevent secretion into the lumen.

The volume should be limited in a high-output stoma (>1500 ml/24 h), each litre input will have an extra litre output. Pharmaceutical influence like diphenoxylate-atropine, loperamide, codeine and opium to limit the output can be useful, but will have to be evaluated in the individual patient. Because of the gastrocolic response, antidiarrhoeals are most effective when administered 30–60 min before a meal (Matarese, 2013).

Studies comparing dietary supplements have also shown no beneficial effects of elemental diets in absorptive capacity (McIntyre *et al.*, 1986). Non-polymeric feeds have the disadvantage of being both hyperosmolar and containing a minimal amount of sodium, which will exacerbate stoma water and sodium losses (Newton *et al.*, 1985). If enteral nutrition should be provided, the use of polymeric iso-osmotic formulas is advised with additional sodium (total 6 g sodium/litre formula) (Thompson *et al.*, 2012).

Carbohydrates

Simple sugars like fructose and sucrose will increase the osmotic load and will ferment in the small bowel causing osmotic diarrhoea. Especially fruit juices are high in osmolarity and fermenting fructose should be limited.

Lactose can be used in normal quantities (maximum 400 ml of milk divided over the day) as lactose is digested in the proximal jejunum which is still present in most short bowel patients. The use of lactose-free milk, soy milk or sour milk products like yoghurt and buttermilk is to be advised if normal milk causes diarrhoea.

It is preferred to use complex carbohydrates (e.g. bread, pasta, potatoes and rice). If the colon is present, limited fat intake (20–30% of energy intake) should be replaced by carbohydrates (50–60% of energy intake).

Insoluble fibres can absorb fluids and decrease transit time. These fibres can be used in normal food like bread or as a supplement (Metamucil®). Soluble fibres (from fruits and vegetables) can increase diarrhoea due to the production of gas by intestinal bacteria. Patients should avoid the use of large amounts of fruits (also because of the fructose; limited to 1–2 pieces/day, no fruit juices) and uncooked vegetables. Specific vegetables that are not chewed well (maize, carrots, peas) can be identified in the stools and this can raise questions from the patient. This can be explained by referring to the time the patient had normal stools but also these vegetables were visible. Fermentation of carbohydrate to short-chain fatty acids in the colon may provide up to 1000 kcal/day (Nordgaard *et al.*, 1996).

Fat

Most long-chain triacylglycerols (LCTs) are absorbed in the distal ileum. Most patients with short bowel lack this part of the bowel. The colon can adapt and absorb LCTs but this can take a while. In patients with a colon *in situ*, a fat-restricted diet is advised (20–30% of energy intake). As these patients should eat a hypercaloric diet to maintain their nutritional status, this can cause conflicts. To ensure the intake of sufficient calories the use of medium-chain triacylglycerols (MCTs) could cover the lacking caloric load. MCTs should be introduced slowly as margarine on bread or in the main cooked meals. They can also be used as a supplemented MCT emulsion drink (2–3 times/day, 30 ml, 50% MCT/50% water). The toleration could differ in each patient. In patients with a high-output stoma there is no need for fat restriction in the diet. The use of a normal intake of fat will not stimulate the output, so as fat intake increases there is an increased amount of fat in the stoma effluent. This does not seem to be harmful, although increased fat excretion may reduce the absorption of calcium and magnesium (Hessov *et al.*, 1982; Woolf *et al.*, 1983). High-fat diets have the benefit of increasing energy intake and palatability.

Micronutrients

If the colon is still in continuity unabsorbed fatty acids and bile salts reduce water and sodium absorption (Ammon and Philips, 1973), bind calcium and magnesium and contribute to the formation of calcium oxalate renal stones (Nightingale *et al.*, 1992b). Patients with short bowel with colon in continuity should be recommended a low-oxalate diet (avoidance of beetroot, rhubarb and spinach) (Tomson, 2001).

Vitamins

The intake of vitamins should be monitored, with special care for vitamins that are normally absorbed in the terminal ileum. If the patient is using TPN with added vitamins still routinely, these should be evaluated. Especially the fat-soluble vitamins A, D, E and K and vitamin B_{12} (cobalamin) could cause deficiencies.

Vitamin B_{12} can be supplemented by intramuscular bolus every 1–2 months. Vitamins A and D could be supplemented by high oral doses (vitamin A 1500 µg/day (5000 IU/day), vitamin D 1250 µg/week (50,000 IU/week)). Not all vitamin supplements contain vitamin K. This could be supplemented intravenously or orally on monitoring the international normalized ratio (INR).

In order to ensure that the micronutrient status of the patient who is weaned from TPN will be sufficient, all patients should be prescribed an oral multivitamin/mineral supplement.

Electrolytes and trace elements

Electrolytes (sodium, potassium, magnesium, calcium and phosphorus) and trace elements (zinc, chromium, copper, selenium and iron) should be routinely evaluated. In the case of low serum levels supplementation should be intravenously if possible. If the intravenous route is terminated, these electrolytes and trace elements will have to be supplemented by the oral/enteral route. This is not easy in normal foods and pharmacological supplementation is advised. All patients should be advised to use sufficient sodium.

Examples of oral supplementation are as follows.

- Calcium and vitamin D: tablets or drink.
- Magnesium: tablets or suspension. Magnesium causes diarrhoea.
- Potassium: tablets or drink (1 mmol/ml).
- Phosphate: drink or tablets.
- Sodium bicarbonate: tablets or intravenous solution (8.4% as a drink).
- Chromium, selenium, zinc: tablets or drink.
- Iron: tablets or drink. An intravenous bolus is recommended for low serum levels.

Most of these products will not be reimbursed in most countries. Drugstores will have cheap products of good content.

Hydration status

Patients with short bowel syndrome frequently have excessive losses of fluid and electrolytes from jejunostomy and/or fistula. While additional fluid and electrolytes can be provided via the parenteral nutrition, advice on the management of hydration status, including oral fluid intake, is important. Patients should be educated to recognize the symptoms of dehydration (postural hypotension, dizziness, thirst and reduced urine output) and given practical day-to-day management guidance. This should include recommendations on increasing the intravenous fluid administration or use of fluid restriction (500–1000 ml/day), administration of an oral glucose/electrolyte (ORS) solution (with a sodium content >90 mmol/l; Nightingale *et al.*, 1992a), medication to reduce stoma losses and additional intravenous saline, as required.

In contrast to patients with a colon in continuity, requirements for fluid, electrolytes and nutrients is not likely to change over time in those with a jejunostomy (Hill *et al.*, 1974; Nightingale *et al.*, 1990).

Intestinal Failure without a Short Bowel

Patients suffering from pseudo-obstruction, motility disorders or scleroderma are another group of HPN users. These patients may have significantly reduced oral intakes and can suffer from malabsorption. Support should be given to optimize oral nutrition and a modified dietary consistency/composition may be required. If no intravenous nutritional support is given, oral supplements of vitamins, minerals and trace elements are advised.

Paediatric HPN Patients

The use of TPN in paediatric patients is more complicated than the use in adults. Where in adults the goal is an optimal nutritional status, the goal in paediatric patients is optimal growth and an optimal nutritional status.

Evaluation of the outcome of TPN should be recorded in growth charts next to the evaluation of anthropometric and biochemical criteria. Growth means the provision of adequate amounts of protein (amino acids) and energy; evaluation of micronutrients and electrolytes should also be according to weight and age. As there are no specific ready-to-use TPN formulas for paediatric patients, a specialized (hospital) pharmacy is a requirement to provide good care. There is a large group of paediatric patients with acute intestinal failure suffered from birth (neonatal necrotizing enterocolitis, gastroschisis), who are independent on TPN from the first months until years after birth. Rehabilitation of the bowel by slowly increasing the intake of enteral nutrition can also be provided at home nowadays.

Most paediatric patients in need of long-term or chronic home TPN have a motility dysfunction, in contrast with adults where most patients suffer from short bowel. Weaning of TPN is an intensive process, starting with use of (hypoallergenic) infant formula 2–10 ml/h and trying to increase the enteral intake in order to stop the intravenous need for nutrients. If the enteral nutrition is well tolerated, the introduction of oral food can start. Most of these patients do not know how or what to eat and need special eating therapy to be able to have a good enteral intake.

Role of the Dietician in HPN and Intestinal Failure

To conclude, a dietician has a central role to play in the assessment and prospective monitoring of patients receiving HPN. This heterogeneous population requires individualized treatment based on remnants of the gastrointestinal anatomy. The main goal is to prevent complications related to the formula or the delivery route. The final goal should always be to decrease the parenteral nutrition to the greatest extent possible. Appropriate oral and/or entral nutrition could help in this process. Enteral nutrition has a trophic effect on the gut mucosa and can prevent hepatobiliary complications, while positively influencing the quality of life of the patient. A clear understanding of the patient's anatomy is imperative to advise the patient on appropriate diet and fluid intake, while liaising with the multidisciplinary team to ensure the nutritional adequacy of the parenteral nutrition regimen.

Summary

The dietician should be part of the multidisciplinary team facilitating HPN (TPN) and can have the role of the case manager in these specific patients. Depending on the role in the home TPN team, the dietician can be in charge of informing the patient about the consequences of HPN and the transition to home can be started by ordering nursing care, defining and ordering the parenteral formula, pumps, utensils and supplements for home use. After discharge the dietician will have a role in the monitoring of the patient at home. This can be nutritional assessment (body composition, evaluation of nutritional status, output (stools, stoma) and blood results) and the transition of TPN to oral or enteral nutrition.

References

Ammon, H.V. and Philips, S.F. (1973) Inhibition of colonic water and electrolyte absorption by fatty acids in man. *Journal of Clinical Investigation* 65, 744–749.

Blackburn, G.L., Bristrian, B.R. and Maini, B.S. (1977) Nutritional and metabolic assessment of the hospitalised patient. *JPEN Journal of Parenteral and Enteral Nutrition* 1, 11–22.

Cober, M.P., Killu, G., Brattain, A., Welch, K.B., Kunisaki, S.M. and Teitelbaum, D.H. (2012) Intravenous fat emulsions reduction for patients with parenteral nutrition-associated liver disease. *Journal of Pediatrics* 160, 421–427.

Dewys, W.D., Begg, C., Lavin, P.T., Band, P.R., Bennett, J.M., Bertino, J.R., Cohen, M.H., Douglass, H.O., Engstrom, P.F., Ezdinli, E.Z., Horton, J., Johnson, G.J., Moertel, C.G., Oken, M.M., Perlia, C., Rosenbaum, C., Silverstein, M., Skeel, R.T., Sponzo, R. and Tormey, D.C. (1980) Prognostic effect of weight loss prior to chemotherapy in cancer patients. *American Journal of Medicine* 69, 491–497.

DiBaise, J.K., Matarese, L.E., Messing, B. and Steiger, E. (2006) Strategies for parenteral nutrition weaning in adult patients with short bowel syndrome. *Journal of Clinical Gastroenterology* 40, 94–98.

Earthman, C., Traughber, D., Dobratz, J. and Howell, W. (2007) Bioimpedance spectroscopy for clinical assessment of fluid distribution and body cell mass. *Nutrition in Clinical Practice* 22, 389–405.

Frisancho, A.R. (1981) New norms of upper limb fat and muscle areas for assessment of nutritional status. *American Journal of Clinical Nutrition* 34, 2540–2545.

Guglielmi, F.W., Moran Penco, J.M., Gentile, A., Capogna, D., Messanelli, R., Regano, N., Panella, C. and Francavilla, A. (2001) Hepatobiliary complications of long term parenteral nutrition. *Clinical Nutrition* 20, 51–56.

Hall, J.C., O'Quigley, J., Giles, G.R., Appleton, N. and Stocks, H. (1980) Upper limb anthropometry: the value of measurements variance studies. *American Journal of Clinical Nutrition* 33, 1846–1851.

Hessov, I., Andersson, H. and Isaksson, B. (1982) The use of low-fat diet on mineral absorption in small-bowel disease. *Scandinavian Journal of Gastroenterology* 18, 551–554.

Hill, G.L., Mair, W.S.J. and Goligher, J.C. (1974) Impairment of 'ileostomy adaptation' in patients after ileal resection. *Gut* 15, 982–987.

Howard, J.P., Jonkers-Schuitcann, C.F. and Kyle, V. (1999) The role of the nutritional support dietitian in Europe. *Clinical Nutrition* 18, 379–383.

Jelliffe, D.B. (1966) The assessment of the nutritional status of the community: with specific reference to field surveys in developing regions of the world. *World Health Organization Monograph Series* 53, 1–271.

Kinney, J.M. (1988) The influence of calorie and nitrogen balance on weight loss. *British Journal of Clinical Practice* 63, 114–120.

Koletzko, B., Goulet, O., Hunt, J., Krohn, K., Shamir, R.; Parenteral Nutrition Guidelines Working Group; European Society for Clinical Nutrition and Metabolism; European Society of Paediatric Gastroenterology, Hepatology and Nutrition (ESPGHAN); European Society of Paediatric Research (ESPR) (2006) ESPEN/ESPGHAN Guidelines on paediatric parenteral nutrition. *Clinical Nutrition* 25, 177–360.

Lumen, W. and Shaffer, J.L. (2002) Prevalence, outcome and associated factors of deranged liver function tests in patients on home parenteral nutrition. *Clinical Nutrition* 21, 337–343.
Matarese, L.E. (2013) Nutrition and fluid optimization for patients with short bowel syndrome. *JPEN Journal of Parenteral and Enteral Nutrition* 37, 161–170.
McIntyre, P.B., Fitchew, M. and Lennard-Jones, J.E. (1986) Patients with a high jejunostomy do not need a special diet. *Gastronenterology* 91, 25–33.
Messing, B., Crenn, P., Beau, P., Boutron-Ruault, M.C., Rambaud, J.C. and Matuchansky, C. (1999) Long-term survival and parenteral nutrition dependence in adult patients with the short bowel syndrome. *Gastroenterology* 117, 1043–1050.
Newton, C.R., Gonvers, J.J., McIntyrre, P.B., Preston, D.M. and Lennard-Jones, J.E. (1985) Effect of different drinks on fluid and electrolyte losses from a jejunostomy. *Journal of the Royal Society of Medicine* 78, 27–34.
Nightingale, J.M.D., Lennard-Jones, J.E., Walker, E.R. and Farthing, M.J.G. (1990) Jejunal efflux in short bowel syndrome. *The Lancet* 336, 765–768.
Nightingale, J.M.D., Lennard-Jones, J.E., Walker, E.R. and Farthing, M.J.G. (1992a) Oral salt supplements to compensate for jejunostomy losses: comparison of sodium chloride capsules, glucose electrolyte solution and glucose polymer electrolyte solution (Maxijul). *Gut* 33, 759–761.
Nightingale, J.M.D., Lennard-Jones, J.E., Gertner, D.J., Wood, S.R. and Bartum, C.I. (1992b) Colonic preservation reduces need for parenteral therapy, increases incidence of renal stones, but does not change high prevalence of gall stones in patients with a short bowel. *Gut* 33, 1493–1497.
Nordgaard, I., Hansen, B.S. and Mortensen, P.B. (1996) Importance of colonic support for energy absorption as short-bowel failure proceeds. *American Journal of Clinical Nutrition* 64, 222–231.
Norman, K., Stobaus, N., Gonzalez, M.C., Schulzke, J.D. and Pirlich, M. (2010) Hand grip strength: outcome predictor and marker of nutritional status. *Clinical Nutrition* 30, 135–142.
Prado, R.A., Márquez, H.A. and Moya, D.A. (eds) (2012) *Nutricion Enteral y Parenteral*, 2nd edn. McGraw-Hill, New York, pp. 484–496.
Roche, A.F. (1981) Grading body fatness from limited anthropometric data. *American Journal of Clinical Nutrition* 34, 2831–2838.
Stratton, R.J. and Elia, M. (1999) The effects of enteral tube feeding and parenteral nutrition on appetite sensations and food intake in health and disease. *Clinical Nutrition* 18, 63–70.
Thompson, J.S., Rochling, F.A., Weseman, R.A. and Mercer, D.F. (2012) Current management of short bowel syndrome. *Current Problems in Surgery* 49, 52–115.
Tomson, C.R.V. (2001) Nephrocalcinosis and nephrolithiasis. In: Nightingale, J.M.D. (ed.) *Intestinal Failure*. Greenwich Medical, London, pp. 52–115.
Wierdsma, N.J., Peters, J.H., Weijs, P.J., Keur, M.B., Girbes, A.R., van Bodegraven, A.A. and Beishuizen, A. (2011) Malabsorption and nutritional balance in the ICU: fecal weight as a biomarker: a prospective observational pilot study. *Critical Care* 15, R264.
Woolf, G.M., Miller, C., Kurian, R. and Jeejeebhoy, K.N. (1983) Diet for patients with a short bowel: high fat or high carbohydrate? *Gastroenterology* 84, 823–828.
World Health Organization (2006) *Growth Standards: Length/Height-for-Age, Weight-for-Age, Weight-for-Length, Weight-for-Height and Body Mass Index-for-Age. Methods and Development.* WHO, Geneva, Switzerland. Available at: http://www.who.int/childgrowth/standards (accessed 23 July 2014).
World Health Organization (2007) Growth Reference Data for Children from 5 to 19 Years. Available at: http://www.who.int/growthref/en (accessed 23 July 2014).
Zamboni, M., Mazzali, G., Fantin, F., Rossi, A. and Di Francesco, V. (2008) Sarcopenic obesity: a new category of obesity in the elderly. *Nutrition, Metabolism and Cardiovascular Diseases* 18, 388–395.

V Paediatrics

33 Home Parenteral Nutrition in Children

Virginie Colomb[1], Cécile Lambe[2] and Olivier Goulet[2*]

[1]*French Association against Cystic Fibrosis 'Vaincre la mucoviscidose', Paris, France;* [2]*Pediatric Gastroenterology and Nutrition, Hôpital Necker-Enfants Malades, Paris, France*

Key Points

- Home parenteral nutrition (HPN) should be considered in all children who depend on long-term parenteral nutrition (PN), if clinical and familial criteria are fulfilled.
- Parents and other caregivers should undergo a structured teaching and training programme conducted by a specialized nurse from the paediatric HPN centre's nutrition team.
- PN solutions providing macro- and micronutrients for paediatric HPN should be prescribed and compounded according to individual patients' needs.
- Alternatively, if industrial standardized solutions are preferred for some children on HPN, only specific paediatric premixes should be delivered to children on HPN.
- Centres caring for infants and children on HPN must have adequate expertise and resources.

Introduction

In the late 1960s in the USA, Dudrick and Wilmore demonstrated that long-term administration of a hypertonic mixture of glucose, protein hydrolysate, electrolytes, minerals and vitamins through a central venous catheter (CVC) made it possible to achieve normal growth and development in an infant with short bowel (Dudrick *et al.*, 1968, Wilmore and Dudrick, 1968). In children, as in adult patients, long-term total or complementary parenteral nutrition (PN) is needed to preserve nutritional status, especially in a variety of paediatric digestive and

*E-mail: olivier.goulet@nck.aphp.fr

non-digestive diseases responsible for chronic intestinal failure (IF), i.e. when oral or enteral nutrition cannot meet protein–energy needs.

When a child depends on long-term PN, home PN (HPN) is the only alternative to prolonged hospitalization. Whatever the duration of PN and the prognosis of the disease, HPN has been recognized for more than 30 years as the best option for improving the quality of life (QoL) of these children and their families within the constraints of the disease (Vargas *et al.*, 1987; Ricour *et al.*, 1990; Wong *et al.*, 2000; Gottrand *et al.*, 2005; Colomb *et al.*, 2007) and as the most cost-effective way of care (Howard *et al.*, 1995). In 2005, the expert working groups gathered under the auspices of the European Society of Paediatric Gastroenterology, Hepatology and Nutrition (ESPGHAN) and the European Society for Clinical Nutrition and Metabolism (ESPEN) provided guidelines on paediatric parenteral nutrition (ESPGHAN-ESPEN, 2005). These guidelines included recommendations regarding indications and organization of paediatric HPN and stated that 'all children who depend on long-term HPN should be discharged on HPN if familial criteria are fulfilled'. The prevalence of paediatric HPN all over Europe is hardly assessed, due to the lack of registers. Recently, a British study conducted by the members of the British Society of Paediatric Gastroenterology, Hepatology and Nutrition and participants in the British Intestinal Failure Survey reported 139 children on HPN, this number representing a fourfold increase since the study performed by the British Paediatric Surveillance Unit in 1993, with a mean HPN prevalence of 13.7 patients per million (Beath *et al.*, 2011). In France, the number of HPN paediatric patients has also increased over the last 10 years from 74 in 2003 to about 200 in 2012 (personal data).

Indications and Contraindications

Most indications for prolonged PN and thus HPN in children are primary digestive diseases (Table 33.1), of which most are congenital or acquired neonatal diseases causing chronic or lifelong IF (Goulet and Ruemmele, 2006). Short bowel syndrome (SBS) (Sondheimer *et al.*, 1998a; Goulet *et al.*, 2013), mainly congenital, is the largest group, accounting for 30% to more than 50% of the indications for HPN in the major published surveys (Vargas *et al.*, 1987; Colomb *et al.*, 2007; Gandullia *et al.*, 2011). The other main digestive indications are chronic intestinal pseudo-obstruction syndrome (CIPOS) (Goulet *et al.*, 1999) and congenital mucosal disorders, so-called untreatable diarrhoea of infancy – especially tufting enteropathy (Goulet *et al.*, 2007) and microvillus inclusion disease (Halac *et al.*, 2011). Because of the therapeutic advances over the last 10 years, inflammatory bowel diseases (IBDs), especially severe Crohn's disease either extensive and/or with multiple surgery, have become rare indications for prolonged PN. The need for HPN in primary non-digestive indications such as immune deficiency, cancers or metabolic diseases is less common and HPN programmes are usually shorter than for primary digestive diseases.

Children eligible for HPN should be in a stable, safe condition. This includes stability of the underlying disease in the short term, stable fluid and electrolyte requirements, tolerance to cyclic PN and a safe central venous access. Age for

Table 33.1. Indications for HPN in children.

Primary digestive diseases	Non-primary digestive diseases
SBS	AIDS
Intestinal atresia	Cancer
Gastroschisis	Cystic fibrosis
Necrotizing enterocolitis in neonates	Hereditary immune deficiency
Mesenteric volvulus resulting in gut necrosis	Mitochondrial disease
IBD	Chronic organ failure including preparation prior to transplantation
Intestinal wall damage	
Congenital mucosal disorders (untreatable diarrhoea)	
IBD	
Radiation enteropathy	
Motility disorders	
CIPOS	
Long-segment Hirschsprung disease	
Other indications	
Intestinal fistulas	
Protein-losing enteropathy after failure of oral/enteral feeding	

safely commencing HPN depends on the individual child's clinical condition. Most paediatric HPN programmes cater for children under 1 year old and even include babies <6 months of age (Vargas *et al.*, 1987; ESPGHAN-ESPEN, 2005; Colomb *et al.*, 2007).

Techniques

Venous access

Paediatric HPN requires a central venous access, which allows for infusion of hypertonic solutions. Selection of the most appropriate central venous access device (CVAD) is based on the patient's vascular access history, the venous anatomy, the nature of the underlying disease, the child's development and body image concerns.

Types of CVAD

PARTIALLY IMPLANTED DEVICES OR TUNNELLED CATHETERS As for adults, these central venous catheters (CVC), so-called Broviac-type CVCs, are placed percutaneously, under general or regional anaesthesia, in a central vein. The CVC is usually inserted into the superior vena cava above (or high in) the right cardiac atrium. The most common access point for central venous catheterization is the internal jugular, external jugular or subclavian vein. The CVC is tunnelled from the access site to an exit site usually in the anterior chest wall in the midclavicular line or in the upper abdomen through a jugular or subclavian vein and tunnelled subcutaneously, with one or two Dacron cuffs allowing safe fixation. In the case that these vessels are inaccessible, the CVC is placed in the inferior caval vein through the femoral or saphenous veins and emerges in the lower part of the abdomen.

TOTALLY IMPLANTED DEVICES OR IMPLANTABLE ACCESS PORTS Most available data regarding the use of implanted devices in children have been obtained from haematology and oncology patients (Bucki *et al.*, 2008; Gapany *et al.*, 2011). No data are available to compare the use of implanted ports with Broviac-type CVCs for paediatric HPN use in terms of lifespan, complications and QoL (ESPGHAN-ESPEN, 2005). Tunnelled CVCs are usually preferred in young children and in children who need daily PN infusion, due to the psychological and technical problems related to daily puncture of the implanted port.

Other access

Rarely, arteriovenous fistulae can be used for long-term HPN programmes, especially in the case of repeated complications related to CVCs (Ricour *et al.*, 1990).

Infusions

Fluids and electrolytes

PN is not merely an energy and protein supply. It is inseparable from fluids and electrolytes. Like for macro- and micronutrients, water and electrolyte requirements vary depending on age, weight, underlying disease, hydration status and environmental conditions (Table 33.2) (ESPGHAN-ESPEN, 2005). When PN is not the sole source of protein–energy intake, the absorptive capacities of the intestine should be estimated. Digestive tract losses due to diarrhoea or from stomas should be measured (volume and sodium concentration), replaced and the patient should be on a stable regime before starting an HPN programme.

Carbohydrates

Dextrose (D-glucose) is the sole source of carbohydrate used for PN. One gram of dextrose provides 3.4 kcal. It should provide at least 70% of the non-protein energy supply in children on long term-PN (Table 33.3) (ESPGHAN-ESPEN, 2005). The maximum rate of glucose oxidation (RGO) differs strongly among patients according to age and clinical status. In term infants or babies on long-term TPN, the maximal RGO is about 12 mg/kg body weight/min or 18 g/kg body weight/day (Bresson *et al.*, 1991). When glucose is administered in excess of the amount that can be directly oxidized for energy production and glycogen production, the excess is directed to lipogenesis and promotes fat deposition. The rate of parenteral glucose delivery should be progressively increased and should not exceed 1.2–1.4 g/kg body weight/h in an infant, 1.0–1.2 g/kg body weight/h in a child aged 1–10 years and 0.5–0.8 g/kg body weight/h in an adolescent. The total glucose supply should not exceed 400 g/day in an adolescent receiving cyclic 10/24 h or 12/24 h infusion. Therefore, particular attention must be paid to glucose tolerance (hyperglycaemia, glycosuria) in children on cyclic HPN. In such

Table 33.2. Daily requirements for fluids and electrolytes.

Age (years)	Fluid (ml/kg body weight/day)	Na (mmol/kg body weight/day)	K (mmol/kg body weight/day)
<1	120–150	2–3	1–3
1–2	80–120	1–3	1–3
3–5	80–100	1–3	1–3
6–12	60–80	1–3	1–3
13–18	50–70	1–3	1–3

Table 33.3. Energy and macronutrient requirements.

Age (years)	Glucose (g/kg body weight/day)	Lipids (g/kg body weight/day)	Amino acids (g/kg body weight/day)	Total non-protein energy (kcal/kg body weight/day)
<1	12–18	2–3	2–3	90–100
1–7	8–12	1–2	1–2	75–90
7–12	8–12	1–2	1–2	60–75
13–18	5–7	1–2	1–2	30–60

patients on stable long-term PN, glucosuria may reveal a stressful event, particularly infection, which impairs sensitivity to insulin.

Lipids

Lipids should be given to children on HPN. Intravenous lipid emulsions (ILEs) are a source of essential fatty acids and a highly concentrated source of energy (9 kcal/g). The use of ILEs also enables a diversified energy input, with a reduction in the deleterious consequences of excessive glucose supply. A lipid supply of 1–3 g ILE/kg body weight/day, according to age and clinical status, is recommended (ESPGHAN-ESPEN, 2005) (Table 33.2). The first ILEs for PN use were based solely on soybean or safflower oil which contain a high concentration of the *n*-6 polyunsaturated fatty acid (PUFA), linoleic acid, and lower concentration of the *n*-3 PUFA, α-linolenic acid. Such ILEs have been strongly suspected to be involved in the so-called PN-associated liver disease (PNALD) (Colomb *et al.*, 2000b). Alternative sources of lipids are currently available, i.e. medium-chain triacylglycerols, olive oil and fish oil. Further studies are needed to assess the optimal lipid intake in children on long-term PN.

ILEs may be infused either on a Y-line in association with continuous inflow of glucose and amino acids, or as a ternary 'all-in-one' mixture.

Amino acids

Solutions of L-amino acids are the sole source of nitrogen for paediatric PN. Amino acid requirements in PN depend on age, weight and underlying disease. There is a larger number of essential amino acids in infants than in adults. Cysteine, taurine, tyrosine, histidine, glutamic acid and aspartic acid can be ranked among the essential amino acids. Therefore, the composition of amino acid solutions for infants and young children differs from those used in adult patients (Shelton *et al.*, 2010). Paediatric amino acid mixtures containing essential amino acids for infants and toddlers have been shown to be effective in clinical use, providing appropriate nitrogen utilization and retention (Storm and Helms, 2007). A nitrogen supply of 250–450 mg/kg body weight/day, according to clinical status, is recommended and the optimal ratio of energy to nitrogen in children is about 200–250:1 (ESPGHAN-ESPEN, 2005) (Table 33.2).

Vitamins and trace elements

Each PN infusion should provide water-soluble and fat-soluble vitamins as well as trace elements, according to the patient's age, weight and specific needs. The vitamin requirements in children differ from those of adults. The major differences concern the fat-soluble vitamins (Green *et al.*, 1988). The most widely used vitamin solutions in children up to 11 years of age are Soluvit® (water-soluble vitamins) and Vitalipid Infant® (fat-soluble vitamins). Preparations used for children over 11 years of age include Soluvit®, Vitalipid Adult® and Cernevit® (water- and fat-soluble vitamins without vitamin K, which should be given separately). In certain circumstances, e.g. a patient who depends on a limited PN intake, vitamins and minerals may be given enterally. Vitamins will need to be given separately if stability of the PN admixture with vitamins included is not guaranteed, e.g. if PN bags can only be delivered to the patient's home on a monthly basis (Ben Hariz *et al.*, 1993a).

Some of the trace elements are routinely provided in PN solutions, e.g. Peditrace® (Zn, Cu, Mn, Se and F) for children weighing up to 15 kg, or Addamel® (Cr, Cu, Fe, Mn, I, F, Mo, Se, Zn) for children weighing over 15 kg.

Iron

Iron supplementation should be provided periodically (intramuscularly or intravenously) to children receiving long-term PN (>3 weeks). In infants and young children, the standard iron supply is 100 μg/kg body weight/day. Using this dose in long-term PN, an accumulation of excess iron can be observed (Ben Hariz *et al.*, 1993b). Therefore, ferritin plasma concentration should be monitored in children on long-term PN. Provision of iron should be decreased at ferritin concentration of 500 ng/ml and stopped completely at 1000 ng/ml (Ben Hariz *et al.*, 1993b).

Phosphate

Organic phosphate solutions (Glycophos®, Phocytan®) are more often used than inorganic ones, as in young children a small volume of a PN admixture may contain a high concentration of ions – especially calcium and phosphate – which can precipitate. The reaction may be prevented by the use of organic phosphate solutions.

Organization and Technical Aspects

Centres caring for infants and children on HPN must have adequate expertise and resources to ensure a good standard of care, including multidisciplinary nutrition support teams that include physician(s), pharmacist(s), nurse(s), dietician(s), social worker(s) and psychologist(s) (Agostoni *et al.*, 2005). Physicians should be trained and qualified to be responsible for use and prescription of HPN in children (ESPGHAN-ESPEN, 2005; Colomb *et al.*, 2007). Nurses who are responsible for parents' teaching and training should evaluate their capacities to deal with all medical and technical issues related to the child's treatment.

Social and familial requirements for HPN

Whatever the medical indication, several social and familial criteria have to be fulfilled before a child's HPN programme is organized. Parents have to be informed, motivated and should be able to cope with all medical, emotional and technical problems related to HPN. Family suitability for HPN should be carefully assessed by the healthcare team, with the assistance of a social worker, before discharge. This may include visiting the home, to examine practical details such as space for a dedicated refrigerator, electricity supply and bathroom facilities (Puntis, 1995; Colomb *et al.*, 2007). In other cases, the professional status of both parents needs to be carefully examined, for occasionally one of them has to stop working. In one-parent households, the mother is usually the parent responsible for administering HPN. A single-parent family is not always a contraindication for HPN, but social help and home nursing assistance may become necessary (Ricour *et al.*, 1990). Separated parents who share the child's care should be trained providing they each connect/disconnect the PN at least once per week to maintain their skills.

Preparation of a paediatric HPN programme

Parents' training

Prior to discharge, parents must undergo structured training in all aspects of care and complications (Puntis, 1995; ESPGHAN-ESPEN, 2005; Colomb *et al.*, 2007). The teaching programme should begin as soon as the decision to proceed to HPN has been taken. It is best undertaken during the period when at least one parent, or preferably both, is resident in the hospital, especially if the family lives far from the HPN centre. The mean duration of a complete teaching programme is about 2 weeks (Ricour *et al.*, 1990; Colomb *et al.*, 2007), but the duration needs to be tailored to each family's needs. The structured teaching programme must have a written plan, step-by-step instructions and a method to record competence comprising theoretical and practical aspects. Written and audio-visual tools may be used. Each session is limited to learning one particular skill, and a new subject should be introduced only when parents are competent and confident in the previous one. A written record of progress should be kept. Parents' skills and knowledge should be checked prior to home discharge (ESPGHAN-ESPEN, 2005). When parents cannot be autonomous, especially in the case of a single-parent family, the help of a community nurse is required (Ricour *et al.*, 1990; Puntis, 1995). In some countries, candidates for HPN can be referred to outside service organizations, which employ nurses who sometimes meet the family in the hospital for the first encounter and then visit the patient at home to complete the training given at the hospital. Community health professionals should be involved in all aspects of discharge planning and subsequent shared care (Meadows, 1997; Smith and Daughtrey, 2000; ESPGHAN-ESPEN, 2005). The physicians and the teaching nurses from the HPN centre should also inform staff from the patient's local hospital about emergency guidelines (ESPGHAN-ESPEN, 2005; Colomb *et al.*, 2007). This may be done by holding a discharge planning meeting attended by parents and all professionals involved in the child's care. It is best held at the patient's local hospital. Those attending may include the child (if old enough), parents, members of the specialist nutrition team, the local paediatrician and a nurse from the local hospital, a community nurse and the patient's general practitioner.

Rhythm of infusion

HPN is based on cyclical (10–18/24 h) parenteral infusion of a nutrient formula (Ricour *et al.*, 1990; Colomb *et al.*, 2007). Children, like adults, almost always tolerate a nocturnal infusion over a period of 10–12 h, especially when oral or enteral feeding is possible. Cyclic infusion has metabolic (Lienhardt *et al.*, 1998), physical and psychological advantages. However, in infants, especially when enteral feeding is not tolerated, or in children with major digestive fluid and electrolyte losses, a longer period of infusion (14–18 h) may be necessary.

When PN is commenced in the hospital ward, all children are infused continuously 24/24 h before undergoing a period of adaptation, during which time the rate of infusion is gradually increased and the infusion period generally decreased, usually from 24/24 h to 12/24 h and at most 18/24 h per day in exceptional circumstances. According to the patient's condition, a progressive increase and decrease in infusion rate during the initial and final hours of infusion should be considered to avoid hypoglycaemia and hyperglycaemia (Ricour *et al.*, 1990; Colomb *et al.*, 2007).

Equipment

Pumps

A pump is indispensable for PN infusion in children. Pumps for children's HPN should achieve a good compromise between safety and comfort. The main requirements for safety are: (i) volumetric accuracy over a wide range of flow rates; (ii) no risk of sudden discontinuation of infusion (reliable battery); (iii) no risk of free flow; (iv) 'keep vein open' status; (v) audible and written alarms (e.g. for air bubbles in line, empty container, occlusion, change in pressure, dose limit or low battery); and (vi) lockable settings (Meadows, 1997; ESPGHAN-ESPEN, 2005).

Other requirements are also important for the QoL: (i) simplicity in priming the set; (ii) clean ambient air; (iii) pre-selection of infusion rates; (iv) programmed stepwise increased and decreased flow rates at the onset and end of the infusion times; (v) minimum number of false alarms; (vi) minimum motor noise; and (v) minimum weight and volume with carrying handle and binding on intravenous poles. Portable pumps are now more widely available and can have a major impact on improving QoL. Any faulty pump should be replaced within a reasonable timespan (e.g. 4h), or a second pump should be available in the home. Pumps should be serviced annually. The supply of equipment and ancillaries should be delivered to the home (Meadows, 1997).

Filters

The aim of filtration to reduce the risk of precipitates reaching the patient has been emphasized (Bethune *et al.*, 2001; ESPGHAN-ESPEN, 2005). Filters should be 1.2 μm, air-eliminating filters when an all-in-one, lipid-containing formula is delivered, in contrast to 0.22 μm, air-eliminating filters suitable for non-lipid-containing PN.

Nutrition mixtures for paediatric HPN

Binary mixtures including glucose, amino acids, electrolytes, trace elements and vitamins (lipids being administered separately on a Y-line) or all-in-one mixtures are provided to children on HPN. Mixtures may be manufactured and delivered to patients with ancillary equipment weekly, fortnightly or monthly. Vitamins or drugs added to nutrient mixtures might impair their stability and, on the other hand, availability of drugs and vitamins might be reduced when introduced into PN mixtures (Ben Hariz *et al.*, 1993a). Thus, depending on these limiting factors, the 'safe' duration of PN bag storage varies from about 8 days to up to (exceptionally) 30 days. Bags should be stored at 4°C from their production to their delivery to the patients. Home care companies should provide the families with dedicated refrigerators for PN bag storage.

Special mixtures should be prepared according to individual children's requirements (Ricour *et al.*, 1990; ESPGHAN-ESPEN, 2005; Colomb *et al.*, 2007). The use of non-paediatric standardized PN formulations in children at home can lead to severe metabolic complications. Recently, standardized PN formulations (so-called premixes) have been designed for children (Colomb *et al.*, 2012). However, children on HPN, i.e. who depend on long-term PN, require PN that fits optimally their individual needs. Therefore, the use of standardized premixes should be restricted to children who do not depend on total PN, e.g. children who experience intestinal adaptation and tolerate oral/enteral feeding.

Complications

Catheter-related sepsis

Although the incidence of catheter-related sepsis (CRS) in HPN patients is usually lower than in hospitalized patients (Melville *et al.*, 1997; Hojsak *et al.*, 2012), CRS is the most frequent complication of HPN in children. Its incidence varies from 1 to more than 4 per 1000 HPN-days among series published by expert centres (Colomb *et al.*, 2000a; Ferroni *et al.*, 2006; Mohammed *et al.*, 2011; Chu *et al.*, 2012; Cordero Cruz *et al.*, 2012; Hojsak *et al.*, 2012; Wiskin *et al.*, 2012). The risk of CRS is higher at young ages (Schmidt-Sommerfeld *et al.*, 1990; Moukarzel *et al.*, 1994; Melville *et al.*, 1997), especially during the first 2 years of HPN as compared with later years. All studies have shown that some children have more than one infection over the period of study while others remain infection free. Risk factors, except for young age, are uncertain. Underlying disease, ostomy and the socio-economic level of the family have not appeared to be discriminant. A study showed that the increase in HPN duration was associated with a lower incidence of CRS and suggested that early occurrence of the first episode of CRS after starting HPN was a predictive factor for later infections (Colomb *et al.*, 2000a). Coagulase-negative staphylococci accounted for at least 60% of sepsis in several large studies (Schmidt-Sommerfeld *et al.*, 1990; Colomb *et al.*, 2000a; Ferroni *et al.*, 2006). However, the incidence of *Staphylococcus aureus*, Gram-negative bacilli and fungal catheter infections was higher in other paediatric surveys (Moukarzel *et al.*, 1994; Melville *et al.*, 1997; Cordero Cruz *et al.*, 2012). Prevention of CRS requires strict asepsis during both CVC insertion and changes of filter and infusion sets (ESPGHAN-ESPEN, 2005). Daily care of the skin at the CVC exit site is of great importance. PN solutions must be prepared under strict aseptic conditions. The care of the child should be undertaken by physicians and nurses who have been specifically trained in this technique. Parents should be taught about the signs of CRS. They have to contact their general practitioner and the hospital (referring local hospital and/or HPN centre) in case of fever or any signs of infection. Fever or clinical signs suggestive of CRS should lead to a thorough search for a source of sepsis, together with blood exams such as a white blood cell count, C-reactive protein and procalcitonin. Samples for blood cultures should be taken via the catheter and from a peripheral vein. According to the clinical and biological assessment, broad-spectrum antibiotic therapy may be started (ESPGHAN-ESPEN, 2005), including antibiotics against *Staphylococcus*. Removal of the catheter should be systematically considered in case of fungal infection, infection due to *S. aureus* with cutaneous infection, or if the patient continues to deteriorate even when appropriate antibiotic therapy has been started. In patients who present with repeated CRS, the use of taurolidine, a catheter lock solution that prevents biofilm formation and has broad-spectrum bactericidal and antifungal action, might be proposed, although its paediatric use in HPN patients is still limited (Bradshaw and Puntis, 2008; Chu *et al.*, 2012).

PNALD

Hepatobiliary complications of PN in children are well recognized and documented (Kelly, 2006). Many PN-related and patient-related risk factors have been identified. The underlying digestive disease plays a prominent role. This is especially the case in SBS (Peyret *et al.*, 2011), with the disruption of bile acid enterohepatic circulation due to ileal amputation, impairment in choleresis when oral feeding is impossible, bacterial overgrowth due to bowel obstruction, stasis and lack of ileocaecal valvula, which are all factors thought to contribute to PN-associated cholestasis (Goulet *et al.*, 2009). Interestingly, children with intractable diarrhoea of infancy have been recently shown to be significantly more likely to develop liver disease than patients with other digestive diseases, including SBS (Colomb *et al.*, 2007). Recurrent septic episodes, either catheter related (Gram-positive bacteria) or digestive related (Gram-negative sepsis from intraluminal bacterial overgrowth), also contribute to liver injury (Sondheimer *et al.*, 1998b; Hermans *et al.*, 2007; Peyret *et al.*, 2011). Multiple risk factors are also directly related to the composition of the PN admixtures, such as amino acid content of PN solutions, aluminium overload, excessive glucose intake and deficiency of essential fatty acids. However, with the progress in knowledge and in the quality of PN admixtures, the main concern related to PNALD is lipid intake.

Various mechanisms have been suspected for the possible role of ILEs in PNALD, especially those based solely on soybean or safflower oil, which contain a high concentration of the *n*-6 PUFA linoleic acid and lower concentration of the *n*-3 PUFA α-linolenic acid. In a paediatric cohort of patients with PN-associated cholestasis, the temporary decrease or discontinuation in ILE administration was attempted in 20/23 cholestasis episodes and led to normalization of bilirubin in 18 episodes. In most cases plasma bilirubin decrease was rapid within the first month, reaching a normal concentration by 3.2 ± 2.0 months (Colomb *et al.*, 2000b). Excessive intake of linoleic acid, which is converted to arachidonic acid, a precursor of pro-inflammatory agents, might have adverse effects on the liver. Oxidative stress is also considered one of the possible causes of liver injury resulting from lipids (Roma and Sanchez Pozzi, 2008). Another major concern is related to the plant sterol – also called phytosterol – content of soybean ILE (Kurvinen *et al.*, 2011). In children, chronic administration of ILE might also overload reticular endoplasmic complexes and induce their acute or chronic activation, leading to haematological disorders, accompanied by liver dysfunction, especially cholestasis (Goulet *et al.*, 1986). Fish oil has theoretical advantages over soybean oil, i.e. a high concentration of α-tocopherol (four- to eightfold that in soybean) and no phytosterol. Fish oil is also a source of docosahexaenoic acid, which is important for neurodevelopment and visual function, and also a source of eicosapentaenoic acid, which favourably modulates inflammation. The first reports of the compassionate use of parenteral fish oil (Omegaven®) as the sole lipid source (1 g/kg body weight/day) in infants with chronic IF and severe IF-associated liver disease were provided recently (Gura *et al.*, 2006; Diamond *et al.*, 2008; Puder *et al.*, 2009; Fuchs *et al.*, 2011). In most of these studies, a high dose of soybean-based emulsion was replaced by 1 g fish oil/kg body weight. Therefore, one might wonder whether reversal of cholestasis was the effect of decreasing or stopping the soybean load or the effect of the fish oil itself (including the high α-tocopherol load) or both (Koletzko and Goulet, 2010).

The earliest and most sensitive, but not specific, laboratory markers are plasma alkaline phosphatase and γ-glutamyl transferase activities, while hyperbilirubinaemia is the latest marker of cholestasis to appear. Careful monitoring of hepatic function is important to in order to minimize factors responsible for liver disease (ESPGHAN-ESPEN, 2005). Liver biopsy is still the most reliable tool to assess liver impairment in children on HPN. Steatosis, associated with clinical liver enlargement, may appear early after PN onset as a result of either excessive glucose supply leading to lipogenesis, or the deposition of exogenous fatty acids. It is the first-non specific histological abnormality, followed by cholestasis and portal and periportal cell infiltration. Fibrosis indicates severe liver disease, which can lead to cirrhosis and liver failure, but is fortunately rare if the multidisciplinary management of chronic IF is performed correctly (Colomb *et al.*, 2007).

PN-related bone disease

PN-related metabolic bone disease (MBD) with a decrease in bone mineral density (BMD), osteoporosis, pain and fractures has been described in adults on long-term PN, while a few data exist in children (Diamanti *et al.*, 2010; Pastore *et al.*, 2012). The so-called PN-related bone disease resembles rickets, with fractures of the limbs which are sometimes asymptomatic and are discovered only after routine X-ray examination. Diagnosis of bone disease relies primarily on the measure of BMD, which can be performed by dual-energy X-ray absorptiometry. The most constant laboratory features are an elevated alkaline phosphatase activity and hypercalciuria, with normal or subnormal levels of vitamin D metabolites and parathyroid hormone. Bone histology shows osteomalacia-like changes with reduced mineralization and excess of osteoid tissue. MBD has been shown even in children weaned from long-term PN (Leonberg *et al.*, 1998). The cause of MBD is probably multifactorial including both underlying disease and PN-related mechanisms: excess vitamin D, phosphorus, nitrogen and energy imbalance, excess amino acid and aluminium contaminations (Advenier *et al.*, 2003). Hypercalciuria may be reduced by ensuring balanced supplies of phosphorus, nitrogen and energy, while reducing the supply of amino acids, especially the sulfur-containing amino acids. Regular measurements of urinary calcium, plasma calcium, plasma phosphorus, plasma parathyroid hormone and vitamin D concentrations, and serum alkaline phosphatase activity should be performed (ESPGHAN-ESPEN, 2005). Treatment with pamidronate for osteoporosis might be discussed on an individual basis (Pastore *et al.*, 2012).

Other complications

Central venous thrombosis and pulmonary embolism are rare complications in children on HPN (Van Ommen and Tabbers, 2010). Symptoms of vein thrombosis or thromboembolism should be reported immediately to the reference HPN centre

(ESPGHAN-ESPEN, 2005). With good technique, leakage, displacement or obstruction of the catheter can be avoided. Children and caregivers should be educated about the safety of the catheter (ESPGHAN-ESPEN, 2005). Some repair kits have been developed and may often be used to repair the damaged portion, thus avoiding replacement of the catheter (ESPGHAN-ESPEN 2005).

Long-term Outcome: The Role of Centralized HPN Expert Centres

The largest paediatric surveys (Vargas *et al.*, 1987; Ricour *et al.*, 1990; Colomb *et al.*, 2007; Gandullia *et al.*, 2011) reported a mean HPN duration of about 2 years with an upper duration longer than 15 years. Children on HPN have better survival rates than older patients (Pironi *et al.*, 2011, 2012). About 50% of paediatric patients can be weaned from HPN, the functional prognosis being better for congenital SBS than for other indications (Colomb *et al.*, 2007). Ethical dilemmas may arise with children with chronic IF that does not allow weaning off PN, such as extensive gastrointestinal resection, microvillus atrophy or severe CIPOS. Small bowel transplantation (SBTx) might be an alternative to lifelong HPN in such patients, according to each individual situation (complications of long-term PN, tolerance of the family) (Sauvat *et al.*, 2008; Pironi *et al.*, 2011, 2012). Since the first isolated SBTx using cyclosporine A, major advances have resulted from the use of new immunosuppressive treatments (Goulet *et al.*, 2000). When liver structure and function are impaired by long-term PN, a combined SBTx and liver transplantation should be considered. However, the timing of referral and criteria for isolated intestinal or combined transplantation are still a matter of debate (Kaufman *et al.*, 2001; Kocoshis *et al.*, 2004; Pironi *et al.*, 2011, 2012). The role of expert centralized HPN centres is to improve the quality of HPN and thus to decrease the number of transplantations that are due to, or precipitated by, PN-associated complications. Therefore, early referral of patients on long-term PN to specialized HPN centres, especially before irreversible liver failure occurs, might increase their QoL and survival and reduce the cost of care (ESPGHAN-ESPEN, 2005).

Monitoring

Once discharged from hospital, a regular outpatient follow-up should be planned in order to check clinical and biological parameters (Table 33.4). Visits are planned on a regular basis, according to each individual situation, initially at monthly intervals, more frequently if necessary, especially in infants. A close connection with general practitioners and local non-specialized hospital units is indispensable in an emergency.

Summary

HPN is the best alternative to prolonged hospitalization in children with chronic IF who depend on long-term PN. Early referral of such patients on long-term PN

Table 33.4. Laboratory monitoring.

Laboratory parameters	Baseline	Optional baseline	Weekly × 2	Monthly × 3	Every 3–6 months	Every 6–12 months
Blood count, prothrombin time	x		x	x		x
Blood electrolytes (Ca, P, Mg, bicarbonate), blood urea, creatinine	x		x	x	x	
Urine electrolytes (Na, K)	x		x	x	x	
Glucose, protein, albumin	x		x	x	x	
Liver tests	x		x	x	x	
Iron, ferritin	x				x	
Vitamin B_{12}, folate		x				x

to specialized HPN centres is mandatory, in order to increase their QoL and survival and reduce the cost of care; and also in order to decrease the number of transplantations that are due to, or precipitated, by PN-associated complications.

References

Advenier, E., Landry, C., Colomb, V., Cognon, C., Pradeau, D., Florent, M., Goulet, O., Ricour, C. and Corriol, O. (2003) Aluminium contamination of parenteral nutrition and aluminium loading in children on long-term parenteral nutrition. *Journal of Pediatric Gastroenterology and Nutrition* 36, 448–453.

Agostoni, C., Axelson, I., Colomb, V., Goulet, O., Koletzko, B., Michaelsen, K.F., Puntis, J.W., Rigo, J., Shamir, R., Szajewska, H. and Turck, D.; ESPGHAN Committee on Nutrition; European Society for Paediatric Gastroenterology (2005) The need for nutrition support teams in pediatric units: a commentary by the ESPGHAN committee on nutrition. *Journal of Pediatric Gastroenterology and Nutrition* 41, 8–11. Erratum in: *Journal of Pediatric Gastroenterology and Nutrition* 41, 267–271.

Beath, S.V., Gowen, H. and Puntis, J.W. (2011) Trends in paediatric home parenteral nutrition and implications for service development. *Clinical Nutrition* 30, 499–502.

Ben Hariz, M., De Potter, S., Corriol, O., Goulet, O., Chaumont, P., Forget, D. and Ricour, C. (1993a) Home parenteral nutrition in children: bioavailability of vitamins in binary mixtures stored for 8 days. *Clinical Nutrition* 12, 147–152.

Ben Hariz, M., Goulet, O., De Potter, S., Girot, R., Rambaud, C., Colomb, V., Corriol, O. and Ricour, C. (1993b) Iron overload in children receiving prolonged parenteral nutrition. *Journal of Pediatrics* 123, 238–241.

Bethune, K., Allwood, M., Grainger, C. and Wormleighton, C. (2001) Use of filters during the preparation and administration of parenteral nutrition: position paper and guidelines prepared by a British pharmaceutical nutrition group working party. *Nutrition* 17, 403–408.

Bradshaw, J.H. and Puntis, J.W. (2008) Taurolidine and catheter-related bloodstream infection: a systematic review of the literature. *Journal of Pediatric Gastroenterology and Nutrition* 47, 179–186.

Bresson, J.L., Bader, B., Rocchiccioli, F., Mariotti, A., Ricour, C., Sachs, C. and Rey, J. (1991) Protein-metabolism kinetics and energy-substrate utilization in infants fed parenteral solutions with different glucose–fat ratios. *American Journal of Clinical Nutrition* 54, 370–376.

Bucki, B., Tomaszewska, R., Karpe, J., Stoksik, P., Sonta-Jakimczyk, D. and Szczepanski, T. (2008) Central venous access ports in children treated for hematopoietic malignancies. *Journal of Pediatric Hematology/Oncology* 25, 751–755.

Chu, H.P., Brind, J., Tomar, R. and Hill, S. (2012) Significant reduction in central venous catheter-related bloodstream infections in children on HPN after starting treatment with taurolidine line lock. *Journal of Pediatric Gastroenterology and Nutrition* 55, 403–407.

Colomb, V., Fabeiro, M., Dabbas, M., Goulet, O., Merckx, J. and Ricour, C. (2000a) Central venous catheter-related infections in children on long-term home parenteral nutrition: incidence and risk factors. *Clinical Nutrition* 19, 355–359.

Colomb, V., Jobert-Giraud, A., Lacaille, F., Goulet, O., Fournet, J.C. and Ricour, C. (2000b) Role of lipid emulsions in cholestasis associated to long term-parenteral nutrition in children. *JPEN Journal of Parenteral and Enteral Nutrition* 24, 345–350.

Colomb, V., Dabbas-Tyan, M., Taupin, P., Révillon, Y., Jan, D., De Potter, S., Gorski-Colin, A.M., Talbotec, C., Lamor, M., Herreman, K., Corriol, O., Landais, P., Ricour, C. and Goulet, O. (2007) Long-term outcome of children on home parenteral nutrition. The 20 year-experience of a single center in 302 patients. *Journal of Pediatric Gastroenterology and Nutrition* 44, 347–353.

Colomb, V., Marlowe, M.L., Bonnot, D. and Rigo, J. (2012) Practical use of a new three-chamber bag for parenteral nutrition in pediatric patients. *e-SPEN Journal* 7, e93–e99.

Cordero Cruz, A.M., Aguilella Vizcaíno, M.J., González Fuentes, C., Rubio Murillo, M., Moreno Villares, J.M., Gomis Muñoz, P. and Herreros de Tejada, A. (2012) Home parenteral nutrition in infants and children in a tertiary level hospital between 1993 and 2009. *Nutrición Hospitalaria* 27, 262–265.

Diamanti, A., Bizzarri, C., Basso, M.S., Gambarara, M., Cappa, M., Daniele, A., Noto, C. and Castro, M. (2010) How does long-term parenteral nutrition impact the bone mineral status of children with intestinal failure? *Journal of Bone and Mineral Metabolism* 28, 351–358.

Diamond, I.R., Sterescu, A., Pencharz, P.B. and Wales, P.W. (2008) The rationale for the use of parenteral omega-3 lipids in children with short bowel syndrome and liver disease. *Pediatric Surgery International* 24, 773–778.

Dudrick, S.J., Wilmore, D.W., Vars, H.M. and Rhoads, J.E. (1968) Long-term total parenteral nutrition with growth, development and positive nitrogen balance. *Surgery* 64, 134–142.

ESPGHAN-ESPEN (2005) Guidelines on Paediatric Parenteral Nutrition of the European Society of Paediatric Gastroenterology, Hepatology and Nutrition (ESPGHAN) and the European Society for Clinical Nutrition and Metabolism (ESPEN), supported by the European Society of Paediatric Research (ESPR). *Journal of Pediatric Gastroenterology and Nutrition* 41(Suppl. 2), 1–87.

Ferroni, A., Moumile, K., Pasquier, A., Berche, P. and Colomb, V. (2006) Evaluation of the gram stain–acridine orange leukocyte cytospin test for diagnosis of catheter-related bloodstream infection in children on long-term parenteral nutrition. *European Journal of Clinical Microbiology & Infectious Diseases* 25, 199–201.

Fuchs, J., Fallon, E.M., Gura, K. and Puder, M. (2011) Use of an omega-3 fatty acid-based emulsion in the treatment of parenteral nutrition-induced cholestasis in patients with microvillous inclusion disease. *Journal of Pediatric Surgery* 46, 2376–2382.

Gandullia, P., Lugani, F., Costabello, L., Arrigo, S., Calvi, A., Castellano, E., Vignola, S., Pistorio, A. and Barabino, A.V. (2011) Long-term home parenteral nutrition in children with chronic intestinal failure: a 15-year experience at a single Italian centre. *Digestive and Liver Diseases* 43, 28–33.

Gapany, C., Tercier, S., Diezi, M., Clement, C., Lemay, K. and Joseph, J.M. (2011) Frequent accesses to totally implanted vascular ports in pediatric oncology patients are associated with higher infection rates. *Journal of Vascular Access* 12, 207–210.

Gottrand, F., Staszewski, P., Colomb, V., Loras-Duclaux, I., Guimber, D., Marinier, E., Breton, A. and Magnificat, S. (2005) Satisfaction in different life domains in children receiving home parenteral nutrition and their families. *Journal of Pediatrics* 146, 793–797.

Goulet, O. and Ruemmele, F. (2006) Causes and management of intestinal failure in children. *Gastroenterology* 130(2 Suppl. 1), 16–28.

Goulet, O., Girot, R., Maier-Redelsperger, M., Bougle, D., Virelizier, J.L. and Ricour, C. (1986) Hematologic disorders following prolonged use of intravenous fat in children. *JPEN Journal of Parenteral and Enteral Nutrition* 10, 284–288.

Goulet, O., Jobert-Giraud, A., Michel, J.L., Jaubert, F., Lortat-Jacob, S., Colomb, V., Cuenod-Jabri, B., Jan, D., Brousse, N., Gaillard, D., Nihoul-Fékéte, C. and Ricour, C. (1999) Chronic intestinal pseudo-obstruction syndrome in pediatric patients. *European Journal of Pediatric Surgery* 9, 83–89.

Goulet, O., Lacaille, F., Jan, D. and Ricour, C. (2000) Intestinal transplantation: indications, results and strategy. *Current Opinion in Clinical Nutrition & Metabolic Care* 3, 329–338.

Goulet, O., Salomon, J., Ruemmele, F., de Serres, N.P. and Brousse, N. (2007) Intestinal epithelial dysplasia (tufting enteropathy). *Orphanet Journal of Rare Diseases* 20, 2–20.

Goulet, O., Joly, F., Corriol, O. and Colomb-Jung, V. (2009) Some new insights in intestinal failure-associated liver disease. *Current Opinion in Organ Transplantation* 14, 256–261.

Goulet, O., Olieman, J., Ksiazyk, J., Spolidoro, J., Tibboe, D., Köhler, H., Yagci, R.V., Falconer, J., Grimble, G. and Beattie, R.M. (2013) Neonatal short bowel syndrome as a model of intestinal failure: physiological background for enteral feeding. *Clinical Nutrition* 32, 162–171.

Greene, H.L., Hambidge, K.M., Schanler, R. and Tsang, R.C. (1988) Guidelines for the use of vitamins, trace elements, calcium, magnesium, and phosphorus in infants and children receiving total parenteral nutrition: report of the Subcommittee on Pediatric Parenteral Nutrient Requirements from the Committee on Clinical Practice Issues of the American Society for Clinical Nutrition. *American Journal of Clinical Nutrition* 48, 1324–1342. (Erratum in: *American Journal of Clinical Nutrition* 1989, 49, 1332; *American Journal of Clinical Nutrition* 1989, 50, 560.)

Gura, K.M., Duggan, C.P., Collier, S.B., Jennings, R.W., Folkman, J., Bistrian, B.R. and Puder, M. (2006) Reversal of parenteral nutrition-associated liver disease in two infants with short bowel syndrome using parenteral fish oil: implications for future management. *Pediatrics* 118, e197–e201.

Halac, U., Lacaille, F., Joly, F., Hugot, J.P., Talbotec, C., Colomb, V., Ruemmele, F.M. and Goulet, O. (2011) Microvillous inclusion disease: how to improve the prognosis of a severe congenital enterocyte disorder. *Journal of Pediatric Gastroenterology and Nutrition* 52, 460–465.

Hermans, D., Talbotec, C., Lacaille, F., Goulet, O., Ricour, C. and Colomb, V. (2007) Influence of early infections on the liver in children on long-term parenteral nutrition. *Journal of Pediatric Gastroenterology and Nutrition* 44, 459–463.

Hojsak, I., Strizic, H., Misak, Z., Rimac, I,. Bukovina, G., Prlic, H. and Kolacek, S. (2012) Central venous catheter related sepsis in children on parenteral nutrition: a 21-year single-center experience. *Clinical Nutrition* 31, 672–675.

Howard, L., Ament, M., Fleming, C.R., Shike, M. and Steiger, E. (1995) Current use and clinical outcome of home parenteral and enteral nutrition therapies in the United States. *Gastroenterology* 109, 355–365.

Kaufman, S.S., Atkinson, J.B., Bianchi, A., Goulet, O., Grant, D., Langnas, A., McDiarmid, S., Mittal, N., Reyes, J. and Tzakis, A., for the American Society of Transplantation (2001) Indications for pediatric intestinal transplantation: a position paper of the American Society of Transplantation. *Pediatric Transplantation* 5, 80–87.

Kelly, D.A. (2006) Intestinal failure-associated liver disease: what do we know today? *Gastroenterology* 130, 70–77.

Kocoshis, S.A, Beath, S.V., Booth, I.W., Garcia Oliva, C.A., Goulet, O., Kaufman, S.S., Lai, H.S., Luque, C. and Ohtsuka, Y.; North American Society for Gastroenterology, Hepatology and Nutrition (2004) Intestinal failure and small bowel transplantation, including clinical nutrition: working group report of the Second World Congress of Pediatric Gastroenterology, Hepatology, and Nutrition. *Journal of Pediatric Gastroenterology and Nutrition* 39, 655–661.

Koletzko, B. and Goulet, O. (2010) Fish oil containing intravenous lipid emulsions in parenteral nutrition-associated cholestatic liver disease. *Current Opinion in Clinical Nutrition & Metabolic Care* 13, 321–326.

Kurvinen, A., Nissinen, M.J., Gylling, H., Miettinen, T.A., Lampela, H., Koivusalo, A.I., Rintala, R.J. and Pakarinen, M. (2011) Effects of long-term parenteral nutrition on serum lipids, plant sterols, cholesterol metabolism, and liver histology in pediatric intestinal failure. *Journal of Pediatric Gastroenterology and Nutrition* 53, 440–446.

Leonberg, B., Chuang, E., Eicher, P., Teshakovec, A., Leonard, L. and Stallings, V. (1998) Long-term growth and development in children after home parenteral nutrition. *Journal of Pediatrics* 132, 461–466.

Lienhardt, A., Rakotoambinina, B., Colomb, V., Souissi, S., Sadoun, E., Goulet, O., Robert, J.J. and Ricour, C. (1998) Insulin secretion and sensitivity in children on cyclic total parenteral nutrition. *JPEN Journal of Parenteral and Enteral Nutrition* 22, 382–386.

Meadows, N. (1997) Home parenteral nutrition in children. *Baillière's Clinical Paediatrics* 5, 189–199.

Melville, C.A.S., Bisset, W.M., Long, S. and Milla, P.J. (1997) Counting the cost: hospital versus home central venous catheter survival. *Journal of Hospital Infection* 35, 197–205.

Mohammed, A., Grant, F.K., Zhao, V.M., Shane, A.L., Ziegler, T.R. and Cole, C.R. (2011) Characterization of posthospital bloodstream infections in children requiring home parenteral nutrition. *JPEN Journal of Parenteral and Enteral Nutrition* 35, 581–587.

Moukarzel, A.A., Haddad, I., Ament, M.E., Buchman, A.L., Reyen, L., Maggioni, A., Baron, H.I. and Vargas, J. (1994) 230 patient years of experience, with home long-term parenteral nutrition in childhood: natural history and life of central venous catheters. *Journal of Pediatric Surgery* 29, 1323–1327.

Pastore, S., Londero, M., Barbieri, F., Di Leo, G., Paparazzo, R. and Ventura, A. (2012) Treatment with pamidronate for osteoporosis complicating long-term intestinal failure. *Journal of Pediatric Gastroenterology and Nutrition* 55, 615–618.

Peyret, B., Collardeau, S., Touzet, S., Loras-Duclaux, I., Yantren, H., Michalski, M.C., Chaix, J., Restier-Miron, L., Bouvier, R., Lachaux, A. and Peretti, N. (2011) Prevalence of liver complications in children receiving long-term parenteral nutrition. *European Journal of Clinical Nutrition* 65, 743–749.

Pironi, L., Joly, F., Forbes, A., Colomb, V., Lyszkowska, M., Baxter, J., Gabe, S., Hébuterne, X., Gambarara, M., Gottrand, F., Cuerda, C., Thul, P., Messing, B., Goulet, O., Staun, M. and Van Gossum, A.; Home Artificial Nutrition & Chronic Intestinal Failure Working Group of the European Society for Clinical Nutrition and Metabolism (ESPEN) (2011) Long-term follow-up of patients on home parenteral nutrition in Europe: implications for intestinal transplantation. *Gut* 60, 17–25.

Pironi, L., Goulet, O., Buchman, A., Messing, B., Gabe, S., Candusso, M., Bond, G., Gupte, G., Pertkiewicz, M., Steiger, E., Forbes, A., Van Gossum, A. and Pinna, A.D.; Home Artificial Nutrition and Chronic Intestinal Failure Working Group of ESPEN (2012) Outcome on home parenteral nutrition for benign intestinal failure: a review of the literature and benchmarking with the European prospective survey of ESPEN. *Clinical Nutrition* 31, 831–845.

Puder, M., Valim, C., Meisel, J.A., Le, H.D., de Meijer, V.E., Robinson, E.M., Zhou, J., Duggan, C. and Gura, M. (2009) Parenteral fish oil improves outcome in patients with parenteral nutrition-associated liver injury. *Annals of Surgery* 250, 395–402.

Puntis, J.W.L. (1995) Home parenteral nutrition. *Archives of Disease in Childhood* 72, 186–190.

Ricour, C., Gorski, A.M., Goulet, O., De Potter, S., Corriol, O., Postaire, M., Nihoul-Fékété, C., Jan, D., Révillon, Y., Lortat-Jacob, S. and Pellerin, D. (1990) Home parenteral nutrition in children: 8 years of experience with 112 patients. *Clinical Nutrition* 9, 65–71.
Roma, M.G. and Sanchez Pozzi, E.G. (2008) Oxidative stress: a radical way to stop making bile. *Annals of Hepatology* 7, 16–33.
Sauvat, F., Fusaro, F., Lacaille, F., Dupic, L., Bourdaud, N., Colomb, V., Hugot, J.P., Aigrain, Y., Goulet, O. and Revillon, Y. (2008) Is intestinal transplantation the future of children with definitive intestinal insufficiency? *European Journal of Pediatric Surgery* 18, 368–371.
Schmidt-Sommerfeld, E., Snyder, G., Rossi, T.M. and Lebenthal, E. (1990) Catheter-related complications in 35 children and adolescents with gastrointestinal disease on home parenteral nutrition. *JPEN Journal of Parenteral and Enteral Nutrition* 14, 148–151.
Shelton, C.M., Clark, A.J., Storm, M.C. and Helms, R.A. (2010) Plasma amino acid concentrations in 108 children receiving a pediatric amino acid formulation as part of parenteral nutrition. *Journal of Pediatric Pharmacology and Therapeutics* 15, 110–118.
Smith, L. and Daughtrey, H. (2000) Weaving the seamless web of care: an analysis of parents' perceptions of their needs following discharge of their child from hospital. *Journal of Advanced Nursing* 31, 812–820.
Sondheimer, J.M., Cadnapaphornchai, M., Sontag, M. and Zerbe, G.O. (1998a) Predicting the duration of dependence on parenteral nutrition after neonatal intestinal resection. *Journal of Pediatrics* 132, 80–84.
Sondheimer, J.M., Asturias, E. and Cadnapaphornchai, M. (1998b) Infection and cholestasis in neonates with intestinal resection and long-term parenteral nutrition. *Journal of Pediatric Gastroenterology and Nutrition* 27, 131–137.
Storm, M.C. and Helms, R.A. (2007) Normalizing plasma amino acid levels in pediatric patients requiring parenteral nutrition. *Nutrition in Clinical Practice* 22, 194–203.
Van Ommen, C.H. and Tabbers, M.M. (2010) Catheter-related thrombosis in children with intestinal failure and long-term parenteral nutrition: how to treat and to prevent? *Thrombosis Research* 126, 465–470.
Vargas, J.H., Ament, M.E. and Berquist, W.E. (1987) Long-term home parenteral nutrition in pediatrics: ten years of experience in 102 patients. *Journal of Pediatric Gastroenterology and Nutrition* 6, 24–32.
Wilmore, D.M. and Dudrick, S.J. (1968) Growth and development of an infant receiving all nutrients by vein. *Journal of the American Medical Association* 203, 860–864.
Wiskin, A.E., Cole, C., Owens, D.R., Morgan, M., Burge, D.M. and Beattie, R.M. (2012) Ten-year experience of home parenteral nutrition in a single centre. *Acta Paediatrica* 101, 524–527.
Wong, C., Akobeng, A.K., Miller, V. and Thomas, A.G. (2000) Quality of life of parents of children on home parenteral nutrition. *Gut* 46, 294–295.

34 Home Parenteral Nutrition: Quality of Life and Psychosocial Issues

Janet P. Baxter[1]* and Jose Manuel Moreno Villares[2]

[1]*Ninewells Hospital and Medical School, Dundee, UK;* [2]*Unidad de Nutrición Clínica, Hospital Universitario 12 de Octubre, Madrid, Spain*

Key Points

- One of the main aims of home parenteral nutrition (HPN) is to improve quality of life (QoL).
- HPN inevitably impacts QoL – either positively or negatively.
- HPN affects the patient as well as his/her family or caregiver.
- QoL assessment should be part of routine clinical monitoring.

Introduction

Home parenteral nutrition (HPN) remains the treatment of choice for patients with severe intestinal failure. The provision of equipment and services to allow treatment to be delivered at home aims to rehabilitate patients as far as possible to restore function, comfort and health. To meet the aims of therapy, patients and carers must be equipped with the knowledge, skills and confidence to manage this complex therapy in a safe and competent manner. According to Van Gossum *et al.* (1996) most centres in Europe train patients to manage their HPN while in hospital, 67% using standard protocols. Data from the British Artificial Nutrition Survey (Smith *et al.*, 2011) report that 97.4% of adult HPN patients were discharged to their own home; 60.1% of newly discharged patients in 2010 were described as independent compared with 52.0% in 2009 and 53.5% in 2008. Independence levels improve following discharge and 71% of established patients were described as fully independent. Approximately 40% of new registrations require 'some help' or 'total help' but only 29% of established cases require such help.

HPN has been described by patient groups as an 'enabling therapy' (Ehrenpreis and Hilf, 1998). Although considered a life-saving therapy, HPN radically

*E-mail: janetbaxter@nhs.net

changes life as patients are faced with the ongoing symptoms of the underlying condition and also with leading a complex, technology-dependent life. It is a time-consuming and invasive procedure and as well as facing physical problems, patients face difficulties in their everyday lives including a wide range of psychosocial problems. There are psychological issues for patients related to living with a central venous catheter and with the lifestyle restrictions that HPN poses (Stern, 2006). HPN puts great demands on patients and so inevitably has an impact on their quality of life (QoL). The alternatives are to die from malnutrition or dehydration, or to have lifelong parenteral nutrition in the hospital setting, which not only would be intolerable to patients but also an unacceptable use of healthcare resources. Therefore, patients and/or their carers need to be trained to administer parenteral nutrition at home safely to prevent potentially life-threatening complications such as intravenous catheter-related infections.

QoL in HPN

There is no universally accepted definition of QoL with different meanings depending on the application and context in which it is measured. The World Health Organization (1948) defined it as 'A state of complete physical, mental and social well-being, and not merely the absence of disease'.

Moving patients from hospital to home with HPN has improved QoL (Detsky *et al.*, 1986), but in some patients it is still associated with a substantial reduction in QoL (Winkler, 2005; Baxter *et al.*, 2006). HPN dependency can therefore have a detrimental effect on patients' social function as well as employment status, with unemployment rates of up to 86% reported. Thus, while HPN may offer many patients a lifeline, dependency can have a detrimental effect on QoL.

A review by Baxter *et al.* (2006) described a variety of studies of QoL among HPN patients with benign disease. Some have demonstrated positive effects and some have demonstrated negative effects. The differences in results may relate to the method of comparison. Some studies have, for example, compared pre-HPN with HPN-dependent status, and some have compared HPN with the situation after successful intestinal transplantation. Because of the growing number of centres successfully offering intestinal transplantation, data in this field are required to demonstrate patients' subjective perceptions of health and QoL. Despite the fact that an improvement in QoL is one of the main aims of HPN, studies addressing this important topic are relatively rare. In a bibliographic study of patient-assessed health-outcome measures, no instruments were reported that looked at QoL among patients receiving HPN, although 100 reports covered 'gastrointestinal disease' (Borgaonkar and Irvine, 2000). One study found the best QoL to be among young patients with a long duration of treatment, with high self-esteem, in good personal relationships, and with wealth and employment (Richards and Irving, 1997). The worst QoL was observed in older patients, those addicted to narcotics, those who were less affluent, single or unemployed, and those who had a short duration of treatment (Richards and Irving, 1997). The initiation of HPN does not remove or reduce the systemic symptoms associated with the underlying diseases. Indeed, because of the nature of HPN therapy, a new set of problems, such as physical and social functioning and family and relationship problems, often develop. It is therefore not surprising that QoL on HPN does not appear good when compared with that of the normal population. When compared with the pre-HPN state, however, QoL appears likely to improve.

Malignant disease

In the USA (Howard *et al.*, 1991) malignancy is the main indication for HPN, accounting for 46% of patients. However, there is considerable variance in the prevalence of HPN in incurable cancer across Europe. Van Gossum *et al.* (1996) found the prevalence to range from 60% in the Netherlands to the lowest of 5% in the UK. There may be ethical and cultural differences as well as variance in healthcare provision.

It is interesting to note that in an Italian study (Bozzetti *et al.*, 2002) only 43% of patients were aware of their diagnosis and <1% of their prognosis, whereas in the UK diagnosis and prognosis are usually fully disclosed. The evidence of improved QoL on HPN in advanced cancer remains poor but the dilemma for clinicians still exists – should we burden the patient/caregiver with the complexity of HPN technology or should we let the patient die with dignity (McKinlay, 2004) without the added risk of complications?

The duration of HPN for the majority of patients is short lived. King *et al.* (1993) recorded a median duration of 66.5 days for patients with gynaecological cancers. Other studies have demonstrated a median duration of 4 months (Cozzaglio *et al.*, 1997; Bozzetti *et al.*, 2002). King *et al.* (1993) reported an HPN-related complication rate of 9%, mainly catheter-related sepsis, and there was a readmission rate of 4% over the entire HPN period – meaning that HPN was relatively safe and readmission rate to hospital acceptable.

King *et al.* (1993) showed an overall improvement in QoL compared with that pre-HPN. Morale and social interactions improved as did gastrointestinal discomfort, nausea, vomiting and fatigue. Sixteen per cent of patients worked outside the home and 6.6% undertook recreational travel. However, in this study the perception of patients' QoL was based on the impressions of clinicians who had undertaken a retrospective case note review. Cozzaglio *et al.* (1997) also reported and improved QoL for patients who survived more than 3 months, but it was also based on clinical judgement rather than on direct evidence from patients.

Bozzetti *et al.* (2002) studied 69 Italian patients, measuring QoL using the Rotterdam Symptom Checklist (RSCL), a validated cancer-specific tool, at the start of HPN followed by monthly intervals. Fifty per cent of patients complained of worries, tension and desperate feelings about the future. Anorexia, tiredness, lack of energy and decreased sexual interest were evident. Most were unable to do housekeeping, climb stairs, do odd jobs, walk outside and go to work, or they needed help with these activities. After 1 month on HPN, approximately 50% of patients had deteriorated, 40% had improved and the rest remained the same in assessment of physical, psychological functions and activity.

Cozzaglio *et al.* (1997) and Bozzetti *et al.* (2002) have demonstrated improved or stabilized QoL for patients surviving longer than 3 months, although this deteriorated during the final 2 months of life. This indicates that, for HPN to impact positively on QoL, a patient needs to survive for at least 3 months. Both studies used the Karnofsky performance status (KPS), which is a score that measures a functional score (range from 100 = normal to 10 = moribund) to follow the course of a patient's illness. Those with the highest score at the time of the tumour diagnosis tended to have the best survival and quality of life over the course of their illness. Patients starting HPN with a KPS score >50 survived longer than those with a lower score.

Illness beliefs

Until a study in 2005 was published by Fortune *et al.* (2005), little was known about illness beliefs held by HPN patients. Sixty-one patients were assessed regarding their beliefs about causes of their condition, consequences, symptoms experiences, personal and treatment control and recurrence, and feelings of anger, upset, anxiety, low mood and fear. They found that emotional effects on patients were affected by how well they understand their illness and how much their treatment makes sense to them. The relationship between psychological factors, disease and illness is important for optimizing treatments and evaluating outcomes.

Eating and drinking

The requirement for intravenous feeding is obviously based on the fact that insufficient food/fluid is absorbed to maintain nutrition/fluid status. Some patients continue to eat and drink while others take nothing orally. The eating behaviour of HPN patients is not frequently assessed. Using a questionnaire to assess appetite and intake, Oz *et al.* (2008) studied the QoL in relation to eating habits of HPN patients in Israel. They found the oral intake of HPN patients to be significantly impaired and this correlated with physical activity and QoL. Winkler *et al.* (2010) further studied the relationship between food intake and QoL in HPN patients by interviewing patients about their eating habits. Three patterns of eating emerged: (i) eating for survival; (ii) eating for health benefits; and (iii) eating for social pleasure. They concluded that clinicians should ensure that attention is paid to the emotional context of eating in this population.

Technology dependence

The need for dependence on the technology associated with nutrient infusion impacts on the QoL of patients. The complexity of HPN is related to the requirement for a central venous catheter, an infusion pump, drip stand and the ancillary items required for safe delivery of the feeding. Patients need to have a dedicated area at home to store equipment and have a refrigerator store their HPN bags. It has been suggested (Winkler *et al.*, 2006) that more work is needed to prepare patients for the technology-dependent lifestyle.

Psychosocial complaints

HPN does not exist alone – there are often multifactorial issues including the symptoms of the underlying illness and the problems related to leading a technology-dependent life. There is an inevitable impact on lifestyle associated with treatment (Baxter *et al.*, 2006). As well as the technical issues they have to deal with, patients also have psychosocial complaints. For HPN to be effective and to allow patients to remain out of the acute care setting there has to be careful training of the patient and his/her family or caregiver. The most significant complication of HPN is catheter-related bloodstream infection (CRBSI), which carries significant morbidity and mortality. Anxiety and fear are common reactions to the realistic threat of life-threatening complications of treatment including severe infection, thrombosis and liver damage (Persoon *et al.*, 2005; Huisman-de Waal *et al.*, 2007). Depression, anger, negative self-image and social limitations are frequently reported (Baxter *et al.*, 2006). Depression is seen in up to 65% and may have serious consequences as it has been shown to lead to less careful catheter care and social impairment in 55% (Persoon *et al.*, 2005), all of which correlate with QoL.

The most frequently reported physical problems that HPN patients report are muscle cramps (Elphick *et al.*, 2009) and depression and fatigue (Huisman-de Waal *et al.*, 2011). Although reported as a 'minor' complication compared with CRBSI, central vein thrombosis or liver disease, cramps have a distressing effect on patients and affect QoL. Severe fatigue has been reported as one of the most frequent complaints – in up to 63% of HPN patients (Huisman-de-Waal *et al.*, 2011). Despite its lowering effect on QoL, its recognition and treatment remain suboptimal.

QoL Assessment

Assessment of QoL on HPN is vital to guide clinicians and healthcare providers in strategies to optimize and improve patient care. A primary problem with existing QoL data in the HPN population is the inability to determine whether any effects on QoL are a direct result of HPN itself or a consequence of the underlying disease.

The assessment of QoL needs to produce clinically relevant data on patient-derived issues as a means of facilitating communication to identify a range of problems that HPN patients experience. They can then be in a position to more easily share problems with their HPN clinician and nutrition support team, and can also provide information to other patients to allow better understanding of HPN-related issues. QoL is a patient-reported outcome that is usually measured with carefully designed and validated instruments such as questionnaires. It should be measured from the patient's perspective as the clinician, family member or caregiver is likely to provide inaccurate results. In the context of HPN, this requirement is fulfilled by the development of the HPN-QOL© (Baxter *et al.*, 2010).

The HPN-QOL© has been developed in response to the recognition that a treatment-specific instrument did not exist to assess the QoL of HPN patients.

Using published guidelines, the development of the HPN-QOL© involved qualitative research methodology, semi-structured interviews with health professionals and patients and then pilot testing. The questionnaire was then subject to clinical and psychometric validation to make sure that it was fit for purpose and acceptable to the HPN patient population. It has been translated into seven European languages – Danish, Dutch, French, German, Italian, Polish and Spanish (Baxter *et al.*, 2008). Further work was completed to allow the French version to be suitable for use in Belgium and French-speaking Canada and the English version slightly adapted for use in the USA.

QoL in Children Receiving HPN and Their Families

A major aim of providing parenteral nutrition in the home setting is to minimize morbidity and maximize survival and QoL. In children, QoL is defined as a multidimensional situation that is composed of social, emotional and physical functions of the child/adolescent and the family (Kostac, 2006). When compared with adults there are theoretical and practical differences in defining QoL in children. QoL in children depends on the complex connections between the children and their social environment. Environment factors include families, peers, neighbours, school and healthcare organizations. Children go to school, play games and participate in sport activities and social events. In adolescence, chronic illness may play a great role in the development of independence or in body image.

Paediatric HPN patients and their families benefit psychologically by being at home and resuming relatively normal lives. A major difference between children and adults is the important role of families in providing and improving health care. The families are accepting a huge responsibility by becoming both parents and medical providers. Then, when we evaluate QoL in children it seems mandatory to evaluate their parents' QoL as well.

Young children cannot define their own health-related QoL so it needs to be done by their parents. But measurement should be done from the child's perspective. This is even clearer in older children and adolescents.

Tools to evaluate QoL in children

QoL measurements have been used increasingly in the evaluation of medical care for chronic illness. Health-related QoL scales developed for adults are not appropriate for children (Bullinger *et al.*, 2002). In a systematic review published in 2006, the authors found 28 generic and 47 condition-specific tools to evaluate QoL in children (Pane *et al.*, 2006). Most of them were developed as multidimensional and based on a psychometric model. Domains include emotional, social and physical health, and well-being. Items commonly assessed difficulties, intensity and frequency of feelings and symptoms, in contrast to positive aspects of life and happiness (Davis *et al.*, 2006). Unfortunately, there are no specific questionnaires for either HPN or short bowel syndrome in children and their families.

QoL in paediatric HPN patients

Initial studies on the effects HPN had on lifestyle were focused on growth and development and returning to school or participating in peer-group activities. Only in the last few years have general or specific QoL questionnaires been evaluated both in children and families. An excellent review has been recently published on QoL in adults and children on HPN (Chambers, 2011). Table 34.1 summarizes the QoL studies in children on HPN.

Table 34.1. QoL studies in children on HPN. (From Chambers, 2011.)

Author	QoL assessment	Outcome
Dudrick *et al.* (1969)	Clinical parameters	Normal growth and development and faster restoration to productive life
Filler *et al.* (1969)	Clinical parameters	Reduced length of hospital stay and acceptable growth
Strobel *et al.* (1978)	Peer-group activities	Majority attend full-time classes Improved state of general well-being
Strobel *et al.* (1979)	Peer group activities (HPN in Crohn's)	Majority attend full-time classes Improved state of general well-being
Byrne *et al.* (1979)	Clinical parameters Peer-group activities	Sufficient growth Improved school attendance Normal lives at home
Cannon *et al.* (1980)	Clinical parameters Development assessment Gesell evaluations	Appropriate development during the first 2 years of HPN
Wolfe *et al.* (1983)	Clinical parameters	Depressive symptoms were common Satisfactory growth and development
Ralston *et al.* (1984)	Clinical parameters Gesell evaluations	Adequate growth and development within the first 3 years of life
Ricour *et al.* (1985)	None stated	QoL near normal
Amarnath *et al.* (1987)	Medical interviews	Good general sense of well-being
O'Connor *et al.* (1988)	Weschsler Preschool and Primary Scale of Intelligence Beery Buktenica Developmental Test of Visual-Motor Integration	Average intelligence with perceptual-motor delays and some problems of attention
Gorski *et al.* (1989)	None stated	Satisfactory growth and QoL
Ricour *et al.* (1990)	Medical and socio-psychological interviews	Remarkable improvement in QoL
Weber *et al.* (1991)	None stated	Excellent growth, development and QoL
Bissett *et al.* (1992)	Griffiths Mental Development Scales Wechsler Preschool and Primary Scale of Intelligence	Normal growth and development

Continued

Table 34.1. *Continued.*

Author	QoL assessment	Outcome
O'Hanrahan and Irving (1992)	School attendance and development	Satisfactory lifestyle
Loras Duclaux *et al.* (1993)	Medical and socio-psychological interviews	Normal school attendance Decreased physical activity Difficulties in eating behaviours
Candusso *et al.* (1995)	None stated	Presence of behaviour disorders
Leonberg *et al.* (1998)	Clinical parameters Expressive and receptive language, auditory memory and visual-motor function	Normal development Discrepancies between language and perceptual-motor performance
Candusso *et al.* (2001)	None stated	Presence of psychological disability
Engstrom *et al.* (2003)	Child Behaviour Checklist questionnaires Interview Schedule of Social Interaction	More psychological and emotional problems than peers
Gottrand *et al.* (2005)	Qualin Questionnaire, Auquei Questionnaire and OK.ado Questionnaire	QoL not different from healthy children
Colomb *et al.* (2007)	None stated	Repeated hospitalizations have a serious impact on QoL
Emedo *et al.* (2010)	Medical and psycho-social interviews	Good resilience, maintain a positive outlook and cope well with illness-related demands

When considering studying QoL, most published studies have typically involved parents' ratings of their children's QoL. Usually parents rate lower scores than adolescents or older children when referred to the children's QoL. Recently two studies have attempted to evaluate the QoL asking the children. The study by Gottrand *et al.* (2005), a multicentre study involving 72 patients presenting a digestive disease requiring HPN, 90 siblings, 67 fathers and 69 mothers, showed that QoL of HPN-dependent children and siblings was not different from that of healthy children, suggesting that they actually use effective coping strategies. On the contrary, the study by Engstrom *et al.* (2003) in 20 families pointed out that children and adolescents on HPN were quite distressed psychologically. When individually questioned about their lifestyle and health, patients on HPN cope well with the technique but are troubled when complications of the underlying disease arise. Mainly the burdens of life with intravenous nutrition appear to be less significant than living with a chronic disease. As has been shown by Baxter *et al.* (2010) in the adult population, there is a need to analyse differently the burdens from the technique and the ones from the underlying disease. This is one of the focuses of the Home Artificial Working Group of the European Society for Parenteral and Enteral Nutrition (ESPEN), and the topic of several ongoing studies (http://www.espen.org/homeartificialnutrition.html).

Quality of life in the families caring for a child on HPN

Having a child on HPN has a major impact on the QoL of the parents and other siblings. Initial studies on QoL in children on HPN were devoted to consequences in family lifestyle and constraints (Loras Duclaux *et al.*, 1993). Although parents have been shown to provide a high quality of HPN care, they are aware that the survival of their child is dependent on their skill in providing the right care, and many find this a great burden. Most studies show a significant deterioration for social life, family life, sex life and work when compared with healthy families. They are also more likely to be physically tired and to have difficulties in taking holidays, going shopping and spending time with partners (Wong *et al.*, 2000). Mothers of HPN children had lower QoL scores than reference mother populations and lower than fathers' scores for items related to work, inner life and freedom. Interestingly, mothers' QoL scores were not significantly correlated with their children's scores. Siblings, on the contrary, and different from expected, had a QoL similar to their peers. But this aspect has been scarcely studied.

There are many sources of stress including: (i) general uncertainty about child's future; (ii) the unpredictability of complications that may occur; (iii) the need to balance domestic and employment responsibilities; and (iv) physical exhaustion associated with sleepless nights/sleep disturbance (Brook, 1998; Baxter *et al.*, 2008).

One question that arises from the results of the published studies is whether the psychological distress of the families of children on HPN can be reduced or prevented. A major factor in reducing the psychological distress is reducing the worry about complications related to the technique. A multi-professional and close team approach can help in this issue. To cope with the burdens of HPN as well as having a child with a chronic condition, the joining of an association of families or patients with the same problem may help. There are some good experiences in participating in summer camps with other patients with the same condition (http://www.oley.org/links).

Healthcare professionals should be aware of these problems and offer the necessary support to families providing this demanding care for their children.

Summary

HPN allows patients with intestinal failure to survive and lead relatively normal lives at home, but their QoL remains impaired by the dependence on intravenous infusions and loss of control over their treatment and condition.

HPN is associated with numerous complications, all of which increase morbidity and mortality. The provision of parenteral nutrition raises challenging ethical questions, increasing in recent years as the indication for treatment has come to be considered life-enhancing as well as life-extending. The psychological impact has to be considered when assessing the appropriateness of treatment, together with detecting the potential problems and concerns that face patients and families. Long-term HPN patients may have improved symptoms from their underlying illnesses, but they need continued nutrition support. This may lead to problems of psychological adaptation as they try to come to terms with the prospect of a lifelong therapy. Apart from the relief of symptoms, there may be other issues affecting QoL, such as fatigue, worry or lack of clinical support.

There has been much more interest in health-related QoL in recent years as, along with survival, it is used as a key clinical outcome. As current healthcare moves to a 'patient centred' approach, we need to incorporate assessment of QoL as a patient-reported outcome – along with patient satisfaction. Embedding QoL measurement into routine practice is a challenge, but is one that should be addressed according to ESPEN guidelines.

References

Amarnath, R.P., Fleming, C.R. and Perrault, J. (1987) Home parenteral nutrition in chronic intestinal diseases: its effect on growth and development. *Journal of Pediatric Gastroenterology and Nutrition* 6, 89–95.

Baxter, J.P., Fayers, P.M. and McKinlay, A.W. (2006) A review of the quality of life of adult patients treated with long-term parenteral nutrition. *Clinical Nutrition* 25, 543–553.

Baxter, J.P., Fayers, P.M. and McKinlay, A.W. (2008) The development and translation of a treatment-specific quality of life questionnaire for adult patients on home parenteral nutrition. *e-SPEN Journal* 3(1), e22–e28.

Baxter, J.P., Fayers, P.M. and McKinlay, A.W. (2010) The clinical and psychometric validation of a questionnaire to assess the quality of life of adult patients treated with long term parenteral nutrition. *JPEN Journal of Parenteral and Enteral Nutrition* 34, 131–142.

Bissett, W.M., Stapleford, P., Long, S., Chamberlain, A., Sokel, B. and Milla, P.J. (1992) Home parenteral nutrition in chronic intestinal failure. *Archives of Diseases in Childhood* 67, 109–114.

Borgaonkar, M.R. and Irvine, E.J. (2000) Quality of life measurement in gastrointestinal and liver disorders. *Gut* 47, 444–454.

Bozzetti, F., Cozzaglio, L., Biganzoli, E., Chiavenna, G., De Cicco, M., Donati, D., Gilli, G., Percolla, S. and Pironi, L. (2002) Quality of life and length of survival in advanced cancer patients on home parenteral nutrition. *Clinical Nutrition* 21, 281–287.

Brook, G. (1998) Quality of life issues: parenteral nutrition to small bowel transplantation – a review. *Nutrition* 14, 813–816.

Bullinger, M., Schmidt, S., Peterson, C. and The Disabkids Group (2002) Assessing quality of life of children with chronic health conditions and disabilities: a European approach. *International Journal of Rehabilitation Research* 25, 197–206.

Byrne, W.J., Ament, M.E., Burke, M. and Fonkalsrud, E. (1979) Home parenteral nutrition. *Surgical Gynecology and Obstetrics* 149, 593–599.

Candusso, M., Giglio, L. and Faraguna, D. (1995) Long-term parenteral nutrition in children. *Clinical Nutrition* 14(Suppl. 1), 28–32.

Candusso, M., Faraguna, D., Dileo, G. and Loganes, C. (2001) Home parenteral nutrition in children. *Clinical Nutrition* 20(Suppl. 2), 7–10.

Cannon, R.A., Byrne, W.J., Ament, M.E., Gates, B., O'Connor, M. and Fonkalsrud, E. (1980) Home parenteral nutrition in infants. *Journal of Pediatrics* 96, 1098–1104.

Chambers, A. (2011) Quality of life in intestinal failure. PhD thesis, Queen Mary College University of London, London.

Colomb, V., Dabbas-Tyan, M., Taupin, P., Talbotec, C., Revillon, Y. and Jand, D. (2007) Long-term outcome of children receiving home parenteral nutrition: a 20-year single center experience in 302 patients. *Journal of Pediatric Gastroenterology and Nutrition* 44, 347–353.

Cozzaglio, L., Balzola, F., Cosetino, F., Cicco, M., Fellagara, P., Gaggiotti, G., Gallitelli, L., Giacosa, A., Fadda, M., Gavazzi, C., Pirovano, F. and Bozzetti, F. (1997) Outcome of cancer patients receiving home parenteral nutrition. *JPEN Journal of Parenteral and Enteral Nutrition* 21, 339–342.

Davis, E., Waters, E., Mackinnon, A., Reddihough, D., Graham, D.K., Mehmet-Radji, O. and Boyd, R. (2006) Paediatric quality of life instruments: a review of the impact of the conceptual framework on outcomes. *Developmental Medicine & Child Neurology* 48, 311–318.

Detsky, A.S., McLaughlin, J.R., Abrams, H.B., Abbe, K., Whitwell, J., Bombadier, C. and Jeejeebhoy, K. (1986) Quality of life of patients on long term parenteral nutrition at home. *Journal of Internal Medicine* 1, 26–33.

Dudrick, S.J., Wilmore, D.W., Vars, H.M. and Rhoads, J.E. (1969) Can intravenous feeding as the sole means of nutrition support growth in the child and restore weight loss in an adult? An affirmative answer. *Annals of Surgery* 169, 974–984.

Ehrenpreis, B. and Hilf, A. (1998) Home parenteral nutrition; the consumer's perspective. *Lifeline Letter* November/December, 1–3.

Elphick, D.A., Baker, M., Baxter, J.P., Nightingale, J.M., Bowling, T., Page, K.B. and McAlindon, M.E. (2009) Muscle cramps are the commonest side effect of home parenteral nutrition. *Clinical Nutrition* 28, 351–361.

Emedo, M.J., Godfrey, E.I. and Hill, S.M. (2010) A qualitative study of the quality of life of children receiving intravenous nutrition at home. *Journal of Pediatric Gastroenterology and Nutrition* 50, 431–440.

Engstrom, I., Bjornestam, B. and Finkel, Y. (2003) Psychological distress associated with home parenteral nutrition in Swedish children, adolescents, and their parents: preliminary results. *Journal of Pediatric Gastroenterology and Nutrition* 37, 246–250.

Filler, F.M., Eraklis, A.J., Rubin, V.G. and Das, J.B. (1969) Long term total parenteral nutrition in infants. *New England Journal of Medicine* 281, 589–594.

Fortune, D.G., Varden, J., Parker, S., Harper, L., Richards, H.L. and Shaffer, J.L. (2005) Illness beliefs of patients on home parenteral nutrition (HPN) and their relation to emotional distress. *Clinical Nutrition* 24, 896–903.

Gorski, A.M., Goulet, O., Lamor, M., Postaire, M., Lalondrelle, F., Corriol, O., Cauchefer, V., Nihoul-Fekete, C., Revillon, Y. and Jan, D. (1989) Home parenteral nutrition in children. Evaluation after 8 years' activity with 88 patients. *Archives of French Pediatrics* 46, 323–329.

Gottrand, F., Staszewski, P., Colomb, V., Loras-Duclaux, I., Guimber, D. and Marinier, E. (2005) Satisfaction in different life domains in children receiving home parenteral nutrition and their families. *Journal of Pediatrics* 146, 793–797.

Howard, L., Heaphey, L., Fleming, C.R., Lininger, L. and Steiger, E. (1991) Four years of North American registry: home parenteral nutrition outcome data and their implications for patient management. *JPEN Journal of Parenteral and Enteral Nutrition* 15, 384–393.

Huisman-de Waal, G., Schoonhoven, L., Jansen, J. and Wanten, G. (2007) The impact of home parenteral nutrition on daily life – a review. *Clinical Nutrition* 26, 275–288.

Huisman-de Waal, G., Versleijen, M., van Achterberg, T., Jansen, J.B., Sauerwein, H., Schoonhoven, L. and Wanten, G. (2011) Psychosocial complaints are associated with venous access-device related complications in patients on home parenteral nutrition. *JPEN Journal of Parenteral and Enteral Nutrition* 5, 588–595.

King, L.A., Carson, L.F., Konstantinides, N., House, M.S., Adcock, L.L., Prem, K.A., Twiggs, L.B. and Cerra, F.B. (1993) Outcome assessment of home parenteral nutrition in patients with

gynaecological malignancies: what have we learned in a decade of experience? *Gynaecological Oncology* 51, 377–382.
Kostac, M. (2006) Measuring the quality of life in children. *Biotechnology & Biotechnology Equipment* 20, 142–144.
Leonberg, B.L., Chuang, E., Eicher, P., Tershakoves, A.M., Leonard, L. and Stallings, V.A. (1998) Long-term growth and development in children after home parenteral nutrition. *Journal of Pediatrics* 132, 461–466.
Loras Duclaux, I., De Potter, S., Pharaon, I., Olives, J.P. and Hernier, M. (1993) Qualité de vie des enfants en nutrition parentérale à domicile et de leurs parents. *Pédiatrie* 7/8, 555–560.
McKinlay, A. (2004) Nutrition support in patients with advanced cancer: permission to fall out? *Proceedings of the Nutrition Society* 63, 431–435.
O'Connor, M., Ralston, C.W. and Ament, M.E. (1988) Intellectual and perceptual-motor performance of children receiving prolonged home parenteral nutrition. *Pediatrics* 81, 231–236.
O'Hanrahan, T. and Irving, M.H. (1992) Home parenteral nutrition in the United Kingdom and Ireland. *Clinical Nutrition* 11, 331–336.
Oz, V., Theilla, M. and Singer, P. (2008) Eating habits of patients on long term parenteral nutrition in Israel. *Clinical Nutrition* 27, 95–99.
Pane, S., Solans, M., Gaite, L., Serra-Sutton, V., Estrada, M.D. and Rajmil, L. (2006) *Instrumentos de calidad relacionada con la salud en la edad pediátrica. Revisión sistemática de la literatura: actualización.* Agència d'Avaluació de Tecnologia i Recerca Mèdiques and Red YRYSS, Barcelona, Spain.
Persoon, A., Huisman-de Waal, G., Naber, T., Schoonhoven, L., Tirzah, T., Sauerwein, H. and van Achterberg, T. (2005) Impact of long-term HPN on daily life in adults. *Clinical Nutrition* 24, 304–313.
Ralston, C.W., O'Connor, M., Ament, M.E., Berquist, W. and Parmelee, A.H. Jr (1984) Somatic growth and developmental functioning in children receiving prolonged home parenteral nutrition. *Journal of Pediatrics* 195, 842–846.
Richards, D.M. and Irving, M.H. (1997) Assessing the quality of life of patients with intestinal failure on home parenteral nutrition. *Gut* 40, 218–222.
Ricour, C., Duhamel, J.F., Arnaud-Battendier, F., Collar, Y., Revillon, Y. and Nihoul-Fekete, C. (1985) Enteral and parenteral nutrition in the short bowel syndrome in children. *World Journal of Surgery* 9, 310–315.
Ricour, C., Gorski, A.M., Goulet, O., Potter, S., Corriol, O. and Postaire, M. (1990) Home parenteral nutrition in children: 8 years of experience with 112 patients. *Clinical Nutrition* 9, 65–71.
Smith, T., Micklewright, A., Hirst, A., Stratton, R. and Baxter, J. (2011) *BANS Annual Report, 2011. Artificial Nutrition Support in the UK 2000–2010.* BAPEN, Redditch, UK. Available at: http://www.bapen.org.uk/pdfs/bans_reports/bans_report_11.pdf
Stern, J. (2006) Home parenteral nutrition and the psyche: psychological challenges for patient and family. *Proceedings of the Nutrition Society* 65, 222–226.
Strobel, C.T., Byrne, W.J., Fonkalsrud, E.W. and Ament, M.E. (1978) Home parenteral nutrition: results in 34 pediatric patients. *Annals of Surgery* 188, 394–403.
Strobel, C.T., Byrne, W.J. and Ament, M.E. (1979) Home parenteral nutrition in children with Crohn's disease: an effective management alternative. *Gastroenterology* 77, 272–279.
Van Gossum, A., Bakker, H., De Francesco, A., Ladefoged, K., Leon-Sanz, M., Messing, B., Pironi, L., Pertkiewicz, M. and Shaffer, J. (1996) Home parenteral nutrition in adults: a multicentre survey in Europe in 1993. ESPEN-Home Artificial Working Group. *Clinical Nutrition* 15, 53–59.
Weber, T.R., Tracy, T. Jr and Connors, R.H. (1991) Short-bowel syndrome in children. Quality of life in an era of improved survival. *Archives of Surgery* 126, 841–846.

Winkler, M.F. (2005) Quality of life in adult home parenteral nutrition patients. *JPEN Journal of Parenteral and Enteral Nutrition* 29, 162–170.
Winkler, M.F., Ross, V.M., Piamjariyakul, U., Gajewski, B. and Smith, C.E. (2006) Technology dependence in home care: impact on patients and their family caregivers. *Nutrition in Clinical Practice* 21, 544–556.
Winkler, M.F., Wetle, T., Smith, C., Hagan, E., O'Sullivan Maillet, J. and Touger-Decker, R. (2010) The meaning of food and eating among home parenteral nutrition adults with intestinal failure: a qualitative inquiry. *Journal of the American Dietetic Association* 110, 1676–1683.
Wolfe, B.M., Beer, W.H., Hayashi, J.T., Halsted, C.H., Cannon, R.A. and Cox, K.L. (1983) Experience with home parenteral nutrition. *American Journal of Surgery* 146, 7–14.
Wong, C., Akoberng, A.K., Miller, V. and Thomas, A.G. (2000) Quality of life of parents of children on home parenteral nutrition. *Gut* 46, 294–295.
World Health Organization (1948) Preamble to the Constitution of the World Health Organization as adopted by the International Health Conference, New York, 19–22 June, 1946; signed on 22 July 1946 by the representatives of 61 States (*Official Records of the World Health Organization*, no. 2, p. 100) and entered into force on 7 April 1948.

VI Miscellaneous Aspects of Home Parenteral Nutrition

35 Ethical and Legal Aspects of Home Parenteral Nutrition

Federico Bozzetti[1]* and Simon Allison[2]

[1]*Faculty of Medicine, University of Milan, Milan, Italy;* [2]*Clinical Nutrition Unit, University Hospital, Queen's Medical Centre, Nottingham, UK*

Key Points

- Follow the four moral principles of beneficence, non-maleficence, respect for autonomy and justice.
- No one of them has supremacy over the others.
- Always try to defend the best interests and wishes of the patient.
- Consider morally equivalent the withholding and the withdrawing of home parenteral nutrition.
- Be aware that the concept of medical futility is ethically invalid and pragmatically ineffectual.
- Discuss frankly with the patient and family the pros and cons of every deliberation; this will help to avoid conflict and will pre-empt them from an excessive emotional impact.

Introduction

Ethical codes of caring professions include not only minimal standards of behaviour and morality but also ideals, and have been described as the 'collective conscience of our profession'. The law, on the other hand, defends individual rights and liberties and sets minimal standards below which conduct can be regarded as lacking in care, negligent or downright criminal. It also protects those who are unable or incompetent to make their own decisions. The legal frameworks may differ, in detail, from one country to another, but in European countries is based largely on a common ethical tradition. For these reasons, this chapter focuses mainly on the main principles underlying all of medical ethics (Lennard Jones,

*E-mail: federicobozzetti@gmail.com

1988; MacFie, 2000; Allison, 2004) rather than on legal issues that may be different in various countries.

Especially, clinical decisions regarding patients undergoing home parenteral nutrition (HPN) for conditions of intestinal failure associated with a severe basic disease may be fraught with ethical and sometimes legal implications. Reasons for this include: (i) the ability of medicine to prolong 'biological' life through the use of technology; (ii) the global acceptance, in Western countries, that the competent patient is empowered to take part in medical decisions; and (iii) concerns about financial constraints and cost containments. In some sense, the benefits of medical advance and social progress have introduced a new set of burdens.

Principles of Moral Reasoning

The four classic clusters of principles as proposed by Beauchamp and Childress (2001) are: (i) beneficence; (ii) non-maleficence (both originally propounded by Hippocrates); (iii) respect for autonomy; and (iv) justice. No one principle automatically enjoys supremacy over the others but overreliance on them can be simplistic; rather, ethical decisions require weighing and balancing the various principles against one another in each specific situation.

1. *Beneficence.* Aim to do some good, foster the interests and happiness of the patient. This entails not only good intentions but also the necessity to first, be equipped with the latest published knowledge concerning the benefits and risks of HPN and, second, support or take part in the research needed to obtain such knowledge.

2. *Non-maleficence.* Aim to avoid doing harm. Ask the question 'is HPN really in the patient's interests, or do the likely risks outweigh any possible benefits?'

3. *Respect for autonomy.* The Nuremberg code in 1945 added to the first two Hippocratic principles the principle of autonomy, recognizing the patient's human right to take all decisions concerning the management of his/her condition. This concept was confirmed in the Helsinki Declaration and the International Covenant on Civil and Political Rights. The mentally competent patient, therefore, not only has the ethical but also the legal right to refuse treatment. In numerous legal cases the courts consistently have reaffirmed that the refusal of treatment by a competent individual must be respected.

The converse of this is that, in Europe at least, no doctor can be forced by the patient, the patient's family or by anyone else to give treatment that he or she believes be futile or against the patient's interest.

In relation to the patient's competence, the British Medical Association and the Law Society have published clear guidelines on the assessment of mental capacity. A person should be able to:

- understand in simple language what the medical treatment (or research intervention) is, its purpose and nature and why it is proposed;
- understand its principal benefits, risks and alternatives;
- understand in broad terms what the consequences of not receiving the proposed treatment will be;

- retain the information for long enough to make an effective decision; and
- make a free choice (without pressure).

As a consequence, if there is a programme of starting short-term HPN or withdrawing an already ongoing HPN programme in an incurable patient, an open discussion with the patient helps to decipher his/her exact wishes/expectations about the future and allow him/her to maintain dignity as a moral autonomous agent.

4. *Justice*. This concept, which has evolved through the 20th century, demands that there should be equal access to healthcare for all. However, the increasing complexity and cost of treatment technology, exemplified by HPN, faces all societies with the problem of satisfying increasing demands from finite resources (Kitzhaber, 1993).

The above principles, while appearing straightforward in many cases, can also involve a duty to society to husband resources and use them effectively. Although we should be wary of allowing ourselves to be swayed by short-term administrative, business or political considerations that have little to do with clinical benefit or justice, nonetheless every healthcare system operates under some rationing constraints, by ability to pay, reimbursement, waiting lists or political decisions concerning state funding (Hermann, 1999).

Examples

Some practical examples concerning HPN will illustrate the role of ethical and legal considerations. Short-term hospital care is not discussed and the focus is mainly on the treatment of patients in their own home. It will be relevant, however, to consider long-term care in community institutions such as nursing homes for the elderly.

HPN is essentially the treatment of gastrointestinal failure that is permanent or likely to last for many months before it is corrected by definitive treatment. In most cases, the clinical, ethical and legal decisions are straightforward. In some cases, however, there may be some doubt concerning the patient's capacity to cope with the technical demands of this treatment without a high risk of serious and possibly life-threatening complications. This may be due to mental or emotional limitations or to the lack of resources in the patient's home. Doubt may be resolved by a well-supervised and time-limited trial of treatment, with agreement to withdraw treatment if complications prove prohibitive. The doctor should also consider carefully whether he and his team have the requisite resources, training and experience to carry out HPN in an optimal way (Allison, 1992) or whether the patient should be referred to the nearest specialist centre. To carry out treatment without such considerations could be construed as unethical or even negligent. In this respect, it is the duty of treatment centres to keep careful records of their outcomes and complication rates in order that adequate judgements of risk can be made. Difficulties arise in the case of frail elderly patients living on their own, although, with some extra support, it is remarkable how some patients manage. In other cases however, the risks prove so great that alternative, if less nutritionally effective approaches are appropriate, including optimal oral and drug therapy combined with subcutaneous fluid and electrolyte administration (Martinez-Riquelme *et al.*, 2005). It may also be possible in some cases to use less risky enteral nutrition to provide at least part of the patient's needs. In every instance the issues should be discussed fully with the patient, the family and other carers, before coming to a final judgement in which clinical and ethical issues are closely involved.

Three additional principles were proposed in the European bioethics and biolaw conference (Kemp *et al.*, 2000; Rendtorff, 2002) to enrich the clinical meaning and interpretation of the classic bioethical principles:

1. *The principle of dignity*. This principle implies that a person has an innate right to respect and ethical treatment.
2. *The principle of integrity*. This principle implies respect of the wholeness of the human person.
3. *The principle of vulnerability*. This principle refers to the fragility of an intact but destructible human totality and takes into account the biological, social and cultural characteristics of the person living in the modern technological world. It expresses the finitude of the human condition.

Ethical Dilemmas

Despite the wide acceptance of the above-mentioned principles, controversy may frequently arise, especially in severely ill patients, depending on the different perspective of the individuals involved in the ethical debate.

Patients and their families might consider nutritional support a basic need that not only sustains life but provides comfort as well and is associated with respect of human dignity.

The person mainly concerned with the intrinsic merits or otherwise of a medical initiative rather than with its consequences, the 'duty-based moralist', will tend to feed always the patient regardless of the final outcome because this is the 'mission' of the physician.

The 'utilitarian moralist' is more concerned with the consequences of an act rather than the act itself and would privilege the indication for an HPN programme on the basis of the scientific evidence.

Finally, the 'rights-based moralist' mainly relies for any deliberation on the free choice of the patient who has to be adequately informed.

Nowadays few people would agree with a rigid position of a wholly committed 'duty-based moralist' supporting the sanctity of life at all costs. The Roman Catholic Church too has the following position on the use of artificial nutrition and hydration near the end of life: 'There should be a presumption in favour of providing nutrition and hydration to all patients who require medically-assisted nutrition and hydration' and this approach is warranted only as long as 'there is sufficient benefit to outweigh the burden to the patient' (United States Conference of Catholic Bishops, 2009).

The 'utilitarian moralist' will accept an indication for HPN in incurable preterminal patients only if there is an evidence-based demonstration of its effectiveness. He tends to consider nutrition as a drug, starting from the original definition of drug as 'any chemical agent which affects living processes' (Goodman and Gilman, 1941). He ignores the guidelines of the American Society for Parenteral and Enteral Nutrition (A.S.P.E.N. Board of Directors and the Clinical Guideline Task Force, 2002) which state:

> a major distinction between therapeutic trials of efficacy of a drug or a procedure and the feeding of nutrients known to be essential to maintenance of human health and survival must be made. Withholding a drug or an invasive procedure will not produce disease in otherwise healthy humans, whereas essential nutrients must be provided to both healthy and ill people.

He also disregards the fact that 'the ethics of clinical research requires a state of genuine uncertainty on the part of the clinical investigator or the expert community regarding the comparative therapeutic merits of each arm in a trial' (Freedman, 1987) and that, consequently, if you are taking care of malnourished aphagic people, it is unacceptable to have a control group which is randomized to 'no nutrition'. In other words, it is almost impossible to get an evidence-based proof of effectiveness if the treatment you are investigating may represent a life-saving/prolonging procedure.

The 'rights-based moralist' will mainly rely for his deliberation on the wishes of the patient. Although in the USA and in most European countries total parenteral nutrition (TPN) is now considered a medical treatment as opposed to a simple basic care, and hence subject to the same ethical constraints as regards initiation and withdrawal, the debate on this issue is still open (Bozzetti, 2003).

Autonomy, which is the pre-eminent theme in law in most democratic states, implies that the patient is aware about the diagnosis and prognosis of his/her disease and, more important, his/her wishes are constant with time. However, Chochinov *et al.* (1999) have clearly shown that there is a substantial variation in the will-to-live score during 1 day, 1 week or 1 month in terminal cancer patients. Similarly there is a low percentage (10–14%) of individuals who having survived a suicide attempt, commit suicide during the following 10 years (Diekstra and Garnefski, 1995). Therefore, the assessment of the patient's will to live should be repeated several times and only if answers are consistent should this information be utilized to determine whether to initiate or withdraw a life-prolonging treatment such as HPN in patients affected by malignant diseases.

Finally, some patients prefer to avoid the trauma of a frank disclosure of the diagnosis and prognosis, depending on the different cultural background and religious traditions of various countries.

If we accept the principle of self-determination as a right and duty of the individual, we have also to respect his/her wish not to know the diagnosis and/or the prognosis. The Council of Europe states in Chapter III, Article 10, paragraph 2 of the Convention of Human Rights and Biomedicine, which came into force on 10 September 1996, that: 'everyone is entitled to know any information collected about his/her health. However, the wish of individuals not to be so informed shall be observed.'

Futile care

The patient should be able to differentiate between benefit (i.e. treatment conferring a net gain or advantage) and the simple effect to have an improvement in some physiological functions.

This raises the problem of the 'futile care': an action that cannot achieve the goals that are intended by the action, no matter how long it lasts or how often it is repeated. Futility has two aspects, one quantitative and the other qualitative. The first focuses on the probability that HPN can achieve the expected outcome, but who is entitled to judge the threshold below which it is no longer worthwhile to attempt it (i.e. it is futile)? The second is the qualitative dimension of an effect/benefit. For instance, who can decide whether the benefit in quality of life associated with HPN is valuable or is futile? Although ethics and law place a premium on patient autonomy, nevertheless we agree with ethicists who believe that 'futile care is ethically unjustifiable, as it holds autonomy as an absolute in all situations and ignores other valid principles, such as nonmaleficience and justice' (Pawlik and Curley, 2005). The concept of medical futility is, therefore, ethically invalid and pragmatically ineffectual (Hinshaw *et al.*, 2003).

When there is a conflict between the option of the physician and that of the patient, it is worth asking for wider consultation or considering a time-limited trial of nutritional support. In these, definite goals are agreed and shared among the patient, relatives and medical staff, and outcome is carefully monitored over a previously determined period of time.

As has been emphasized by MacFie (2005), many studies have shown that ethical dilemmas can be emotionally pre-empted if they have been previously discussed with the patient, relatives and the healthcare team.

Withholding and withdrawing nutritional support

Most ethicists believe that the distinction between withholding and withdrawing treatment is conceptually and morally incoherent, because treatment always can be withdrawn permissibly if it can be withheld permissibly; hence they employ the term 'forgoing' for both, recognizing that withdrawing is more emotionally laden than withholding, especially within specific cultures. However, many clinicians, patients and relatives believe that such a distinction exists ethically and legally.

It is true, however, that many physicians feel ethically justified in withholding treatments that they never initiated, but not in withdrawing treatments that already started. In addition, they find it harder to withdraw a life-sustaining or long-standing treatment such as nutrition and hydration rather than to limit resuscitative efforts or recently instituted interventions. Again, clinicians prefer to withdraw a treatment that supports organs failing for natural reasons rather than for iatrogenic factors (Christakis and Asch, 1993; Dowdy *et al.*, 1998). One should also consider that withholding or withdrawing TPN does not mean that patients do not receive any fluids: home subcutaneous fluids can be sometimes used in truly terminal conditions or in patients unable to cope with HPN and whose main problem is recurrent fluid and electrolyte deficit due to gastrointestinal losses (Martinez-Riquelme *et al.*, 2005).

The majority of terminally ill patients will reach a point in their illness where they refuse food or are unable to take nutrition orally. Families may feel a moral duty and an emotional need to provide food and water to their dying loved ones. It is thus important to discuss with patients and families that loss of the desire to eat and drink is a natural part of the dying process. The risks, benefits and burdens of HPN in these patients, along with cultural and religious values and patient and family preferences and values, must be weighed in each individual case (Hallenbeck, 2005).

Hence the decision to forgo nutritional support in these patients remains a challenging dilemma and requires clinicians and health professionals in general to integrate scientific knowledge together with legal, cultural, religious, ethical as well as emotional considerations.

Conclusion

It is often difficult to determine which principle pertains to any given situation and how the principle should be applied, especially when there is a conflict between the four principles of autonomy, beneficence, non-maleficence and justice, and the subsequent principles of dignity, integrity and vulnerability, and among different individuals' perspectives on ethical debate.

Although this decision-making process is complex, time intensive and resource consuming, it is essential to try to build with the patient and his/her kin the most meaningful plan of care in a morally responsible way.

We would like to conclude with the very appropriate considerations by MacFie (2005):

> These conflicts serve to emphasize that ethics is a process of reasoning whereby a morally respectable and defensible position can be reached, which protects the best interests of the patient. There are no absolutely satisfactory resolutions of ethical dilemmas and the most that one can hope to achieve is a balance between the conflicting interests and goals of different individuals involved in patient care.

We would add that it is extremely important that any crucial deliberation concerning the start or withdrawal of HPN follows an effective communication between physicians, nurses, the patient and family to discover what are the best interests and wishes of the patient. It has been demonstrated that components for a 'good death' as they are perceived by patients are not the same ones deemed so important to their physicians (Steinhauser *et al.*, 2000a,b). Therefore it is only within a relationship of empathy and sensitivity with the patient that the physician can help him/her to prolonging life or prepare him/her for the process of dying.

Summary

The main principles of moral reasoning (respect for autonomy, justice, beneficience, non-maleficience) and potential onset of conflicts among them are discussed. No one principle enjoys automatic supremacy over the others and blind overreliance on them can be simplistic and detrimental. Rather, ethical decisions require weighing and balancing the various principles against one another in each specific situation.

Since HPN is a life-prolonging treatment, it is not possible to reach, in severely ill patients with malignant intestinal failure, an evidence-based demonstration of efficiency or non-efficiency, which usually relies on clinical trials that randomize nutritional support versus non-nutrition.

The concept of futile care, which proves to be ethically invalid and pragmatically ineffectual, has been discussed.

Any distinction between withholding and withdrawing HPN is conceptually and morally incoherent.

The authors emphasize the concept of a frank and open discussion of the medical staff with patient and family to understand the deeply held wishes of the patient that have to be respected and to pre-empt from emotional conflict any potential ethical controversy.

References

Allison, S.P. (1992) The uses and limitations of nutritional support. *Clinical Nutrition* 11, 319–325.

Allison, S.P. (2004) Organisation of nutritional support: ethical and legal aspects. In: Sobotka, L. (ed.) *Basics of Clinical Nutrition.* Galen, Prague, pp. 139–148.

A.S.P.E.N. Board of Directors and the Clinical Guideline Task Force (2002) Guidelines for the use of parenteral and enteral nutrition in adult and pediatric patients. *JPEN Journal of Parenteral and Enteral Nutrition* 26(1 Suppl.), 1SA–138SA.

Beauchamp, T.L. and Childress, J.F. (2001) *Principles of Biomedical Ethics*, 5th edn. Oxford University Press, Oxford.

Bozzetti, F. (2003) Home parenteral nutrition in incurable cancer patients: a therapy, a basic humane care or something in between? *Clinical Nutrition* 22, 109–111.

Chochinov, H.M., Tataryn, D., Clinch, J.J. and Dudgeon, D. (1999) Will to live in the terminally ill. *The Lancet* 354, 816–819.

Christakis, N.A. and Asch, D.A. (1993) Biases in how physicians choose to withdraw life support. *The Lancet* 342, 642–646.

Diekstra, R.F. and Garnefski, N. (1995) On the nature, magnitude, and causality of suicidal behaviours: an international perspective on the epidemiology and prevalence of suicide. *Suicide Life Threat Behaviour* 25, 36–57.

Dowdy, M.D., Robertson, C. and Bander, J.A. (1998) A study of proactive ethics consultation for critically ill and terminally ill patients with extended lengths of stay. *Critical Care Medicine* 26, 252–259.

Freedman, B. (1987) Equipoise and the ethics of clinical research. *New England Medical Journal* 317, 141–145.

Goodman, L.S. and Gilman, A. (1941) *The Pharmacologic Basis of Therapeutics.* Macmillan, London/Toronto.

Hallenbeck, J. (2005) Fast Facts and Concepts #10; Tube Feed or Not Tube Feed?, 2nd edn. End-of-life Physician Education Resource Center (http://www.eperc.mcw.edu).

Herrmann, V.M. (1999) Nutrition support: ethical or expedient and who will choose? Presidential address to A.S.P.E.N.. *JPEN Journal of Parenteral and Enteral Nutrition* 23, 195–202.

Hinshaw, D.B., Pawlik, T., Mosenthal, A.A., Civetta, J.M. and Hallenbeck, J. (2003) When do we stop, and how do we do? Medical futility and withdrawal of care. *Journal of the American College of Surgeons* 196, 621–651.

Kemp, P., Rendtorff, J.D. and Mattson, N. (2000) *Bioethics and Biolaw*, vols 1 and 2. Rhodos, Copenhagen.

Kitzhaber, J.A. (1993) Prioritizing health services in an era of limits: the Oregon experience. *British Medical Journal* 307, 373–377.

Lennard Jones, J.E. (ed.) (1988) *Ethical and Legal Aspects of Clinical Hydration and Nutritional Support. BAPEN Report.* BAPEN, Maidenhead, UK.

MacFie, J. (2000) Ethics and legal considerations in the provision of nutritional support to the perioperative patient. *Current Opinion in Clinical Nutrition and Metabolic Care* 3, 23–29.

MacFie, J. (2005) Ethics and nutrition. In: Gibney, M.J., Elia, M., Ljunqvist, O. and Dowsett, J. (eds) *Clinical Nutrition.* Blackwell, Oxford, pp. 132–145.

Martinez-Riquelme, A., Rawlings, J., Morley, S., Kendall, J., Hosking, D. and Allison, S.P. (2005) Self-administered subcutaneous fluid infusion at home in the management of fluid depletion and hypomagnesemia in gastrointestinal disease. *Clinical Nutrition* 24, 158–163.

Pawlik, T.M. and Curley, S.A. (2005) Ethical issues in surgical palliative care: am I killing the patient by 'letting him go'? *Surgical Clinics of North America* 85, 273–286.

Rendtorff, J.D. (2002) Basic ethical principles in European bioethics and biolaw: autonomy, dignity, integrity and vulnerability – towards a foundation for bioethics and biolaw. *Medical Healthcare Philosophy* 5, 235–244.

Steinhauser, K.E., Christakis, N.A. and Clipp, E.C. (2000a) Factors considered important at the end of life by patients, family, physicians, and other care providers. *Journal of the American Medical Association* 284, 2476–2482.

Steinhauser, K.E., Clipp, C.E. and McNeilly, M. (2000b) In search of a good death: observations of patients, families, and providers. *Annals of Internal Medicine* 132, 825–832.

United States Conference of Catholic Bishops (2009) *Ethical and Religious Directives for Catholic Health Care Services, Fifth Edition. Issued by USCCB, November 17, 2009.* United States Conference of Catholic Bishops, Washington, DC.

36 Surgical Alternatives to Intestinal Transplantation in Patients with Short Bowel Syndrome

Laura Beyer-Berjot[1], Léon Maggiori[1], Francisca Joly[2,3], Olivier Corcos[2], Bernard Messing[2] and Yves Panis[1]*

[1]Department of Colorectal Surgery, Beaujon Hospital, Assistance Publique – Hôpitaux de Paris, Université Paris VII, Clichy, France; [2]Department of Gastroenterology and Nutrition Support, Beaujon Hospital, Assistance Publique – Hôpitaux de Paris, Université Paris VII, Clichy, France; [3]Gastrointestinal and Metabolic Dysfunctions in Nutritional Pathologies, Inserm UMR 1149, Centre de Recherche sur l'Inflammation Paris Montmartre – UFR de Médecine Paris Diderot, Paris, France

Key Points

- Parenteral nutrition (PN) is the primary treatment for intestinal failure and intestinal transplantation (IT) is considered only when life-threatening PN complications, especially chronic liver failures, occur.
- Five-year survival rates are 62–78% after long-term PN and 40–60% after IT.
- Conservative surgical options for 'permanent' PN dependency are: intestinal lengthening and tapering, segmental reversal of the small bowel (SRSB), artificial intestinal valve construction and colonic interposition. They aim to improve the function of the existing small bowel remnant by either expanding the intestinal surface area or slowing transit time.
- Intestinal lengthening and SRSB are the most described procedures. They have similar weaning (42–59%) and morbidity rates.
- Intestinal lengthening can only be performed on dilated small bowels, preferably with a diameter ≥4 cm, whereas SRSB can be performed regardless of the small bowel diameter.

*E-mail: yves.panis@bjn.aphp.fr

- In a recent study, SRSB improved patients' nutritional status in 97% of the cases, by either weaning (45%) or reducing PN intakes. SRSB also had a better 5-year survival rate than both long-term PN and IT (84%).
- SRBS is associated with higher chances of weaning if reversal is performed shortly after enterectomy, ideally at the time of intestinal continuity restoration.

Introduction

Short bowel syndrome (SBS) is defined as diarrhoea with malabsorption, fluid and electrolyte disorders, progressive malnutrition and weight loss after extensive resection of the small bowel. Bowel adaptation is generally observed within the first months after an extensive small bowel resection (Thompson *et al.*, 1995a). In adults, SBS is likely to be associated with permanent parenteral nutrition (PN) dependency if the length of the remnant small bowel is under 60–80 cm (Gouttebel *et al.*, 1986), in patients lacking an ileocolonic junction (ICJ) and/or with partial colectomy (Bond *et al.*, 1980; Galea *et al.*, 1992; Panis *et al.*, 1997). In the infant, the length of remaining intestine is a more controversial prognostic factor (Thompson *et al.*, 1995a), but a length of less than 30 cm in the absence of the ICJ leaves the infant at high risk for permanent intestinal insufficiency.

The introduction of home parenteral nutrition (HPN) and intestinal transplantation (IT) has revolutionized the care of SBS patients. HPN is the primary treatment for intestinal failure (Pironi *et al.*, 2011). Although long-term survival is possible in patients with permanent HPN, this therapy is still associated with high cost, poor quality of life and specific morbidities (Thompson, 1992; Shanbhogue and Molenaar, 1994) that (with the exception of cirrhosis) are reversible after weaning (Sudan *et al.*, 2005). Indeed, patients receiving long-term HPN are exposed to catheter-related complications, bone disease, cholelithiasis or liver failure. Furthermore, HPN impairs work and social activities and costs over US$70,000 per year (Messing *et al.*, 1995). Moreover, the 5-year survival rate in long-term HPN patients ranges between 62 and 78%, with 10% mortality related to the HPN itself (Messing *et al.*, 1995; Thompson *et al.*, 1995a; Vantini *et al.*, 2004).

IT is the radical treatment for SBS: first developed in the 1960s, it was not until the early 1990s that IT finally came into its own after the introduction of new immunosuppressive therapies such as tacrolimus (Hoffman *et al.*, 1990); by 2011, over 2600 patients had undergone IT worldwide (40% adults, 60% children at 79 centres). Prior to IT, most transplanted patients (80% of adults and 65% of children) had been at home on waiting lists prior to their transplantation (Intestine Transplant Association Registry Report, 2011). While short-term survival has improved dramatically in recent years, the long-term results have not shown much progress (5-year survival in the range of 40–60%) (Sudan, 2007; Ueno and Fukuzawa, 2010), and the indications for transplantation as well as the type of graft to employ remain topics of active debate (Ueno and Fukuzawa, 2010; Pironi *et al.*, 2011). Although essential, both HPN and IT have serious limitations, and IT should still be considered an extreme procedure that could be proposed only when life-threatening HPN complications, especially chronic liver failure, occur (Pironi *et al.*, 2011). Non-transplant surgical procedures should therefore be evaluated as alternatives in the light of the recent results reported for HPN and IT.

First proposed in the early 1960s, surgical 'rehabilitation' of the intestine aims to improve the function of the existing small bowel remnant by either expanding the intestinal surface area or slowing transit time (Thompson, 2004). The choice of surgical treatment is influenced by the existing bowel length, function and diameter (DiBaise *et al.*, 2004). Besides restoring intestinal continuity (which is clearly beneficial in order to recruit small bowel and colonic segments) and relieving obstruction (by stricturoplasty or limited resection), several non-transplant surgical alternatives have been described, including: (i) tapering (i.e. reducing the circumference of the intestine by either overlapping or excising the bowel wall along the antimesenteric border); (ii) isoperistaltic intestinal lengthening (i.e. longitudinal transection of the intestine between the mesenteric and antimesenteric edges and anastomosis of these segments); (iii) artificial intestinal valve construction; (iv) colonic interposition; and (v) segmental reversal of the small bowel (SRSB). The best-known procedures are SRSB and lengthening, either by Bianchi (1980) or by serial transverse enteroplasty (STEP) (Kim *et al.*, 2003). However, lengthening and tapering can only be performed on dilated intestines. Artificial valve and colonic interposition remain marginal procedures in SBS treatment, with only a few series (mainly of paediatric patients) being reported to date. Moreover, few case series have assessed non-transplant SBS surgery in adults and most studies have examined both paediatric and adult patients (Thompson *et al.*, 1995a; Sudan *et al.*, 2007; Andres *et al.*, 2008). To date, the largest series examining non-transplant surgical SBS options in adults included 37 and 20 patients receiving various procedures, such as lengthening, tapering, stricturoplasty, continuity restoration and SRSB (Thompson and Langnas, 1999; Sudan *et al.*, 2005), one series of 38 patients undergoing SRSB (Beyer-Berjot *et al.*, 2012) and one series of 20 patients that compared Bianchi's procedure and STEP (Yannam *et al.*, 2010). For this reason, it is difficult to determine the best conservative procedure for SBS adults.

The aim of this chapter is to report the results of such conservative operations in SBS, with special reference to SRSB, for which we have now an experience of 38 cases.

Segmental Reversal of the Small Bowel

Principles and previously reported experience of the procedure

SRSB may act as an ileocolonic junction (ICJ) (i.e. the valve separating the ileum from the caecum, also called Bauhin's valve) in SBS patients and prolong the transit time and contact between the luminal nutrients and remnant mucosal surface (Panis *et al.*, 1997). It can be performed regardless of the small bowel diameter. Experimental SRSB has been found to result in the lack of a normal hormonal response, persistently altered myoelectrical activity, a transient or permanent increase in transit time and a longer survival period (Stahlgren *et al.*, 1962; Baldwin-Price *et al.*, 1965; Keller *et al.*, 1965; Thompson *et al.*, 1995b). The reversed segment was observed to cause retrograde peristalsis and to disrupt the motility of the proximal intestine (Tanner *et al.*, 1978).

In addition to three series describing eight, six and 38 patients (Panis *et al.*, 1997; Oh *et al.*, 1999; Beyer-Berjot *et al.*, 2012), a few anecdotal reports about SRSB have been published (Gibson *et al.*, 1962; Thomas and Jordan, 1965; Shepard, 1966; Venables *et al.*, 1966; Fink and Olson, 1967; Wilmore and Johnson, 1968; Poth, 1969; Javett and Brooke, 1971; Pertsemlidis and Kark, 1974; Hakami *et al.*, 1975; Pigot *et al.*, 1990; Thompson *et al.*, 1995a; Loriau *et al.*, 2005). Most of these reports have included one or two patients and date back to the 1960s, i.e. before the development of HPN. Approximately 70 cases of SRSB treatment have been reported so far. With the exception of our own series, the results have been varied. This may be explained by the great differences in the length of both the remnant small bowel and the reversed segment, and follow-up. Among the case reports, 75% of the patients appear to have received some benefit from SRSB, but concerns have been raised about the long-term success of the procedure (Wilmore and Johnson, 1968). Our preliminary series of eight patients found reassuring results on this issue: a 50% weaning rate was obtained with a median follow-up of 35 months. Our recent study based on 38 patients found a 45% weaning rate and an 84% survival rate at the 5-year follow-up, which is superior to both HPN and IT.

There is general agreement that SRSB should not be performed at the time of the initial resection because of the possibility of intestinal adaptation (Thompson, 1993). However, our study demonstrated that a short time between enterectomy and SRSB was associated with higher chances of weaning ($P=0.036$) even in the case of an extremely short bowel (Beyer-Berjot *et al.*, 2012). We therefore recommend performing SRSB at the time of intestinal continuity restoration, with a delay of 4–6 months after the subtotal enterectomy, to assess the possibility of intestinal adaptation.

The optimal length of the reversed segment had not been determined thus far, and defining this length has been one of the principal issues discussed in the previous SRSB case reports (Stahlgren *et al.*, 1962; Baldwin-Price *et al.*, 1965; Wilmore and Johnson, 1968; Pertsemlidis and Kark, 1974). Questions have been raised about the happy medium between a segment that is too short, which would be inefficient, and a segment that is too long, which may be responsible for chronic obstruction (Baldwin-Price *et al.*, 1965). The results of our study showed that a length of over 10 cm (i.e. between 10 and 12 cm) should be ideal ($P=0.024$) (Beyer-Berjot *et al.*, 2012). In addition, to achieve optimal benefit, the reversed segment should be located in the most distal part of the small bowel. However, SRSB has three limitations. The first is the presence of an extremely short remnant small bowel, which may not allow sacrificing a reversed segment. This length threshold has previously been defined as 40 cm (Sudan *et al.*, 2005), but in our series the smallest length associated with post-operative weaning was 25 cm. Therefore, we recommend a threshold of 25 cm. The second limitation is chronic liver failure, in which case IT combined with liver transplantation should be chosen as the best treatment. Furthermore, in patients older than 60 years who may not be candidates for IT, SRSB could be proposed as a satisfactory alternative.

Finally, despite careful attention during the operation, SRSB has been told to exceptionally expose the risks of ischaemia and anastomotic leakage (Shanbhogue and Molenaar, 1994).

The Beaujon Intestinal Failure Centre experience

The following data have been previously published (Beyer-Berjot *et al.*, 2012). At our institution, SRSB was indicated in patients with the two following conditions: (i) SBS with a permanent PN dependency (usually with a post-duodenal small bowel remnant under 80 cm and without ICJ); and (ii) an indication for jejuno-colic continuity restoration. Preoperative evaluations were performed to exclude the patients with end-stage liver disease or complications from cirrhosis, who were likely to be better candidates for IT. All patients fulfilling the stated criteria for SRSB underwent this procedure.

Between 1985 and 2010, 38 patients underwent SRSB for SBS in our department. The most frequent causes of SBS were mesenteric infarctions in 20 patients and radiation enteritis in four patients (Table 36.1). Endocrine tumour was responsible for SBS in two patients and Crohn's disease in one patient. The other non-neoplastic causes consisted of three iterative small bowel obstructions, two gunshots, two traffic accidents, two desmoid tumours, one case of ulcerative colitis and one iatrogenic fistula with multiple operations. No patient had received a previous intestine or liver transplant.

With one exception, all of the patients were permanently dependent on PN before undergoing SRSB; 34 out of 38 patients had received PN on 7 days per

Table 36.1. Demographic and disease characteristics of the 38 patients undergoing SRSB for SBS. (From Beyer-Berjot *et al.*, 2012.)

	Overall	Weaned from HPN	Not weaned from HPN	*P*
n	38	17	21	–
Age (years)	55.5 (18–76)	50.0 (24–70)	55.5 (18–76)	0.75
Gender female (*n*)	12	5	7	0.80
BMI (kg/m^2)	22 (16–37)	22 (18–37)	22 (16–33)	0.53
ASA score (*n*)				
1–2	20	9	11	0.49
3–4	15	5	10	0.49
SBS aetiology (*n*)				
Mesenteric infarction	20	11	9	0.18
Radiation enteritis	4	0	4	0.11
Cancer	2	1	1	1
Crohn's disease	1	0	1	1
Other benign disease	11	5	6	1
No. of operations	2 (1–10)	2 (1–4)	2 (1–10)	0.45

BMI, body mass index; ASA, American Society of Anesthesiology.
Data are reported as number or median (range).

week, while the three other patients received PN on 6 ($n=2$) or 5 ($n=1$) days per week. One patient underwent SRSB at the time of subtotal enterectomy: he had undergone surgery for a desmoid tumour 6 years after a subtotal colectomy for familial adenomatous polyposis.

Operative procedure

The technique was previously described (Panis *et al.*, 1997). Briefly, the first step of SRSB consisted of preparing a short segment of the distal remnant small bowel: it was separated from the remaining small bowel, leaving its blood supply intact, and then reversed. Next, the segment was re-anastomosed, proximally to the remaining small bowel and distally to the remaining colon (Fig. 36.1). Complete 360° mesenteric rotation was avoided by correct positioning of the proximal and distal parts of the intestine before anastomosis (rotation of both segments was approximately of 90°). This meant that the necessary mesenteric rotation of the reversed segment was only of about 180°. During the procedure, the remnant small bowel was measured along the antimesenteric border from the ligament of Treitz to the enterocolonic anastomosis.

In our series, mean length of the remnant small bowel, before SRSB, was 49 cm (range 20–140 cm). The ICJ had been effectively removed in all but one patient. Three patients had no remaining colon, but the other 35 had a partial colectomy only or no colectomy at all (Table 36.2). The mean length of the segment used for SRSB was 10 cm (range 6–15 cm). Thirty-three patients had jejunocolic anastomoses, two patients had enteroenteral anastomoses, two had jejunorectal anastomoses and one had the reversed jejunal segment anastomosed to an ileal J pouch.

Post-operative morbidity and mortality

Six patients presented with major complications, including four patients who required early reoperation. One patient received additional surgery for haemorrhage, during which the SRSB was removed and a new jejunocolostomy was created. He died from acute renal failure at day 26; this was the only post-operative death. The three remaining patients received additional surgery for haemorrhage at day 4, sepsis of unknown origin at day 2 and acute acalculous cholecystitis at day 21. The other major complications were an enterocutaneous fistula and a subphrenic abscess for which additional surgery was not required. The median length of stay was 14.5 days (range 6–53 days) in surgery followed by 19 days (range 0–60 days) in the nutrition unit.

Long-term results

The median follow-up was 57.7 months (range 1–304 months). Overall, 18 patients out of 38 have been followed more than 5 years. During the entire follow-up period, the patients were placed on an unrestricted oral diet and were encouraged to eat as much as they could.

At the 5-year follow-up, 17 patients had been weaned off PN (45%), including the patient who had a proximal SRSB. The median weaning time was 14 months (range 4–60 months). Among the weaned patients, two patients required electrolyte infusions (either 2 or 3 days per week). According to the Kaplan–Meier

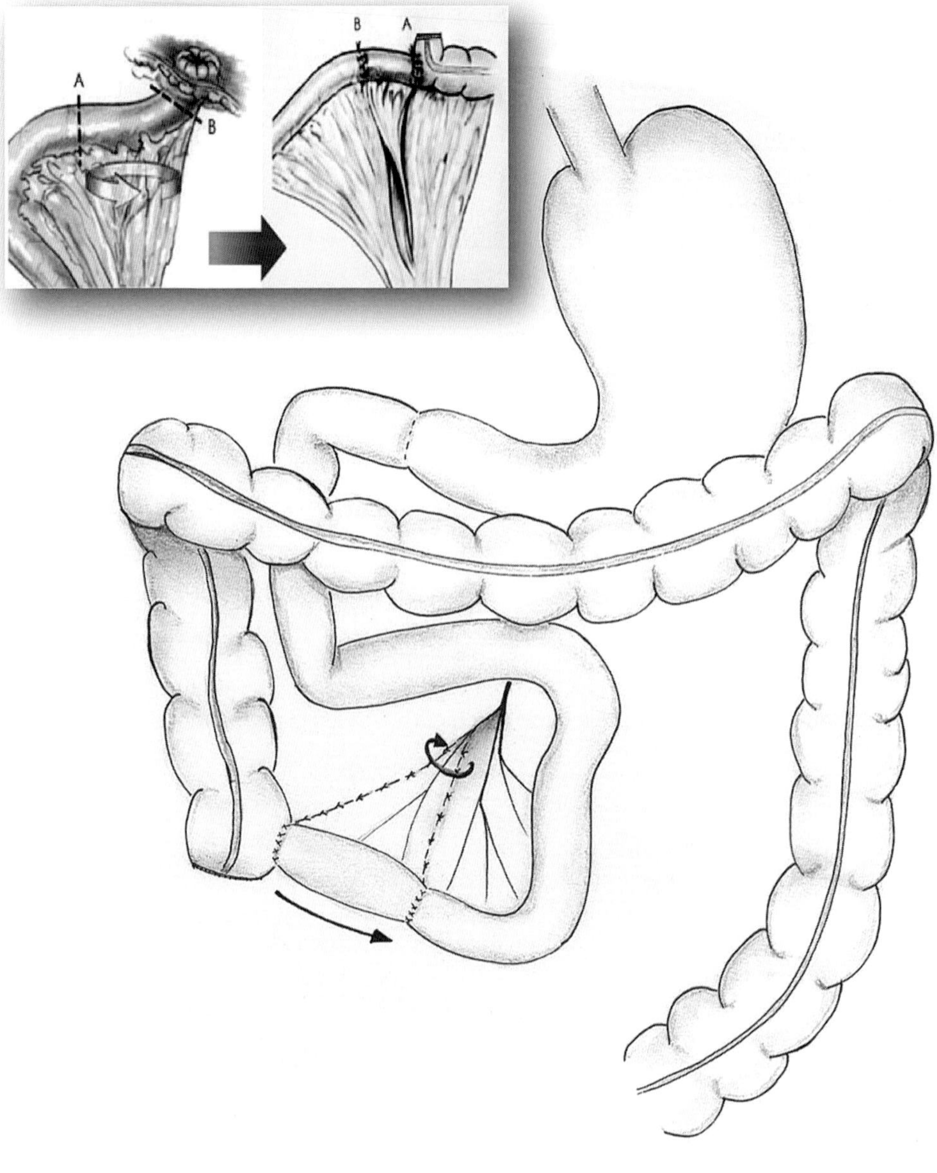

Fig. 36.1. SRSB with jejunocolic anastomosis at the time of continuity restoration.

analysis, the probability of PN weaning increased from 22% at 12 months to 52% at 60 months (Fig. 36.2).

Although the remaining 20 patients still required PN at the 5-year follow-up, the median PN dependency in days per week decreased from 7 (range 0–7) to 4 (range 2–6) ($P < 0.001$). Overall, 37/38 of the patients (excluding the patient who died post-operatively) had improved their nutritional status after the SRSB.

Table 36.2. Perioperative characteristics and short-term outcomes of the 38 patients undergoing SRSB for SBS.

	Overall	Weaned from HPN	Not weaned from HPN	*P*
n	38	17	21	–
Preoperative intestinal status (*n*)				
Jejunocolostomy	15	6	9	0.93
Jejunocolostomy + colon closed in the abdomen	6	3	3	0.66
Jejunocolic anastomosis	3	0	3	0.25
Other	3	4	1	0.55
Length of small bowel (cm)	49 (20–140)	50 (25–70)	48 (20–140)	0.84
Time between subtotal enterectomy and SRSB (months)	6 (0–168)	4 (0–14)	7 (3–168)	0.036
Ileal remnant (*n*)	4	2	2	1
ICJ (*n*)	1	1	0	0.45
Remnant colon (*n*)				
Whole	4	2	2	1
Right/left	1	0	1	1
Transverse/left	26	13	13	0.34
Left	4	1	3	0.61
Total colectomy	3	1	2	1
Length of reversed segment (cm)	10 (6–15)	10 (7–15)	10 (6–12)	0.102
Length of hospital stay (days)				
In surgery	14.5 (6–53)	15 (6–36)	14 (9–53)	0.73
In nutrition unit	19 (0–60)	32 (0–60)	7 (0–39)	0.035

Data are reported as number or median (range).

At the 5-year follow-up, six patients had undergone delayed repeat surgery (for cholangitis and acute biliary pancreatitis among the weaned patients, and for intra-abdominal sepsis among the patients who were not weaned). No patient required later IT. The overall 5-year survival rate was 84%. Five of the patients died during the late post-operative course: three patients who had not been weaned from PN died from septic shock (line sepsis), pulmonary embolism or cerebrovascular accident; and two patients who had been weaned died from septic shock or renal failure.

In a second study published by our centre matching SRSB with controls, SRSB allowed a gain in macronutrient absorption with significantly higher intestinal absorption for total calories (69.5% versus 58.0%), fat (48.4% versus 33.2%) and protein (62.7% versus 53.4%) (Layec *et al.*, 2013).

Prognostic factors of weaning

In the univariate analysis, the factors significantly associated with weaning in our study were a short time between subtotal enterectomy and SRSB ($P = 0.036$) and a longer than typical stay in the nutrition unit ($P = 0.035$) (Table 36.2). A segmental reversal longer than 10 cm was associated with more rapid weaning ($P = 0.024$, log-rank test).

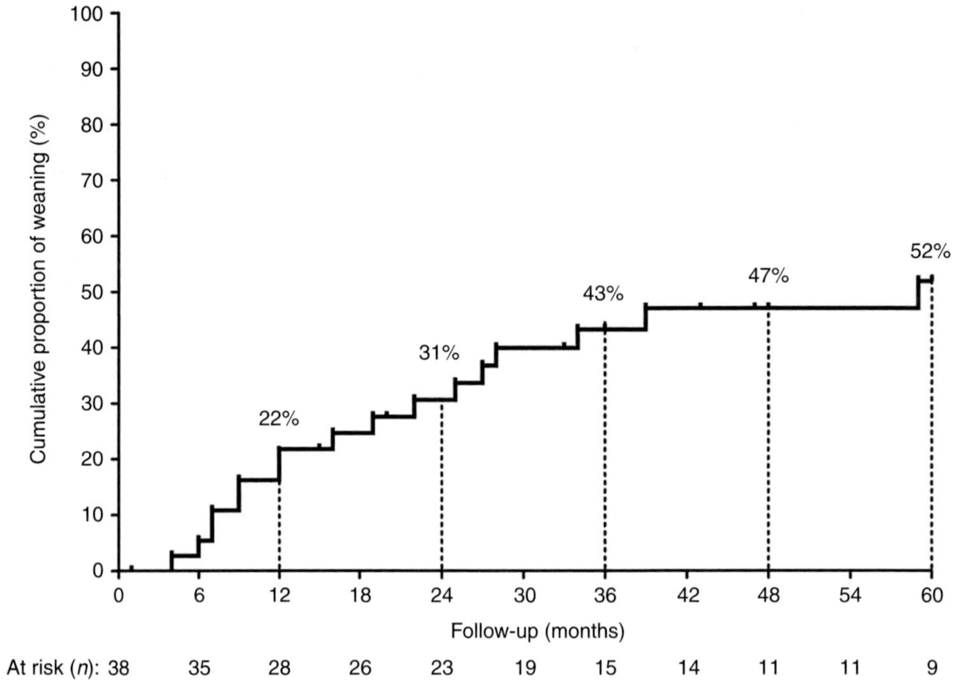

Fig. 36.2. Kaplan–Meier analysis of time to weaning from PN in 38 patients with SRSB for SBS. (From Beyer-Berjot *et al.*, 2012.)

Other Conservative Surgical Procedures for SBS

Small bowel lengthening

Lengthening, either by Bianchi or STEP, is the most described non-transplant operation (Fig. 36.3). Both lengthening techniques result in weaning rates similar to those of SRSB (42–59%) (Sudan *et al.*, 2005, 2007; Yannam *et al.*, 2010). However, these weaning rates cannot be rigorously compared because the patients are not similar. First, only those patients with dilated small bowels, preferably with a diameter ≥4 cm (Thompson *et al.*, 1995a; Sudan *et al.*, 2007), can undergo a lengthening procedure, whereas SRSB can be performed regardless of the small bowel diameter. Second, and most importantly, with the exception of the adult series by Yannam *et al.* (2010) which reported a 42% weaning rate, lengthening studies have mixed adult and paediatric series, which usually have large majorities of infants (Thompson *et al.*, 1995a; Sudan *et al.*, 2005, 2007; Andres *et al.*, 2008). The abundance of paediatric patients explains the ability to perform lengthening procedures. Indeed, most children with SBS have a dilated small bowel, whereas adults (who usually have a stoma) do not. Lengthening procedures have similar complication rates to those of SRSB. However, specific complications have been described after Bianchi's lengthening, such as interloop fistulas (Huskisson *et al.*, 1993; Sudan *et al.*, 2005, 2007) and anastomotic stenoses (Sudan *et al.*, 2007).

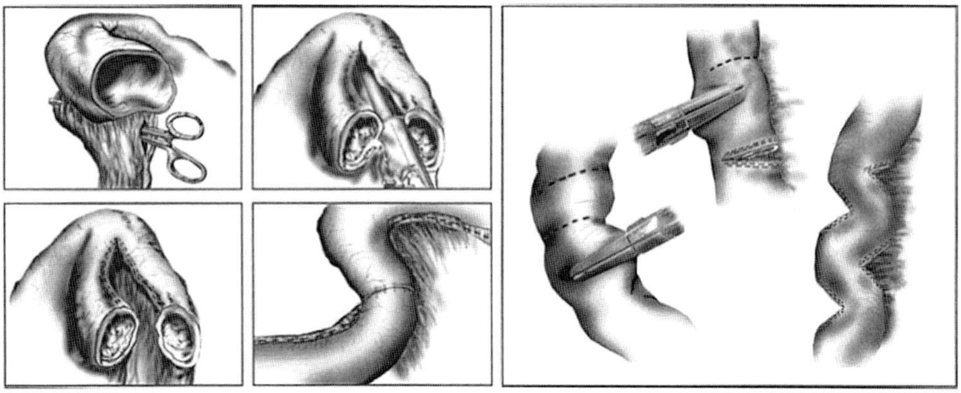

Bianchi STEP

Fig. 36.3. Intestinal lengthening procedures: Binachi and STEP. (From Sudan *et al.*, 2007.)

Proximal colonic interposition

Proximal colonic interposition has been performed in 12 infants and in only one adult (Brolin, 1986). It may be a useful technique in cases when the small bowel is too short to be used for reversal. Poor results have been reported for anti-peristaltic distal colonic interposition (Carner and Raju, 1981), which resulted in increased morbidity, even though some improved absorption was obtained.

Intestinal valve

The creation of intestinal valves by constricting intestine externally and intussuscepting an intestinal segment has also been proposed (Chardavoyne *et al.*, 1984). Numerous techniques have been described, which prevents a homogeneous assessment (Chardavoyne *et al.*, 1984; Zurita *et al.*, 2004). Thompson reported good results of artificial valve in one adult and one child with rapid transit time, with reduced ostomy output, and discontinuing HPN after 2 months for one patient. The other remained off HPN for 4 years (Thompson, 1993).

Conclusion

After massive small bowel resection in adults, permanent PN dependency can be anticipated if the post-duodenal length of the remaining small bowel is less than 60–80 cm, together with the absence of an ICJ and a partial colonic resection. Our experience suggests that SRSB could be safely proposed for these patients with a very short remnant small bowel requiring definitive HPN. Despite a significant morbidity rate (16%), SRSB allowed almost 50% of the patients to be free of HPN and improved the nutritional status in 97% of the cases, with a better survival rate than both IT and HPN. Lengthening procedures allow similar weaning rates and morbidity. Finally, we believe that SRSB, as well as other conservative surgical procedures (i.e. tapering, lengthening, artificial intestinal valve construction, colonic interposition), for which reported experience remains however very small, could be proposed early in the course of SBS, before life-threatening HPN-related complications arise. In the future, tissue engineering (i.e. fabrication of 'new' intestine with biodegradable organoid units containing multicellular units derived from neonatal rat intestine) could constitute a new way to treat patients with SBS (Grikscheit *et al.*, 2004).

Summary

SBS requiring permanent HPN can be expected if less than 60 cm of the small bowel (with absence of ICJ) remains after surgery. In these cases, conservative surgical procedures such as SRSB or lengthening could be proposed at the time of continuity restoration. They are indeed safe and appealing options before life-threatening HPN complications arise and intestinal transplantation is needed. Small series have demonstrated weaning rates of almost 50% in case of 'permanent' HPN dependency.

References

Andres, A.M., Thompson, J.S., Grant, W., Botha, J., Sunderman, B., Antonson, D., Langnas, A. and Sudan, D. (2008) Repeat surgical bowel lengthening with the STEP procedure. *Transplantation* 85, 1294–1299.

Baldwin-Price, H.K., Copp, D. and Singleton, A.O. Jr (1965) Reversed intestinal segments in the management of anenteric malabsorption syndrome. *Annals of Surgery* 161, 225–230.

Beyer-Berjot, L., Joly, F., Maggiori, L., Corcos, O., Bouhnik, Y., Bretagnol, F. and Panis, Y. (2012) Segmental reversal of the small bowel can end permanent parenteral nutrition dependency: an experience of 38 adults with short bowel syndrome. *Annals of Surgery* 256, 739–744.

Bianchi, A. (1980) Intestinal loop lengthening – a technique for increasing small intestinal length. *Journal of Pediatric Surgery* 15, 145–151.

Bond, J.H., Currier, B.E., Buchwald, H. and Levitt, M.D. (1980) Colonic conservation of malabsorbed carbohydrate. *Gastroenterology* 78, 444–447.

Brolin, R.E. (1986) Colon interposition for extreme short bowel syndrome: a case report. *Surgery* 100, 576–580.

Carner, D.V. and Raju, S. (1981) Failure of antiperistaltic colon interposition to ameliorate short-bowel syndrome. *American Surgeon* 47, 538–540.

Chardavoyne, R., Isenberg, H.D., Tindel, M., Stein, T.A., Sampson-Scherer, J. and Wise, L. (1984) Microbiologic efficacy of a surgically constructed nipple valve. *American Journal of Surgery* 147, 230–233.

DiBaise, J.K., Young, R.J. and Vanderhoof, J.A. (2004) Intestinal rehabilitation and the short bowel syndrome: part 2. *American Journal of Surgery* 99, 1823–1832.

Fink, W.J. and Olson, J.D. (1967) The massive bowel resection syndrome. Treatment with reversed intestinal segments. *Archives of Surgery* 94, 700–706.

Galea, M.H., Holliday, H., Carachi, R. and Kapila, L. (1992) Short-bowel syndrome: a collective review. *Journal of Pediatric Surgery* 27, 592–596.

Gibson, L.D., Carter, R. and Hinshaw, D.B. (1962) Segmental reversal of small intestine after massive bowel resection. Successful case with follow-up examination. *Journal of the American Medical Association* 182, 952–954.
Gouttebel, M.C., Saint-Aubert, B., Astre, C. and Joyeux, H. (1986) Total parenteral nutrition needs in different types of short bowel syndrome. *Digestive Diseases and Sciences* 31, 718–723.
Grikscheit, T.C., Siddique, A., Ochoa, E.R., Srinivasan, A., Alsberg, E., Hodin, R.A. and Vacanti, J.P. (2004) Tissue-engineered small intestine improves recovery after massive small bowel resection. *Annals of Surgery* 240, 748–754.
Hakami, M., Moslehy, A. and Mosavy, S.H. (1975) Reversed jejunal segment used to treat the short bowel syndrome. *American Surgeon* 41, 432–435.
Hoffman, A.L., Makowka, L., Banner, B., Cai, X., Cramer, D.V., Pascualone, A., Todo, S. and Starzl, T.E. (1990) The use of FK-506 for small intestine allotransplantation. Inhibition of acute rejection and prevention of fatal graft-versus-host disease. *Transplantation* 49, 483–490.
Huskisson, L.J., Brereton, R.J., Kiely, E.M. and Spitz, L. (1993) Problems with intestinal lengthening. *Journal of Pediatric Surgery* 28, 720–722.
Intestine Transplant Association Registry Report (2011) 2011 – ISBTS 2011 Symposium (Washington, DC, USA). Available at: http://www.tts.org/component/tts/?view=presentations&meeting=27&Itemid=655 (accessed 31 July 2014).
Javett, S.L. and Brooke, B.N. (1971) Reversed ileal segment or ileostomy diarrhoea. *The Lancet* 1, 291.
Keller, J.W., Stewart, W.R.C., Westerheide, R. and Pace, W.G. (1965) Prolonged survival with paired reversed segment after massive intestinal resection. *Archives of Surgery* 91, 174–179.
Kim, H.B., Fauza, D., Garza, J., Oh, J.T., Nurko, S. and Jaksic, T. (2003) Serial transverse enteroplasty (STEP): a novel bowel lengthening procedure. *Journal of Pediatric Surgery* 38, 425–429.
Layec, S., Beyer, L., Corcos, O., Alves, A., Dray, X., Amiot, A., Stefanescu, C., Coffin, B., Bretagnol, F., Bouhnik, Y., Messing, B., Panis, Y., Kapel, N. and Joly, F. (2013) Increased intestinal absorption by segmental reversal of the small bowel in adult patients with short-bowel syndrome: a case–control study. *American Journal of Clinical Nutrition* 97, 100–108.
Loriau, J., Benoist, S., Panis, Y., Joly, F., Messing, B. and Valleur, P. (2005) Salvage of ileal pouch-anal anastomosis by a reversed jejunal segment. *Surgery* 137, 111–113.
Messing, B., Lemann, M., Landais, P., Gouttebel, M.C., Gerard-Boncompain, M., Saudin, F., Vangossum, A., Beau, P., Guedon, C., Barnoud, D., Beliah, M., Joyeux, H., Bouletreau, P., Robert, D., Matuchansky, C., Leverve, X., Lerebours, E., Carpentier, Y. and Rambaud, J.-C. (1995) Prognosis of patients with nonmalignant chronic intestinal failure receiving long-term home parenteral nutrition. *Gastroenterology* 108, 1005–1010.
Oh, N.G., Kang, I.S., Song, G.A. and Sim, M.S. (1999) Antiperistaltic ileostomy using the long terminal ileal segment. *Diseases of the Colon and Rectum* 42, 1330–1333.
Panis, Y., Messing, B., Rivet, P., Coffin, B., Hautefeuille, P., Matuchansky, C., Rambaud, J.C. and Valleur, P. (1997) Segmental reversal of the small bowel as an alternative to intestinal transplantation in patients with short bowel syndrome. *Annals of Surgery* 225, 401–407.
Pertsemlidis, D. and Kark, A.E. (1974) Antiperistaltic segments for the treatment of short bowel syndrome. *American Journal of Gastroenterology* 62, 526–530.
Pigot, F., Messing, B., Chaussade, S., Pfeiffer, A., Pouliquen, X. and Jian, R. (1990) Severe short bowel syndrome with a surgically reversed small bowel segment. *Digestive Diseases and Sciences* 35, 137–144.
Pironi, L., Joly, F., Forbes, A., Colomb, V., Lyszkowska, M., Baxter, J., Gabe, S., Hebuterne, X., Gambarara, M., Gottrand, F., Cuerda, C., Thul, P., Messing, B., Goulet, O., Staun, M. and

Van Gossum, A. (2011) Long-term follow-up of patients on home parenteral nutrition in Europe: implications for intestinal transplantation. *Gut* 60, 17–25.

Poth, E.J. (1969) Use of gastrointestinal reversal in surgical procedures. *American Journal of Surgery* 118, 893–899.

Shanbhogue, L.K.R. and Molenaar, J.C. (1994) Short bowel syndrome: metabolic and surgical management. *British Journal of Surgery* 81, 486–499.

Shepard, D. (1966) Antiperistaltic bowel segment in the treatment of the short bowel syndrome. *Annals of Surgery* 163, 850–855.

Stahlgren, L.H., Umana, G., Roy, R. and Donnelly, J. (1962) A study of intestinal absorption in dogs following massive small intestinal resection and insertion of an antiperistaltic segment. *Annals of Surgery* 156, 483–492.

Sudan, D.L. (2007) Treatment of intestinal failure: intestinal transplantation. *National Clinical Practice. Gastroenterology & Hepatology* 4, 503–510.

Sudan, D., DiBaise, J., Torres, C., Thompson, J., Raynor, S., Gilroy, R., Horslen, S., Grant, W., Botha, J. and Langnas, A. (2005) A multidisciplinary approach to the treatment of intestinal failure. *Journal of Gastrointestinal Surgery* 9, 165–176.

Sudan, D., Thompson, J., Botha, J., Grant, W., Antonson, D., Raynor, S. and Langnas, A. (2007) Comparison of intestinal lengthening procedures for patients with short bowel syndrome. *Annals of Surgery* 246, 593–601.

Tanner, W.A., O'Leary, J.F., Byrne, P.J. and Hennessy, T.P. (1978) The effect of reversed jejunal segments on the myoelectrical activity of the small bowel. *British Journal of Surgery* 65, 567–571.

Thomas, J.F. and Jordan, G.L. Jr (1965) Massive resection of small bowel and total colectomy: use of reversed segment. *Archives of Surgery* 90, 781–786.

Thompson, J.S. (1992) Reoperation in patients with the short bowel syndrome. *American Journal of Surgery* 164, 453–456.

Thompson, J.S. (1993) Surgical considerations in the short bowel syndrome. *Surgery, Gynecology & Obstetrics* 176, 89–101.

Thompson, J.S. (2004) Surgical rehabilitation of intestine in short bowel syndrome. *Surgery* 135, 465–470.

Thompson, J.S. and Langnas, A.N. (1999) Surgical approaches to improving intestinal function in the short-bowel syndrome. *Archives of Surgery* 134, 706–711.

Thompson, J.S., Langnas, A.N., Pinch, L.W., Kaufman, S., Quigley, E.M. and Vanderhoof, J.A. (1995a) Surgical approach to short-bowel syndrome. Experience in a population of 160 patients. *Annals of Surgery* 222, 600–605.

Thompson, J.S., Quigley, E.M. and Adrian, T.E. (1995b) Effect of reversed intestinal segments on intestinal structure and function. *Journal of Surgical Research* 58, 19–27.

Ueno, T. and Fukuzawa, M. (2010) Current status of intestinal transplantation. *Surgery Today* 40, 1112–1122.

Vantini, I., Benini, L., Bonfante, F., Talamini, G., Sembenini, C., Chiarioni, G., Maragnolli, O., Benini, F. and Capra, F. (2004) Survival rate and prognostic factors in patients with intestinal failure. *Digestive and Liver Disease* 36, 46–55.

Venables, C.W., Ellis, H. and Smith, A.D. (1966) Antiperistaltic segments after massive intestinal resections. *The Lancet* 2, 1390–1394.

Wilmore, D.W. and Johnson, C.J. (1968) Metabolic effects of small bowel reversal in treatment of the short bowel syndrome. *Archives of Surgery* 97, 784–791.

Yannam, G.R., Sudan, D.L., Grant, W., Botha, J., Langnas, A. and Thompson, J.S. (2010) Intestinal lengthening in adult patients with short bowel syndrome. *Journal of Gastrointestinal Surgery* 14, 1931–1936.

Zurita, M., Raurich, J.M., Ramirez, A., Gil, J. and Darder, J. (2004) A new neovalve type in short bowel syndrome surgery. *Revista Espanola de Enfermedades Digestivas* 96, 110–118.

37 The Use of Hormonal Factors to Promote Intestinal Function in Short Bowel Syndrome

Palle B. Jeppesen*

Department of Medical Gastroenterology, Rigshospitalet, Denmark

Key Points

- High-dose growth hormone treatment in patients with short bowel syndrome (SBS) may have a positive effect on intestinal wet-weight absorption, but the use is often associated with significant side-effects.
- Low-dose growth hormone has been demonstrated to have beneficial effect on intestinal energy absorption in a single study, but partly this effect may be due to a stimulatory effect on oral energy intake.
- The positive effects of growth hormone are described mainly in SBS patients with a colon in continuity.
- Glucagon-like peptide-2 and the degradation-resistant analogue, teduglutide, mainly increase intestinal wet-weight absorption, whereas effects on energy absorption are less predominant. Effects are seen in short bowel patients with and without a colon in continuity.
- Since the effects of growth factors are present only during treatments, long-term treatments are required. A careful surveillance of these SBS patients is suggested in order to detect possible adverse effects in relation to long-term treatment.

Introduction

Malabsorption of non-essential and essential nutrients, fluids and electrolytes, if not compensated for by increased intake, will lead to diminished body stores and subclinical and (eventually) clinical deficiencies. By definition, intestinal failure prevails when parenteral support (PS) is necessary to maintain fluid, electrolyte, trace element, vitamin and nutrient balances. After intestinal resection, adaptation

*E-mail: Bekker@dadlnet.dk

– a progressive recovery from the malabsorptive disorder – may be evident. This chapter describes factors responsible for the morphological, structural and functional changes in the adaptive processes and presents published results of clinical trials that have employed growth hormones, glutamine, glucagon-like peptide-2 (GLP-2) or the analogue, teduglutide, in the treatment of short bowel patients.

Intestinal Adaptation

The term 'intestinal adaptation' may be applied to the progressive recovery from intestinal insufficiency or failure that follows a loss of intestinal length. Figure 37.1 illustrates a theoretical graphical presentation of intestinal function in relation to time after intestinal resection. A 'spontaneous adaption', or recovery of intestinal function, is generally described, reaching a plateau at a certain time ('SA' in Fig. 37.1). When trying to improve intestinal adaptation, therapies could either reach a higher plateau phase ('hyperadaptation', 'HA' in Fig. 37.1) or reduce the time period until the plateau is reached ('accelerated adaptation', 'AA', or 'accelerated hyperadaptation', 'AHA' in Fig. 37.1). The time issue may be relevant in patients who are difficult to maintain on parenteral nutrition (PN). However, the maximal increase in the functional absorptive capacity obtained by hyperadaptation, represented by the level of the plateau, is the aim when trying to wean stable patients from PS.

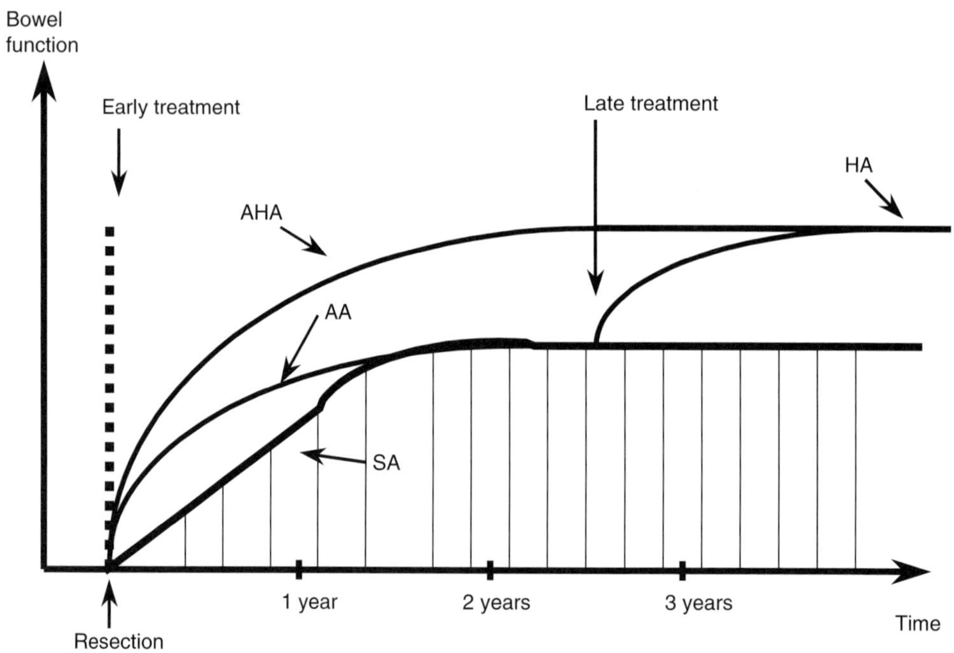

Fig. 37.1. Schematic presentation of intestinal adaptation. SA, spontaneous adaptation; AA, accelerated adaptation; HA, hyperadaptation; AHA, accelerated hyperadaptation.

Morphological, biochemical, hormonal and neural systems appear to be involved in intestinal adaptation. Data supporting this are derived mainly from studies on animals in which the process of compensatory hyperplasia is extraordinary in some species. It is important to realize that an overall translation of these data to humans cannot be presumed. In the rat, the ileal villi grow to their fully adapted height within about 2 weeks when the jejunum is resected (Forrester, 1972). In humans, this process has been demonstrated in patients with jejunoileal bypass operations after which villus height increased and reached a plateau in 1 year (Friedman *et al.*, 1978). Most animal and human resection studies describe jejunal changes in short bowels with colon in continuity. Thus, conclusions drawn may not hold for patients with a jejunostomy.

The process of epithelial turnover is highly dynamic in the intestine. Thus, within 3–6 days, the epithelial cells proliferate within the crypts at the base of the villi, mature, differentiate and move upward towards the tip of a villus, from which they are shed into the bowel lumen (Eastwood, 1977). Adaptation is characterized by cellular hyperplasia that increases the crypt depth and villus size (Booth *et al.*, 1958; Porus, 1965; Dowling and Booth, 1967; Nygaard, 1967; Obertop *et al.*, 1977). The morphological changes are more marked in the mucosal surface area, but changes are also seen in the submucosa or muscularis layers (Hanson *et al.*, 1977).

The intensity of the adaptive response is greater in the distal small bowel following proximal resection compared with the proximal bowel after distal resection (Dowling and Booth, 1967; Nygaard, 1967; Tilson and Wright, 1970; Weser and Hernandez, 1971; Eastwood, 1977; Hanson *et al.*, 1977). Adaptive hyperplasia of colonic mucosa occurs after both jejunal and ileal resection (Tilson *et al.*, 1976; Nundy *et al.*, 1977; Solhaug and Tvete, 1978; Williamson *et al.*, 1978). The adaptive response also occurs in the jejunal remnant after ileal resection, but it is less dramatic, more variable and may partly be related to adaptive changes in food intake (Young and Weser, 1974). Finally, ileal mucosa may also undergo hyperplasia after colectomy (Wright *et al.*, 1969; Woo and Nygaard, 1978).

Only a few longitudinal studies have been performed in humans with respect to functional changes following intestinal resection. However, it is the clinical experience that short bowel patients with an intact colon show improved absorption with time, whereas patients with jejunostomy do not (Nightingale and Lennard-Jones, 1993). A diminished faecal water loss and increased absorption of glucose, galactose, amino acids and fats during the time after extensive small bowel resection have been described in two patients with preserved colon (Dowling and Booth, 1966). The jejunal absorptive capacity of short bowel patients has also been examined by segmental perfusion techniques, and the absorption of glucose, water and sodium was increased per unit of length compared with that of control subjects (Dowling and Booth, 1966; Weinstein *et al.*, 1969). Ileostomy adaptation does occur within a period of 6 months; however, this response is lacking in 'ileostomists' who have had an ileal resection (Hill *et al.*, 1974). Thus, the preservation of the terminal ileum and the colon seems to be of importance in the adaptive response following intestinal resection. The time required to maximum adaptation is not certain. Studies of calcium absorption have suggested that it may continue for more than 2 years (Gouttebel *et al.*, 1989), although the main adaptive response seems to take place within a few months.

It seems that the increase in intestinal function with time following intestinal resection may simply be related to the morphologically demonstrated villus hyperplasia, because only minor changes in the activity of specific intestinal disaccharidases, hydrolases, enterokinase and Na^+/K^+-ATPase have been demonstrated (Weser and Hernandez, 1971; Tilson and Wright, 1971; McCarthy and Kim, 1973). However, functional adaptation may also involve a trend towards normalization of the gastric hypersecretion, gastric emptying and rapid intestinal transit reported in short bowel syndrome (SBS) (Remington *et al.*, 1983).

The signals and precise mechanisms that trigger the hyperplastic adaptive response after small bowel resection are not completely understood. The main factors thought to influence intestinal adaptation are exposure of the remaining mucosa to luminal nutrients and non-nutritive components of the diet, various factors related to the provision of enteral feedings (e.g. pancreatic-biliary secretions and enteric hormones) and possibly various growth factors and hormones not secreted from the intestine.

Hormonal Stimulation of Intestinal Adaptation

Two major hormonal candidates – growth hormones and GLP-2 – have been suggested and employed in the treatment of patients with SBS. The overall aim of any given treatment in short bowel patients is to improve their quality of life. Quality of life may be estimated by the use of standardized questionnaires; however, at present, it is difficult to establish what numerical improvement on the disease-specific questionnaires or non-disease specific scales would justify the introduction of a new treatment.

The main focus of research performed in short bowel has been to increase the absolute intestinal absorption. However, in most studies assessing the effects of pharmacological interventions, the dietary intake has been fixed during balance studies. Therefore, in contrast to these 'physiological studies', the effect on the dietary intake of these interventions, and thereby on the true absolute absorption, has not been established *in vivo* in the everyday settings of the patients. For instance, pharmacological agents could (i.e. due to an effect on the gastric emptying) induce a sensation of satiety, thereby also reducing the overall dietary intake.

Even in studies in which a true increase in the intestinal absorption has been established, the outcomes may differ in individual patients. It is possible that an improved energy and macronutrient balance in some patients may lead to changes in body weight and composition and, in others, to a change in basal metabolic rate, whereas some may increase their physical activity. Improved fluid and electrolyte balance may allow for increased perspiration and production of urine and sweat. Thus, to get a more precise picture of the individual short bowel patient, each of these parameters ideally should be measured in long-term experiments. Because of the vast requirements and efforts to conduct such experiments, the ability to wean patients off PS has been used as a surrogate marker of an effect of given treatments. However, unless the pre-treatment need for PS has been verified, such an end point is invalid. Most home PS patients can be reduced in PS for shorter or longer periods. This is especially true for patients with a preserved colon, who are not as prone to dehydration as patients with a jejunostomy. In patients with true intestinal failure, in whom attempts of weaning from PS are made, the patients may in the short run compensate for these changes in the energy, macronutrient, fluid and electrolyte balances either by increasing their oral intake or their metabolism may be down-regulated. However, eventually, they become malnourished or dehydrated and need to be put on PS again.

In spite of these difficulties, the search for factors to enhance bowel adaptation and increase the assimilation of macronutrients and absorption of wet weight, thereby decreasing the need for PS, is intensive. Hence, a comparison of the results obtained in clinical trials employing growth hormone, glutamine, GLP-2 and teduglutide is presented.

Effects of Growth Hormone, Glutamine, GLP-2 and Teduglutide in Clinical Studies

Wet-weight absorption

Byrne and Wilmore were the first to introduce the concept of 'bowel rehabilitation' with the introduction of high-dose (0.14 mg/kg body weight/day) growth hormone, glutamine and a high-carbohydrate diet in the treatment of short bowel patients (Byrne *et al.*, 1995a,b). In the first study published by Byrne and Wilmore, the wet-weight absorption increased from 1.7 to 2.4 kg/day and sodium absorption increased from 74 to 113 mmol/day over 5 weeks of treatment. From the baseline absorptive parameters, the actual need for parenteral fluid and sodium could be questioned in the majority of the patients in that study, according to the guidelines of intestinal failure defined by Jeppesen and Mortensen (2000). All eight patients in the Byrne and Wilmore study had a colon in continuity, and in addition to dietary changes towards a high-carbohydrate diet, they were also given oral rehydration solutions as a part of the 'rehabilitation'.

Despite claims to the contrary, the effects may, in fact, be related to dietary changes and rehydration solutions, rather than growth hormones and glutamine. Although significant, the effect of growth hormones (0.13 mg/kg body weight/day) and oral glutamine on intestinal sodium and potassium absorption was less than 5 mmol/day in the placebo-controlled, double-blind study by Scolapio *et al.* (1997). In contrast, growth hormone (0.11 mg/kg body weight/day) and glutamine, both orally and parenterally administered, tended to decrease wet-weight absorption and increase faecal excretion of sodium and potassium, which reached significance ($P < 0.05$) in comparison with baseline values from the study of Szkudlarek *et al.* (2000). However, these findings were contrasted by clinical findings of generalized oedema, increased body weight, a need for diuretics and a reduction in parenteral saline during treatment. The patients were probably in the process of excreting water and sodium accumulated during the treatment at the time of the post-treatment balance studies 5 days after termination of treatment. In the lower-dose studies from Ellegård *et al.* (1997) (growth hormone

0.024 mg/kg body weight/day) and Seguy *et al.* (2003) (0.05 mg/kg body weight/day), no significant positive effects on either wet-weight or sodium absorption were seen.

The efficacy data of somatotropin (0.1 mg/kg body weight/day for 4 weeks) in a randomized, double-blind parallel-group study of 41 patients with SBS (mainly with a preserved colon and stool volume less than 3 l/day) who were dependent on PN have been obtained from the manufacturer's prescribing information (Byrne *et al.*, 2005). The protocol for weaning from PS is not given, but it mainly seems to be based on body weight, measurement of total body water by bioelectrical impedance analysis (BIA) and measurements of serum sodium, potassium and bicarbonate. A significantly greater reduction from baseline in total parenteral volume occurred in recipients of somatropin (Zorptive™) plus glutamine or somatropin (Zorptive™) alone than in placebo plus glutamine recipients (−7.7 and −5.9 versus −3.8 l/week). Thus, the effect of somatropin (Zorptive™) and glutamine averages 557 ml/day. Balance studies on intestinal absorption were not performed and the results on urinary excretions are not given (Byrne *et al.*, 2005).

The effects of growth hormone are global and not specific for the intestine. It has been reported that growth hormone increases extracellular volume by stimulating sodium reabsorption in the distal nephron and preventing pressure natriuresis (Johannsson *et al.*, 2002). Therefore, when employing BIA in the weaning from PS, it should be considered that the effects of growth hormone on fluid balance in short bowel patients may be related to effects on the kidneys and the extracellular space rather than on the intestine.

The effects of GLP-2 and teduglutide (Gattex™ and Revestive™) are presumed to be more specific for the intestine. In the first study with native GLP-2 by Jeppesen *et al.*, eight patients were treated with 400 µg of native GLP-2 twice daily, given subcutaneously for 35 days, in an open-label study (corresponding to 0.013 ± 0.002 mg/kg body weight/day, a range of 0.011–0.017 mg/kg body weight/day) (Jeppesen *et al.*, 2001a). Four patients with a mean residual jejunum of 83 cm received home parenteral nutrition (HPN), whereas four patients with a mean ileum resection of 106 cm did not. None of the patients had colon in continuity. Their average wet-weight absorption was 1.2 ± 1.7 kg/day at baseline and the wet-weight absorption increased by 420 ± 480 g/day ($P = 0.04$), whereas the effect on sodium absorption did not quite reach statistical significance (33 ± 49 mmol/day; $P = 0.10$).

In a subsequent open-label, pilot phase 2 study employing a dipeptidyl peptidase IV-resistant GLP-2 analogue, teduglutide, at doses of 0.03–0.15 mg/kg body weight/day in 16 short bowel patients (six with remnant parts of the colon), wet-weight absorption increased by 743 ± 477 g/day ($P < 0.001$), thereby significantly increasing urine weight (555 ± 485 g/day; $P < 0.001$) and sodium excretion (53 ± 40 mmol/day; $P < 0.001$) (Jeppesen *et al.*, 2005).

Having illustrated that increases in wet-weight absorption were paralleled by increases in urine production, the ability to reduce PS according to increases in urine production served as the end point in the phase 3 development of teduglutide. In the first phase 3 study, patients with SBS were randomized to a 0.05 mg/kg body weight/day dose ($n = 35$), a 0.10 mg/kg body weight/day dose ($n = 32$) or placebo ($n=16$) for up to 24 weeks (Jeppesen *et al.*, 2011). In the primary efficacy analysis of the study, no statistically significant difference between the group on teduglutide 0.10 mg/kg body weight/day and the placebo group was shown, while the proportion of patients receiving the recommended dose of 0.05 mg/kg body weight/day who achieved at least a 20% reduction of PS at weeks 20 and 24 was significantly higher versus placebo (46% versus 6%; $P<0.01$). At week 24, teduglutide treatment resulted in a 2.5 l/week reduction in PS requirements from 9.6 l/week at baseline. In this study, teduglutide also induced expansion of the intestinal mucosa. Sixty-five patients opted to enter an open-label, 28-week extension study. In the patients who received one year of continuous teduglutide treatment, the mean reduction of weekly PS volume was 4.9 l/week, equivalent to a 52% reduction from baseline levels. After modifications of the study protocol allowing for earlier (at week 2 versus week 4) and more aggressive PS weaning (10% versus 10–30%), a second pivotal, phase 3 study was performed (Jeppesen *et al.*, 2012). Forty-three SBS patients were randomized to a teduglutide dose of 0.05 mg/kg body weight/day and 43 patients received placebo for up to 24 weeks. The proportion of teduglutide-treated patients achieving a 20–100% reduction of PS at weeks 20 and 24 was statistically significantly higher compared with placebo (27 out of 43 patients, 62.8%, versus 13 out of 43 patients, 30.2%; $P=0.002$). Teduglutide treatment resulted in a 4.4 l/week reduction in PS volume from a pre-treatment baseline of 12.9 l/week, versus 2.3 l/week from a pre-treatment baseline of 13.2 l/week for placebo, at week 24. In patients completing the study, 21 patients treated with teduglutide (54%) versus nine on placebo (23%) achieved at least a one-day reduction in PS administration ($P=0.005$).

Energy absorption

In studies using growth hormone, there have been conflicting results on intestinal energy and macronutrient absorption. In the study by Byrne and Wilmore, the baseline dietary energy intake was 2692 kcal/day (~12,269 kJ/day) and 1618 kcal/day (~6773 kJ/day; 60%) was absorbed (Byrne *et al.*, 1995b). Thus, according to the guidelines that define intestinal failure suggested by Jeppesen and Mortensen (2000), the majority of these patients did not need parenteral energy. After 3 weeks of treatment, the intake and absorption were 2367 kcal/day (9908 kJ/day) and 1759 kcal/day (~7363 kJ/day; 74%), respectively, which was a significant improvement in percentage ($P<0.003$) but an increase of only 141 kcal/day (~590 kJ/day) in absolute amount. In this study by Byrne and Wilmore, all eight short bowel patients had a colon in continuity. As stated, the 'rehabilitation' included a high-carbohydrate, low-fat diet, which in itself is known to increase the energy absorption in this segment of short bowel patients. Supporting the hypothesis that diet alone resulted in this effect, intestinal fat absorption did not improve. In the study by Scolapio *et al.* (1997), where only two of eight patients had a colon in continuity, high-carbohydrate diets were provided in both the placebo and treatment arms. Energy absorption was not measured, but no changes were observed regarding nitrogen or fat absorption. In the studies by Ellegård *et al.* (1997) and Szkudlarek *et al.* (2000), no changes were found in intestinal energy or in fat or nitrogen absorption. In the study by Seguy *et al.* (2003), growth hormone (0.05 mg/kg body weight/day, nine of 12 patients with colon in continuity) and an unrestricted hyperphagic diet increased intestinal absorption of nitrogen by 146% ($P<0.040$), carbohydrates by 104% ($P<0.040$) and energy by 155% ($P<0.002$), which in absolute terms was 427 kcal/day (~1787 kJ/day). Fat absorption was unaffected by the treatment. During growth hormone treatment the mean dietary energy intake was 192 kcal/day (~804 kJ/day) higher. In the study on somatropin (Zorptive™), the mean reductions from baseline in total parenteral calories were significantly greater in recipients of somatropin (Zorptive™) plus glutamine or somatropin (Zorptive™) alone than in recipients of placebo plus glutamine: 5751 and 4338 versus 2633 kcal/week (~24,074 and ~18,159 versus ~11,022 kJ/week) (Byrne *et al.*, 2005). Thus, the effect of the combined therapy of somatropin (Zorptive™) plus glutamine would correspond to an effect of 445 kcal/day (~1863 kJ/day). Apparently, there were no changes in the dietary energy intake in the three parallel study groups.

In the study with native GLP-2, the absolute energy absorption tended to increase by 441 ± 634 kJ/day (105 ± 151 kcal/day; $P=0.09$). Treatment with GLP-2 increased the energy absorption by 3.5 ± 4.0%, from 49.9 ± 20.3% to 53.4 ± 18.1% ($P=0.04$), which was equivalent to an increase of 13.1 ± 22.3% in the percentage of absorption at baseline (49.9%). Absorption of carbohydrates improved by 347 ± 444 kJ/day (83 ± 106 kcal/day; $P=0.06$), which was borderline significant, whereas the relative absorption showed a non-significant increasing trend of 4.4 ± 7.5% ($P=0.14$) from 69.7 ± 22.0% to 74.1 ± 15.9%. Excretion of protein (nitrogen) decreased by 143 ± 127 kJ/day (34 ± 30 kcal/day; $P=0.02$), but the effect on the absolute absorption did not reach statistical significance ($P=0.16$). This was in contrast to the improvement in the relative absorption of protein, which increased by 4.7 ± 5.4% from 47.4 ± 29.3% to 52.1 ± 28.4% ($P=0.04$). The effect of GLP-2 on fat absorption was not significant. The improvement in the absolute amount of energy absorbed was obtained in spite of a non-significant decrease in intake of 173 kJ/day (~41 kcal/day), which means that the reduction in the energy malabsorbed (equal to the stomal excretion) was proportionally larger (617 kJ/day; ~147 kcal/day).

In the study employing the dipeptidyl peptidase IV-resistant GLP-2 analogue, teduglutide, in doses of 0.03–0.15 mg/kg body weight/day in 16 short bowel patients (six with remnant parts of the colon), faecal energy excretion was reduced by 808 ± 1453 kJ/day (193 ± 347 kcal/day; $P=0.04$), but this translated into a significant increase in intestinal absorption (963 ± 1290 kJ/day (230 ± 308 kcal/day); $P<0.05$) only in a subset of patients with high dietary compliance during balance studies. No significant changes were seen in the absolute absorption of individual macronutrients (Jeppesen *et al.*, 2005).

The reduction in parenteral energy supply was reported only in the first of the two phase 3 teduglutide studies. Reductions in parenteral energy at week 24 of 243 ± 450 kJ/day (58 ± 108 kcal/day; $P=0.056$), 447 ± 1051 kJ/day (107 ± 251 kcal/day; $P=0.030$) and 912 ± 1333 kJ/day (218 ± 318 kcal/day; $P=0.001$), respectively, were seen in the placebo group, teduglutide 0.10 mg/kg body weight/day group and the teduglutide 0.05 mg/kg body weight/day group, respectively, compared with baseline. However, the reductions in parenteral energy were not significant between active teduglutide (0.10 mg/kg body weight/day and 0.05 mg/kg body weight/day) and placebo ($P = 0.11$) (Jeppesen *et al.*, 2011).

Body weight, composition and urine creatinine excretion

In the growth hormone study by Byrne *et al.* (1995b) a weight gain of 5.4 ± 1.2 kg was described in the eight patients after 21 days of treatment. Occurrence of oedema was not reported, but increases in body weight are difficult to explain considering the magnitude of the effect on energy balance of approximately 12.4 MJ (590 kJ/day) (~2962 kcal (~141 kcal/day)) over the 21 days of treatment. In this study neither body composition nor urine creatinine excretion was measured.

In the 8-week growth hormone (0.024 mg/kg body weight/day) study by Ellegård *et al.* (1997), an increase in lean body mass of 2.5 kg and a decrease in fat mass of 0.1 kg were found. Total body potassium increased by 4.7%, equivalent to 1.1 ± 0.4 kg of body cell mass, which was parallel to the 5.6% increase in lean body mass measured by dual energy X-ray absorptiometry (DEXA). Ellegård *et al.* (1997) concluded that the increase in lean body mass was derived from both increased body cell mass and extracellular water.

Using DEXA measurements, Scolapio *et al.* (1997) found an increase in lean body mass of 3.96 ± 0.5 kg and a decrease in the percentage body fat of 2.51 ± 0.4%, which corresponded to approximately 1.0 kg compared with placebo (Scolapio, 1999). Scolapio *et al.* (1997) concluded that the increased body weight during treatment with high doses of growth hormone was caused mainly by the increase in extracellular water and the presence of peripheral oedema, which was encountered in all eight patients treated.

In the study by Szkudlarek *et al.* (2000), a weight gain of 1.0 ± 0.3 kg ($P < 0.050$) was measured daily for 5 days after 4 weeks of treatment. DEXA evaluation indicated that lean body mass increased by 2.9 kg ($P < 0.001$) and fat mass decreased by 2.4 kg ($P < 0.001$) compared with baseline, whereas the changes were not significant in comparison to placebo. No changes were seen in urinary creatinine excretion (Jeppesen *et al.*, 2001b).

The most likely explanation for the rather modest weight gain and increase in lean body mass in the study of Szkudlarek *et al.* (2000) could be the timing of measurements. The patients had been off growth hormone and glutamine for 5 days when the DEXA-scan measurements were performed. At this time, generalized oedemas, which occurred in all eight patients, were on the decline. In the other studies, lean body mass was measured while patients were still receiving treatment. In the study by Seguy *et al.* (2003) body weight increased by 2.0 kg ($P < 0.003$) and the lean body mass, measured by BIA, increased by 2.2 kg ($P < 0.006$). No adverse events of the growth hormone treatment were encountered.

In the study on somatropin (Zorptive™), a body weight loss of 5.2 kg (from 63.9 kg to 58.7 kg) was observed from week 2 (pre-treatment) to week 18 (12 weeks post-treatment) in patients treated with the combined therapy of somatropin (Zorptive™) plus glutamine. This weight loss closely reflects the anticipated weight loss derived by calculation of the energy deficit obtained by reduction of the parenteral energy support of 1863 kJ/day (~445 kcal/day) (Byrne *et al.*, 2005).

In the 35-day study with native GLP-2 treatment, the overall increase in energy absorption of 15 MJ translated into a significant increase in body weight of 1.2 ± 1.0 kg (P = 0.010) (Jeppesen *et al.*, 2001a). Lean body mass improved by 2.9 ± 1.9 kg (P = 0.004) and fat mass decreased by 1.8 ± 1.3 kg (P = 0.007). The study demonstrated positive findings on urine creatinine excretion (0.7 ± 0.7 mmol/day; P = 0.02), which suggests an increase in muscle mass or increase in renal function in relation to the GLP-2 treatment.

In all of the clinical teduglutide studies, numerical increases in body weight were seen: 0.9 ± 2.1 kg at week 3 (Jeppesen *et al.*, 2005); 1.4 ± 2.5 kg with teduglutide 0.10 mg/kg body weight/day and 1.2 ± 2.8 kg with teduglutide 0.05 mg/kg body weight/day at week 24 (Jeppesen *et al.*, 2011); and 1.0 ± 2.8 kg with teduglutide 0.05 mg/kg body weight/day at week 24 (Jeppesen *et al.*, 2012). However, none of these reached statistical significance compared with placebo.

Conclusion

In recent years, increased attention has been addressed to the pharmacological enhancement of bowel adaptation aimed at improving remnant bowel function, limiting symptoms of malabsorption and the burden and risks of PS in SBS patients with intestinal failure, thereby providing the best possible quality of life (Jeppesen *et al.*, 1999). Both growth hormone and teduglutide have been approved for the treatment of patients with SBS and intestinal failure. However, when implementing new treatment strategies, it is prudent to evaluate and balance the benefit or clinical meaningfulness of the intervention versus the inconveniences, adverse effects and risks.

Although the initial trials employing growth hormone and glutamine were positive, the subsequent controlled trials demonstrated conflicting findings. Regarding improvements in wet-weight absorption, the largest effects were in studies employing the highest doses and mainly in short bowel patients with a preserved colon. The maximum effect reported on wet-weight absorption was approximately 700 g/day, but it is not possible to determine if this effect is due to the combination of growth hormone and glutamine and a high-carbohydrate low-fat diet, oral rehydration solutions or the combination. The effect on wet-weight absorption in jejunostomy short bowel patients without a colon in continuity seems limited. Regarding the intestinal energy absorption, the effects seem to be limited in the high-dose studies, whereas the low-dose study of Seguy *et al.* (2003) demonstrated an impressive effect of 427 kcal/day (~1787 kJ/day). This effect was, however, obtained at a higher dietary intake (192 kcal/day, ~ 804 kJ/day) possibly reducing the true effect to about 200 kcal/day (~ 1000 kJ/day). The indirectly demonstrated effect on energy absorption by weaning from parenteral energy support in relation to somatropin (Zorptive™) treatment was 445 kcal/day (~ 1863 kJ/day), but the significant 5.2 kg weight loss after weaning from PS has raised concern. The overall impression is that the effects of high doses of growth hormone are related to the wet-weight absorption (or fluid retention) and mainly in patients with a preserved colon, whereas the effects on energy absorption are minor. In the lower doses of growth hormone there may be an effect on energy absorption in short bowel patients with a colon in continuity, whereas an effect on wet-weight absorption regardless of intestinal anatomy seems minimal. This may restrict the benefit of this therapy, since a large fraction of the SBS patients in an HPN population are jejunostomy patients without a colon in continuity. Since none of the studies have demonstrated ongoing effects after termination of treatment, there is a need for sustained treatment. The risk of acromegaly and the presence and severity of adverse events is a concern. The myalgia, arthralgia, gynaecomastia, carpal tunnel syndrome, nightmares and insomnia reported in many growth hormone studies in short bowel patients may also jeopardize the positive effects on quality of life, which should be the ultimate goal of such treatment.

Therefore, hopes have been directed towards GLP-2 and the analogue, teduglutide (Gattex™ and Revestive™), because the physiological effects appear rather specific for the gut, which is concordant with the localization of the GLP-2 receptor. These peptides have intestinotrophic, antisecretory and transit-modulating effects in short bowel patients. Initially, the effects of native GLP-2 were not clinically dramatic: an increase in energy absorption of 105 kcal/day (~441 kJ/day) and in wet-weight absorption of 420 g/day, but in the first human trial, the dose of GLP-2 and the duration of therapy were chosen arbitrarily. The GLP-2 analogue, teduglutide, which is more slowly degraded (Drucker *et al.*, 1997), doubled the effects seen in the study employing native GLP-2, increasing the energy absorption by 189 kcal/day (~792 kJ/day) and the wet-weight absorption by 743 g/day (Jeppesen *et al.*, 2005). Equivalent effects were demonstrated in the phase 3 development programme, where reduction in PS was the primary end point. Days off PS were seen in 54% of the patients (Jeppesen *et al.*, 2012). The optimal dosage and administration of this new treatment to short bowel patients to induce beneficial effects on intestinal secretion, motility, morphology and (most important) absorption is not known, but since the effect is seen in both short bowel with and without a colon in continuity, it may eventually result in long-term improvements in nutritional status and independence from PN in a large fraction of the borderline short bowel patients.

The phase 3 teduglutide studies have revealed that teduglutide treatment may be associated with adverse events, mainly of gastrointestinal origin (abdominal distension, abdominal pain, nausea and stoma enlargement), due to its pharmacological mode of action. However, it was reassuring that only two patients in the teduglutide group and three in the placebo group terminated the second phase 3 study owing to treatment-emergent adverse events. A carefully monitored down-titration of the daily dose may be considered for some patients with adverse events to optimize tolerability of teduglutide treatment. As a precaution for the development of neoplasia (Thulesen *et al.*, 2004), a colonoscopy with removal of polyps should be performed at the start of treatment with teduglutide. Adherence to follow-up guidelines is recommended. In the case of neoplasia of the liver, gallbladder, pancreas or gastrointestinal tract, teduglutide treatment should be discontinued. In general, teduglutide should not be prescribed to patients with malignancies within the last 5 years. Cases of cholecystitis, cholangitis, cholelithiasis and pancreatitis have been reported in the clinical studies, and therefore in such cases continued teduglutide treatment should be reassessed. Causes of intestinal obstruction have been described in clinical studies, and in such incidences continued teduglutide treatment should be reassessed. Due to the increased fluid absorption in relation to teduglutide, patients with cardiovascular disease should be monitored for cardiac insufficiency or hypertension, especially during initiation of treatment. Patients receiving medicinal products with a narrow therapeutic index should also be monitored due to the potential for increased absorption.

In the years to come, it is anticipated that more novel agents will be investigated to provide further incremental improvement in the care of SBS patients with intestinal failure. The recent successful setup, design and conduct of trials has revealed that drug approval indeed is possible in this heterogeneous patient population, establishing statistical significance, clinical efficacy and safety of the investigated treatments. The appropriate selection of end points, usage of strict criteria for inclusion and exclusion, optimization and stabilization of patients along with strong collaboration between medical centres of excellence with an interest in SBS patients with intestinal failure will help produce powerful clinical trials with informative results, which will substantially aid in the management of patients with this chronic debilitating disease.

Summary

So far, the conventional pharmacological treatments in short bowel patients have mainly included antisecretory and antidiarrhoeal agents. However, over the past decades, it has become increasingly clear that mucosal nerve ends and endocrine cells within the gastrointestinal tract pass information via the enteric nervous system in response to the passing of luminal contents, thereby regulating the highly coordinated processes of nutrient assimilation. The neuro-endocrine feedback mechanisms often referred to as the 'gastric, ileal or colonic brake' may be disrupted by intestinal resections or mucosal disease. The attenuation of the meal-stimulated secretion of hormones may result in some of the pathophysiological features of SBS: accelerated gastrointestinal motility, gastric and intestinal hypersecretion, diminished intestinal blood flow, disturbed immunological and barrier functions, impaired mucosal replacement, repair and adaptation. These observations have instigated the use of hormonal factors in the intestinal rehabilitation of SBS patients. Thus, somatropin (Zorptive™) and teduglutide (Revestive™ and Gattex™ in Europe and the USA, respectively) have gained marketing approval for the treatment of SBS patients. These modern treatments aim to maximize remnant intestinal absorption, decrease malabsorption and accompanying symptoms, reduce the need, burdens and complications related to PS, and ultimately to improve the health-related quality of life in SBS patients with intestinal failure.

References

Booth, C.C., Evans, K.T., Menzies, T. and Street, D.F. (1958) Intestinal hypertrophy following partial resection of the small bowel in the rat. *British Journal of Surgery* 46, 403–410.

Byrne, T.A., Morrissey, T.B., Nattakom, T.V., Ziegler, T.R. and Wilmore D.W. (1995a) Growth hormone, glutamine, and a modified diet enhance nutrient absorption in patients with severe short bowel syndrome. *JPEN Journal of Parenteral and Enteral Nutrition* 19, 296–302.

Byrne, T.A., Persinger, R.L., Young, L.S., Ziegler, T.R. and Wilmore, D.W. (1995b) A new treatment for patients with short-bowel syndrome. Growth hormone, glutamine, and a modified diet. *Annals of Surgery* 222, 243–254

Byrne, T.A., Wilmore, D.W., Iyer, K., DiBaise, J., Robinson, M.K., Chang, P., Getner, J.M. and Lautz, D. (2005) Growth hormone, glutamine, and an optimal diet reduces parenteral nutrition in patients with short bowel syndrome: a prospective, randomized, placebo-controlled, double-blind clinical trial. *Annals of Surgery* 242, 655–661.

Dowling, R.H. and Booth, C.C. (1966) Functional compensation after small-bowel resection in man. Demonstration by direct measurement. *The Lancet* 2, 146–147.

Dowling, R.H. and Booth, C.C. (1967) Structural and functional changes following small intestinal resection in the rat. *Clinical Science* 32, 139–149.

Drucker, D.J., Shi, Q., Crivici, A., Sumner-Smith, M., Tavares, W., Hill, M., DeForest, L., Cooper, S. and Brubaker, P.L. (1997) Regulation of the biological activity of glucagon-like peptide 2 *in vivo* by dipeptidyl peptidase IV. *Nature Biotechnology* 15, 673–677.

Eastwood, G.L. (1977) Gastrointestinal epithelial renewal. *Gastroenterology* 72, 962–975.

Ellegård, L., Bosaeus, I., Nordgren, S. and Bengtsson, B.A. (1997) Low-dose recombinant human growth hormone increases body weight and lean body mass in patients with short bowel syndrome. *Annals of Surgery* 225, 88–96.

Forrester, J.M. (1972) The number of villi in rat's jejunum and ileum: effect of normal growth, partial enterectomy, and tube feeding. *Journal of Anatomy* 111, 283–291.

Friedman, H.I., Chandler, J.G., Peck, C.C., Nemeth, T.J. and Odum, S.K. (1978) Alterations in intestinal structure, fat absorption and body weight after intestinal bypass for morbid obesity. *Surgery, Gynecology & Obstetrics* 146, 757–767.

Gouttebel, M.C., Saint Aubert, B., Colette, C., Astre, C., Monnier, L.H. and Joyeux, H. (1989) Intestinal adaptation in patients with short bowel syndrome. Measurement by calcium absorption. *Digestive Diseases and Sciences* 34, 709–715.

Hanson, W.R., Osborne, J.W. and Sharp, J.G. (1977) Compensation by the residual intestine after intestinal resection in the rat. I. Influence of amount of tissue removed. *Gastroenterology* 72, 692–705.

Hill, G.L., Mair, W.S. and Goligher, J.C. (1974) Impairment of 'ileostomy adaptation' in patients after ileal resection. *Gut* 15, 982–987.

Jeppesen, P.B. and Mortensen, P.B. (2000) Intestinal failure defined by measurements of intestinal energy and wet weight absorption. *Gut* 46, 701–706.

Jeppesen, P.B., Langholz, E. and Mortensen, P.B. (1999) Quality of life in patients receiving home parenteral nutrition. *Gut* 44, 844–852.

Jeppesen, P.B., Hartmann, B., Thulesen, J., Graff, J., Lohmann, J. and Hansen, B.S., Tofteng, F., Poulsen, S.S., Madsen, J.L., Holst, J.J. and Mortensen, P.B. (2001a) Glucagon-like peptide 2 improves nutrient absorption and nutritional status in short-bowel patients with no colon. *Gastroenterology* 120, 806–815.

Jeppesen, P.B., Szkudlarek, J., Hoy, C.E. and Mortensen, P.B. (2001b) Effect of high-dose growth hormone and glutamine on body composition, urine creatinine excretion, fatty acid absorption, and essential fatty acids status in short bowel patients: a randomized, double-blind, crossover, placebo-controlled study. *Scandinavian Journal of Gastroenterology* 36, 48–54.

Jeppesen, P.B., Sanguinetti, E.L., Buchman, A., Howard, L., Scolapio, J.S., Ziegler, T.R., Gregory, J., Tappenden, K.A., Holst, J. and Mortensen, P.B. (2005) Teduglutide (ALX-0600), a dipeptidyl peptidase IV resistant glucagons-like peptide 2 analogue, improves intestinal function in short bowel syndrome patients. *Gut* 54, 1224–1231.

Jeppesen, P.B., Gilroy, R., Pertkiewicz, M., Allard, J.P., Messing, B. and O'Keefe, S.J. (2011) Randomised placebo-controlled trial of teduglutide in reducing parenteral nutrition and/or intravenous fluid requirements in patients with short bowel syndrome. *Gut* 60, 902–914.

Jeppesen, P.B., Pertkiewicz, M., Messing, B., Iyer, K., Seidner, D.L., O'Keefe, S.J., Forbes, A., Heinze, H. and Joelsson, B. (2012) Teduglutide reduces the need for parenteral support among patients with short bowel syndrome with intestinal failure. *Gastroenterology* 143, 1473–1481.

Johannsson, G., Sverrisdottir, Y.B., Ellegard, L., Lundberg, P.A. and Herlitz, H. (2002) GH increases extracellular volume by stimulating sodium reabsorption in the distal nephron and preventing pressure natriuresis. *Journal of Clinical Endocrinology and Metabolism* 87, 1743–1749.

McCarthy, D.M. and Kim, Y.S. (1973) Changes in sucrase, enterokinase, and peptide hydrolase after intestinal resection. The association of cellular hyperplasia and adaptation. *Journal of Clinical Investigation* 52, 942–951.

Nightingale, J.M. and Lennard-Jones, J.E. (1993) The short bowel syndrome: what's new and old? *Digestive Diseases* 11, 12–31.

Nundy, S., Malamud, D., Obertop, H., Sczerban, J. and Malt, R.A. (1977) Onset of cell proliferation in the shortened gut. Colonic hyperplasia after ileal resection. *Gastroenterology* 72, 263–266.

Nygaard, K. (1967) Resection of the small intestine in rats. 3. Morphological changes in the intestinal tract. *Acta Chirurgica Scandinavica* 133, 233–248.

Obertop, H., Nundy, S., Malamud, D. and Malt, R.A. (1977) Onset of cell proliferation in the shortened gut. Rapid hyperplasia after jejunal resection. *Gastroenterology* 72, 267–270.

Porus, R.L. (1965) Epithelial hyperplasia following massive small bowel resection in man. *Gastroenterology* 48, 753–757.

Remington, M., Malagelada, J.R., Zinsmeister, A. and Fleming, C.R. (1983) Abnormalities in gastrointestinal motor activity in patients with short bowels: effect of a synthetic opiate. *Gastroenterology* 85, 629–636.

Scolapio, J.S. (1999) Effect of growth hormone, glutamine, and diet on body composition in short bowel syndrome: a randomized, controlled study. *JPEN Journal of Parenteral and Enteral Nutrition* 23, 309–313.

Scolapio, J.S., Camilleri, M., Fleming, C.R., Oenning, L.V., Burton, D.D., Sebo, T.J., Batts, K.P. and Kelly, D.G. (1997) Effect of growth hormone, glutamine, and diet on adaptation in short-bowel syndrome: a randomized, controlled study. *Gastroenterology* 113, 1074–1081.

Seguy, D., Vahedi, K., Kapel, N., Souberbielle, J.C. and Messing, B. (2003) Low-dose growth hormone in adult home parenteral nutrition-dependent short bowel syndrome patients: a positive study. *Gastroenterology* 124, 293–302.

Solhaug, J.H. and Tvete, S. (1978) Adaptative changes in the small intestine following bypass operation for obesity. A radiological and histological study. *Scandinavian Journal of Gastroenterology* 13, 401–408.

Szkudlarek, J., Jeppesen, P.B. and Mortensen, P.B. (2000) Effect of high dose growth hormone with glutamine and no change in diet on intestinal absorption in short bowel patients: a randomised, double blind, crossover, placebo controlled study. *Gut* 47, 199–205.

Thulesen, J., Hartmann, B., Hare, K.J., Kissow, H., Orskov, C., Holst, J.J. and Poulsen, S.S. (2004) Glucagon-like peptide 2 (GLP-2) accelerates the growth of colonic neoplasms in mice. *Gut* 53, 1145–1150.

Tilson, M.D. and Wright, H.K. (1970) Adaptation of functioning and bypassed segments of ileum during compensatory hypertrophy of the gut. *Surgery* 67, 687–693.

Tilson, M.D. and Wright, H.K. (1971) An adaptive change in ileal Na-K-ATPase activity after jejunectomy or jejunal transposition. *Surgery* 70, 421–424.

Tilson, M.D., Michaud, J.T. and Livstone, E.M. (1976) Early proliferative activity in the left colon of the rat after partial small-bowel resection. *Surgical Forum* 27, 445–446.

Weinstein, L.D., Shoemaker, C.P., Hersh. T. and Wright, H.K. (1969) Enhanced intestinal absorption after small bowel resection in man. *Archives of Surgery* 99, 560–562.

Weser, E. and Hernandez, M.H. (1971) Studies of small bowel adaptation after intestinal resection in the rat. *Gastroenterology* 60, 69–75.

Williamson, R.C., Bauer, F.L., Ross, J.S. and Malt, R.A. (1978) Proximal enterectomy stimulates distal hyperplasia more than bypass or pancreaticobiliary diversion. *Gastroenterology* 74, 16–23.

Woo, Z.H. and Nygaard, K. (1978) Small-bowel adaptation after colectomy in rats. *Scandinavian Journal of Gastroenterology* 13, 903–910.

Wright, H.K., Poskitt, T., Cleveland, J.C. and Herskovic, T. (1969) The effect of total colectomy on morphology and absorptive capacity of ileum in the rat. *Journal of Surgical Research* 9, 301–304.

Young, E.A. and Weser, E. (1974) Nutritional adaptation after small bowel resection in rats. *Journal of Nutrition* 104, 994–1001.

38 Indications for Intestinal Transplantation

Loris Pironi*

Center for Chronic Intestinal Failure, Department of Medical and Surgical Science, University of Bologna, Bologna, Italy

Key Points

- Home parenteral nutrition (HPN) is the primary treatment for patients with chronic intestinal failure. These patients have a high probability of long-term survival, but they may have also an increased risk of death due to factors related to parenteral nutrition or the underlying disease that caused the intestinal failure. Intestinal rehabilitation programmes based on medical treatments and non-transplant surgery can reverse intestinal failure in about half of them. The risk of death after intestinal transplantation (ITx) is higher than on HPN, mainly because of complications related to immunosuppressive therapy and of acute cellular rejection.
- A European prospective study on the survival probability and causes of death on long-term HPN has identified liver failure, due to intestinal failure/parenteral nutrition-associated liver disease, and invasive intra-abdominal desmoids as the only conditions associated with an increased risk of death on HPN and, therefore, the only indications for a life-saving ITx. The other major complications of HPN, as well as the other causes of intestinal failure, were not associated with a statistically significant increased risk of death on HPN. For these conditions, a rehabilitative ITx could be offered on a case-by-case basis, carefully selecting patients to avoid the risk of premature death following a transplant.
- The probability of survival after ITx is increased in patients who are admitted directly from home to undergo transplantation, younger patients, those who receive a first transplant and those who receive antibody induction therapy or maintenance sirolimus. These findings emphasize the importance of early referral of patients who are well enough to await transplantation at home.

*E-mail: loris.pironi@unibo.it

- In order to maximize the opportunity of weaning from HPN, prevent major complications of the treatment and ensure timely ITx when this is needed, an early referral of patients to intestinal rehabilitation centres with expertise in both medical and surgical treatment for intestinal failure is recommended.

Introduction

Intestinal failure is defined as a reduction in the functioning gut mass below the minimum amount necessary for adequate digestion and absorption of nutrients to achieve and maintain normal nutritional status (Fleming and Remington, 1981). It results from obstruction, dysmotility, surgical resection, congenital defect or disease-associated loss of absorption, and is characterized by the inability to maintain protein–energy, fluid, electrolyte or micronutrient balance (O'Keefe *et al.*, 2006). Intestinal failure can be classified into four major pathophysiological conditions: (i) short bowel syndrome (SBS); (ii) chronic intestinal pseudo-obstruction; (iii) small bowel parenchymal disease; and (iv) intestinal fistula, which may originate from various gastrointestinal or systemic diseases (Pironi *et al.*, 2006). Intestinal failure may be an acute or a chronic condition and can be associated with the presence of a benign disease or an active cancer. Long-term home parenteral nutrition (HPN) is the 'artificial gut' for the medical treatment of chronic intestinal failure (CIF) due to benign disease. Intestinal rehabilitation programmes based on dietary and medical therapy and on surgical reconstruction can improve intestinal function and allow the patient to be weaned off HPN (Shatnawei *et al.*, 2010).

Patients with irreversible CIF are destined to remain on lifelong HPN or to undergo intestinal transplantation (ITx). The mean survival rates on HPN at 1, 5 and 10 years have been reported to be 91%, 70% and 55% in adults, and 96%, 89% and 81% in children, respectively. Deaths related to HPN complications were 14% of the total deaths in adults and up to 70% in babies younger than a year old (Pironi *et al.*, 2012a). The 2011 International Transplant Registry report showed a 5-year patient survival rate after ITx of 40% in adults and 50% in children (Grant *et al.*, 2005; http://www.tts.org). Similar data were reported in the 2009 annual report of the US Organ Procurement and Transplantation Network, which showed a wide range between transplant centres (30–72%) with the best result achieved in the most experienced centres (UNOS Report, 2009). The database showed that almost all of the deaths after ITx were related to the treatment.

On the basis of data on safety and efficacy, HPN is considered the primary treatment for CIF. In 2001, the indications for ITx were defined by two documents and were categorized as life-threatening complications related to HPN (USA Center for Medicare and Medicaid Services) (Buchman *et al.*, 2003) and high risk of death or very poor quality of life related to the underlying intestinal failure (American Society of Transplantation position paper on paediatric ITx) (Kaufman *et al.*, 2001):

1. Failure of HPN
   - Impending (total bilirubin above 3–6 mg/dl (54–108 µmol/l), progressive thrombocytopenia and progressive splenomegaly) or overt liver

failure (portal hypertension, hepatosplenomegaly, hepatic fibrosis or cirrhosis) because of parenteral nutrition-associated liver injury.
- Central venous catheter (CVC)-related thrombosis of two or more central veins.
- Frequent central line sepsis: two or more episodes per year of systemic sepsis secondary to line infections requiring hospitalization; a single episode of line-related fungaemia; septic shock and/or acute respiratory distress syndrome.
- Frequent episodes of severe dehydration despite intravenous fluid in addition to HPN.

2. High risk of death attributable to the underlying disease
- Desmoid tumours associated with familial adenomatous polyposis.
- Congenital mucosal disorders (i.e. microvillus inclusion disease, tufting enteropathy).
- Ultra-short bowel (gastrostomy, duodenostomy, residual small bowel <10 cm in infants and <20 cm in adults).

3. Intestinal failure with high morbidity or low acceptance of HPN
- Intestinal failure with high morbidity (frequent hospitalization, narcotic dependency) or inability to function (i.e. pseudo-obstruction, high-output stoma).
- Patient's unwillingness to accept long-term HPN (i.e. young patients).

Those documents were based on retrospective analyses of national and international registries, individual centre experience and case reports. Some indications for ITx were a matter of debate (Buchman *et al.*, 2003). In 2004, the Home Artificial Nutrition and Chronic Intestinal Failure working group of the European Society for Clinical Nutrition (ESPEN) carried out a 5-year comparative study to evaluate their appropriateness. Two cohorts of patients on HPN for CIF were compared: (i) 165 candidates for ITx (108 adults and 57 children, having an indication and no contraindication for ITx); and (ii) 418 non-candidates (322 adults and 96 children, having neither an indication nor a contraindication for ITx) (Pironi *et al.*, 2006, 2008, 2011). Contraindications for ITx were taken from the guidelines for patients eligible for solid organ transplantation (Steinman *et al.*, 2001) and were categorized as: (i) absolute (non-resectable malignancy, severe immunological deficiencies, advanced cardiopulmonary disease, advanced neurological dysfunction, sepsis with multisystem organ failure, major psychiatric illness, demonstrated patient non-compliance with medical recommendations, insufficient vascular patency for central venous access for up to 6 months following ITx); or (ii) relative (depending on clinical judgement: age over 65 years, history of cancer in the past 5 years, physical debilitation, lack of family support). In the 165 candidates the indications for ITx were: liver failure, 29; multiple CVC-related deep-vein thrombosis, 37; frequent CVC-related sepsis, 15; frequent dehydration, 2; desmoid tumours, 7; congenital mucosal disorders, 19; ultra-short bowel, 36; intestinal failure with high morbidity or unwillingness to continue HPN, 20.

The 5-year survival rate on HPN was 87% in non-candidates, 74% in candidates with HPN failure, 84% in those with high-risk underlying disease and 100%

in those with high-morbidity intestinal failure/low acceptance of HPN (Pironi *et al.*, 2011). The analysis of the risk of death on HPN and the causes of death associated with each indication showed that only the patients with liver failure due to intestinal failure/parenteral nutrition-associated liver disease (IF/PNALD) or invasive intra-abdominal desmoids had an actual increased risk of death on HPN. In these patients, death on HPN was primarily related to the indication for ITx. For these indications a life-saving role of ITx was confirmed. On the contrary, none of the other indications for ITx showed a statistically significant increased risk of death on HPN, and most of the deaths that occurred in patients with these indications were not related to the underlying disease or to HPN. Furthermore, the 5-year survival rate of the candidates designated because of CVC-related complications or ultra-short bowel did not differ between those who remained on HPN (83%) and those who underwent ITx (78%), the latter being similar to the results obtained by the most experienced US transplant centres (Abu-Elmagd *et al.*, 2012). Therefore, ITx could not have a life-saving role for every patient having these indications, but it might have a pre-emptive/rehabilitative role for patients carefully selected on a case-by-case basis and appropriately informed patients (Table 38.1).

Referral for Life-saving Intestinal Transplantation

A particular issue is represented by the criteria for referral of patients with liver failure due to IF/PNALD. In recent years prevention and treatment of IF/PNALD have improved, allowing liver disease to be reversed and avoiding the need for transplantation in a consistent number of patients (Shatnawei *et al.*, 2010). When medical treatment fails, the issues of the timing of referral for transplantation and of the type of transplantation arise. The definition of impending and overt liver failure due to IF/PNALD used for the USA Medicare indications for ITx are derived from studies in children but apply well also to adults. Persistent hyperbilirubinaemia

Table 38.1. Five-year relative risk of death and causes of death on HPN associated with each indication for ITx: implications for the role of ITx. (From Pironi, 2012a.)

	Hazard ratio		Deaths on HPN due to an indication for	
Indications for ITx	RR	*P* value	ITx (%)	Role for ITx
Intra-abdominal invasive desmoids	7.1	<0.001	91.7	Life saving
Liver failure	3.2	0.002		
CVC – thrombosis (multiple)	2.1	0.058	38.5	Pre-emptive
CVC – sepsis (multiple and severe)	1.1	0.929		Rehabilitative
Ultra-short bowel	0.8	0.763		??
Congenital mucosal disease	0.4	0.374		
Intestinal failure with high morbidity or low acceptance of HPN	0.0		No death	

RR, relative risk.

from 3 to 6 mg/dl (50–100 μmol/l) is a criterion for referral to an intestinal failure rehabilitation unit, whereas a persistent concentration >6 g/dl is a criterion for consultation or referral for ITx assessment (Beath *et al.*, 2008). The prevalence of IF/PNALD is estimated to be approximately 40–60% in infants and up to 85% in neonates who are receiving HPN for intestinal failure, but only 15% of patients on long-term HPN eventually develop an end-stage liver disease, which leads to combined intestinal and liver transplant (Nathan *et al.*, 2007).

The Intestinal Transplant Registry shows that combined liver and intestinal transplantation, either small bowel alone or multivisceral, has the same patient survival probability as ITx without liver, but a higher probability of graft survival (http://www.tts.org/images/stories/ITA/curren_update_worldwide_experience.pdf). In experienced centres, combined liver and intestine transplants approach a 2-year patient and graft survival rate of over 90% (Mazariegos *et al.*, 2006). After successful engraftment of an isolated intestinal transplant, early liver disease may regress with the cessation of parenteral therapy. Recently a case regression of liver cirrhosis has also been reported in adults (Fiel *et al.*, 2009). However, liver function that is preserved at the time of intestinal resection often deteriorates rapidly in small children, accounting for the relatively larger proportion of children who receive combined organ transplants (Fishbein, 2009). On the other hand, it has been reported that isolated liver transplantation in children with liver failure as a result of SBS, who have favourable prognostic features for full enteral adaptation, is feasible with satisfactory long-term survival (Botha *et al.*, 2006; Dell-Olio *et al.*, 2009). According to their results Dell-Olio *et al.* (2009) suggested the following criteria for isolated liver transplantation in children with SBS and liver failure: (i) established intestinal failure-associated liver disease (serum bilirubin >200 μmol/l, moderate/severe fibrosis, portal hypertension); (ii) at least 50 cm functional small bowel remaining intact in the absence of an ileocaecal valve or 30 cm with an ileocaecal valve; (iii) at least 50% of the estimated daily energy requirement was tolerated as enteral feeds for at least 4 weeks before the development of liver disease and was associated with an increase in weight; and (iv) in children with dilated and dysmotile bowel who had minimal line infections (<6 in 12 months). Whether these criteria would be applicable to adults as well is not known. To date, the exact extent of liver damage associated with IF/PNALD that would indicate the need for a liver transplant as well as the type of transplantation remain a matter of judgement.

In patients with invasive intra-abdominal desmoids, survival has been observed to be negatively affected by the presence of pain, the dimension of the tumour (e.g. >10 cm) and the requirement for long-term HPN (Quintini *et al.*, 2012). Patients requiring HPN were more likely to have advanced-stage disease and significantly higher incidence of chronic abdominal pain, narcotic dependency, bowel obstruction, ureteral obstruction, deep-vein thrombosis, pulmonary embolism, fistulae and sepsis. Even though the duration of HPN did not affect mortality, the need for HPN represented a strong predictor of mortality and represented an independent poor prognostic factor associated with high morbidity and mortality. ITx would offer the advantages of making removal of the tumour easier and more complete and is a potentially life-saving therapy for early referred patients (Shatnawei *et al.*, 2013).

Issues with Pre-emptive/Rehabilitative Intestinal Transplantation

The information to be given to a patient asking for a rehabilitative ITx should consider the survival rate, the safety, the morbidity and the quality of life of both HPN and ITx, as well as the timing of referral in order to have the highest probability of a successful ITx (Table 38.2). The 5-year survival probability might be similar provided that ITx is performed in an experienced centre, but over a longer period of time the probability of survival on HPN should be considered higher than after ITx (Abu-Elmagd *et al.*, 2012; Pironi *et al.*, 2012a). Whatever the survival rate, the safety of HPN must be considered greater than that of ITx; the treatment-related death, as well as late morbidity rate, being higher after ITx. Considering

Table 38.2. Factors to be considered for a case-by-case referral for pre-emptive/rehabilitative ITx.

Issue	HPN	ITx
Probability of survival	Higher than after ITx	Higher when performed at most experienced centres
Safety (treatment-related death; % of total deaths)	Adults and children: about 14%	Adults and children: about 85%
	Infants <1 year: up to 70%	
Safety (late morbidity)		
Osteoporosis	41% of patients	42% of patients
Acute cellular rejection		40% of patients
De novo cancer	Rare	17% of patients
Diabetes	Rare	17% of patients
Renal dialysis or kidney transplant		9% of patients
PTLD		4% of patients
Liver disease (biochemistry)	15–85% of patients	Rare
CVC – sepsis	0.14–0.48/year of CVC	
CVC – thrombosis	0.02–0.09/year	
Efficacy	Good nutritional status in almost all patients	Full intestinal autonomy: about 80% Need of intravenous hydration, HPN or re-transplantation: about 20%
Quality of life	After successful ITx: better score in ability to holiday/travel, fatigue, gastrointestinal symptoms, stoma management/bowel movements, ability to eat/drink and global health status/quality of life	
Timing for ITx	Patient clinical status: Higher survival after ITx in patients at home than in patients hospitalized (clinically unstable) at time of calling for the transplantation Patient age: Higher survival in children >1 year and in adults <35 years Lower survival in adults >50 years	

PTLD, post-transplantation lymphoproliferative disorder.

the treatment efficacy, patients should know that in about 20% of ITx recipients a graft failure occurs, primarily because of chronic cellular rejection, and intravenous hydration, HPN or re-transplantation are needed. Only a few studies have compared the quality of life on HPN and after ITx. One of these used the same tool to investigate adult patients, finding that after successful ITx there was a better score in those domains related to gastrointestinal symptoms, food intake and ability to travel (Pironi *et al.*, 2012b). The timing of patient referral for ITx is a key factor for the probability of survival after transplantation, because a late referral is associated with an increased risk of death. Data from the Intestinal Transplant Registry show that survival rate is higher in patients who are in good clinical status at the time of calling for the transplantation (Grant *et al.*, 2005; http://www.tts.org). Also the patient's age is important, especially for adult candidates, with those after the fourth decade having a decreased survival probability (UNOS Report, 2009). Furthermore, those recipients who have received a first transplant, and those who receive antibody induction therapy or maintenance sirolimus, are most likely to survive (Fishbein, 2009).

Summary

The progress in intestinal rehabilitation therapy has modified the strategy of treatment of CIF, moving from straight referral for ITx of any patients with a potential risk of death on HPN to early referral of patients to intestinal rehabilitation centres with expertise in both medical and surgical treatment for intestinal failure, in order to maximize the opportunity of weaning from HPN, prevent HPN failure and ensure timely ITx when this is needed. According to this, an expert consensus recommended that primary caregivers managing intestinal failure patients should establish a link with intestinal failure programmes early and that collaboration with intestinal failure programmes should be initiated for patients whose parenteral nutrition requirements are anticipated to be more than 50% three months after initiating HPN (Beath *et al.*, 2008).

References

Abu-Elmagd, K.M., Kosmach-Park, B., Costa, G., Zenati, M., Martin, L., Koritsky, D.A., Emerling, M., Murase, N., Bond, G.J., Soltys, K., Sogawa, H., Lunz, J., Al Samman, M., Shaefer, N., Sindhi, R. and Mazariegos, G.V. (2012) Long-term survival, nutritional autonomy, and quality of life after intestinal and multivisceral transplantation. *Annals of Surgery* 256, 494–508.

Beath, S., Pironi, L., Gabe, S., Horslen, S., Sudan, D., Mazeriegos, G., Steiger, E., Goulet, O. and Fryer, J. (2008) Collaborative strategies to reduce mortality and morbidity in patients with chronic intestinal failure including those who are referred for small bowel transplantation. *Transplantation* 85, 1378–1384.

Botha, J.F., Grant, W.J., Torres, C., Iverson, A.K., Sudan, D.L., Shaw, B.W. Jr and Langnas, A.N. (2006) Isolated liver transplantation in infants with end-stage liver disease due to short bowel syndrome. *Liver Transplantation* 12, 1062–1066.

Buchman, A.L., Scolapio, J. and Fryer, J. (2003) AGA technical review on short bowel syndrome and intestinal transplantation. *Gastroenterology* 124, 1111–1134.

Dell-Olio, D., Beath, S.V., de Ville de Goyet, J., Clarke, S., Davies, P., Lloyd, C., Protheroe, S., Millar, A.J., Kelly, D.A. and Gupte, G.L. (2009) Isolated liver transplant in infants with short bowel syndrome: insights into outcomes and prognostic factors. *Journal of Pediatric Gastroenterology and Nutrition* 48, 334–340.

Fiel, M.I., Wu, H.S., Iyer, K., Rodriguez-Laiz, G. and Schiano, T.D. (2009) Rapid reversal of parenteral-nutrition-associated cirrhosis following isolated intestinal transplantation. *Journal of Gastrointestinal Surgery* 13, 1717–1723.

Fishbein, T.M. (2009) Intestinal transplantation. *New England Journal of Medicine* 361, 998–1008.

Fleming, C.R. and Remington, M. (1981) Intestinal failure. In: Hill, G.I. (ed.) *Nutrition and the Surgical Patient.* Churchill Livingstone, Edinburgh, pp. 219–235.

Grant, D., Abu-Elmagd, K., Reyes, J., Tzakis, A., Langnas, A., Fishbein, T., Goulet, O. and Farmer, D.; Intestine Transplant Registry (2005) 2003 report of the intestine transplant registry: a new era has dawned. *Annals of Surgery* 241, 607–613.

Kaufman, S.S., Atkinson, J.B., Bianchi, A., Goulet, O.J., Grant, D., Langnas, A.N., McDiarmid, S.V., Mittal, N., Reyes, J. and Tzakis, A.G.; American Society of Transplantation (2001) Indications for pediatric intestinal transplantation: a position paper of the American Society of Transplantation. *Pediatric Transplantation* 5, 80–87.

Mazariegos, G.V., Soltys, K.A., Bond, G.J., Squires, R.H. and Sindhi, R. (2006) Isolated liver transplantation in infants with short gut syndrome: is less better? *Liver Transplantation* 12, 1040–1041.

Nathan, J.D., Rudolph, J.A., Kocoshis, S.A., Alonso, M.H., Ryckman, F.C. and Tiao, G.M. (2007) Isolated liver and multivisceral transplantation for total parenteral nutrition-related end-stage liver disease. *Journal of Pediatric Surgery* 42, 143–147.

O'Keefe, S.J., Buchman, A.L., Fishbein, T.M., Jeejeebhoy, K.N., Jeppesen, P.B. and Shaffer, J. (2006) Short bowel syndrome and intestinal failure: consensus definitions and overview. *Clinical Gastroenterology and Hepatology* 4, 6–10.

Pironi, L., Hébuterne, X., Van Gossum, A., Messing, B., Lyszkowska, M., Colomb, V., Forbes, A., Micklewright, A., Villares, J.M., Thul, P., Bozzetti, F., Goulet, O. and Staun, M. (2006) Candidates for intestinal transplantation: a multicenter survey in Europe. *American Journal of Gastroenterology* 101, 1633–1643.

Pironi, L., Forbes, A., Joly, F., Colomb, V., Lyszkowska, M., Van Gossum, A., Baxter, J., Thul, P., Hébuterne, X., Gambarara, M., Gottrand, F., Moreno Villares, J.M., Messing, B., Goulet, O. and Staun, M.; Home Artificial Nutrition Working Group of the European Society for Clinical Nutrition and Metabolism (ESPEN) (2008) Survival of patients identified as candidates for intestinal transplantation: a 3-year prospective follow-up. *Gastroenterology* 135, 61–71.

Pironi, L., Joly, F., Forbes, A., Colomb, V., Lyszkowska, M., Baxter, J., Gabe, S., Hébuterne, X., Gambarara, M., Gottrand, F., Cuerda, C., Thul, P., Messing, B., Goulet, O., Staun, M. and Van Gossum, A.; Home Artificial Nutrition & Chronic Intestinal Failure Working Group of the European Society for Clinical Nutrition and Metabolism (ESPEN) (2011) Long-term follow-up of patients on home parenteral nutrition in Europe: implications for intestinal transplantation. *Gut* 60, 17–25.

Pironi, L., Goulet, O., Buchman, A., Messing, B., Gabe, S., Candusso, M., Bond, G., Gupte, G., Pertkiewicz, M., Steiger, E., Forbes, A., Van Gossum, A. and Pinna, A.D.; Home Artificial Nutrition and Chronic Intestinal Failure Working Group of ESPEN (2012a) Outcome on home parenteral nutrition for benign intestinal failure: a review of the literature and benchmarking with the European prospective survey of ESPEN. *Clinical Nutrition* 31, 831–845.

Pironi, L., Baxter, J.P., Lauro, A., Guidetti, M., Agostini, F., Zanfi, C. and Pinna, A.D. (2012b) Assessment of quality of life on home parenteral nutrition and after intestinal transplantation using treatment-specific questionnaires. *American Journal of Transplantation* 12(Suppl. 4), S60–S66.

Quintini, C., Ward, G., Shatnawei, A., Xhaja, X., Hashimoto, K., Steiger, E., Hammel, J., Diago Uso, T., Burke, C.A. and Church, J.M. (2012) Mortality of intra-abdominal desmoid tumors in patients with familial adenomatous polyposis: a single center review of 154 patients. *Annals of Surgery* 255, 511–516.

Shatnawei, A., Parekh, N.R., Rhoda, K.M., Speerhas, R., Stafford, J., Dasari, V., Quintini, C., Kirby, D.F. and Steiger, E. (2010) Intestinal failure management at the Cleveland Clinic. *Archives of Surgery* 145, 521–527.

Shatnawei, A., Habib, M., Hamilton, C., Steiger, E., Kirby, D.F., Speerhas, R. and Quintini, C. (2013) The association between home parenteral nutrition and patients with FAP-associated intra-abdominal desmoids: a retrospective study. *JPEN Journal of Parenteral and Enteral Nutrition* 37, 683–688.

Steinman, T.I., Becker, B.N., Frost, A.E., Olthoff, K.M., Smart, F.W., Suki, W.N. and Wilkinson, A.H.; Clinical Practice Committee, American Society of Transplantation (2001) Guidelines for the referral and management of patients eligible for solid organ transplantation. *Transplantation* 71, 1189–1204.

UNOS Report (2009) *2009 Annual Report of the US Organ Procurement and Transplantation Network and the Scientific Registry of Transplant Recipients: Transplant Data 1998–2007.* Department of Health and Human Services, Health Resources and Services Administration, Healthcare Systems Bureau, Division of Transplantation, Rockville, Maryland; United Network for Organ Sharing, Richmond, Virginia; and University Renal Research and Education Association, Ann Arbor, Michigan.

39 Intestinal Transplantation

Antonio D. Pinna[1]*, Loris Pironi[2], Augusto Lauro[1] and Andreas G. Tzakis[3]

[1]*Liver and Multiorgan Transplant Unit, University of Bologna, St Orsola-Malpighi Hospital, Bologna, Italy;* [2]*Center for Chronic Intestinal Failure, Department of Medical and Surgical Science, University of Bologna, Bologna, Italy;* [3]*Division of General Surgery, Cleveland Clinic Florida, Weston, Florida, USA*

Key Points

- Intestinal transplantation has become a therapeutic option for complicated patients on home parenteral nutrition (HPN) affected by benign chronic intestinal failure, when the rescue of the native bowel is not feasible.
- Short-term outcome is excellent, while long-term results remain suboptimal.
- Higher-volume centres tend to achieve better survival rates and recipients with a liver component do best.
- Further improvement in survival is expected from a timely patient referral from HPN centres and from defining a better timing for re-transplantation.

Introduction

Intestinal transplantation (ITx) has become a therapeutic option for irreversible chronic intestinal failure associated with life-threatening complications due to long-term home parenteral nutrition (HPN). It is a relatively new procedure, performed worldwide in 2611 patients up until 2011 (Grant, 2011), and an expensive operation, costing up to US$1,206,000 in the USA: nearly US$800,000 of this total cost goes towards hospital administration and admission fees, while another US$150,000 are used in the days following the surgery and while the patient is in recovery. In 1958, Lillehei *et al.* performed the first experimental transplant of an isolated small bowel in a dog (Lillehei *et al.*, 1959). Shortly after, Starzl and Kaupp (1960) performed the first multivisceral transplant, including liver with stomach, duodenum, pancreas and intestine, also in a dog. Their results were catastrophic due to the high rejection rate. Researchers thus realized that the intestine compared with the liver or kidney is very immunogenic. From 1967

*E-mail: antoniodaniele.pinna@aosp.bo.it

to 1987 a dozen patients underwent ITx in different centres, but the outcome was disappointing. In November 1987, Starzl *et al.* (1989) performed the first successful multivisceral transplant with liver in a human recipient. The patient was a 3-year-old child who survived 6 months after the transplant, but died because of the onset of lymphoma. In 1988, other centres started clinical trials in ITx. The first isolated small bowel transplant was described by Goulet *et al.* (1988) in a child recipient, who had a good outcome. After the introduction of tacrolimus (FK-506) in 1989 (Ochiai *et al.*, 1987; Hoffman *et al.*, 1990), an ITx programme started in Pittsburgh, USA. Five patients underwent transplantation at this centre in 1990: four patients received a combined liver–intestine and one an isolated graft. Improving results were obtained by a series from London, Ontario, Canada (Grant *et al.*, 1990): one patient underwent multivisceral transplant with liver and another two received a combined intestine–liver graft, with the best survival up to 5 years. In the following years, many intestinal transplant centres started their activities, accounting for a total of 79 programmes as of 2011. In 1994, the Intestinal Transplant Registry (ITR) was set up; it collects data from all over the world and organizes a biannual international symposium (International Small Bowel Transplant Symposium; ISBTS) reporting a data collection update.

Nomenclature

The current experience on ITx can be synthesized into four types of transplant (Abu Elmagd, 2011):

1. *Isolated small bowel transplant*, including jejunum and ileum (Fig. 39.1). A subtype could include en bloc the colon and/or the pancreas and/or the kidney for clinical reasons.
2. *Multivisceral transplant*, including stomach, pancreas, duodenum, jejunum and ileum (Fig. 39.2). A subtype could include the native pancreaticoduodenal complex and/or spleen for technical reasons.
3. *Combined liver–intestine transplant*, including liver with jejunum and ileum (Fig. 39.3). A subtype could include the donor pancreaticoduodenal complex for technical reasons.
4. *Liver–multivisceral transplant*, including the liver with the multivisceral graft (Fig. 39.4).

Indications

The indication for isolated small bowel transplantation is irreversible intestinal failure without any possibility of bowel rehabilitation and with normal liver function, associated with one or more of the other HPN-related life-threatening complications (Fishbein *et al.*, 2003a).

The indication for multivisceral transplantation is irreversible intestinal failure without any possibility of bowel rehabilitation, associated with HPN-related complications and disorders involving the upper gastrointestinal tract.

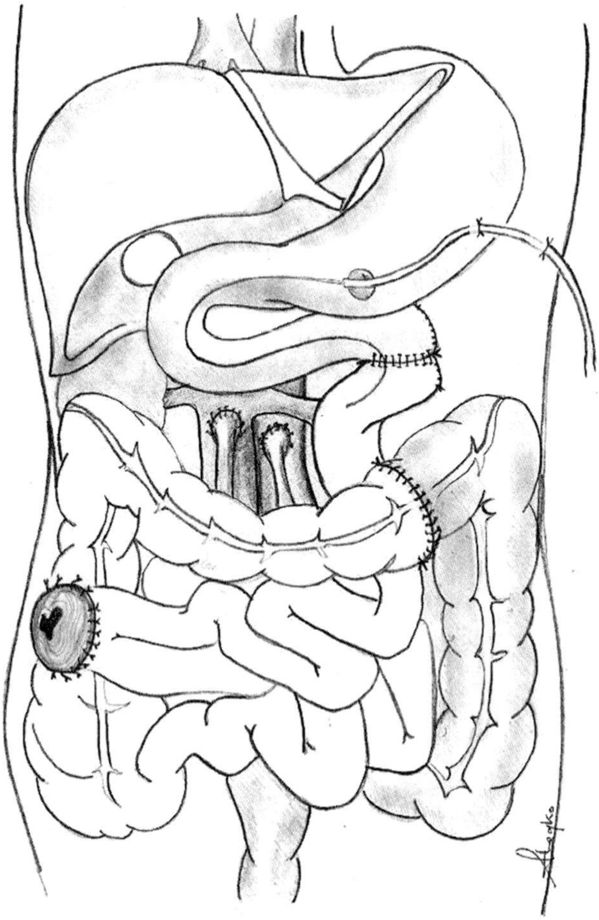

Fig. 39.1. Isolated small bowel transplant, including jejunum and ileum.

The indication for combined liver–intestinal transplantation is irreversible intestinal failure associated with irreversible liver failure or irreversible liver failure associated with superior mesenteric vein thrombosis.

The indication for liver–multivisceral transplantation is irreversible liver failure associated with irreversible intestinal failure and upper gastrointestinal disorders or splanchnic thrombosis.

The US Center for Medicare and Medicaid Services has approved the payment for ITx when the following life-threatening complications related to HPN occur (Buchman *et al.*, 2003):

1. Impending or overt liver failure (elevated serum bilirubin and/or liver enzymes, splenomegaly, thrombocytopenia, gastro-oesophageal varices, coagulopathy, stomal bleeding, hepatic fibrosis or cirrhosis).
2. Thrombosis of two or more major central venous channels (thrombosis in the subclavian, jugular or femoral vein).

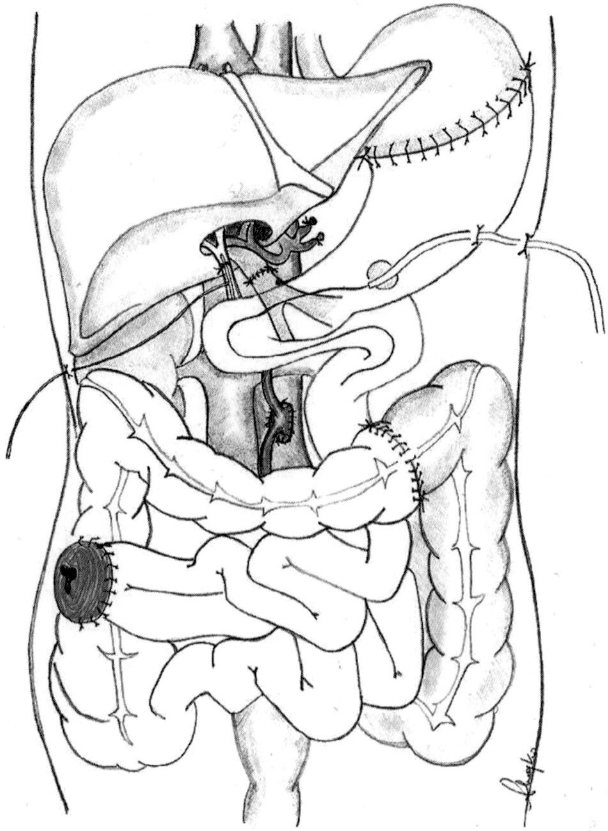

Fig. 39.2. Multivisceral transplant, including stomach, pancreas, duodenum, jejunum and ileum.

3. Frequent central line sepsis (two or more episodes of systemic sepsis secondary to line infections per year; one episode of line-related fungaemia; septic shock or acute respiratory distress syndrome).
4. Frequent severe dehydration.

The American Society of Transplantation position paper on paediatric ITx considers candidates for ITx also those patients with high risk of death or with very poor quality of life related to the following underlying intestinal failure conditions (Kaufman *et al.*, 2001):

1. Locally invasive tumours (e.g. desmoids in familial polyposis).
2. Extremely short bowel (less than 10 cm jejunum in children).
3. Congenital intractable mucosal disorders (microvillus inclusion disease, tufting enteropathy).
4. Intestinal failure with high morbidity and poor quality of life (e.g. severe chronic intestinal pseudo-obstruction, high-output stoma).

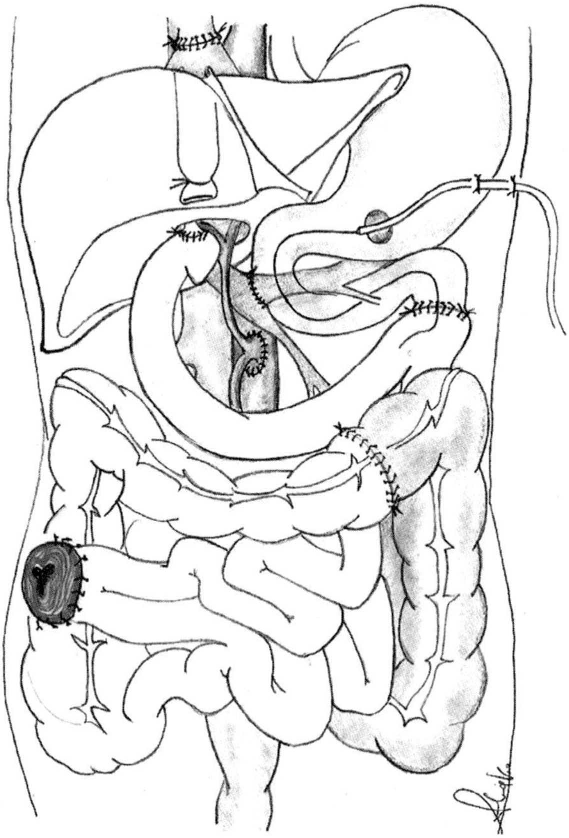

Fig. 39.3. Combined liver–intestine transplant, including liver with jejunum and ileum.

A multicentre survey in Europe evaluated the prevalence of candidacy for ITx on the basis of the Medicare and the American Society of Transplantation indication criteria. Forty-one HPN centres from nine countries enrolled 688 adult (>18 years) and 166 paediatric patients. Candidacy was 15.7% in adults and 34.3% in paediatric patients and was due to HPN failure in 62.1% and 28.1%, high-risk gastrointestinal disease in 25.9% and 59.6% and high-morbidity intestinal failure in 12.0% and 12.3%, respectively. Among the major contributing countries, the prevalence of candidacy ranged from 0.3 to 0.8 per million inhabitants for adults and from 0.9 to 2.0 per million inhabitants aged ≤18 years for the paediatric patients (Pironi *et al.*, 2006).

The gastrointestinal diseases and the causes of intestinal failure of the recipients differ between children and adults (Grant *et al.*, 2005). In children, gastroschisis (21%), necrotizing enterocolitis (12%) and intestinal volvulus (19%) can lead to a short bowel syndrome that accounts for 50% of paediatric transplants. Other minor diseases are represented by intestinal atresia (8%) and motility

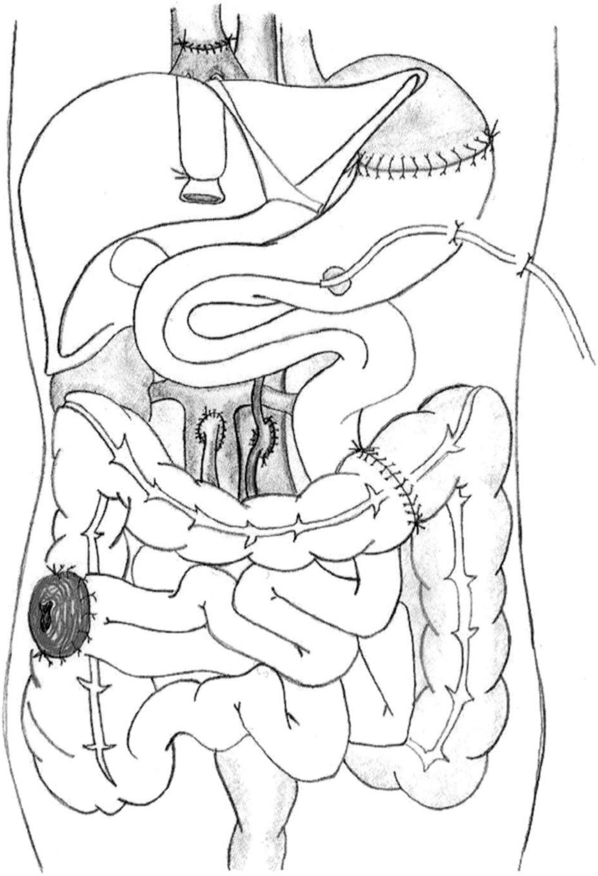

Fig. 39.4. Liver–multivisceral transplant, including liver with the multivisceral graft.

disorders, like intestinal pseudo-obstruction (9%) and aganglionosis/Hirshsprung's disease (7%). In adults the main indication is short bowel syndrome due to intestinal ischaemia (23%), trauma (10%), volvulus (7%) and Crohn's disease (14%). Motility disorders account for 8% of transplants. Desmoid/Gardner syndrome, responsible for 12% of procedures, and abdominal neurofibromatosis are rare indications, requiring an isolated intestinal transplant if the tumour is confined to the mesentery, or a multivisceral transplant if the other upper gastrointestinal organs are affected. A specific indication for a combined liver–intestine transplant is mesenteric vein thrombosis associated with protein-S or protein-C deficit, because a transplant could correct this deficiency. The main contraindications for ITx are advanced cardiopulmonary disease and non-resectable malignancy (local or metastatic). Patients with an active infection should be put on 'hold' as candidates for transplantation.

Referral for transplantation should be considered as soon as HPN-related complications occur, because a late referral may increase mortality rates among those on the waiting list or following ITx. An early referral can grant a greater chance for the patient to be transplanted and to have a better survival, because of the better clinical pre-transplant condition. This is important especially in children with liver failure, due to the risk of a quick and progressive hepatic damage leading to multi-organ failure and sepsis. A late referral could result in patients dying on the waiting list. The United Network for Organ Sharing (UNOS) report showed that the death rate on the waiting list for intestinal transplants is significantly higher than the mortality for any other solid organ in a transplant waiting list (Lao *et al.*, 2010); Pironi *et al.* (2011) reported that an early referral for a life-saving ITx is mandatory for patients with HPN-associated liver failure or invasive intra-abdominal desmoids. Central venous catheter-related major complications and ultra-short bowel might be indications for a pre-emptive/rehabilitative ITx in patients selected on a case-by-case basis.

Pre-transplant Evaluation

All potential candidates for ITx must undergo a multidisciplinary assessment evaluating the gastrointestinal tract, the nutritional status and the hepatic, renal, cardiopulmonary, haematological and immunological functions as well as infectious diseases. Also, a psychosocial assessment must be done. A final anaesthesiology evaluation is performed. The aetiology, extent and severity of the primary disease must be accurately assessed in every patient. A radiological and an endoscopic (with biopsies) examination of the remaining native gastrointestinal tract are carried out to plan the appropriate surgical strategy. When needed, gastrointestinal motility tests and an angiography should be added. A computer tomography (CT) scan should be performed to evaluate the extent of the neoplastic lesions of Gardner's syndrome or abdominal neurofibromatosis and, in some cases, to properly evaluate the abdominal cavity and the remnant space in relation to donor/recipient weight matching.

Donor Selection and Organ Procurement

Donor evaluation is the first step to reach good results. Donors should be young people, haemodynamically stable with minimal amine support, because the intestine is very sensitive to ischaemia. ABO compatibility is mandatory, while the ratio between the donor's weight and the recipient's weight should not exceed 1.1. The organ should be evaluated intraoperatively for appearance, motility and integrity. Organ harvesting (Di Benedetto *et al.*, 2004) requires superior mesenteric vessel isolation for an isolated intestinal graft, and includes aorta and vena cava for a multivisceral graft. Half of the colon, close to the medium colic vein, is harvested with the graft, which is preserved with cold University of Winsconsin or Celsior solution. The difficulty with the donor/recipient matching is the main cause for a long stay on the waiting list.

Surgical Technique

Isolated small bowel transplantation can be summarized in four surgical steps:

1. The diseased organ is removed and a proper space for the allograft is created; during this step, access to aorta and vena cava is gained.
2. The vascular anastomoses are performed, either orthotopic on mesenteric vessels or eterotopic on aorta and vena cava; occasionally a vascular graft extension is needed.
3. The upper and lower intestinal anastomoses are completed; an ileostomy is performed and a gastrostomy tube is positioned.
4. The abdominal wall is closed. In some patients this can be very difficult, thus requiring an abdominal wall transplant (Levi *et al.*, 2003) or the use of miocutaneous flap (Alexandrides *et al.*, 2000).

Multivisceral transplant requires the resection of all the tributary organs to the portal vein, like the stomach, intestine, pancreas and spleen, so that the portal vein of the graft is anastomosed to the recipient portal vein. Arterial blood flow is supplied by an aortic conduit (from the thoracic aorta of the donor) anastomosed to the recipient aorta and subsequently to a patch comprehensive of the mesenteric and coeliac artery of the graft. Biliary reconstruction could be in a duct-to-duct fashion or by Roux-en-Y loop bilio-jejunostomy.

Combined liver–intestine and liver–multivisceral transplants have the venous outflow into the recipient hepatic veins.

Living Donor Intestinal Transplantation

Living donation can be suitable for ITx too. Between the 1990s and the first half of the 2000s, more than 30 patients underwent living donor ITx but the procedure has been decreasing constantly since then. Donor evaluation is comprehensive of infective and gastrointestinal assessment with particular attention to absorption tests, abdominal CT scan and selective superior mesenteric angiography or 3D angio-CT scan. The intestinal graft is a segment of the ileum of 150–200 cm, resected 20 cm proximal to the ileocoecal valve. Ileum is actually preferred to a jejunal segment. A distal segment of the superior mesenteric artery and a proximal segment of the superior mesenteric vein represent the arterial inflow and vein outflow, reconstructed on the recipient aorta and vena cava (Gruessner and Sharp, 1997; Testa *et al.*, 2004).

Reduced Size Organs

The critical shortage of size-matched donor organs for infants and small children needing isolated small bowel or combined liver and intestine transplantation has led to long waiting times and a high risk of dying before transplantation. Utilizing grafts from larger donors could alleviate this problem, but using larger composite grafts in small children has been challenging and unsuccessful in the past. The ability to create suitably reduced-in-size small bowel or liver grafts (in the case of a combined transplant) from adult cadaveric donors has been reported in many studies (Bueno *et al.*, 2000; Delriviere *et al.*, 2000; de Ville de Goyet *et al.*, 2000).

Clinical Management

The immediate post-operative period is the most difficult with intestinal transplant recipients. Close surveillance is required to prevent or treat in a timely manner those complications that may put at risk survival of the graft and the patient, like rejections and infections. Also, re-laparotomies are often required and post-transplant lymphoproliferative disease (PTLD) can develop (Kato *et al.*, 2002). All of these complications, which can be very harmful in the immediate post-operative period, can occur even years after transplantation.

Early Post-operative Complications

Surgical complications are represented by anastomotic stenosis or leak, arterial or venous thrombosis, intestinal malrotation, bleeding, small bowel compression, eventration, abdominal collections and stoma infarction. Treatment of these complications is obviously managed by surgeons or interventional radiologists.

The most frequent medical complications, which may require intensive care support, are renal and respiratory failure.

Renal failure is mainly caused by two factors, negative fluid balance and immunosuppression toxicity. In intestinal transplant, fluid balance is an extremely important landmark. Post-operatively, the small bowel is oedematous and the patient may require abdominal decompression in order to breathe properly. At the same time, during ITx the fluid loss is extremely high. After the operation, starting immunosuppression with calcineurin inhibitors can damage the kidney and precipitate an acute renal failure. Thus, optimal post-operative fluid support is mandatory in order to maintain a normal urinary output.

Respiratory failure can be due to post-operative pneumonia, oedema, pneumothorax, pleural effusion, lung atelectasia or the final picture of sepsis and multi-organ failure. Management is based on large-spectrum antibiotics, diuretics, thoracic drainages and operative broncoscopy. Intubation and ventilator support may be necessary.

Neurological complications also can occur after ITx, mainly related to immunosuppressive therapy with calcineurin inhibitors (primarily FK-506) whose toxic effect may be a direct one or secondary to high blood concentrations. The neurological impairment may be of various degrees up to coma.

Rejection and Immunosuppression

In the early intestinal transplant era, rejection was a very severe complication, because it was very frequently the cause of graft losses and patient deaths. The introduction of new immunosuppressive drugs and induction agents has significantly decreased the rejection rate and improved the graft survival. The ITR data reports show that in more than 50% of patients, the immunosuppressive regimens were based on induction protocols, using daclizumab, basiliximab, alemtuzumab or thymoglobulin (Grant, 2011). Immunosuppression is maintained with FK-506 at high doses, intravenously and through the gastrostomy tube during the first post-operative days, but a few days later the oral route remains the only way of administration. The FK-506 blood concentrations should be monitored daily, because of the rapid improvement of the drug's absorption by the graft and the frequent variation of renal failure and fluid balance that can change FK-506 pharmacokinetics. FK-506 is frequently administered together with steroids. The ITR data show that sirolimus and mycophenolate mofetil were also given to 19.2% and 11.4% of the recipients, respectively (Grant, 2011). In the case of relapsing rejections or ongoing renal toxicity, sirolimus has been reported to be very effective in association with or in place of tacrolimus (Fishbein *et al.*, 2003b). The monitoring of the intestinal mucosa has a key role for the early detection of graft rejection and for its timely treatment. The temporary ileostomy allows frequent ileoscopies and mucosal biopsies and a direct view of the intestinal mucosa. The histological evaluation of the biopsies takes into account the apoptotic index, the cryptal injury and the presence of haemorrhages and inflammatory cells (Lee *et al.*, 1996; Ruiz *et al.*, 2003). A diagnosis of rejection is made when all the three aspects are present. According to the extent of the alterations, acute cellular rejection is classified as mild, moderate and severe, the last being diagnosed when necrosis of the intestinal mucosa is observed. The zoom endoscopy and the histological findings must be evaluated considering the clinical symptoms too. Clinical signs of acute intestinal rejection are fever, nausea, vomiting, high stomal output, mucosal oedema and intestinal bleeding in the case of severe rejection. Chronic rejection is clinically represented by diarrhoea, abdominal pain, progressive weight loss and intermittent intestinal bleeding. Treatment of rejection episodes has to be made according to the histological degree and the clinical feature. The first choice is steroid bolus and tapering, increasing FK-506 dosage. In the case of steroid resistance or severe rejection, monoclonal or polyclonal antibodies, such as OKT-3, infliximab, alemtuzumab or thymoglobulin are given. Rejection, if not treated, can lead to graft removal. Graft versus host disease was a frequent complication in the early days of ITx, represented clinically by skin rash. Nowadays, due to the selective immunosuppression, it is a less frequent finding.

Infections

This category of patients is at high risk of infections for many reasons:

- heavy immunosuppression;
- presence of a central line, in the first post-operative period;
- bacterial translocation, especially in the case of rejection;
- aggressive abdominal surgery;

- malnutrition; and
- renal failure.

Infections are the primary cause of death after ITx. Thus, prophylaxis for bacterial, viral and fungal agents is mandatory. Gut decontamination through the gastrostomy tube, with a solution containing nystatin, gentamicin and polymyxin E, prevents intraluminal bacterial overgrowth. Intravenous antibiotic prophylaxis with ampicillin is administered too. Pneumonia and intra-abdominal abscesses are the most frequent life-threatening infections. In the case of fever, after having excluded a rejection, chest X-ray and CT scan should be performed in order to search for these foci. The most frequent germs are enterobacteria, staphylococci and streptococci. Fungal infections are rare and represented mainly by oral or oesophageal candidiasis, responsive to fluconazole; pulmonary localization (*Aspergillus*) and fungaemia are harmful and require aggressive treatment.

Viral pre-emptive therapy is based on ganciclovir given intravenously during the first post-operative month and then by the oral route, and on immunoglobulin G anti-cytomegalovirus (CMV) during the first month as well. Viruses like CMV and Epstein–Barr virus (EBV) are responsible for enteritis and pulmonary infections. EBV is also associated with PTLD. PTLD can be treated by monoclonal antibodies like rituximab and local ablative surgery (Tzakis *et al.*, 2002). EBV PCR and CMV antigen in blood as well as CMV and EBV PCR in mucosal biopsies should be routinely searched, a positive test requiring prompt treatment. The incidence of severe viral infections has dropped thanks to these early detection methods. Haemodynamic and infective complications are often related to each other. Hypotension, if not related to fluid imbalance, is often an expression of a sepsis and requires the use of intravenous pressor agents, like dopamine, noradrenaline or adrenaline.

Nutritional Management

In the early post-operative days, nutritional support is achieved through parenteral nutrition, until the graft function allows nutritional autonomy. Enteral feeding begins at day 1 after the transplant to maintain mucosal integrity and function. First, a 5% dextrose solution is administered through the gastrostomy tube, later replaced by an isotonic enteral diet. As soon as bowel movement appears through ileostomy, a regular oral diet is encouraged. The parenteral nutrition is discontinued when the patient is able to maintain the nutrition status by the gastrointestinal route alone. The main metabolic complication is represented by a metabolic acidosis due to the systemic consumption and gastrointestinal loss of bases, requiring bicarbonate support by the intravenous or the oral route.

Results and Update

The last report from the ITR (Grant, 2011) showed that, between 1985 and 2011, 79 centres performed 2611 transplants, 43.9% with an isolated small bowel graft and with an increasing re-transplant rate. The number of cases per year increased over time up until 2005; since then it has been constantly decreasing due to the wider use of autologous native intestinal reconstruction and bowel lengthening techniques. The paediatric population (≤18 years) represented the majority of the recipients, 1441 transplants (55.1%); the combined graft (liver plus intestine) represented the majority of the paediatric transplants (47.2%). Overall, the types of grafts were isolated intestine (1148 grafts), combined intestine and liver (845 grafts) and multivisceral with or without liver (619 grafts). Survivors numbered 1341 (51.3%); about 60% of children and 50% of adults were weaned off parenteral nutrition and resumed normal daily activity. The overall patient and graft survival rate at 5 years is stable: 50% for paediatric recipients and 40% for adult patients in the last 'era' (2006–2011), while short-term results are improving steadily over time. Graft removal is mainly due to rejection while death is often related to sepsis. A multivariate analysis of cases transplanted after 1998 revealed that transplantation of patients waiting at home, recipient age (better in younger patients), presence of liver component and centre experience with at least ten cases were associated with improved patient survival.

Conclusions

ITx has become a therapeutic option for irreversible benign chronic intestinal failure associated with life-threatening complications of long-term HPN or high risk of death due to the underlying gastrointestinal disease. Four transplant types can be performed: (i) isolated small bowel transplant; (ii) multivisceral transplant; (iii) combined liver–intestine transplant; and (iv) liver–multivisceral transplant. The Intestine Transplant Registry showed that 2611 transplants were performed between 1985 and 2011, 43.9% with an isolated small bowel graft; however, the number of transplants has decreased constantly since 2005 due to the wider use of autologous native intestinal reconstruction and bowel lengthening techniques. The paediatric population (≤18 years) represented the majority of the recipients. Overall, survivors numbered 1341 (51.3%): about 60% of children and 50% of adults were weaned off parenteral nutrition. The patient and graft survival rate at 5 years is stable: 50% for paediatric recipients and 40% for adult patients in the last 'era' (2006–2011), while short-term results are improving steadily over time. Transplantation of patients waiting at home, recipient age (better in younger patients), presence of liver component and centre experience with at least ten cases were associated with improved patient survival. Recipient and donor selection is a landmark for good graft and patient survival and further improvement in survival is expected from a timely patient referral. The main complications encountered after ITx are rejections, infections and PTLD. Complications account for most of the post-transplant patient deaths and graft failures.

Summary

ITx is the therapeutic option for irreversible benign chronic intestinal failure associated with life-threatening complications of long-term HPN or high risk of death due to the underlying gastrointestinal disease. Recipient and donor selection is a landmark for good graft and patient survival and further improvement in survival is expected from a timely patient referral.

Transplantation of patients waiting at home, recipient age (better in younger patients), presence of liver component and centre experience with at least ten cases are associated with improved patient survival. Donors should be young people, haemodynamically stable with minimal amine support. ABO compatibility is mandatory, while the donor weight/recipient weight ratio should not exceed 1.1. The difficulty with donor/recipient matching is the main cause for a long stay on the waiting list and the high mortality rate, especially for patients who are candidates for a combined liver–intestinal transplantation.

Acknowledgements

The authors wish to thank Dr Alessandro Dazzi, MD for support in writing the manuscript and Dr Alessandro Cucchetti, MD for the drawings.

References

Abu Elmagd, K. (2011) The small bowel containing allografts: existing and proposed nomenclature. *American Journal of Transplantation* 11, 184–185.

Alexandrides, I.J., Liu, P., Marshall, D.M., Nery, J.R., Tzakis, A.G. and Thaller, S.R. (2000) Abdominal wall closure after intestinal transplantation. *Plastic & Reconstructive Surgery* 106, 805–812.

Buchman, A.L., Scolapio, J. and Fryer, J. (2003) AGA technical review on short bowel syndrome and intestinal transplantation. *Gastroenterology* 124, 1111–1134.

Bueno, J., Abu-Elmagd, K., Mazariegos, G., Madariaga, J., Fung, J. and Reyes, J. (2000) Composite liver–small bowel allografts with preservation of donor duodenum and hepatic biliary system in children. *Journal of Pediatric Surgery* 35, 291–295.

Delriviere, L., Muiesan, P., Marshall, M., Davenport, M., Dhawan, A., Kane, P., Karani, J., Rela, M. and Heaton, N. (2000) Size reduction of small bowels from adult cadaveric donors to alleviate the scarcity of pediatric size-matched organs: an anatomical and feasibility study. *Transplantation* 15, 1392–1396.

de Ville de Goyet, J., Mitchell, A., Mayer, A.D., Beath, S.V., McKiernan, P.J., Kelly, D.A., Mirza, D. and Buckles, J.A. (2000) En block combined reduced-liver and small bowel transplants: from large donors to small children. *Transplantation* 69, 555–559.

Di Benedetto, F., Quintini, C., Lauro, A., Masetti, M., Cautero, N., De Ruvo, N., Sassi, S., Diago Uso, T., Di Francesco, F., Romano, A., Dalla Valle, R., Boggi, U., Risaliti, A., Ramacciato, G. and Pinna, A.D. (2004) Outcome of isolated small bowel and pancreas transplants retrieved from multiorgan donor: the *in vivo* technique. *Transplantation Proceedings* 36, 437–438.

Fishbein, T.M., Gondolesi, G.E. and Kaufman, S.S. (2003a) Intestinal transplantation for gut failure. *Gastroenterology* 124, 1615–1628.

Fishbein, T.M., Kaufman, S.S., Florman, S.S., Gondolesi, G.E., Schiano, T., Kim-Schluger, L., Magid, M., Harpaz, N., Tschernia, A., Leibowitz, A. and LeLeiko, N.S. (2003b) Isolated intestinal transplantation: proof of clinical efficacy. *Transplantation* 76, 636–640.

Goulet, O.J., Revillon, Y., Cerf-Bensussan, N., Nezelof, C., Fischer, A., Buisson, C., Hubert, P., Lokiec, F., Martelli, H., Niaudet, P., Jan, D., Pellerin, D. and Ricour, C. (1988) Small intestinal transplantation in a child using cyclosporine. *Transplantation Proceedings* 20(3), 288–296.

Grant, D. (2011) Intestinal Transplant Registry (ITR) 2011 report. *International Small Bowel Transplant Symposium (ISBTS),* Washington, DC. Available at: www.intestinaltransplant.org.

Grant, D., Wall, W., Mimeault, R., Zhong, R., Ghent, C., Garcia, B., Stiller, C. and Duff, J. (1990) Successful small-bowel/liver transplantation. *The Lancet* 335, 181–184.

Grant, D., Abu-Elmagd, K., Reyes, J., Tzakis, A., Langnas, A., Fishbein, T., Goulet, O. and Farmer, D. on behalf of the Intestine Transplant Registry (2005) 2003 Report of the intestine transplant registry. A new era has dawned. *Annals of Surgery* 241, 607–613.

Gruessner, R.W. and Sharp, H.L. (1997) Living-related intestinal transplantation: first report of a standardized surgical technique. *Transplantation* 64, 1605–1607.

Hoffman, A.L., Makowka, L., Cai, X., Banner, B., Cramer, D.V., Pascualone, A., Todo, S. and Starzl, T.E. (1990) The effect of FK 506 on small intestine allotransplantation in the rat. *Transplantation Proceedings* 22, 76–77.

Kato, T., Ruiz, P., Thompson, J.F., Eskind, L.B., Weppler, D., Khan, F.A., Pinna, A.D., Nery, J.R. and Tzakis, A.G. (2002) Intestinal and multivisceral transplantation. *World Journal of Surgery* 26, 226–237.

Kaufman, S.S., Atkinson, J.B., Bianchi, A., Goulet, O.J., Langnas, A.N., McDiarmid, S.V., Mittal, N., Reyes, J. and Tzakis, A.G. (2001) Indications for pediatric intestinal transplantation: a position paper of the American Society of Transplantation. *Pediatric Transplantation* 5, 80–87.

Lao, O.B., Healey, P.J., Perkins, J.D., Reyes, J.D. and Goldin, A.B. (2010) Outcomes in children with intestinal failure following listing for intestinal transplant. *Journal of Pediatric Surgery* 45, 100–107.

Lee, R.G., Nakamura, K., Tsamandas, A.C., Abu-Elmagd, K., Furukawa, H., Hutson, W.R., Reyes, J., Tabasco-Minguillan, J.S., Todo, S. and Demetris, A.J. (1996) Pathology of human intestinal transplantation. *Gastroenterology* 110, 1820–1832.

Levi, D.M., Tzakis, A.G., Kato, T., Madariaga, J., Mittal, N.K., Nery, J., Nishida, S. and Ruiz, P. (2003) Transplantation of the abdominal wall. *The Lancet* 361, 2173–2176.

Lillehei, R.C., Goott, B. and Miller, F.A. (1959) The physiologic response of the small bowel of the dog to ischemia including prolonged in vitro preservation of the bowel with successful replacement and survival. *Annals of Surgery* 150, 543–560.

Ochiai, T., Nakajima, K., Nagata, M., Suzuki, T., Asano, T., Uematsu, T., Goto, T., Hori, S., Kenmochi, T., Nakagoori, T. and Isono, K. (1987) Effect of a new immunosuppressive agent, FK 506, on heterotopic cardiac allotransplantation in the rat. *Transplantation Proceedings* 19, 1284–1286.

Pironi, L., Hébuterne, X., Van Gossum, A., Messing, B., Lyszkowska, M., Colomb, V., Forbes, A., Micklewright, A., Villares, J.M., Thul, P., Bozzetti, F., Goulet, O. and Staun, M. (2006) Candidates for intestinal transplantation: a multicenter survey in Europe. *American Journal of Gastroenterology* 101, 1633–1643.

Pironi, L., Joly, F., Forbes, A., Colomb, V., Lyszkowska, M., Baxter, J., Gabe, S., Hébuterne, X., Gambarara, M., Gottrand, F., Cuerda, C., Thul, P., Messing, B., Goulet, O., Staun, M., Van Gossum, A. and Home Artificial Nutrition & Chronic Intestinal Failure Working Group of the ESPEN (2011) Long-term follow-up of patients on home parenteral nutrition in Europe: implications for intestinal transplantation. *Gut* 60, 17–25.

Ruiz, P., Garcia, M., Pappas, P., Berney, T., Esquenazi, V., Kato, T., Mittal, N., Weppler, D., Levi, D., Nishida, S., Nery, J., Miller, J. and Tzakis, A. (2003) Mucosal vascular alterations in isolated small-bowel allografts: relationship to humoral sensitization. *American Journal of Transplantation* 3, 43–49.

Starzl, T.E. and Kaupp, H.A. (1960) Mass homotransplant of abdominal organs in dogs. *Surgical Forum* 11, 28–30.

Starzl, T.E., Rowe, M.I., Todo, S., Jaffe, R., Tzakis, A., Hoffman, A.L., Esquivel, C., Porter, K.A., Venkataramanan, R., Makowka, L. and Duquesnoy, R. (1989) Transplantation of multiple abdominal viscera. *Journal of the American Medical Association* 261, 1449–1457.

Testa, G., Panaro, F., Schena, S., Holterman, M., Abcarian, H. and Benedetti, E. (2004) Living related small bowel transplantation: donor surgical technique. *Annals of Surgery* 240, 779–784.

Tzakis, A.G., Kato, T., Nishida, S., Levi, D.M., Tryphonopoulos, P., Madariaga, J.R., De Faria, W., Nery, J.R., Regev, A., Vianna, R., Miller, J., Esquenazi, V., Weppler, D. and Ruiz, P. (2002) Successful treatment of post-transplant lymphoproliferative disease with prolonged rituximab treatment in intestinal transplant recipients. *Transplantation* 74, 1000–1006.

40 Home Parenteral Nutrition – Perspectives

André Van Gossum*

Clinic of Intestinal Diseases and Clinical Nutrition, Hôpital Erasme, Free University of Brussels, Brussels, Belgium

The administration of parenteral nutrition at home was initiated in the early 1970s for patients with life-threatening intestinal failure. Short bowel syndrome was the major indication for initiating home parenteral nutrition (HPN) in patients with benign underlying diseases. On the basis of the experience that has been collected by some specialized centres in Europe and North America, this method is now routinely practised in industrialized countries around the world (Shils, 2010).

For more than 25 years, the use of HPN has been extended to patients with advanced cancer who are unable to be fed enterally. For this group of patients, the concerns and objectives of HPN are different from those for patients with benign diseases, but in any case, HPN tends to improve the quality of life (Van Gossum and Messing, 1997; Mueller *et al.*, 2010). The specificity of providing HPN in cancer patients – including medical, psychological and ethical issues – should be carefully recognized by the caregivers.

In this book all of the authors – who have considerable expertise in the field of HPN – have presented an update of the best practice in this field.

Nevertheless, we have to admit that the recommendations that are described in the various chapters are more often based on experts' consensus or personal experience than on well-documented, evidence-based medicine. The lack of randomized controlled trials in some areas of HPN is probably related to the difficulty of performing such trials by using a method that has been recognized as being life-saving (Dreesen *et al.*, 2012).

What are the prospects for the field of HPN? First, we should expect some significant changes in terms of underlying diseases and indications. Indeed, although the incidence of newly enrolled HPN patients is increasing continuously in many countries, it is probably not due to an increase in the incidence of

*E-mail: andre.vangossum@erasme.ulb.ac.be

underlying diseases but to a better usage of HPN, at least for patients with benign diseases (Ireton-Jones and De Legge, 2005).

It is clearly evident that the number of patients with Crohn's disease – which used to be the most frequent underlying disease – who might require HPN is decreasing sharply. This trend is related to an improving therapeutic strategy, especially the development of biologics such as anti-TNF-α medication.

Even if it is not yet apparent in epidemiological surveys, we could also expect to observe a decreased incidence of vascular mesenteric infarction due to a better prevention of cardiovascular diseases and a decrease in the habit of cigarette smoking.

On the contrary, the use of HPN will continue to grow for cancer patients; this is related to the ever-growing incidence of cancer as well as to the development of more aggressive multimodal therapies for cancer (Bozzetti, 2013).

Independently of the underlying diseases, the use of HPN will progressively increase in the future in relation to political and economic trends. Indeed, a major effort is made in all of the industrialized countries to control the cost of the health system by limiting the duration of hospitalizations. In parallel, we observe the expanding development of home care services (Tappenden, 2012). We also hope that the use of HPN will be initiated in countries in which this option is not yet available for medical and economic reasons.

Second, the growing use of HPN should continue to assure and even improve the quality of care. Indeed, epidemiological surveys have raised some concerns about the growing number of HPN centres with only limited experience. It is suspected that complications and mortality rates are negatively related to the level of experience. However, a recent report stated that HPN practised at a non-specialist district general hospital achieved complication rates comparable to those of large, specialist centres (Freshwater *et al.*, 2005).

Moreover, for patients with advanced cancer, home care services which are handled by private companies – and which are very beneficial for logistical support – should not substitute specialized HPN teams. In the same way, the use of the tri-chamber bags should not hide the need for prescription of 'tailored' parenteral support in patients on long-term HPN.

In other words, the difficulty of running an HPN programme should not be minimized; HPN needs to be performed by an expert, multidisciplinary team. Teaching and continuous education in the field of HPN is mandatory. We should also encourage transferring our expertise to newly qualified HPN centres in emerging countries.

Third, we also may expect striking improvement in the medical management of chronic intestinal failure by improvements in the different mechanisms of adaptation: the remaining small bowel, the colon (when possible) and the patient (hyperphagia) (Brown and DiBaise, 2004).

In the area of intestinal adaptation, research is ongoing on the potential benefits of specific nutrients (glutamine, citrulline, etc.) and on growth-hormone factors (Jeppesen, 2012; Dibb *et al.*, 2013).

Fourth, the progress in intestinal transplantation as well as the improved life expectancy of small bowel-transplanted patients should also encourage HPN teams to improve the quality of their programme (Pironi *et al.*, 2012). Indeed, up to now, intestinal transplantation has been reserved mainly for HPN patients who had developed HPN-related complications. In the future, we may consider earlier organ transplantation in HPN patients who cannot be weaned off parenteral nutrition.

Furthermore, although still a matter of debate, research into cloning cells, or cell therapy using autologous stem cells, could be revolutionary – as for other organ failure – for palliation of intestinal failure (Stange, 2013, Barker, 2014).

References

Barker, N. (2014) Adult intestinal stem cells: critical drivers of epithelial homeostasis and regeneration. *Nature Reviews. Molecular Cell Biology* 15, 19–33.

Bozzetti, F. (2013) Nutritional support of the oncology patient. *Critical Reviews in Oncology/Hematology* 87, 172–200.

Brown, C.R. and DiBaise, J.K. (2004) Intestinal rehabilitation: a management program for short-bowel syndrome. *Progress in Transplantation* 14, 290–296.

Dibb, M., Teubner, A., Theis, V., Shaffer, J. and Lal, S. (2013) Review article: The management of long-term parenteral nutrition. *Alimentary Pharmacology & Therapeutics* 37, 587–603.

Dreesen, M., Foulon, V., Vanhaecht, K., De Pourcq, L., Hiele, M. and Willems, L. (2012) Guidelines recommendations on care of adult patients receiving home parenteral nutrition: a systematic review of global practices. *Clinical Nutrition* 31, 602–608.

Freshwater, D., Saadeddin, A., Dell-Smith, P., Digger, T. and Jones, B.J. (2005) Can home parenteral nutrition be provided by non-specialized centres? 2300 weeks of experience at a district general hospital in the United Kingdom. *Clinical Nutrition* 24, 229–235.

Ireton-Jones, C. and De Legge, M. (2005) Home parenteral nutrition registry: a five-year retrospective evaluation of outcomes of patients receiving home parenteral nutrition support. *Nutrition* 21, 156–160.

Jeppesen, P.B. (2012) Teduglutide, a novel glucagon-like peptide 2 analog, in the treatment of patients with short bowel syndrome. *Therapeutic Advances in Gastroenterology* 5, 159–171.

Mueller, M., Lohmann, S., Thul, P., Weimann, A. and Grill, E. (2010) Functioning and health in patients with cancer on home-parenteral nutrition: a qualitative study. *Health and Quality of Life Outcomes* 8, 41.

Pironi, L., Goulet, O., Buchman, A., Messing, B., Gabe, S., Candusso, M., Bond, G., Gupte, G., Pertkiewicz, M., Steiger, E., Forbes, A., Van Gossum, A. and Pinna, A.D.; Home Artificial Nutrition and Chronic Intestinal Failure Working Group of ESPEN (2012) Outcome on home parenteral nutrition for benign intestinal failure: a review of the literature and benchmarking with the European prospective survey of ESPEN. *Clinical Nutrition* 31, 831–845.

Shils, M.E. (2010) The advent of home parenteral nutrition support. *Annual Review of Nutrition* 30, 1–12.

Stange, D.E. (2013) Intestinal stem cells. *Digestive Diseases* 31, 293–298.

Tappenden, K.A. (2012) A challenge to providers of clinical nutrition therapy. *JPEN Journal of Parenteral and Enteral Nutrition* 36, 377.

Van Gossum, A. and Messing, B. (1997) Home parenteral nutrition in adults: new trends raise new questions. *Nutrition* 13, 479–480.

Index

Page numbers in **bold** refer to figures and tables